Breast Cancer

A Multidisciplinary Approach
to Diagnosis and Management

Current Multidisciplinary Oncology

Breast Cancer
A Multidisciplinary Approach to Diagnosis and Management

EDITED BY

Alphonse G. Taghian, MD, PhD

Associate Professor of Radiation Oncology,
Harvard Medical School
Chief of Breast Service
Department of Radiation Oncology
Massachusetts General Hospital
Boston, Massachusetts

Barbara L. Smith, MD, PhD

Associate Professor of Surgery,
Harvard Medical School
Director Breast Program
Massachusetts General Hospital
Boston, Massachusetts

John K. Erban, MD

Associate Professor of Medicine
Harvard Medical School
Director, Clinical Programs and
Co-Director, Gillette Center for Breast Cancer
Massachusetts General Hospital
Boston, Massachusetts

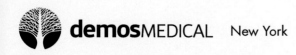 **demos**MEDICAL   New York

Acquisitions Editor: Richard Winters
Cover Design: Joe Tenerelli
Compositor: NewGen North America
Printer: King Printing

Visit our website at www.demosmedpub.com

Library of Congress Cataloging-in-Publication Data
Breast cancer / edited by Alphonse G. Taghian, Barbara L. Smith, John K. Erban.
　　p. ; cm.—(Current multidisciplinary oncology)
　　Includes bibliographical references and index.
　　ISBN 978-1-933864-44-0
　1. Breast—Cancer. I. Taghian, Alphonse G. II. Smith, Barbara Lynn. III. Erban, John K.
IV. Series: Current multidisciplinary oncology.
　[DNLM: 1. Breast Neoplasms—therapy. WP 870 2010]
　RC280.B8B6655624　2010
　616.99'449—dc22　　　　　　　　　　　　　　　　　　　2009034462

Medicine is an ever-changing science. Research and clinical experience are continually expanding our knowledge, in particular our understanding of proper treatment and drug therapy. The authors, editors, and publisher have made every effort to ensure that all information in this book is in accordance with the state of knowledge at the time of production of the book. Nevertheless, the authors, editors, and publisher are not responsible for errors or omissions or for any consequences from application of the information in this book and make no warranty, express or implied, with respect to the contents of the publication. Every reader should examine carefully the package inserts accompanying each drug and should carefully check whether the dosage schedules mentioned therein or the contraindications stated by the manufacturer differ from the statements made in this book. Such examination is particularly important with drugs that are either rarely used or have been newly released on the market.

Special discounts on bulk quantities of Demos Medical Publishing books are available to corporations, professional associations, pharmaceutical companies, health care organizations, and other qualifying groups. For details, please contact:

Special Sales Department
Demos Medical Publishing
11W. 42nd Street, 15th Floor
New York, NY 10036
Phone: 800–532–8663 or 212–683–0072
Fax: 212–941–7842
Email: rsantana@demosmedpub.com

Made in the United States of America
09 10 11 12 13　　5 4 3 2 1

I dedicate this book to my wife Danielle, and my children Nadine, Gabriella, and Alexa. Without their great unending support and love, it would have been impossible to accomplish this work.

I also dedicate this book to the individuals who have provided me with guidance and support throughout my life and career. To my parents, who despite their short lives, inspired me by their great sacrifice to assure me the best education possible; Dr. A. Radi, Germany, my best friend for his support over the years; Professor D. Chassagne, Institut Gustave Roussy, France, who urged me to seek out research and the opportunity to study in the United States; Professor P. Bey, Centre Alexis Vautrin, France, who instilled within me the skills and passion for a career in radiation oncology; Dr. H. Suit, who provided me the opportunity to do research in his lab and to practice at the Massachusetts General Hospital; and Dr. J. Loeffler for his continuous support, which greatly impacted my career in the Department of Radiation Oncology at Massachusetts General Hospital.

—Alphonse Taghian, MD, PhD

To my husband Steve and daughter Kaleigh for their unfailing support and ongoing inspiration.

—Barbara Smith, MD, PhD

To my wife Lisa and my children, Laura, John, and Stephen, for their loving support.

I am also deeply indebted to Drs. Robert Schwartz, Jane Desforges, Denisa Wagner, and Nicholas Robert for their guidance and training early in my career, and for friendship and advice since.

—John K. Erban, MD

Contents

Foreword   ix
Preface   xi
Acknowledgments   xiii
Contributors   xv

1   Importance of the Multidisciplinary Approach to
Breast Cancer   1
*John K. Erban, Barbara L. Smith,
and Alphonse G. Taghian*

2   Multidisciplinary Approach to the Prevention and
Screening of Breast Cancer

   Identification of High-Risk Patients   3
   Kristen Mahoney Shannon and Paula D. Ryan

   Screening for Breast Cancer: Mammography
   and Other Modalities   18
   Phoebe E. Freer and Daniel B. Kopans

3   Intake of New Patients for Multidisciplinary
Clinics   37
Martha Lake and Gwendolyn Mitchell

4   Multidisciplinary Issues for Newly
Diagnosed Patients

   Biopsy Techniques   41
   Elizabeth A. Rafferty

   Surgical Pathology   50
   Elena F. Brachtel

   Multidisciplinary Approach to Breast Cancer   64
   Jerry Younger

   Diagnosis and Initial Evaluation   68
   Elizabeth A. Guancial and Steven J. Isakoff

   Fertility and Pregnancy Considerations   76
   Kathryn J. Ruddy and Ann H. Partridge

5   Medical and Surgical Management of Atypical
Hyperplasia and Lobular Carcinoma in situ   83
*Prakash K. Pandalai, Verónica C. Mariciani,
Melinda F. Lerwill, Constance A. Roche,
and Kevin S. Hughes*

6   Multidisciplinary Approach in the Treatment of
Ductal Carcinoma in situ

   Surgical Management of DCIS   93
   Michelle Specht

   Radiation Treatment of DCIS   99
   *Margarita Racsa, Ariel E. Hirsch,
   and Shannon M. MacDonald*

   Medical Oncology Treatment of DCIS   111
   Janet E. Murphy and Beverly Moy

7   Multidisciplinary Approach in the Treatment
of Early Breast Cancer

   Surgical Management   117
   Barbara L. Smith

   Radiation Treatment of Early-Stage
   Breast Cancer   125
   Jennifer R. Bellon

   Medical Oncology Treatment of Early-Stage
   Breast Cancer   132
   Julie Gold and Harold J. Burstein

8   Multidisciplinary Approach in the Treatment of
     Locally Advanced Breast Cancer

     Surgical Treatment of Locally Advanced
     Breast Cancer   145
     Barbara L. Smith

     Radiation Treatment of Locally Advanced
     Breast Cancer   152
     *Mohamed A. Alm El-Din and
     Alphonse G. Taghian*

     Medical Oncology Treatment of Locally
     Advanced Breast Cancer   165
     Steven J. Isakoff

     Incorporating Translational Research
     in the Treatment of Locally Advanced
     Breast Cancer   174
     Steven J. Isakoff and Leif W. Ellisen

9   Multidisciplinary Approach in Breast
     Reconstruction

     Surgical Considerations in Breast
     Reconstruction   177
     *Liza S. Kim, Anuja Kandanatt Antony,
     Eric C. Liao, and William G. Austen, Jr.*

     Radiation Therapy Considerations in Breast
     Reconstruction   191
     Abram Recht

10   Multidisciplinary Approach in the Treatment
     of Metastatic Disease

     Surgical Management of Metastatic
     Disease   197
     Colleen D. Murphy and Mehra Golshan

     Radiation Management of Metastatic
     Disease   202
     Julia S. Wong

     Medical Oncology Management
     of Metastatic Disease   208
     Nageatte Ibrahim and John K. Erban

     Palliative Care for Metastatic Disease   221
     Marybeth Singer and Catherine Furlani

11   Multidisciplinary Approach in the Management
     of Locally Recurrent Disease

     Surgical and Radiation Management of Locally
     Recurrent Disease   229
     *Laurie Kirstein, Mohamed A. Alm El-Din,
     and Alphonse G. Taghian*

     Medical Oncology Management of Locally
     Recurrent Disease   240
     Irene Kuter

12   Multidisciplinary Approach to the Patient's
     Quality of Life

     Multidisciplinary Approach to Quality
     of Life   247
     Lidia Schapira

     Lymphedema: A Modern Approach to
     Evaluation and Treatment   258
     Jean O'Toole and Tara A. Russell

13   Psychiatric Issues in Breast Cancer   269
     Ilana Monica Braun and Donna Beth Greenberg

14   Multidisciplinary Considerations: Racial
     Disparities in Breast Cancer   277
     Beverly Moy

15   Multidisciplinary Breast Cancer Care in the
     Community   283
     *Karen Krag, Robin Schoenthaler,
     and Jeanne Yu*

16   Future Directions in the Treatment
     of Breast Cancer

     Surgical Innovations in Breast Cancer   289
     Amanda Wheeler and Barbara L. Smith

     Evolving Innovations for Breast
     Radiotherapy   298
     *Shannon M. MacDonald and
     Alphonse G. Taghian*

     Hormonal Therapy in the Treatment
     of Breast Cancer   308
     Kathrin Strasser-Weippl and Paul E. Goss

     Gene Expression Profiling: Personalized
     Treatment   315
     Leif W. Ellisen and Dennis Sgroi

     Future Directions in Breast Cancer
     Clinical Trials   322
     Rachel A. Freedman and Eric P. Winer

Index   329

Foreword

In this inaugural volume of the series *Current Multi-disciplinary Oncology*, devoted to breast cancer, it brings me great pleasure to introduce the practicing clinician to a new resource that will aid in the multidisciplinary approach to solid tumors.

Dr. Alphonse Taghian, a member of the multidisciplinary breast cancer service at Massachusetts General Hospital, has assembled an outstanding group of prolific contributors on the multidisciplinary approach to breast cancer.

Over the past two decades, a myriad of advances in the diagnosis and treatment of breast cancer have occurred. Some of the advances include, but are not limited to, diagnostic molecular tools that may aid in predicting response to certain treatment approaches and/or provide a guide to prognostic outcomes for certain patients.

The very common solid tumor affects women in developed and underdeveloped countries alike and warrants intense efforts to find a cure.

It is clear that Drs. Taghian, Smith, and Erban are examples of the next generation of academic, forward-thinking oncologists who have committed their careers to eradicating breast cancer. Their vision and ability has allowed them to assemble an outstanding group of investigators to create a very coherent treatise on this topic, for which I am most grateful. Like me, I'm sure that you will enjoy this inaugural volume as you seek guidance in the multidisciplinary approach to your patients with breast cancer.

Charles R. Thomas, Jr., MD
Series Editor
Department of Radiation Medicine
Oregon Health and Science University
Knight Cancer Institute
Portland, Oregon

Preface

The organization of this book reflects the importance of the multidisciplinary approach in the treatment of breast cancer. In the last two decades, the treatment of breast cancer has evolved very rapidly, with new scientific and clinical achievements constantly modifying the standard of care and leading to better clinical outcomes. Furthermore, the treatment of breast cancer has become increasingly complex, requiring comprehensive assessment and review of multiple issues including genetics, radiology, surgery, reconstruction, fertility, radiation, and chemotherapy. It is clear that the harmony and communication between these different specialties that is created by a multidisciplinary team approach are crucial for provision of optimal care to patients and are necessary for truly successful treatment.

Moreover, patients are increasingly well informed and know the value of the multidisciplinary approach to treatment. This book is a review for physicians, residents, fellows, nurses, physician assistants, physical therapists, and all health care providers involved in the treatment of breast cancer. It describes an approach for optimal, multidisciplinary care for women who are at higher risk to develop breast cancer or who have been diagnosed with breast cancer. The multidisciplinary team of authors, representing a range of disciplines, has summarized the state-of-the-art issues related to the treatment of breast cancer. The text was written by expert clinicians expressly for the practicing clinician.

The editors are grateful to all the contributors for the time and effort spent to provide the excellent chapters for this book.

Alphonse G. Taghian
Barbara L. Smith
John K. Erban

Acknowledgments

Without the outstanding assistance, steady hand, and calm demeanor of Joyce Maclean, this project would not have been completed. We are also indebted to all the authors who put in time and effort to contribute to this book. Our colleagues, residents, fellows, and staff at the Gillette Center for Breast Cancer at the Massachusetts General Hospital deserve enormous credit for their wonderful support at various times along the way. Finally we wish to thank our patients for the honor of being selected as their caregivers.

Alphonse G. Taghian
Barbara L. Smith
John K. Erban

Contributors

Mohamed A. Alm El-Din, MD
Lecturer of Radiation Oncology
Tanta Faculty of Medicine
Tanta, Egypt
Breast Oncology Fellow
Department of Radiation Oncology
Massachusetts General Hospital
Harvard Medical School
Boston, Massachusetts

Anuja Kandanatt Antony, MD, MPH
Division of Plastic and Reconstructive Surgery
Harvard School of Public Health
Massachusetts General Hospital
Boston, Massachusetts

William G. Austen, Jr., MD
Chief, Division of Plastic and Reconstructive Surgery
Massachusetts General Hospital
Harvard Medical School
Boston, Massachusetts

Jennifer R. Bellon, MD
Department of Radiation Oncology
Dana-Farber Cancer Institute
Brigham and Women's Hospital
Harvard Medical School
Boston, Massachusetts

Elena Brachtel, MD
Assistant Professor of Pathology
Harvard Medical School
Massachusetts General Hospital
Boston, Massachusetts

Ilana Monica Braun, MD
Department of Psychiatry
Massachusetts General Hospital
Boston, Massachusetts

Harold J. Burstein, MD, PhD
Associate Professor of Medicine
Harvard Medical School
Breast Oncology Center
Dana-Farber Cancer Institute
Boston, Massachusetts

Leif W. Ellisen, MD
Associate Professor of Medicine
Harvard Medical School
Massachusetts General Hospital
Boston, Massachusetts

John K. Erban, MD
Associate Professor of Medicine
Harvard Medical School
Director, Clinical Programs and
Co-Director, Gillette Center for Breast Cancer
Massachusetts General Hospital
Boston, Massachusetts

Rachel A. Freedman, MD, MPH
Instructor in Medicine
Harvard Medical School
Dana-Farber Cancer Institute
Boston, Massachusetts

Phoebe E. Freer, MD
Department of Radiology
Harvard Medical School
Massachusetts General Hospital
Boston, Massachusetts

Catherine Furlani, MSN, FNP, OCN
Oncology Nurse Practitioner
Gillette Center for Breast Cancer
Massachusetts General Hospital
Boston, Massachusetts

Julie Gold, MD
Mount Kisco Medical Group
Northern Westchester Hospital Cancer
    Treatment and Wellness Center
Mount Kisco, New York

Mehra Golshan, MD, FACS
Director of Breast Surgical Services
Brigham and Women's Hospital
Dana-Farber Cancer Institute
Boston, Massachusetts

Paul E. Goss, MD, PhD
Professor of Medicine
Harvard Medical School
Director of Breast Cancer Research
Massachusetts General Hospital
Boston, Massachusetts

Donna Beth Greenberg, MD
Associate Professor of Psychiatry
Harvard Medical School
Program Director
Psychiatric Oncology Service
Massachusetts General Hospital
Boston, Massachusetts

Elizabeth A. Guancial, MD
Clinical Fellow in Hematology/Oncology
Dana-Farber Cancer Institute
Brigham and Women's Hospital
Massachusetts General Hospital
Boston, Masachusetts

Ariel E. Hirsch, MD
Assistant Professor of Radiation Oncology
Boston University School of Medicine
Boston Medical Center
Boston, Massachusetts

Kevin S. Hughes, MD, FACS
Co-Director, Avon Comprehensive
    Breast Evaluation Center
Massachusetts General Hospital
Associate Professor of Surgery
Harvard Medical School
Boston, Massachusetts

Nageatte Ibrahim, MD
Instructor in Medicine
Harvard Medical School
Dana-Farber Cancer Institute
Boston, Massachusetts

Steve J. Isakoff, MD, PhD
Instructor in Medicine
Harvard Medical School
Division of Hematology/Oncology
Massachusetts General Hospital
Boston, Massachusetts

Liza S. Kim, MD
Breast Reconstruction and Aesthetics Fellow
Division of Plastic Surgery
Massachusetts General Hospital
Boston, Massachusetts

Laurie Kirstein, MD
Appel-Venet Breast Center
Beth Israel Medical Center
New York, New York

Daniel B. Kopans, MD, FACR
Professor of Radiology
Harvard Medical School
Senior Radiologist
Breast Imaging Division
Massachusetts General Hospital
Boston, Massachusetts

Karen Krag, MD
Clinical Assistant Professor of Medicine
Harvard Medical School
Division of Hematology/Oncology
Massachusetts General Hospital
Boston, Massachusetts

Irene Kuter, MD, D Phil
Assistant Professor of Medicine
Harvard Medical School
Division of Hematology/Oncology
Department of Medicine
Massachusetts General Hospital
Boston, Massachusetts

Martha Lake, RN, MSN
Nurse Coordinator
Gillette Center for Breast Cancer
Massachusetts General Hospital
Boston, Massachusetts

Melinda F. Lerwill, MD
Assistant Professor of Pathology
Harvard Medical School
Department of Pathology
Massachusetts General Hospital
Boston, Massachusetts

Eric C. Liao, MD, PhD
Instructor in Surgery
Harvard Medical School
Division of Plastic and Reconstructive Surgery
Massachusetts General Hospital
Boston, Massachusetts

Shannon M. MacDonald, MD
Assistant Professor of Radiation Oncology
Harvard Medical School
Department of Radiation Oncology
Massachusetts General Hospital
Boston, Massachusetts

Verónica C. Mariciani, MD
Surgical Oncologist
Hospital Padre Hurtado
Hospital Barros Luco
Santiago, Chile

Gwendolyn Mitchell, LPN, MEd
Nurse Coordinator
Gillette Center for Breast Cancer
Massachusetts General Hospital
Boston, Massachusetts

Beverly Moy, MD, MPH
Assistant Professor of Medicine
Harvard Medical School
Division of Hematology/Oncology
Massachusetts General Hospital
Boston, Massachusetts

Colleen D. Murphy, MD
Instructor in Surgery
Harvard Medical School
Division of Surgical Oncology
Brigham and Women's Hospital
Boston, Massachusetts

Janet E. Murphy, MD
Clinical Fellow in Hematology/Oncology
Dana-Farber Cancer Institute
Brigham and Women's Hospital
Massachusetts General Hospital
Boston, Massachusetts

Jean O'Toole, PT, MPH, CLT-LANA
Clinical Specialist
Physical Therapy Services
Massachusetts General Hospital
Boston, Massachusetts

Prakash K. Pandalai, MD
Surgical Oncology Fellow
Dana-Farber Cancer Institute
Division of Surgical Oncology
Massachusetts General Hospital
Boston, Massachusetts

Ann H. Partridge, MD, MPH
Assistant Professor of Medicine
Harvard Medical School
Division of Medical Oncology
Dana-Farber Cancer Institute and Brigham
   and Women's Hospital
Boston, Massachusetts

Margarita Racsa, MD, MPH
Radiation Oncologist
Massachusetts General Hospital
North Shore Medical Center
Peabody, Massachusetts

Elizabeth A. Rafferty, MD
Director of Breast Imaging
Department of Radiology
Massachusetts General Hospital
Boston, Massachusetts

Abram Recht, MD
Professor of Radiation Oncology
Harvard Medical School
Deputy Chief and Senior Radiation Oncologist
Beth Israel Deaconess Medical Center
Boston, Massachusetts

Constance A. Roche, MSN, ANP-BC
Oncology Nurse Practitioner
Avon Comprehensive Breast Center
Massachusetts General Hospital
Boston, Massachusetts

Kathryn J. Ruddy, MD, MPH
Instructor in Medicine
Harvard Medical School
Dana-Farber Cancer Institute
Brigham and Women's Hospital
Boston, Massachusetts

Tara A. Russell, MPH
Clinical Research Program Manager
Lymphedema Studies Program
Department of Radiation Oncology
Massachusetts General Hospital
Boston, Massachusetts

Paula D. Ryan, MD, PhD
Assistant Professor of Medicine
Harvard Medical School
Director, Breast and Ovarian Cancer Genetics
    and Risk Assessment Clinic
Division of Hematology Oncology
Massachusetts General Hospital
Boston, Massachusetts

Lidia Schapira, MD
Assistant Professor of Medicine
Harvard Medical School
Division of Hematology Oncology
Massachusetts General Hospital
Boston, Massachusetts

Robin Schoenthaler, MD
Instructor in Radiation Oncology
Harvard Medical School
Massachusetts General Hospital
Department of Radiation Oncology at
    Emerson Hospital
Concord, Massachusetts

Dennis Sgroi, MD, PhD
Associate Professor of Pathology
Harvard Medical School
Director of Breast Pathology
Department of Pathology
Massachusetts General Hospital
Boston, Massachusetts

Kristen Mahoney Shannon, MS, CGC
Program Manager and Senior Genetic Counselor
Center for Cancer Risk Assessment
Massachusetts General Hospital
Boston, Massachusetts

Marybeth Singer, MSA, APN-BC, AOCN, ACHPN
Oncology Nurse Practitioner
Gillette Center for Breast Cancer
Massachusetts General Hospital
Boston, Massachusetts

Barbara L. Smith, MD, PhD
Associate Professor of Surgery
Harvard Medical School
Director, Breast Program
Massachusetts General Hospital
Boston, Massachusetts

Michelle Specht, MD
Instructor in Surgery,
Harvard Medical School
Division of Surgical Oncology
Massachusetts General Hospital
Boston, Massachusetts

Kathrin Strasser-Weippl, MD
First Medical Department
Medical Oncology
Wilhelminen Hospital
Vienna, Austria

Alphonse G. Taghian, MD, PhD
Associate Professor of Radiation Oncology
Harvard Medical School
Chief of Breast Service
Department of Radiation Oncology
Massachusetts General Hospital
Boston, Massachusetts

Amanda Wheeler, MD
Division of Surgical Oncology
Massachusetts General Hospital
Boston, Massachusetts

Eric P. Winer, MD
Professor of Medicine
Harvard Medical School
Chief, Division of Women's Cancers
Thompson Senior Investigator in Breast Cancer Research
Dana-Farber Cancer Institute
Boston, Massachusetts

Julia S. Wong, MD
Department of Radiation Oncology
Harvard Medical School
Dana-Farber Cancer Institute
Brigham and Women's Hospital
Boston, Massachusetts

Jerry Younger, MD
Assistant Professor of Medicine
Harvard Medical School
Division of Hematology/Oncology
Massachusetts General Hospital
Boston, Massachusetts

Jeanne Yu, MD
Department of Surgical Oncology
Massachusetts General Hospital
Boston, Massachusetts

Breast Cancer

A Multidisciplinary Approach
to Diagnosis and Management

I Importance of the Multidisciplinary Approach to Breast Cancer

JOHN K. ERBAN

BARBARA L. SMITH

ALPHONSE G. TAGHIAN

Arguably, no patient in all of oncology requires input from more experts than the patient newly diagnosed with breast cancer. Since the observations in the 1800s that surgery could improve the health and quality of life of the patient with breast cancer, there has been exponential growth in knowledge guiding the care of patients with this prevalent disease, a disease with a biological spectrum that is indescribably wide. From Halsted to Urban to Fisher, surgery continues to occupy a dominant position in the specialty known as breast oncology. It remains essential for management of the disease and is vibrantly in evolution, through the development of increasingly less invasive procedures and more creative reconstructive techniques. In a nod to interdisciplinary care, surgeons can also be credited with making the first major observations to suggest that the natural history of breast cancer might be altered through biological and nonsurgical means. The observation that oophorectomy altered the rate of progression of many breast cancers was instrumental in providing a rationale for the first targeted therapy in oncology, that being the development of the selective estrogen receptor modulating agent known as tamoxifen. More recently, surgery-inspired research, coupled with increasingly effective radiation technology and expertise, has led to a dramatic increase in the frequency of breast conservation as an option for millions of women choosing less disfiguring surgery without compromising survival. Since the 1970s, increasingly effective methods to detect and treat breast cancer have caused fewer major toxicities for those undergoing evaluation and treatment. The result over the past decade has been a sustained fall in breast cancer–specific mortality, attributable partly to more effective screening modalities and partly to advances in science that have led to more effective treatments.

Accomplishing this has been neither easy nor the product of unidimensional care. Breast cancer treatment started as single-specialty care but has now expanded to a virtual orchestra of expertise that includes surgical oncologists, medical oncologists, radiation oncologists, breast imaging specialists, pathologists versed in anatomic and molecular techniques, reproductive endocrinologists and fertility experts, nutritionists, geneticists, nurses and physicians with symptom management expertise, social service and psychosocial experts, translational researchers, physical therapists with expertise in the science of lymphedema, and reconstructive surgeons. Access to fully half or more of these specialists is not necessary for most nonbreast oncologists, while it is critical for those dealing with breast cancer patients in order to provide state-of-the-art care.

Furthermore, "access" to the specialty expertise outlined above is a concept that requires definition. While sequential and geographically separate consultations are possible in many medical centers, modern breast cancer care requires not only access to these areas of expertise but also careful coordination of all of the parts to provide communication, proper interpretation of data, and efficient and compassionate decision making. Thus the birth of multidisciplinary breast cancer programs in the 1970s, bringing surgeons, medical oncologists, radiation oncologists, pathologists, and radiologists together, was the result of the acknowledgment that specialists dealing with breast cancer required both geographic and programmatic integration. More recently, modern assessment of breast cancer risk, identification of methods of disease prevention, management of symptoms of disease or its treatment, prevention of disfigurement or cosmetic deformity, and preservation of an essential biologic privilege—the ability of a woman to bear children after treatment for cancer—all involve dynamic conversations among specialists and execution in a timely fashion of treatment and research decisions. Multidisciplinary breast cancer evaluations should be considered the standard of care for patients seeking treatment for newly diagnosed breast cancer.

Perhaps the most important and exciting advances in interdisciplinary care have come in the past few decades in both imaging techniques and the evolution of molecular tools. These have included assessments of hormone responsiveness and HER2/neu amplification and genomic profiling of tumors into discrete categories characterized by distinct biological properties and varied risks of recurrence. What was once considered a single disease is now understood to be a heterogeneous family of disorders whose single common trait is the site of origin, namely, the breast. Thus unique combinations of treatments are required for each of these subtypes, making interdisciplinary consultation increasingly important. It is likely that as molecular pathologists become increasingly comfortable with predicting the behavior of individual tumors by gene expression profiles, personalized medicine will embrace even further the type of decision making uniquely possibly through the multidisciplinary approach to breast cancer care.

As important as the dual aims of early identification of tumors and pursuit of cure have been to the origin of the multidisciplinary approach to breast cancer, the recognition that centers of care are also committed to minimizing toxicity of treatment has spawned truly comprehensive integrated care for the overall management of the patient. Efforts over the years to minimize surgical intervention, to diminish the duration and toxicity of chemotherapy, to improve rates of breast preservation through neoadjuvant treatment paradigms, and to decrease duration of radiation treatment and its toxicity through partial breast irradiation protocols have been quite successful and attest to the success of this approach. Exciting efforts are now under way through genomic analysis to move from population-based treatment recommendations to patient-specific predictive models to guide treatment selection. All of these efforts have been based on a strong foundation of cross-disciplinary care with particular emphasis on conversations between specialists to understand where one modality can be synergistic with another or compensatory for its deficiencies.

A particular challenge to the multidisciplinary approach, as treatments become increasingly successful, is how to provide longitudinal follow-up over years and decades to expanding populations of definitively treated patients. Longitudinal follow-up has led to many important observations that have shaped the field and led to major advances in care. A substantial number of patients treated in their thirties to fifties will have 40 or more years of follow-up. Thus the success of radiation techniques in preventing local recurrence, the ability of sentinel node biopsy to prevent lymphedema, and the estimates of cardiomyopathy from newer chemotherapy regimens are all aspects of treatment that require centers to maintain a commitment to longitudinal follow-up. The impetus to change therapies over time in other fields (e.g., treatment of early-stage Hodgkin's disease evolving from radiation to chemotherapy in many cases) has been borne not of inadequacy of therapy but rather of the recognition that later complications of treatment were prohibitive. The multidisciplinary approach to breast cancer care, therefore, must include judicious plans for longitudinal care over decades if risk assessment, toxicity characterization, and prevention of late recurrence are to be fully understood. As pointed out in Chapter 16 fully half or more of the recurrences in estrogen receptor–positive breast cancer may occur five years after diagnosis. Efforts at Massachusetts General Hospital and elsewhere are ongoing to evaluate the best methods of preventing delayed recurrences.

What are the limitations of the multidisciplinary approach? The multidisciplinary approach to breast cancer care does require commitment of time and resources as it is inherently less time efficient than singular practice. All specialists involved in the care of the patient willingly sacrifice a certain amount of independence for improved outcomes. Throughout this text, each modality is introduced, relative to the theme of each chapter, with an eye to describing opportunities for superior care through integration of services. While the exact cost-effectiveness of this approach has not been fully evaluated in the literature, this is likely not to be a serious limitation even in an increasingly resource-conscious world. Surveys have repeatedly emphasized the positive response patients have to this approach.

Where studies on best practices are incomplete—for example, in the use of novel radiation techniques—authors have chosen to discuss the various clinical options available and to emphasize practical recommendations. It is hoped and expected that ongoing trials, including those at our own center, will address outstanding questions that define this most challenging of oncology specialties.

2 Multidisciplinary Approach to the Prevention and Screening of Breast Cancer

Identification of High-Risk Patients

KRISTEN MAHONEY SHANNON

PAULA D. RYAN

The identification of patients at inherited risk for breast cancer has become an integral part of the practice of preventive medicine and oncology. Although only about 5% to 10% of all cases of breast cancer are attributable to a highly penetrant cancer predisposition gene, individuals who carry a cancer susceptibility gene mutation have a significantly higher risk of developing breast cancer, as well as other cancers, over their lifetime than the general population. The ability to distinguish those individuals at high risk allows physicians and other health care providers to intervene with appropriate counseling and education, surveillance, and prevention, with the overall goal of improved survival for these individuals. This chapter will focus on the identification of patients at high risk for breast cancer, beginning with the assessment of risk and the importance of the family history in referral to genetic counselors for genetic testing. This chapter will also provide an overview of the clinical features, cancer risks, causative genes, and medical management for the most clearly described hereditary breast cancer syndromes.

■ RECOGNIZING RISK

The goal of breast cancer risk assessment is to provide an estimate of disease risk that can be used to guide clinical management for women at all levels of risk. Through this process, the likelihood that breast cancer risk is due to a specific genetic susceptibility in *BRCA1* or *BRCA2* can be determined. This allows the appropriate clinical management strategy to be used, with the aim of increasing survival in high-risk women and decreasing cost and complications in low-risk women. Risk assessment has gained

particular importance because specific clinical management strategies for *BRCA1* and *BRCA2* mutation carriers are now well defined.

A number of empirical models are used to estimate a woman's risk of breast cancer (Table 2.1). Two types of models are used for breast cancer risk assessment. The first model type estimates the risk of developing breast cancer over time, with the most commonly used being the Gail and Claus models (1,2), and the second model type estimates the probability of detecting a *BRCA* mutation in affected and unaffected women (3,4). The model of Gail and colleagues (1), derived from a population of unaffected women undergoing screening, estimates breast cancer risk by taking into account a woman's age at menarche, age at first live birth, number of first-degree relatives with breast cancer, and previous biopsies, with specific focus on the presence of atypical hyperplasia. The Gail model underestimates the risk of developing breast cancer if a woman is a carrier of a cancer susceptibility gene mutation and if the woman has a paternal history of cancer, as it does not include breast cancer in non–first-degree relatives or a family history of ovarian cancer (5). This model is more often useful clinically to provide breast cancer risk estimates to individuals who do not have family histories suggestive of a hereditary breast cancer syndrome or who have tested negative for a known genetic mutation. The Gail model is also used to counsel women about the use of tamoxifen or raloxifene as a chemopreventive agent. The tables of Claus and colleagues (2) also determine the risk of breast cancer for unaffected women, taking into consideration the number and age at breast cancer diagnosis of first- and second-degree female relatives. Despite this, the Claus model also underestimates the risk of a women developing breast cancer if she has a hereditary predisposition to develop breast cancer because it does not take into consideration the ethnicity of the proband or the presence of ovarian cancer in the family. It is a more helpful tool in women without a family history suggestive of a known hereditary cancer syndrome.

■ Table 2.1   Models used to predict the risk of breast cancer and the probability of a *BRCA* mutation

Model	Variables in Model	Comments/Limitations
Risk of breast cancer for unaffected women		
Gail et al. (1) • Provides risk of breast cancer by a given age • Available as an interactive tool at www.cancer.gov/bcrisktool	Age, FH of breast cancer, reproductive factors (age at menarche, menopause, and first childbirth and the number of live births), number of breast biopsies, personal history of atypia	Does not incorporate paternal FH of breast or ovarian cancer; does not include breast cancer in non-FDRs; does not consider age of onset of breast cancer in relatives; derived from a population undergoing screening
Claus et al. (2) • Provides 5-yr and lifetime probability of breast cancer • Available for download at www4. utsouthwestern.edu/breasthealth/ cagene/default.asp	Age, FH of breast cancer (first-degree and second-degree relatives)	Limited to specific combinations of affected relatives; does not incorporate risk factors other than family history
Probability of detecting BRCA *mutation (affected and unaffected women)*		
Tyrer-Cuzick (3) • Also provides 10-yr and lifetime probability of breast cancer	Personal or family history of breast and ovarian cancer, Ashkenazi ethnic background	Incomplete validation, especially in nonwhite populations
Frank et al. (6) • Provides empirical experience from one laboratory • Available for download at www. myriadtests.com/provider/ brca-mutation-prevalence.htm	Personal or family history of breast and ovarian cancer, Ashkenazi ethnic background	Empirical model with incomplete validation; does not include unaffected family members
BRCAPRO (4) • Also provides age-specific probability of breast cancer • Available for download at www4. utsouthwestern.edu/breasthealth/ cagene/default.asp	Personal or family history of breast or ovarian cancer, Ashkenazi ethnic background	Requires information on all affected and unaffected family members; incorporates only FDRs and SDRs, may need to change proband to best capture risk; uses high-penetrance estimates

FDR, first-degree relative; FH, family history; SDR, second-degree relative.

A second group of models is designed to estimate the likelihood of identifying a mutation in the *BRCA1* or *BRCA2* gene (3,4,6–8); these models have strengths and limitations that health care providers need to be familiar with to use and interpret them appropriately (9–11). The BRCAPRO model estimates the probability that an individual is a carrier of a *BRCA* mutation using family history and Bayes' theorem (4). However, BRCAPRO incorporates relevant family history only up to second-degree relatives, potentially underestimating the probability of *BRCA* mutations in individuals with an extended family history (e.g., early-onset breast cancer or ovarian cancer in cousins). The BRCAPRO model does not incorporate pancreatic or prostate cancer risk into its risk estimate, thereby leading to a potential underestimate of risk. On the other hand, the BRCAPRO model analysis is based primarily on large, high-penetrance families, and this may lead to overestimation of risk in a more diverse risk assessment clinic.

It is important when using these models to understand the limitations of these risk calculations and to place risk estimates into the appropriate context. It is important to note that risk estimates calculated using different models may vary—a factor that complicates the use of quantitative thresholds for making screening recommendations (12). The health care provider should use clinical judgment in conjunction with estimates from models to provide the most precise risk assessment for an individual patient. There are no statistical models at present that predict the likelihood of identifying mutations in the *PTEN*, *p53*, or *CDH1* genes; thus it is important to be able to recognize other genetic syndromes on the basis of family history.

■ IDENTIFICATION OF INDIVIDUALS AT HIGHEST RISK FOR BREAST CANCER

Most of the aforementioned risk models rely, to various degrees, on family history of cancer, but none is foolproof in the identification of individuals at the highest risk for breast cancer (i.e., those with a mutation in a cancer predisposition gene). The National Comprehensive Cancer Network (NCCN) has established criteria for individuals who need further genetic risk assessment (Table 2.2). If an individual meets these criteria, the NCCN recommends that the individual be referred to a cancer genetics professional for further workup and potential genetic testing (13).

Setting up explicit risk assessment criteria is very important so that individuals with an inherited cancer are identified as such and referred properly. In one study of family practitioners (14), the detail of information present in the individual's medical record was insufficient to permit risk assessment for more than two thirds of individuals with a significant family history of colon cancer. In the same study, the appropriate level of cancer screening was not achieved in half the patients with a family history of colon cancer, individuals at moderate or high cancer risk were not identified as such, and those at high risk were not offered cancer genetics referral. Although no studies such as this are available with regard to breast cancer family history, one could hypothesize that the same phenomenon holds true for that common cancer.

The process of identifying those needing further genetics assessment will vary from institution to institution.

■ Table 2.2 Criteria for referral to a genetics professional for breast cancer risk assessment

- Early-onset breast cancer[a] (<50 yr)
- Two breast primaries or breast and ovarian cancer[b] in a single individual OR two or more breast primaries or breast and ovarian cancers in close relative(s) from the same side of a family (maternal or paternal)
- Clustering of breast cancer with one or more of the following: thyroid cancer, sarcoma, adrenocortical carcinoma, endometrial cancer, pancreatic cancer, brain tumors, dermatologic manifestations, or leukemia/lymphoma on same side of the family
- Member of a family with a known mutation in a cancer susceptibility gene
- Populations at risk[c]
- Any male breast cancer
- Ovarian cancer[b]: one or more on same side of family

[a]Ductal carcinoma in situ included.
[b]Fallopian tube cancer and primary peritoneal cancer included.
[c]For populations at risk, the guidelines may be more tightened (e.g., women of Ashkenazi Jewish ancestry with breast or ovarian cancer at any age).
Source: From Ref. 13.

Some programs will rely on physicians to recognize these risks and refer individuals to cancer genetics. Caution should be used in this approach, however, because the success of this process will rely on multiple factors—the strongest of which is patient inquiry about the need for genetic testing for cancer (15,16). Other institutions will implement a rudimentary screening program and use a "pen and paper" family history questionnaire that is reviewed by a trained staff member to identify and refer for genetic counseling. Still others will use a more complex approach, where a patient inputs his or her personal and family history into a software program, and the software identifies those needing genetic counseling (17,18). Providing family history information via the Internet is a potentially powerful tool for identifying such individuals, and interest in this modality is high (19). Data are lacking, however, on which of these methods is most efficient for identifying individuals at risk (20).

Once an individual is recognized as being at increased risk, it is important that he or she is referred to a cancer genetics professional (13) because the importance of pretest and posttest genetic counseling for cancer susceptibility testing is widely recognized (21). Referral to a cancer genetics professional is also important because the provider ordering the genetic testing must understand the complexities of genetic testing and the appropriate interpretation of the test results. One study reported that patients undergoing genetic testing for *APC* mutations often received inadequate counseling and would have been given incorrectly interpreted results (22). The authors concluded that physicians should be prepared to offer genetic counseling if they order genetic tests. If the physician is not adequately trained in the complexities of cancer genetic testing, a referral to a cancer genetics professional should be made. The genetics professional will obtain a more detailed family history and determine whether genetic testing is appropriate.

■ GENETIC COUNSELING AND RISK ASSESSMENT

The genetics professional will most often begin the assessment by collecting a detailed family history. Typically, a detailed three-generation family history is constructed in the form of a pedigree (23,24). It is important to gather information on both maternal and paternal lineages, with particular focus on individuals with malignancies (affecteds). Table 2.3 illustrates effective questions used by providers in obtaining this information. It is imperative to include those family members without a personal history of cancer (unaffecteds) because the ratio and pattern of affecteds and unaffecteds influence the risk assessment. It

■ **Table 2.3** Useful questions to use when obtaining a family history	
Questions to Ask All Patients	**Questions to Ask Patients Who Have Had Cancer or Regarding Relatives With Cancer**
• Age • Personal history of benign or malignant tumors • Major illnesses • Hospitalizations • Surgeries • Biopsy history • Reproductive history[a] • Cancer surveillance • Environmental exposures	• Organ in which tumor developed • Age at time of diagnosis • Number of tumors[b] • Pathology, stage, and grade of malignant tumors • Pathology of benign tumors • Treatment regimen (surgery, chemotherapy, radiation)

[a]Especially important for women at increased risk of breast, ovarian, or endometrial cancer. Inquire about age at menarche; age at first live birth; history of oral contraceptive use, infertility medications, or hormone replacement therapy, including dosage and duration; and age at menopause.
[b]For patients who have developed more than one tumor, it is important to discriminate whether the additional tumor was a separate primary, a recurrence, or the result of metastatic disease.

Source: From Ref. 31.

is equally important to include the presence of nonmalignant findings in the proband and family members because some inherited cancer syndromes have other physical characteristics associated with them [e.g., trichilemmomas with Cowden's syndrome (CS)].

When the family history is taken, the accuracy of the information obtained from an individual patient should be considered. Many factors can influence an individual's knowledge of his or her family history (Table 2.4). A recent study indicates that individuals are often confident that a family member has had cancer but are typically unsure of the details surrounding that diagnosis (20,25). Reports of breast cancer tend to be accurate, whereas reports of ovarian cancer are less trustworthy (26,27). It is also important to note that family histories can change over time, with new diagnoses arising in family members as time passes.

All these factors must be considered during the consultation, as the risk assessment and differential diagnosis are based primarily on this information. The primary purpose of the risk assessment process is to distinguish a hereditary form of cancer from familial clustering of cancer and sporadic forms of cancer. Features of a family history that are suggestive of a hereditary cancer syndrome include a preponderance of relatives with similar or related cancers; earlier age at onset of cancer; an autosomal dominant pattern of cancer inheritance; the presence of rare cancers; the presence of multifocal, bilateral, or multiple primary cancers in one individual; and the absence of environmental risk factors. When a hereditary form of cancer is suspected, genetic testing should be considered.

Although some published guidelines for genetic testing exist, much of the time the decision to offer genetic testing is based on clinical judgment. The American Society of Clinical Oncology (ASCO) recommends that genetic testing be offered when (a) the individual has personal or

■ **Table 2.4** Challenges to collecting an accurate family history

• Family history is incomplete:
  • Family members live far away
  • Clients are not prepared to answer questions
  • Cancer is not discussed in the family
• Family history information is not available:
  • Lost contact with relatives
  • Estrangement from the family
  • Adoption
• Reported history is false:
  • Mistaken about the cancer diagnosis
  • Confused about the diagnosis
  • Deliberately fabricating history

Source: Adapted from Ref. 130.

family history features suggestive of a genetic cancer susceptibility condition, (b) the test can be adequately interpreted, and (c) the results will aid in diagnosis or influence the medical or surgical management of the patient or family members at hereditary risk of cancer (21). The NCCN provides guidelines for individuals who should be offered genetic testing for hereditary breast/ovarian cancer syndrome, Li-Fraumeni syndrome (LFS), and CS (13). In the end, however, it is up to the individual provider's judgment as to whether genetic testing is indicated.

■ GENETIC TESTING PROCESS

Once it has been determined that genetic testing is appropriate, the next step is to determine which individual in the family should be tested first. If there is no known mutation in a family, testing should begin with a person with the highest probability of having a mutation. Typically, this is a person who has been diagnosed with cancer at an early age. If no such person is available, the person with the highest a priori risk of carrying a mutation in the gene should be tested. If there is a known mutation in the family, testing should begin with the family members with the highest risk of carrying the familial mutation.

Finding the appropriate laboratory to perform the testing is also very important. Genetic testing for most cancer susceptibility genes is available at a variety of laboratories in a variety of settings. Table 2.5 lists the syndromes discussed in this chapter and the clinically certified laboratories that offer testing for these in the United States. It is important to note that many genetic tests can be done in a research lab as well as a clinical laboratory. Clinical certification via the Clinical Laboratory Improvement Amendments (CLIA) of 1988, however, is essential when using DNA tests for clinical management of the individual. When choosing a laboratory, it is important to consider the fact that laboratory techniques (as well as the sensitivity of the technique) vary. Finally, the cost of testing and level of insurance coverage need to be taken into account when choosing a laboratory to perform the genetic test.

Once a laboratory has been identified, it is necessary to obtain informed consent from the individual undergoing the test. The components and process of informed consent for cancer genetic testing have been described thoroughly (28–30) and are presented in Table 2.6. It is important to note that some US states have very specific laws that provide requirements as to what are the necessary components of the informed consent document itself.

The turnaround time for the genetic test will vary by gene and by laboratory. Once the results are available, it is important to disclose the results to the patient in a timely fashion. The provider should review the significance of the

---

■ Table 2.5 Clinical testing laboratories in the United States

Gene	Laboratories
BRCA1/2	Myriad Genetics Laboratories (www.myriad.com)
	New Jersey Medical School (http://njms.umdnj.edu/genesweb2/diagnostic.html)
	UCLA Medical Center (www.pathnet.medsch.ucla.edu/referral/ODT%20Center/odtc_main.htm)
	UCSF (http://labmed.ucsf.edu/mdx2/)
	University of Chicago (http://genes.uchicago.edu/)
	University of North Carolina Hospitals (http://labs.unchealthcare.org/directory/molecular_pathology/index_html)
	University of Pittsburgh Medical Center (http://path.upmc.edu/divisions/mdx/diagnostics.html)
PTEN	Baylor College of Medicine (www.bcm.edu/geneticlabs/)
	Boston University School of Medicine (www.bumc.bu.edu/hg/)
	Emory University School of Medicine (www.genetics.emory.edu/egl/)
	GeneDx (www.genedx.com/)
	Greenwood Genetics Center (www.ggc.org/diagnostic.htm)
	Johns Hopkins Hospital (www.hopkinsmedicine.org/dnadiagnostic/)
	Signature Genomic Laboratories (www.signaturegenomics.com/)
	Ohio State University (www.pathology.med.ohio-state.edu/ext/Divisions/Clinical/molpath/)
	University of Michigan (http://sitemaker.umich.edu/michigan.medical.genetics.laboratories/home)
	University of Oklahoma Health Sciences Center (www.genetics.ouhsc.edu/)
	Yale University School of Medicine (www.genetics.ouhsc.edu/)
p53	Baylor College of Medicine (www.bcm.edu/geneticlabs/)
	Center for Genetic Testing at St. Francis (www.sfh-lab.com/)
	City of Hope National Medical Center (http://mdl.cityofhope.org/)
	Duke University Health System (http://manual.clinlabs.duke.edu/DukeMolecular/default.aspx)
	Emory University School of Medicine (www.genetics.emory.edu/egl/)
	Harvard Medical School (www.hpcgg.org/LMM/)
	Huntington Medical Research Institute (http://home.pacbell.net/genedoc/Eggspage.html)
CDH1	City of Hope National Medical Center (http://mdl.cityofhope.org/)
	Henry Ford Hospital (www.henryford.com/)
	Stanford Clinical Labs (www.stanfordlab.com)

Source: From Ref. 131.

■ **Table 2.6** Components of informed consent

1. Purpose of the test and whom to test
2. General information about the gene(s)
3. Possible test results:
   - Positive result
   - Negative result: no mutation in the family (i.e., uninformative negative)
   - Negative results: known mutation in the family (i.e., true negative)
   - Variant of uncertain significance
4. Likelihood of positive result
5. Technical aspects and accuracy of the test
6. Economic considerations
7. Risks of genetic discrimination
8. Psychosocial aspects:
   - Anticipated reaction to results
   - Timing and readiness for testing
   - Family issues
   - Preparing for results
9. Confidentiality issues
10. Utilization of test results
11. Alternatives to genetic testing
12. Storage and potential reuse of genetic material

Source: Adapted from Ref. 31.

results and quantify the patient's risk for developing cancer, the emotional impact of the test results on the individual, screening recommendations, how the patient's medical management should proceed given the test results, and the importance of sharing the information with his or her relatives; the provider also should offer additional resources such as informational brochures, Web sites, and support group information if appropriate and desired (31).

The importance of maintaining communication between the health care provider and the patient should be stressed (31). For those individuals who are found to carry a mutation in a cancer predisposition gene, the follow-up can ensure that the patient is adhering to appropriate screening recommendations and also that there is dissemination of the test result through the family. For individuals who are found to be "true negative," the future contact can ensure that they understand what is appropriate screening (i.e., neither too much screening nor avoidance of appropriate, general-population screening recommendations). Patients receiving a "variant of uncertain significance" should stay in touch with the ordering provider so that if the variant is reclassified any new information can be communicated quickly to the patient and the family.

Finally, patients receiving an uninformative negative (i.e., a negative result when no mutation has been previously identified in the family) should stay in contact with the ordering provider so that as new tests become available the provider can advise whether these newer techniques

are appropriate for them. This issue has come up twice recently with genetic testing for *BRCA1/2*. In 2002, Myriad Genetics labs introduced a newer technique for detecting mutations in *BRCA1*. Again, in 2005, Myriad Genetics added a technique called "Rearrangement Testing," which brings the sensitivity of the *BRCA1/2* test up to nearly 99%. For women who had testing prior to these newer technologies, it was important to communicate the availability of these tests so that they could decide whether to proceed with the additional test. The most appropriate method to recontact patients has yet to be determined, and interestingly, the uptake of the additional testing was quite low in one study (32). Nonetheless, every attempt to communicate with individuals should be made to ensure that they receive the best care.

■ TIMING OF GENETIC TESTING

For most of the syndromes discussed in this chapter, genetic testing takes 4 to 12 weeks and results are not available early enough to impact the treatment of a newly diagnosed breast cancer patient. There are two very important exceptions to this.

BRCA1/2 genetic test results are typically available within 14 days of the blood draw. The information gleaned from this test has the potential to affect surgical decision making if the results are available prior to definitive surgery. If a woman tests positive for a deleterious mutation, for example, she may choose bilateral mastectomy to treat her cancer and reduce the risk of developing a second breast malignancy. Studies have shown that women are interested in obtaining this information at the time of diagnosis as it may help them plan their choice of surgery (33). However, women who indicate prior to *BRCA* test initiation that they would not consider bilateral mastectomies even with a *BRCA* mutation are likely to proceed with breast-conserving surgery regardless of *BRCA* result (34). For several reasons, it is important that women who are interested in and would use this testing information in their surgical decision making be identified *prior to* any definitive treatment. When women undergo genetic counseling after definitive surgery, they are less likely to consider genetic testing pertinent to them (35). In addition, one study showed that women who had *BRCA1/2* testing and who had initially undergone breast-conserving surgery chose to undergo subsequent bilateral mastectomies prior to receiving radiation therapy (36). This subjects these women to another surgical procedure and all of the associated risks. Finally, women with a family history of breast cancer may be advised to consider bilateral mastectomies for treatment of their newly diagnosed breast cancer. If tested for *BRCA* mutations, most women

■ **Table 2.7** Genes associated with a hereditary predisposition to breast cancer

High-penetrance Gene	Syndrome	Breast Cancer Risk by Age 70 Yr (%)	Major Associated Cancers
BRCA1	Hereditary breast and ovarian cancer	39–87	Breast, ovary
BRCA2	Hereditary breast and ovarian cancer	26–91	Breast, ovary, prostate, pancreatic
p53	Li-Fraumeni syndrome	>90	Soft-tissue sarcoma, osteosarcoma, brain tumors, adrenocortical carcinoma, leukemia, colon cancer
PTEN	Cowden's syndrome; Bannayan-Riley-Ruvalcaba syndrome; Proteus syndrome; Proteus-like syndrome	25–50	Thyroid, endometrial, genitourinary
CDH1	Hereditary diffuse gastric carcinoma	39 (Ref. 124)	Lobular breast and diffuse gastric cancer; other tumors

would find that they are not mutation carriers. It has been reported that women who learn that they are not mutation carriers *after* the prophylactic procedure may question the decision for prophylactic surgery. This, in turn, is often associated with complications and quality of life problems that they never envisioned (37).

Genetic testing for *p53* mutations can take as little as 3 weeks if ordered as an "urgent" test. It is well known that *p53* mutant cells are extremely sensitive to DNA damage (38,39). In vivo studies suggest that DNA-damaging agents (e.g., chemotherapy and radiotherapy) used for treatment of a cancer in an individual with LFS may increase the risk of a second malignancy (40). One study showed that the risk of developing a second cancer after radiotherapy treatment was as high as 57% and that radiotherapy should be avoided in *p53* mutation carriers (41). Although it may not be possible to avoid chemotherapy in many situations, radiotherapy sometimes can be avoided by choosing mastectomy rather than lumpectomy for surgical treatment. When radiation cannot be avoided, it is imperative that treating physicians and the patient remain aware of the risk of a second primary tumor in the radiation field (40,42).

■ **HEREDITARY BREAST CANCER SYNDROMES**

The identification of individuals with cancer predisposition gene mutations affords the mutation carriers the ability to use the information in making medical management decisions. Four of the most clearly described hereditary breast cancer syndromes for which genetic testing is available are the hereditary breast and ovarian cancer syndrome (HBOCS), CS, LFS, and hereditary diffuse gastric carcinoma syndrome (HDGCS) (Table 2.7). All these syndromes are inherited in an autosomal dominant pattern and are associated with other cancers and clinical features. As noted previously in this chapter, genetic testing for each of the genes associated with these syndromes is available through commercial and research laboratories (see Table 2.5), allowing for appropriate clinical care genetic counseling and testing for at-risk individuals.

Hereditary Breast and Ovarian Cancer Syndrome

HBOCS is associated with a significantly increased risk for breast cancer and ovarian cancer compared with the general population risk. Mutations in *BRCA1* and *BRCA2* account for 80% to 90% of cases of hereditary breast and ovarian cancers (43). The probability that a mutation is present in a family increases if the family history includes multiple cases of early-onset breast cancer (women younger than 50 years of age), a high rate of bilateral breast tumors, clustering of breast and ovarian cancers, or male breast cancer. However, even among families with more than four cases of breast cancer, ascertained because of a suspicion of a hereditary predisposition, a mutation in *BRCA1* or *BRCA2* was found in only 65% of the cases (43).

BRCA2-associated breast cancers are similar in phenotype and clinical behavior to sporadic cancers (44,45). *BRCA1*-related breast cancers differ from other breast cancers in that they are often high-grade, aneuploid carcinomas that do not express estrogen receptor, progesterone receptor, or HER2 (also referred to as "triple negative" phenotype). They often express cytokeratins 5 and 14, vimentin, epidermal growth factor receptor (EGFR), and

P-cadherin (CDH3)—features that predict clustering with the basal-like phenotype by gene expression profiling (46). Atypical medullary carcinomas have also been observed more frequently in *BRCA1* carriers, a phenotype with abundant lymphocytic infiltrate and a smooth margin, which may contribute to the poorer sensitivity of mammograms in mutation carriers (47). The risk of a contralateral breast cancer among *BRCA1* and *BRCA2* carriers is substantial (approximately 3% per year) (48). Serous papillary ovarian carcinoma is a key feature of hereditary cancers in *BRCA1* mutation carriers; it is less common in *BRCA2* carriers. Endometrioid and clear cell subtypes of ovarian cancer have been observed (49), but borderline ovarian tumors do not seem to be a part of the phenotype (50). Both primary tumors of the fallopian tubes and the peritoneum occur with increased frequency in mutation carriers (51). The prognosis for ovarian cancer in *BRCA1* and *BRCA2* carriers is better than in age-matched controls (49,52).

BRCA1 and BRCA2 are proteins with multiple functions, including repair of double-strand breaks in DNA by homologous recombination (53). New therapeutic strategies have exploited this cellular function with the use of agents that cause DNA strand breaks that require repair through homologous recombination. Compounds such as PARP1 protein inhibitors, which block base excision repair, are emerging as potential therapeutic agents in cancers developing in *BRCA1* and *BRCA2* mutation carriers (54).

The *BRCA1* and *BRCA2* genes were cloned in 1994 and 1995, respectively (55,56). More than 1200 deleterious mutations have been identified throughout the length of these large genes: *BRCA1*, located on 17q11, encodes an 1863-amino-acid polypeptide (55), and *BRCA2*, located on 13q12–q13, encodes 3418 amino acids (56,57). Most pathogenic *BRCA1* or *BRCA2* mutations block protein production from the mutated allele and have been identified as frameshift or nonsense mutations or large genomic deletions or duplications (58,59). Missense mutations that interfere with critical regions of the gene, such as the RING finger motif or BRCT region of *BRCA1* (60) or the PALB2 gene-binding region of *BRCA2* (61), behave like truncating mutations, whereas most missense mutations remain uncharacterized and are considered variants of uncertain significance (60). *BRCA1* and *BRCA2* mutations are rare in most populations, occurring in approximately 1 in 400 people, but are much more common in the Ashkenazi Jewish population, in which 1 in 40 people carries one of three main disease-causing mutations: two in *BRCA1* (185delAG and 5382insC) and the 6174delT mutation in *BRCA2* (62). The prevalence of nonfounder mutations identified in Jewish women undergoing genetic testing is approximately 2% (63). Other founder mutations have been identified, including the *BRCA2* 999del5 mutation in Iceland, which is associated with an increased risk

for prostate cancer in some kindreds, and specific large *BRCA1* deletions in the Dutch population (64,65).

The penetrance or lifetime risk of developing breast or ovarian cancer remains an active area of research even 15 years after the discovery of *BRCA1* and *BRCA2*. Women with mutations in *BRCA1* have an estimated lifetime risk of breast cancer in the range of 50% to 80%, and for women with *BRCA2* mutations, the range is 40% to 70% (43,66,67). The rates of survival for women with breast cancers associated with *BRCA1* or *BRCA2* are similar to those for women without these mutations (68). The range of breast cancer risk associated with mutations in *BRCA1* and *BRCA2* is influenced by the population under study: Higher risk estimates have come from studies with affected families and somewhat lower risk estimates from studies in populations. The lifetime risk of ovarian cancer is 40% for *BRCA1* mutation carriers and 20% for *BRCA2* carriers (69). The risk of ovarian cancer is not the same for all *BRCA2* mutations, with mutations in the central ovarian cancer cluster region conferring a higher lifetime risk (70). Other factors, such as birth cohort, oral contraceptive use, age at first pregnancy, and exercise, have all been shown to influence penetrance risk in populations (67). The most robust risk modifier in *BRCA1* and *BRCA2* carriers has been prophylactic oophorectomy, which reduces the subsequent lifetime risk of breast cancer by about 50% (71,72). These clinical observations highlight the fact that risk associated with highly penetrant mutations can be modified or reduced by lifestyle factors, exogenous and endogenous hormone exposures, and possible other strategies.

Several studies have shown an association between *BRCA* mutations and increased risks for other cancers. The cancer risks for *BRCA1* carriers are confined largely to the breast and ovary, whereas pancreas, prostate, melanoma, and other cancer risks are associated with *BRCA2* carriers (73–76).

On the basis of genome-wide linkage studies for breast cancer susceptibility genes, it is thought that other genes with a population frequency and risk profile similar to *BRCA1* or *BRCA2* are unlikely to exist (77); however, genome-wide association studies have identified a class of susceptibility genes in 15% to 40% of women with breast cancer that confer a minimal relative risk of breast cancer (78–82). The clinical utility of these findings is unclear, but these common, low-risk alleles may account for a measurable fraction of population risk through gene-gene interactions. Moderate-risk alleles that are rare in most populations and are associated with an approximate relative risk of breast cancer of 2.0 have been identified and include *BRIP1*, *PALB2*, *ATM*, and *CHECK2*. These alleles may be more clinically significant in selected populations. For example, in the case of *CHECK2*, the carrier frequency is approximately 1% for the 1100delC mutation in Dutch and Finnish populations, the S428F mutant in the

Ashkenazi Jewish population, and the founder mutation IVS2+1G→A in Slavic populations (83). Founder mutations in *PALB2* occur in people in Finland and Quebec, Canada (84,85).

Three breast cancer genes, *BRCA2*, *PALB2*, and *BRIP1*, are associated with Fanconi's anemia when present as biallelic mutations (86). Fanconi's anemia is a rare childhood disease that is characterized by skeletal defects, skin pigmentation, short stature, microphthalmia, and, in some subtypes, medulloblastoma and Wilms' tumors. For those children who survive to adulthood, early-onset acute myeloid leukemia and skin tumors are common.

The current recommendations for the screening of women at risk for HBOCS are based on the best available evidence and are expected to change as more specific features of diseases related to *BRCA1* and *BRCA2* become available. Training in breast self-examination with regular monthly practice should begin at age 18, and semiannual clinical breast exams should begin at age 25 (13,87,88). Women should begin having annual mammograms and breast magnetic resonance imaging (MRI) screening at age 25 or on an individualized timetable based on the earliest age of cancer onset in family members (89–91). Risk-reduction mastectomies are an appropriate consideration for women at the highest hereditary risk for breast cancer. Studies have shown a 90% to 95% reduction in breast cancer risk following prophylactic mastectomy (92–95). Discussion of the benefits and risks of mastectomy should include a review of the degree of protection, reconstruction options, and potential psychological impact. The evidence for the use of tamoxifen or raloxifene as a chemopreventive agent in *BRCA* mutation carriers is limited; however, tamoxifen has been shown to reduce the risk of contralateral breast cancers in carriers (96,97).

Risk-reducing bilateral salpingo-oophorectomy (RRBSO), ideally between the ages of 35 and 40 years or on completion of child bearing, is recommended for management of ovarian cancer risk in *BRCA* mutation carriers. Two recent studies support the role of RRBSO: The hazard ratios for ovarian cancer for women who underwent prophylactic surgery and those who chose close surveillance were 0.15 and 0.04, respectively (71,72). Women should be informed about the potential for the subsequent development of peritoneal carcinomatosis, which has been reported up to 15 years after RRBSO (51,98). Individuals who do not elect risk-reducing surgery should undergo concurrent transvaginal ultrasound and CA-125 every 6 months from 35 years of age or from 5 to 10 years younger than the age of first ovarian cancer diagnosis in the family (88). Combination oral contraceptives containing estrogen and progestin have resulted in a protective effect against ovarian cancer in some studies but not in others (99–101). Particularly in *BRCA1* mutation carriers, there remains the concern of a small increased risk of breast cancer related to oral contraceptive use (101).

Male *BRCA* mutation carriers are advised to undergo training in breast self-examination with regular monthly practice, semiannual clinical breast examinations, and workup of any suspicious breast lesions. The NCCN also recommend that a baseline mammogram be considered, with an annual mammogram if gynecomastia or parenchymal/glandular breast density is identified on baseline study (13). The NCCN guidelines recommend that male *BRCA* mutation carriers should begin prostate cancer screening at age 50, or earlier, based on the youngest age of diagnosis in the family, with other guidelines suggesting that *BRCA* mutation carriers should begin screening for prostate cancer at age 40 (13,74).

Li-Fraumeni Syndrome

LFS is a rare cancer predisposition syndrome that accounts for approximately 1% of hereditary breast cancers (102). Germline mutations in the well-known tumor suppressor gene *p53* are the primary cause of LFS. Classic LFS is defined as three first-degree relatives with component tumors diagnosed before the age of 45 years: soft tissue and osteosarcomas, breast cancer, brain tumors, adrenal cortical carcinoma (ACC), and leukemia (103). Subsequently, many additional tumors have been observed to occur with increased frequency in individuals with LFS, including gastric, pancreatic, and other pediatric cancers (104–107).

The cancer risk associated with LFS has been studied extensively. A study of LFS relatives in 159 extended families found the risk for developing cancer among carriers was 12%, 35%, 52%, and 80% by 20, 30, 40, and 50 years of age, respectively (108). A woman with LFS has a breast cancer risk of 56% by age 45 and greater than 90% by age 70, with most diagnoses of breast cancer occurring under the age of 40 (107,109,110).

Li and Fraumeni and colleagues developed the first clinical diagnostic criteria for LFS, based on their study of 24 LFS kindreds, and these criteria have come to be known as the classic or strictest diagnostic criteria (103). In an attempt to determine whom to test for germline mutations associated with LFS, other groups loosened the strict LFS criteria, developing criteria for Li-Fraumeni–like syndrome (LFLS) (111). LFLS is identified when a proband has any childhood cancer or sarcoma, brain cancer, or ACC diagnosed by age 45 years and has a first- or second-degree family member with a typical LFS cancer at any age and another first- or second-degree family member with cancer diagnosed before age 60 years. Another definition of LFLS (112) was two first- or second-degree relatives with a LFS-related tumor diagnosed at any age. Chompret and colleagues (109) recommended that testing for *p53* mutations should be considered in families who meet the following criteria: a proband affected by sarcoma, brain tumor, breast cancer, or ACC before age 36 years, with at least one first- or second-degree relative diagnosed with cancer (other than breast cancer if the proband has breast cancer) before age 46 years or a relative with multiple primary tumors at any age. The largest single report of testing for germline *p53* mutations in 525 consecutive patients whose blood samples were submitted for diagnostic testing was published in 2009 (113). Mutations were identified in 17% of the 525 patients: All families with a *p53* mutation had at least one family member with a sarcoma or breast, brain, or adrenocortical carcinoma; every individual with a choroid plexus tumor (8/8) and 14 of 21 individuals with childhood ACC had a mutation regardless of family history. On the basis of reported personal and family history, 95% of patients with a mutation met either classic LFS or Chompret criteria (Table 2.8).

Management of individuals at risk for LFS is difficult because of the diverse array of tumors and the fact that the rarity of the syndrome has made studies of intensified surveillance logistically difficult. Current breast screening guidelines (13) recommend training and education in breast self-examination and regular monthly breast self-examination starting at age 18, semiannual clinical breast examination starting at ages 20 to 25 or 5 to 10 years before the age at onset of the earliest known breast cancer in the family (whichever is earliest), and annual mammogram and breast MRI screening starting at ages 20 to 25 or individualized based on the earliest age of onset in the family. Options for risk-reducing mastectomy should be discussed on a case-by-case basis and include counseling on the degree of protection, degree of cancer risk, and reconstruction options. Many of the other cancers associated with *p53* mutations do not lend themselves to early

detection. Screening may be considered for cancer survivors with LFS, with annual comprehensive physical examination and colonoscopy every 2 to 5 years starting no later than 25 years of age. Pediatricians should be apprised of the risk of childhood cancers in affected families.

Cowden's Syndrome

CS, also known as multiple hamartoma syndrome, is characterized by the formation of multiple hamartomas that may develop in any organ, with a high risk of benign and malignant tumors of the thyroid, breast, and endometrium. Consensus diagnostic criteria for CS establish three diagnostic categories (114), with pathognomonic criteria including facial trichilemmomas, acral keratoses, papillomatous papules, and mucosal lesions. Major and minor criteria may also be considered, including Lhermitte-Duclos disease and benign lesions of the breast and other organs (Table 2.9). Women with CS have up to a 76% risk for benign breast disease, such as fibroadenomas and fibrocystic breast disease, and a 25% to 50% lifetime risk for breast cancer (115–117). An increased risk of early-onset male breast cancer has also been identified in mutation carriers (118).

The gene for CS, *PTEN*, a tumor suppressor gene, has been mapped to 10q22–23 (119). *PTEN* acts as a tumor suppressor by mediating cell cycle arrest and/or apoptosis (120). Mutations in the *PTEN* gene are also associated with Bannayan-Riley-Ruvalcaba syndrome, Proteus syndrome, and Proteus-like syndrome. Full sequencing and molecular testing by Southern blot are available clinically and on a research basis, respectively. A *PTEN* mutation can be detected in about 80% of patients who meet the strict operational diagnostic criteria for CS (121).

Women who have CS should be screened for breast cancer, with regular monthly breast self-examination beginning at age 18 years, clinical breast examinations beginning at age 25 years or 5 to 10 years earlier than the earliest known breast cancer in the family, and annual mammography and breast MRI beginning at ages 30 to 35 years or 5 to 10 years earlier than the earliest-onset breast cancer diagnosis in the family (whichever is earlier) (13). The American Cancer Society recommends annual breast MRI for individuals with CS and their first-degree relatives (12). Options for prophylactic mastectomy should be discussed on a case-by-case basis. Endometrial carcinoma screening with blind endometrial biopsies should be performed annually in premenopausal women starting at age 35 to 40 years (or 5 years before the earliest endometrial cancer diagnosis in the family), and annual endometrial ultrasonography should be performed in postmenopausal women (13). A comprehensive annual physical examination starting at age 18 years with screening for skin and

---

■ **Table 2.8** Classic and Chompret criteria for Li-Fraumeni syndrome[a]

Classic Li-Fraumeni syndrome:

- Proband with sarcoma diagnosed at age 45 yr or younger, and
- First-degree relative with any cancer diagnosed at age 45 yr or younger, and
- Another first- or second-degree relative in the same lineage diagnosed at age 45 yr or younger with any cancer or a sarcoma at any age

Chompret criteria:

- One first- or second-degree relative with cancer diagnosed before the age of 46 yr
- Multiple primary tumors in the proband, regardless of family history

---

[a]In a study of a cohort of 525 patients undergoing testing for *p53* germline mutations, 95% of patients (71 of 75) with a mutation met either classic or Chompret criteria (113).

Note: See Refs. 103 and 109 for classic and Chrompet criteria, respectively.

■ **Table 2.9** International Cowden Syndrome Consortium operational criteria for diagnosis of Cowden's syndrome

Pathognomonic criteria (mucocutaneous lesions):

- Facial trichilemmomas
- Acral keratoses
- Papillomatous papules
- Mucosal lesions

Major criteria:

- Breast cancer
- Nonmedullary thyroid carcinoma, especially follicular thyroid cancer
- Macrocephaly (occipital frontal circumference ≥95%)
- Endometrial carcinoma
- Lhermitte-Duclos disease

Minor criteria:

- Other thyroid disease (e.g., multinodular goiter or adenoma)
- Mental retardation (IQ ≤75)
- Gastrointestinal hamartomas
- Fibrocystic breast disease
- Lipomas
- Fibromas
- Genitourinary tumors (e.g., renal cell carcinoma)
- Genitourinary malformations
- Uterine fibroids

Operational diagnosis in an individual, any single pathognomonic criterion, but

1. Mucocutaneous lesions alone if there are:
   a. Six or more facial papules, three or more of which must be trichilemmoma, or
   b. Cutaneous facial papules and oral mucosal papillomatous, or
   c. Oral mucosal papillomatosis and acral keratoses, or
   d. Six or more palmoplantar keratoses
2. Two major criteria, but one must be macrocephaly or Lhermitte-Duclos disease
3. One major and three minor criteria
4. Four minor criteria

Operational diagnosis in a family member with a known diagnosis of Cowden's syndrome in the family:

1. A pathognomonic criterion
2. Any one major criterion with or without minor criteria
3. Two minor criteria

Source: Adapted from Ref. 114.

thyroid lesions, including a baseline thyroid ultrasound, is recommended for men and women with CS. Annual dermatological examination should also be considered. An annual urinalysis, with consideration for annual urine cytology and renal ultrasound, should be performed in both men and women if there is a family history of renal carcinoma.

Hereditary Diffuse Gastric Carcinoma Syndrome

HDGCS is an autosomal dominant susceptibility for diffuse gastric cancer. The common familial histology is a poorly differentiated diffuse gastric adenocarcinoma, often with signet ring histology (122). Penetrance of the syndrome is estimated to be 60% to 80%, with the average age of onset being 38 years (range: 14–69 years). Women have an increased risk for breast cancer, especially lobular carcinoma, and early-onset colon cancers have also been reported (123,124). The E-cadherin gene (*CDH1*) is a calcium-dependent cell-cell adhesion molecule expressed in junctions between epithelial cells (125) and is the only gene known to be associated with HDGCS. Mutations in *CDH1* are found in up to 48% of diffuse gastric cancer kindreds (126).

The 5-year survival rate for diffuse gastric cancer is about 10%. Although it has been proposed that individuals who have a *CDH1* mutation undergo routine surveillance for gastric cancer, the optimal management of individuals at risk is uncertain because of the unproven value of surveillance regimens. Options for screening include annual esophagoduodenoscopy with directed biopsies with or without random biopsies, annual endoscopic ultrasonography, and chromoendoscopy. However, the majority of tumors spread submucosally rather than forming a visible mass, so endoscopic biopsies will likely detect less than 50% of infiltrative tumors, and the role of vital dye staining in detecting diffuse gastric carcinoma is unknown. For these reasons, prophylactic gastrectomy has become part of the management of this syndrome. In two published series, intramural gastric cancer was found in 10 of 10 prophylactic gastrectomy specimens from individuals with germline *CDH1* mutations (127,128). These findings suggest that prophylactic gastrectomy is the best preventive measure for individuals who have a *CDH1* mutation; however, the morbidity from this surgery is high. All individuals have long-term morbidity related to rapid intestinal transit, dumping syndrome, diarrhea, and weight loss (129). These factors should be considered in the decision to undergo prophylactic gastrectomy, as well as the risk of developing extragastric cancers such as lobular breast cancer and colorectal cancer. Postgastrectomy screening and follow-up should include breast and colon cancer screening. Although there are no definite screening guidelines, on the basis of the lifetime risk of approximately 40% of developing breast cancer, referral of women with a *CDH1* mutation to a high-risk breast cancer screening program is appropriate, and breast cancer screening should include a clinical breast examination every 6 months, annual mammography, and annual breast MRI.

■ SUMMARY

Cancer genetics has become an integral subspecialty of the practice of preventive medicine and oncology. The discovery of high-risk cancer susceptibility genes has translated into the need for specialized care for individuals who inherit a predisposition to cancer. This care begins with the identification of individuals at high risk and proceeds through the genetic counseling and testing process, culminating in the heightened surveillance and medical management that are often required for high-risk individuals and possibly their family members. Genetic counselors provide the expertise in the attainment of the family history, cancer risk assessment, and guidance for individuals as they pursue genetic testing through the informed consent process. The interpretation of results, and particularly of unclassified variants, can be complex and warrants appropriate pretest and posttest counseling for people who undergo genetic testing. Ultimately, the goal is the appropriate identification and care of high-risk individuals who can benefit from specialized psychosocial and medical support.

■ MULTIDISCIPLINARY CONSIDERATIONS

- Identification of patients who should consider genetic testing is a multidisciplinary process and includes input from primary care physicians, obstetricians, and gynecologists, as well as oncology specialists.
- Patients presenting with a new cancer diagnosis who have a significant risk of carrying a genetic mutation should be referred promptly to genetic counselors (i.e., prior to any definitive surgery) because their surgical options may be altered.
- Genetic counselors must work with a patient's surgeons, radiation oncologists, and medical oncologists when a mutation carrier is identified so that the appropriate surgical, radiotherapy, and chemotherapy treatments are pursued.

■ REFERENCES

1. Gail MH, Brinton LA, Byar DP, et al. Projecting individualized probabilities of developing breast cancer for white females who are being examined annually. *J Natl Cancer Inst.* 1989;81:1879–1886.
2. Claus EB, Risch N, Thompson WD. Autosomal dominant inheritance of early-onset breast cancer. Implications for risk prediction. *Cancer.* 1994;73:643–651.
3. Tyrer J, Duffy SW, Cuzick J. A breast cancer prediction model incorporating familial and personal risk factors. *Stat Med.* 2004; 23:1111–1130.
4. Berry DA, Iversen ES Jr, Gudbjartsson DF, et al. BRCAPRO validation, sensitivity of genetic testing of BRCA1/BRCA2, and prevalence of other breast cancer susceptibility genes. *J Clin Oncol.* 2002;20:2701–2712.
5. MacKarem G, Roche CA, Hughes KS. The effectiveness of the Gail model in estimating risk for development of breast cancer in women under 40 years of age. *Breast J.* 2001;7:34–39.
6. Frank TS, Manley SA, Olopade OI, et al. Sequence analysis of BRCA1 and BRCA2: correlation of mutations with family history and ovarian cancer risk. *J Clin Oncol.* 1998;16:2417–2425.
7. Couch FJ, DeShano ML, Blackwood MA, et al. BRCA1 mutations in women attending clinics that evaluate the risk of breast cancer. *New Engl J Med.* 1997;336:1409–1415.
8. Shattuck-Eidens D, Oliphant A, McClure M, et al. BRCA1 sequence analysis in women at high risk for susceptibility mutations. Risk factor analysis and implications for genetic testing. *JAMA.* 1997;278:1242–1250.
9. Kang HH, Williams R, Leary J, Ringland C, Kirk J, Ward R. Evaluation of models to predict BRCA germline mutations. *Br J Cancer.* 2006;95:914–920.
10. Barcenas CH, Hosain GM, Arun B, et al. Assessing BRCA carrier probabilities in extended families. *J Clin Oncol.* 2006;24: 354–360.
11. James PA, Doherty R, Harris M, et al. Optimal selection of individuals for BRCA mutation testing: a comparison of available methods. *J Clin Oncol.* 2006;24:707–715.
12. Saslow D, Castle PE, Cox JT, et al. American Cancer Society Guideline for human papillomavirus (HPV) vaccine use to prevent cervical cancer and its precursors. *CA Cancer J Clin.* 2007; 57:7–28.
13. NCCN. *NCCN Clinical Practice Guidelines in Oncology: High-Risk Assessment: Breast and Ovarian.* 2008;V.1.2008.
14. Tyler CV Jr, Snyder CW. Cancer risk assessment: examining the family physician's role. *J Am Board Fam Med.* 2006;19:468–477.
15. Sifri R, Myers R, Hyslop T, et al. Use of cancer susceptibility testing among primary care physicians. *Clin Genet.* 2003;64:355–360.
16. Wideroff L, Freedman AN, Olson L, et al. Physician use of genetic testing for cancer susceptibility: results of a national survey. *Cancer Epidemiol Biomarkers Prev.* 2003;12:295–303.
17. Acheson LS, Zyzanski SJ, Stange KC, Deptowicz A, Wiesner GL. Validation of a self-administered, computerized tool for collecting and displaying the family history of cancer. *J Clin Oncol.* 2006;24:5395–5402.
18. Sweet KM, Bradley TL, Westman JA. Identification and referral of families at high risk for cancer susceptibility. *J Clin Oncol.* 2002;20:528–537.
19. Simon C, Acheson L, Burant C, et al. Patient interest in recording family histories of cancer via the Internet. *Genet Med.* 2008; 10:895–902.
20. Reid GT, Walter FM, Brisbane JM, Emery JD. Family history questionnaires designed for clinical use: a systematic review. *Public Health Genomics.* 2009;12:73–83.
21. ASCO. American Society of Clinical Oncology policy statement update: genetic testing for cancer susceptibility. *J Clin Oncol.* 2003; 21:2397–2406.
22. Giardiello FM, Brensinger JD, Petersen GM, et al. The use and interpretation of commercial APC gene testing for familial adenomatous polyposis. *N Engl J Med.* 1997;336:823–827.
23. Bennett RL, French KS, Resta RG, Doyle DL. Standardized human pedigree nomenclature: update and assessment of the recommendations of the National Society of Genetic Counselors. *J Genet Couns.* 2008;17:424–433.
24. Bennett RL, Steinhaus KA, Uhrich SB, et al. Recommendations for standardized human pedigree nomenclature. Pedigree

Standardization Task Force of the National Society of Genetic Counselors. *Am J Hum Genet*. 1995;56:745–752.

25. Jefferies S, Goldgar D, Eeles R. The accuracy of cancer diagnoses as reported in families with head and neck cancer: a case-control study. *Clin Oncol (R Coll Radiol)*. 2008;20:309–314.

26. Murff HJ, Spigel DR, Syngal S. Does this patient have a family history of cancer? An evidence-based analysis of the accuracy of family cancer history. *JAMA*. 2004;292:1480–1489.

27. Chang ET, Smedby KE, Hjalgrim H, Glimelius B, Adami HO. Reliability of self-reported family history of cancer in a large case-control study of lymphoma. *J Natl Cancer Inst*. 2006;98:61–68.

28. Bernhardt BA, Geller G, Strauss M, et al. Toward a model informed consent process for BRCA1 testing: a qualitative assessment of women's attitudes. *J Genet Couns*. 1997;6:207–222.

29. Geller G, Botkin JR, Green MJ, et al. Genetic testing for susceptibility to adult-onset cancer. The process and content of informed consent. *JAMA*. 1997;277:1467–1474.

30. Geller G, Strauss M, Bernhardt BA, Holtzman NA. Decoding informed consent. Insights from women regarding breast cancer susceptibility testing. *Hastings Cent Rep*. 1997;27:28–33.

31. Trepanier A, Ahrens M, McKinnon W, et al. Genetic cancer risk assessment and counseling: recommendations of the National Society of Genetic Counselors. *J Genet Couns*. 2004;13:83–114.

32. Shannon KM, Muzikansky A, Chan-Smutko G, Niendorf KB, Ryan PD. Uptake of BRCA1 rearrangement panel testing: in individuals previously tested for BRCA1/2 mutations. *Genet Med*. 2006;8:740–745.

33. Schwartz MD, Lerman C, Brogan B, et al. Impact of BRCA1/BRCA2 counseling and testing on newly diagnosed breast cancer patients. *J Clin Oncol*. 2004;22:1823–1829.

34. Ray JA, Loescher LJ, Brewer M. Risk-reduction surgery decisions in high-risk women seen for genetic counseling. *J Genet Couns*. 2005;14:473–484.

35. Vadaparampil ST, Quinn GP, Brzosowicz J, Miree CA. Experiences of genetic counseling for BRCA1/2 among recently diagnosed breast cancer patients: a qualitative inquiry. *J Psychosoc Oncol*. 2008;26:33–52.

36. Stolier AJ, Corsetti RL. Newly diagnosed breast cancer patients choose bilateral mastectomy over breast-conserving surgery when testing positive for a BRCA1/2 mutation. *Am Surg*. 2005;71:1031–1033.

37. Silva E. Genetic counseling and clinical management of newly diagnosed breast cancer patients at genetic risk for BRCA germline mutations: perspective of a surgical oncologist. *Fam Cancer*. 2008;7:91–95.

38. Liang L, Shao C, Deng L, Mendonca MS, Stambrook PJ, Tischfield JA. Radiation-induced genetic instability in vivo depends on p53 status. *Mutat Res*. 2002;502:69–80.

39. Shay JW, Tomlinson G, Piatyszek MA, Gollahon LS. Spontaneous in vitro immortalization of breast epithelial cells from a patient with Li-Fraumeni syndrome. *Mol Cell Biol*. 1995;15:425–432.

40. Heyn R, Haeberlen V, Newton WA, et al. Second malignant neoplasms in children treated for rhabdomyosarcoma. Intergroup Rhabdomyosarcoma Study Committee. *J Clin Oncol*. 1993;11:262–270.

41. Hisada M, Garber JE, Fung CY, Fraumeni JF Jr, Li FP. Multiple primary cancers in families with Li-Fraumeni syndrome. *J Natl Cancer Inst*. 1998;90:606–611.

42. Salmon A, Amikam D, Sodha N, et al. Rapid development of post-radiotherapy sarcoma and breast cancer in a patient with a novel germline de-novo TP53 mutation. *Clin Oncol (R Coll Radiol)*. 2007;19:490–493.

43. Ford D, Easton DF, Stratton M, et al. Genetic heterogeneity and penetrance analysis of the BRCA1 and BRCA2 genes in breast cancer families. The Breast Cancer Linkage Consortium. *Am J Hum Genet*. 1998;62:676–689.

44. Chappuis PO, Nethercot V, Foulkes WD. Clinico-pathological characteristics of BRCA1- and BRCA2-related breast cancer. *Semin Surg Oncol*. 2000;18:287–295.

45. Phillips KA, Andrulis IL, Goodwin PJ. Breast carcinomas arising in carriers of mutations in BRCA1 or BRCA2: are they prognostically different? *J Clin Oncol*. 1999;17:3653–3663.

46. Turner NC, Reis-Filho JS. Basal-like breast cancer and the BRCA1 phenotype. *Oncogene*. 2006;25:5846–5853.

47. Eisinger F, Nogues C, Birnbaum D, Jacquemier J, Sobol H. BRCA1 and medullary breast cancer. *JAMA*. 1998;280:1227–1228.

48. Metcalfe K, Lynch HT, Ghadirian P, et al. Contralateral breast cancer in BRCA1 and BRCA2 mutation carriers. *J Clin Oncol*. 2004;22:2328–2335.

49. Boyd J, Sonoda Y, Federici MG, et al. Clinicopathologic features of BRCA-linked and sporadic ovarian cancer. *JAMA*. 2000;283:2260–2265.

50. Lakhani SR, Manek S, Penault-Llorca F, et al. Pathology of ovarian cancers in BRCA1 and BRCA2 carriers. *Clin Cancer Res*. 2004;10:2473–2481.

51. Levine DA, Argenta PA, Yee CJ, et al. Fallopian tube and primary peritoneal carcinomas associated with BRCA mutations. *J Clin Oncol*. 2003;21:4222–4227.

52. Cass I, Baldwin RL, Varkey T, Moslehi R, Narod SA, Karlan BY. Improved survival in women with BRCA-associated ovarian carcinoma. *Cancer*. 2003;97:2187–2195.

53. Venkitaraman AR. Cancer susceptibility and the functions of BRCA1 and BRCA2. *Cell*. 2002;108:171–182.

54. Ashworth A. A synthetic lethal therapeutic approach: poly(ADP) ribose polymerase inhibitors for the treatment of cancers deficient in DNA double-strand break repair. *J Clin Oncol*. 2008;26:3785–3790.

55. Miki Y, Swensen J, Shattuck-Eidens D, et al. A strong candidate for the breast and ovarian cancer susceptibility gene BRCA1. *Science*. 1994;266:66–71.

56. Wooster R, Bignell G, Lancaster J, et al. Identification of the breast cancer susceptibility gene BRCA2. *Nature*. 1995;378:789–792.

57. Wooster R, Neuhausen SL, Mangion J, et al. Localization of a breast cancer susceptibility gene, BRCA2, to chromosome 13q12–13. *Science*. 1994;265:2088–2090.

58. Walsh T, Casadei S, Coats KH, et al. Spectrum of mutations in BRCA1, BRCA2, CHEK2, and TP53 in families at high risk of breast cancer. *JAMA*. 2006;295:1379–1388.

59. Nagy R, Sweet K, Eng C. Highly penetrant hereditary cancer syndromes. *Oncogene*. 2004;23:6445–6470.

60. Easton DF, Deffenbaugh AM, Pruss D, et al. A systematic genetic assessment of 1,433 sequence variants of unknown clinical significance in the BRCA1 and BRCA2 breast cancer-predisposition genes. *Am J Hum Genet*. 2007;81:873–883.

61. Xia B, Sheng Q, Nakanishi K, et al. Control of BRCA2 cellular and clinical functions by a nuclear partner, PALB2. *Mol Cell*. 2006;22:719–729.

62. Struewing JP, Hartge P, Wacholder S, et al. The risk of cancer associated with specific mutations of BRCA1 and BRCA2 among Ashkenazi Jews. *New Engl J Med*. 1997;336:1401–1408.

63. Kauff ND, Perez-Segura P, Robson ME, et al. Incidence of non-founder BRCA1 and BRCA2 mutations in high risk Ashkenazi breast and ovarian cancer families. *J Med Genet*. 2002;39:611–614.

64. Thorlacius S, Olafsdottir G, Tryggvadottir L, et al. A single BRCA2 mutation in male and female breast cancer families from Iceland with varied cancer phenotypes. *Nat Genet*. 1996;13:117–119.

65. Unger MA, Nathanson KL, Calzone K, et al. Screening for genomic rearrangements in families with breast and ovarian cancer identifies BRCA1 mutations previously missed by conformation-sensitive gel electrophoresis or sequencing. *Am J Hum Genet*. 2000;67:841–850.

66. Antoniou A, Pharoah PD, Narod S, et al. Average risks of breast and ovarian cancer associated with BRCA1 or BRCA2 mutations detected in case Series unselected for family history: a combined analysis of 22 studies. *Am J Hum Genet*. 2003;72:1117–1130.

67. King MC, Marks JH, Mandell JB. Breast and ovarian cancer risks due to inherited mutations in BRCA1 and BRCA2. *Science*. 2003;302:643–646.

68. Rennert G, Bisland-Naggan S, Barnett-Griness O, et al. Clinical outcomes of breast cancer in carriers of BRCA1 and BRCA2 mutations. *New Engl J Med*. 2007;357:115–123.

69. Risch HA, McLaughlin JR, Cole DE, et al. Prevalence and penetrance of germline BRCA1 and BRCA2 mutations in a population series of 649 women with ovarian cancer. *Am J Hum Genet*. 2001;68:700–710.

70. Thompson D, Easton D. Variation in cancer risks, by mutation position, in BRCA2 mutation carriers. *Am J Hum Genet*. 2001;68:410–419.

71. Rebbeck TR, Lynch HT, Neuhausen SL, et al. Prophylactic oophorectomy in carriers of BRCA1 or BRCA2 mutations. *New Engl J Med*. 2002;346:1616–1622.

72. Kauff ND, Satagopan JM, Robson ME, et al. Risk-reducing salpingo-oophorectomy in women with a BRCA1 or BRCA2 mutation. *New Engl J Med*. 2002;346:1609–1615.

73. Cancer risks in BRCA2 mutation carriers. The Breast Cancer Linkage Consortium. *J Natl Cancer Inst*. 1999;91:1310–1316.

74. Liede A, Karlan BY, Narod SA. Cancer risks for male carriers of germline mutations in BRCA1 or BRCA2: a review of the literature. *J Clin Oncol*. 2004;22:735–742.

75. Thompson D, Easton DF. Cancer incidence in BRCA1 mutation carriers. *J Natl Cancer Inst*. 2002;94:1358–1365.

76. van Asperen CJ, Brohet RM, Meijers-Heijboer EJ, et al. Cancer risks in BRCA2 families: estimates for sites other than breast and ovary. *J Med Genet*. 2005;42:711–719.

77. Smith P, McGuffog L, Easton DF, et al. A genome wide linkage search for breast cancer susceptibility genes. *Genes Chromosomes Cancer*. 2006;45:646–655.

78. Hunter DJ, Kraft P, Jacobs KB, et al. A genome-wide association study identifies alleles in FGFR2 associated with risk of sporadic postmenopausal breast cancer. *Nat Genet*. 2007;39:870–874.

79. Easton DF, Pooley KA, Dunning AM, et al. Genome-wide association study identifies novel breast cancer susceptibility loci. *Nature*. 2007;447:1087–1093.

80. Stacey SN, Manolescu A, Sulem P, et al. Common variants on chromosomes 2q35 and 16q12 confer susceptibility to estrogen receptor-positive breast cancer. *Nat Genet*. 2007;39:865–869.

81. Frank B, Wiestler M, Kropp S, et al. Association of a common AKAP9 variant with breast cancer risk: a collaborative analysis. *J Natl Cancer Inst*. 2008;100:437–442.

82. Gold B, Kirchhoff T, Stefanov S, et al. Genome-wide association study provides evidence for a breast cancer risk locus at 6q22.33. *Proc Natl Acad Sci U S A*. 2008;105:4340–4345.

83. Nevanlinna H, Bartek J. The CHEK2 gene and inherited breast cancer susceptibility. *Oncogene*. 2006;25:5912–5919.

84. Erkko H, Xia B, Nikkila J, et al. A recurrent mutation in PALB2 in Finnish cancer families. *Nature*. 2007;446:316–319.

85. Foulkes WD, Ghadirian P, Akbari MR, et al. Identification of a novel truncating PALB2 mutation and analysis of its contribution to early-onset breast cancer in French-Canadian women. *Breast Cancer Res*. 2007;9:R83.

86. Tischkowitz MD, Hodgson SV. Fanconi anaemia. *J Med Genet*. 2003;40:1–10.

87. Saslow D, Boetes C, Burke W, et al. American Cancer Society guidelines for breast screening with MRI as an adjunct to mammography. *CA Cancer J Clin*. 2007;57:75–89.

88. Burke W, Daly M, Garber J, et al. Recommendations for follow-up care of individuals with an inherited predisposition to cancer. II. BRCA1 and BRCA2. Cancer Genetics Studies Consortium. *JAMA*. 1997;277:997–1003.

89. Kriege M, Brekelmans CT, Boetes C, et al. Efficacy of MRI and mammography for breast-cancer screening in women with a familial or genetic predisposition. *New Engl J Med*. 2004;351:427–437.

90. Warner E, Plewes DB, Hill KA, et al. Surveillance of BRCA1 and BRCA2 mutation carriers with magnetic resonance imaging, ultrasound, mammography, and clinical breast examination. *JAMA*. 2004;292:1317–1325.

91. Stoutjesdijk MJ, Boetes C, Jager GJ, et al. Magnetic resonance imaging and mammography in women with a hereditary risk of breast cancer. *J Natl Cancer Inst*. 2001;93:1095–1102.

92. Hartmann LC, Sellers TA, Schaid DJ, et al. Efficacy of bilateral prophylactic mastectomy in BRCA1 and BRCA2 gene mutation carriers. *J Natl Cancer Inst*. 2001;93:1633–1637.

93. Rebbeck TR, Friebel T, Lynch HT, et al. Bilateral prophylactic mastectomy reduces breast cancer risk in BRCA1 and BRCA2 mutation carriers: the PROSE Study Group. *J Clin Oncol*. 2004;22:1055–1062.

94. Meijers-Heijboer H, van Geel B, van Putten WL, et al. Breast cancer after prophylactic bilateral mastectomy in women with a BRCA1 or BRCA2 mutation. *New Engl J Med*. 2001;345:159–164.

95. Robson M, Svahn T, McCormick B, et al. Appropriateness of breast-conserving treatment of breast carcinoma in women with germline mutations in BRCA1 or BRCA2: a clinic-based series. *Cancer*. 2005;103:44–51.

96. Narod SA, Brunet JS, Ghadirian P, et al. Tamoxifen and risk of contralateral breast cancer in BRCA1 and BRCA2 mutation carriers: a case-control study. Hereditary Breast Cancer Clinical Study Group. *Lancet*. 2000;356:1876–1881.

97. Gronwald J, Tung N, Foulkes WD, et al. Tamoxifen and contralateral breast cancer in BRCA1 and BRCA2 carriers: an update. *Int J Cancer*. 2006;118:2281–2284.

98. Piver MS, Jishi MF, Tsukada Y, Nava G. Primary peritoneal carcinoma after prophylactic oophorectomy in women with a family history of ovarian cancer. A report of the Gilda Radner Familial Ovarian Cancer Registry. *Cancer*. 1993;71:2751–2755.

99. Modan B, Hartge P, Hirsh-Yechezkel G, et al. Parity, oral contraceptives, and the risk of ovarian cancer among carriers and noncarriers of a BRCA1 or BRCA2 mutation. *New Engl J Med*. 2001;345:235–240.

100. Narod SA, Risch H, Moslehi R, et al. Oral contraceptives and the risk of hereditary ovarian cancer. Hereditary Ovarian Cancer Clinical Study Group. *New Engl J Med*. 1998;339:424–428.

101. Narod SA, Dube MP, Klijn J, et al. Oral contraceptives and the risk of breast cancer in BRCA1 and BRCA2 mutation carriers. *J Natl Cancer Inst*. 2002;94:1773–1779.

102. Sidransky D, Tokino T, Helzlsouer K, et al. Inherited p53 gene mutations in breast cancer. *Cancer Res*. 1992;52:2984–2986.

103. Li FP, Fraumeni JF Jr, Mulvihill JJ, et al. A cancer family syndrome in twenty-four kindreds. *Cancer Res*. 1988;48:5358–5362.

104. Nichols KE, Malkin D, Garber JE, Fraumeni JF Jr, Li FP. Germline p53 mutations predispose to a wide spectrum of early-onset cancers. *Cancer Epidemiol Biomarkers Prev*. 2001;10:83–87.

105. Hartley AL, Birch JM, Marsden HB, Harris M. Malignant melanoma in families of children with osteosarcoma, chondrosarcoma, and adrenal cortical carcinoma. *J Med Genet*. 1987;24:664–668.

106. Jay M, McCartney AC. Familial malignant melanoma of the uvea and p53: a Victorian detective story. *Surv Ophthalmol*. 1993;37:457–462.

107. Birch JM, Alston RD, McNally RJ, et al. Relative frequency and morphology of cancers in carriers of germline TP53 mutations. *Oncogene*. 2001;20:4621–4628.

108. Hwang SJ, Lozano G, Amos CI, Strong LC. Germline p53 mutations in a cohort with childhood sarcoma: sex differences in cancer risk. *Am J Hum Genet*. 2003;72:975–983.

109. Chompret A, Brugieres L, Ronsin M, et al. P53 germline mutations in childhood cancers and cancer risk for carrier individuals. *Br J Cancer*. 2000;82:1932–1937.

110. Le Bihan C, Bonaiti-Pellie C. A method for estimating cancer risk in p53 mutation carriers. *Cancer Detect Prev.* 1994;18:171–178.

111. Birch JM, Hartley AL, Tricker KJ, et al. Prevalence and diversity of constitutional mutations in the p53 gene among 21 Li-Fraumeni families. *Cancer Res.* 1994;54:1298–1304.

112. Eeles RA. Germline mutations in the TP53 gene. *Cancer Surv.* 1995;25:101–124.

113. Gonzalez KD, Noltner KA, Buzin CH, et al. Beyond Li Fraumeni syndrome: clinical characteristics of families with p53 germline mutations. *J Clin Oncol.* 2009;27:1250–1256.

114. Eng C. Will the real Cowden syndrome please stand up: revised diagnostic criteria. *J Med Genet.* 2000;37:828–830.

115. Starink TM, van der Veen JP, Arwert F, et al. The Cowden syndrome: a clinical and genetic study in 21 patients. *Clin Genet.* 1986;29:222–233.

116. Brownstein MH, Wolf M, Bikowski JB. Cowden's disease: a cutaneous marker of breast cancer. *Cancer.* 1978;41:2393–2398.

117. Eng C. PTEN: one gene, many syndromes. *Hum Mutat.* 2003; 22:183–198.

118. Fackenthal JD, Marsh DJ, Richardson AL, et al. Male breast cancer in Cowden syndrome patients with germline PTEN mutations. *J Med Genet.* 2001;38:159–164.

119. Li J, Yen C, Liaw D, et al. PTEN, a putative protein tyrosine phosphatase gene mutated in human brain, breast, and prostate cancer. *Science.* 1997;275:1943–1947.

120. Eng C. Role of PTEN, a lipid phosphatase upstream effector of protein kinase B, in epithelial thyroid carcinogenesis. *Ann N Y Acad Sci.* 2002;968:213–221.

121. Marsh DJ, Kum JB, Lunetta KL, et al. PTEN mutation spectrum and genotype-phenotype correlations in Bannayan-Riley-Ruvalcaba syndrome suggest a single entity with Cowden syndrome. *Hum Mol Genet.* 1999;8:1461–1472.

122. Charlton A, Blair V, Shaw D, Parry S, Guilford P, Martin IG. Hereditary diffuse gastric cancer: predominance of multiple foci of signet ring cell carcinoma in distal stomach and transitional zone. *Gut.* 2004;53:814–820.

123. Guilford PJ, Hopkins JB, Grady WM, et al. E-cadherin germline mutations define an inherited cancer syndrome dominated by diffuse gastric cancer. *Hum Mutat.* 1999;14:249–255.

124. Pharoah PD, Guilford P, Caldas C. Incidence of gastric cancer and breast cancer in CDH1 (E-cadherin) mutation carriers from hereditary diffuse gastric cancer families. *Gastroenterology.* 2001;121:1348–1353.

125. Graziano F, Humar B, Guilford P. The role of the E-cadherin gene (CDH1) in diffuse gastric cancer susceptibility: from the laboratory to clinical practice. *Ann Oncol.* 2003;14:1705–1713.

126. Brooks-Wilson AR, Kaurah P, Suriano G, et al. Germline E-cadherin mutations in hereditary diffuse gastric cancer: assessment of 42 new families and review of genetic screening criteria. *J Med Genet.* 2004;41:508–517.

127. Chun YS, Lindor NM, Smyrk TC, et al. Germline E-cadherin gene mutations: is prophylactic total gastrectomy indicated? *Cancer.* 2001;92:181–187.

128. Huntsman DG, Carneiro F, Lewis FR, et al. Early gastric cancer in young, asymptomatic carriers of germ-line E-cadherin mutations. *New Engl J Med.* 2001;344:1904–1909.

129. Grady WM, Peek RM Jr. Hereditary diffuse gastric cancer: more answers or more questions? *Gastroenterology.* 2002;122:830–831; discussion 831–832.

130. Schneider KA. *Counseling About Cancer: Strategies for Genetic Counseling.* 2nd ed. New York, NY: Wiley-Liss; 2002.

131. GeneTests. Gene Tests 2009; available at www.ncbi.nlm.nih.gov/sites/GeneTests/?db=GeneTests.

Screening for Breast Cancer: Mammography and Other Modalities

PHOEBE E. FREER

DANIEL B. KOPANS

Mammography screening is one of the major medical advances of the past 30 years. Prior to 1990, the death rate from breast cancer had been unchanged for 50 years. By 1984, mammography screening had begun in sufficient numbers to affect national statistics in the United States, reflected in an abrupt increase in recorded breast cancer incidence. Subsequently, as would be expected, in 1990, five to seven years after the introduction of screening, the death rate from breast cancer abruptly began to fall (1). By 2008, the death rate had decreased by almost 30%. Although a small percentage of this decrease has been attributed to improved therapy, repeated studies have shown that most of the reduction in deaths is due to the screening and the earlier detection afforded by mammography (2–4).

Breast cancer is the most common noncutaneous cancer among women and, behind lung cancer, is the second leading cause of cancer deaths among women in the United States. The risk of developing breast cancer for a woman at average risk in the United States is one in seven over her lifetime (5). In 2007, the American Cancer Society (ACS) estimated that more than 178,000 women were diagnosed with invasive breast malignancies, and an additional 62,000 women were diagnosed with ductal carcinoma in situ (DCIS). In 2007, there were approximately 40,000 deaths attributable to breast cancer (3). There is, as yet, no safe method for preventing breast cancer for the general population, and no universal cure is on the horizon. Screening mammography is the single most important factor in the reduction in mortality from breast cancer that has occurred over the past 30 years and is the only test to date which has demonstrated a significant decrease in mortality from breast cancer in randomized controlled trials. It is estimated that participating in screening can reduce a woman's chance of death from breast cancer by as much as 50% (6).

■ SCREENING RECOMMENDATIONS

The ACS, the American College of Radiology (ACR), and other major medical associations recommend that every woman be screened annually with bilateral two-view mammography starting at age 40 (7). For high-risk women, screening may start even earlier and includes additional modalities such as annual magnetic resonance imagining (MRI). Some suggest that a woman who has an inherited genetic predisposition to breast cancer should begin screening at age 25 (8) and a woman whose mother or sister had premenopausal breast cancer should begin screening 5 to 10 years earlier than the age at which the youngest first-degree relative was diagnosed.

As a result of economic constraints and misplaced radiation exposure concerns, some countries have elected to perform mammograms less often or with single-view mammography [mediolateral oblique (MLO) view only], but the data suggest that screening should be with two-view mammography [craniocaudal (CC) view and MLO view] and annual (9,10) to be most effective. If resources require a longer interval between screens, then women should be informed that it is not due to an equivalent benefit but to the economics of screening. Currently, there is no safe method of breast cancer prevention for the general population. Early detection and treatment constitute the only method that has resulted in reducing breast cancer deaths.

In the United States, screening mammography is performed annually with bilateral two-view mammograms, which include an MLO view that images the breast from side to side and a CC view that images the breast from top to bottom (Fig. 2.1). The two views give the radiologist an idea of the three-dimensional structures being imaged. The radiologist looks for masses, areas of architectural distortion, calcifications, and developing asymmetries, among other findings (Fig. 2.2). Compression is used to improve the contrast resolution of the image, decrease motion blur, and reduce the summation shadows of overlying normal breast parenchyma; this makes cancers more easily detectable. It is critical that the patient's breast be pulled out as much as possible and compressed fully to include a larger portion of the breast in the image and improve the image. The inferomedial and posterior breast tissue areas are more often excluded from the image, and each mammogram should be checked for appropriate positioning and for possible motion (motion most often occurs inferiorly on the MLO image and can obscure faint calcifications), and a technical callback should be made if the image is inadequate.

In order to be cost-effective, screening must be done in an efficient fashion. The most efficient method of providing screening is for the woman to attend a screening center, have her mammograms, and leave. Her study will

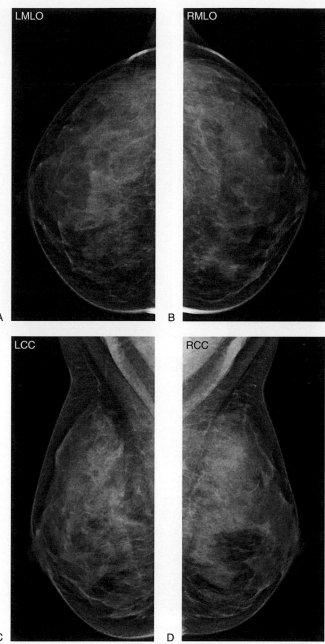

FIGURE 2.1 (A–D) Normal mammogram. The labeling is standardized such that each image has the marker placed at the axilla, giving both the side (right or left) and the view (CC, craniocaudal; MLO, mediolateral oblique). The MLO image should include the pectoralis muscle to the level of the nipple. The amount of tissue imaged posteriorly on the CC image should be within 1 cm of the depth included on the MLO view.

be read subsequently, in batches with others. This facilitates more rapid and accurate review by the radiologist. Although online reading to provide the screened patient with an immediate result sounds desirable, this places a great deal of pressure on the radiologist to read quickly so that patients are not kept waiting, which may then result in increased errors. Delayed, batch reading is safer and preferred.

The purpose of the screening study is to detect findings that may represent early cancers. These include masses, groups of very small calcifications in certain patterns, and areas of architectural distortion (see Fig. 2.2). When possible abnormalities are seen on a screening study, the patient is called back for a diagnostic evaluation. Although mammography is rarely diagnostic in the sense of providing a specific diagnosis, the additional imaging allows the radiologist to determine the significance, if any, of the finding identified at screening and how best to proceed if the finding warrants additional evaluation such as biopsy. A radiologist should be on site for the diagnostic evaluation, which, most commonly, includes additional mammographic views, ultrasound, or both. Women who present with a sign or symptom that warrants imaging evaluation should also be evaluated in the diagnostic setting.

The breasts, as imaged by mammography, change little from year to year. Changes from one year to the next are important for the detection of cancer. Comparison with previous studies allows the radiologist to detect changes (see Fig. 2.2D). Conversely, if a finding is noted, recall for diagnostic evaluation can be reduced if the finding has been present and unchanged on prior mammograms. Women should be encouraged to attend the same screening center every year, but if they change centers, they should bring their previous studies to the new center to permit comparisons.

Screening mammography has been demonstrated to have decreased sensitivity in women with silicone or saline implants because the implant blocks portions of the breast. However, it should still be performed. Two sets of mammograms—one with the implants in place and one with implants displaced from the films toward the chest wall—should be obtained. In addition to assessment for suspicious findings, occasionally implant failure can also be determined by a disruption of the contour of the implant or the visualization of extracapsular silicone. Since the rupture of a saline implant results in a rapid loss of saline, saline implant rupture is a clinical diagnosis and does not require mammography or any other imaging.

Screening and early detection are the keys to survival. It has been shown that women are more likely to undergo mammographic screening when it is recommended to them by their physician, and thus primary care physicians, obstetricians/gynecologists, and other physicians caring for the general population should both recommend and encourage that their female patients obtain annual screening mammography (11). Not all patients are aware of or follow through on these recommendations. Interestingly, even very high-risk women do not always follow through on the recommendations for screening, but they are more likely to follow through when reminded by a physician. For example, in a large cohort study of very high-risk women

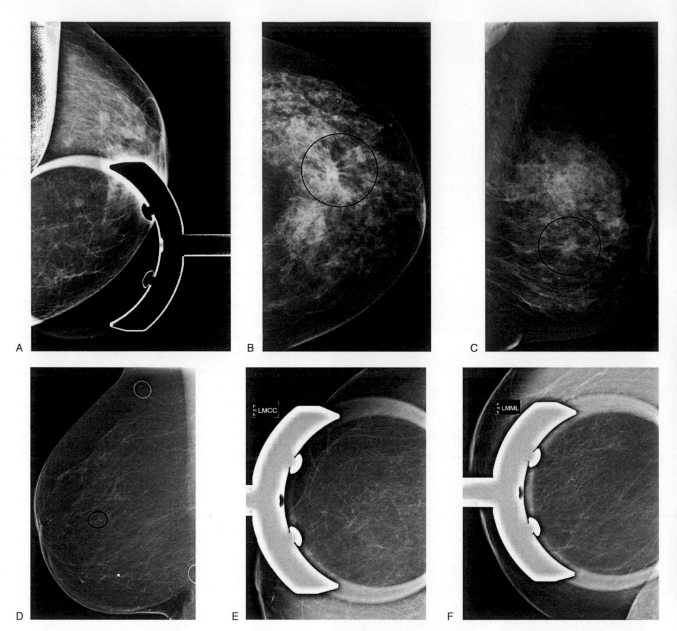

FIGURE 2.2 (A) Right craniocaudal (CC) spot image obtained during a diagnostic workup after the screening mammogram demonstrated a new mass. Biopsy yielded a 5 mm invasive ductal carcinoma. (B,C) Right CC and mediolateral oblique (MLO) images demonstrate an area of architectural distortion in a dense breast that yielded an invasive mammary carcinoma on further workup. (D–F) Diagnostic full-view lateral-medial (LM) spot magnification CC and spot magnification LM images obtained after screening mammography demonstrated new calcifications in the left breast. The additional images confirm a tiny cluster of branching, pleomorphic calcifications with a dot-dash appearance characteristic of the biopsy-proven ductal carcinoma in situ in this patient.

with a history of pediatric malignancy and chest radiation in whom screening is recommended annually at age 25 or 8 to 10 years after treatment, nearly 50% of women aged 25 to 39 had never had a mammogram, and even in women aged 40 to 50, nearly 25% had not had a single mammogram in the previous 2 years (12). However, if the patient's physician had recommended they receive mammographic screening, 76% of these women had obtained at least one mammogram in the previous 2 years, compared with only 17.6% of the women whose physicians had not suggested they receive the screening.

■ SCREENING STANDARDIZATION AND REPORTING

The Mammographic Quality Standards Act (MQSA)

Breast imaging has been at the leading edge of the quality assurance movement within radiology and has been at the forefront of the evidence-based practice movement in medicine. The ACR was first to develop a mammography accreditation program, as well as the Breast Imaging Reporting and Data System (BIRADS) to standardize mammography

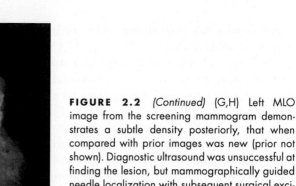

FIGURE 2.2 *(Continued)* (G,H) Left MLO image from the screening mammogram demonstrates a subtle density posteriorly, that when compared with prior images was new (prior not shown). Diagnostic ultrasound was unsuccessful at finding the lesion, but mammographically guided needle localization with subsequent surgical excision was performed. The specimen radiograph clearly shows the small 5 mm irregular mass with spiculated margins that pathology revealed to be a small invasive ductal carcinoma. Without comparison with prior mammography, this tiny developing focal asymmetry might not have been picked up so early.

reporting. Today, all facilities performing mammography in the United States must be certified and practice according to the guidelines of the MQSA, passed by Congress in 1992. The Food and Drug Administration (FDA) was given the responsibility for promulgating and overseeing the requirements defined by the MQSA to regulate and standardize mammographic technique and quality control—from personnel and equipment specifications, to radiation dose, to details of standardized reporting and auditing guidelines. To be accredited, each mammography facility must apply to an FDA-approved accreditation body (either the ACR or a qualifying state government) and undergo periodic review of its clinical images, as well as an annual survey by a medical physicist and a certified MQSA inspector. The MQSA review ensures that each facility meets the federal quality standards. In the United States, only the Department of Veterans Affairs is exempt from the MQSA certification because it has very similar enforced guidelines (13).

Physician Requirements

The MQSA requires that the physicians who interpret mammograms also meet certain standards. In addition to an active state license and certification in an appropriate specialty area approved by the FDA, such as radiology, each interpreting physician must document a minimum of 60 hours of dedicated education in mammography and have interpreted or read, under the supervision of a certified reader, at least 240 mammographic examinations within 6 months prior to certification. Then, within the first 2 years of certification, the interpreting physician must read an additional minimum of 960 mammographic examinations and have taught or completed at least 15 category I continuing medical education units in mammography. Similar strict standards for initial and

continuing medical education are required for mammographic technologists.

Breast Imaging Reporting and Data System (BIRADS)

The ACR, recognizing the need for standardization, clearly defined action-based reporting, and the importance of patient outcome monitoring to assess success and improve future analysis, developed the BIRADS, which continues to be updated and is now in its fourth edition. The ACR also offers a quality assurance program used by all radiology groups performing mammography. The BIRADS provides a standardized reporting guideline with a lexicon portion that clearly defines the terminology of the specialty so that reports can be more easily interpreted and understood by referrers anywhere in the country. In addition, it provides a structure for collecting data to assist the auditing of mammography practices and outcomes measurements. The standardization in mammographic technique as well as in reporting and outcomes measurements in breast imaging is unique not only within radiology but within medicine, and the BIRADS is at the forefront in creating a model of how to practice evidence-based medicine in today's world. A complete discussion of the BIRADS is beyond the scope of this chapter; however, all physicians involved in primary care and breast care should understand the most commonly encountered standardized reports from screening and diagnostic mammography.

Standardized Screening Mammographic Interpretation

All mammographic reports should describe the overall breast composition, divided into one of four categories (from almost entirely fat to extremely dense tissue), as breast density has been shown to inversely correlate with mammographic sensitivity (Fig. 2.3) (14,15). The radiologist assesses each image by looking for masses, certain patterns of calcifications, areas of architectural distortion, and developing densities with comparison to old images. The findings are described, and a BIRADS Final Assessment Category is required at the end of each mammography report to summarize the most important action determined by the interpretation of the mammogram (Table 2.10). By law, every patient receiving a mammogram must receive a

letter stating the overall impression and recommendation in lay terminology.

In addition, guidelines for screening mammography quality assurance benchmarks are provided, recommending that the callback rate (or recall rate) for screening mammography is less than 10%, that the positive predictive value of a positive screening or diagnostic mammogram leading to a biopsy (BIRADS 4 or 5) is more than 25%, and that the average size of diagnosed cancers and percentage of lymph node positivity in diagnosed cancers

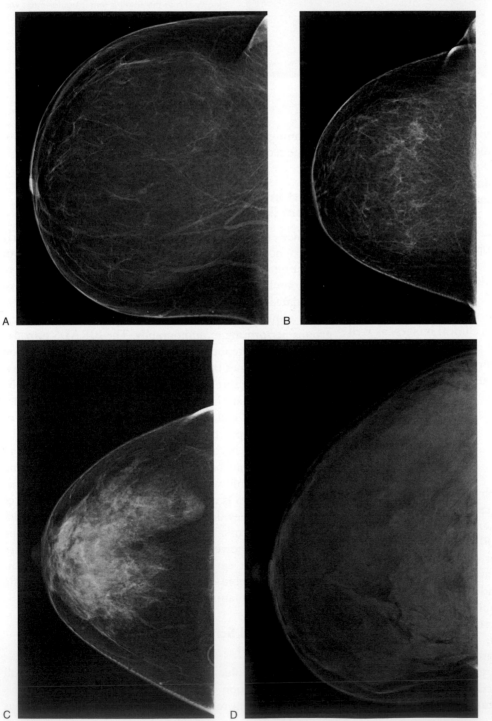

FIGURE 2.3 ACR BIRADS breast density lexicon: (A) almost entirely fat; (B) fatty with scattered fibroglandular densities; (C) heterogeneously dense; (D) extremely dense.

■ **Table 2.10** Breast Imaging Reporting and Data System (BIRADS) assessment categories

BIRADS 0: Needs additional imaging evaluation: Abnormality on screening mammogram for which diagnostic mammogram and/or ultrasound is recommended. May also use this if prior outside comparison is required for interpretation.

BIRADS 1: Negative mammogram: Normal

BIRADS 2: Benign finding: Either characteristic benign appearance or a known prior biopsied lesion

BIRADS 3: Probably benign finding, initial short-term interval follow-up suggested: <2% risk of malignancy; should only be used on diagnostic studies, not straight off of a screening abnormality. Usually performed at 6-month intervals.

BIRADS 4: Suspicious finding, intervention suggested (i.e., biopsy)
    4a: Low suspicion for malignancy, still requiring intervention (e.g., probable fibroadenoma, but biopsy suggested)
    4b: Intermediate suspicion for malignancy
    4c: Moderate concern, but not classic for malignancy

BIRADS 5: Highly suggestive of malignancy. Appropriate action should be taken: Almost certainly malignant; >95% risk of malignancy.

BIRADS 6: Known biopsy-proven malignancy. Appropriate action should be taken: For biopsy-proven lesions prior to definitive therapy; often used for monitoring patients on neoadjuvant chemotherapy or for second opinions.

are sufficiently low, among other benchmarks. In the average-risk population, a breast cancer is detected in 5 to 7 of every 1000 women on their initial baseline screening mammogram. On subsequent annual mammography, cancer is detected in 2 to 3 of every 1000 women, although the incidence will, of course, vary with the prior probability of cancer in the population being screened.

Initially developed to cover screening mammography only, the BIRADS continues to be updated and expanded to include a nearly comprehensive description of the findings and recommendations for all breast imaging studies including mammography, sonography, and MRI.

■ BREAST DENSITY

Breast density is unrelated to the properties of the breast on clinical examination. The firmness of the tissues has no relationship to the density, which is derived from the x-ray attenuation properties of the breast. Fibroglandular breast tissues are dense (radioopaque), whereas adipose tissue is not dense (radiolucent). Since the dense tissues of the breast can hide a breast cancer on mammography by superimposition of tissues, the goal in stating the breast density is to alert the referring physician that, in women with a denser pattern, the sensitivity of mammography is somewhat reduced (see Fig. 2.3). This does not mean that mammography is of no benefit in these women. Many small cancers can still be found in women with radiographically dense breasts, but additional screening modalities such as the clinical examination are likely of increased importance. Much has been written to suggest that women with dense patterns are at increased risk for breast cancer (15). This association remains controversial due to errors in understanding the physics of image generation and analysis (16) and the fact that women with less-dense patterns account for a large number of breast cancers. Even if there is a slight increased risk among those with dense patterns, there are no data to support concentrating on women with dense patterns to the exclusion of those with fatty patterns.

As discussed in the next section, there are some data to suggest that women with dense breasts may benefit more from annual mammography using a digital technique rather than an analog technique, but this remains inconclusive. Depending on other risk factors, women with dense breasts may benefit from screening with supplemental screening techniques of clinical breast exams, annual MRI, or both in addition to mammography, but this too needs to be confirmed in scientific trials.

■ DIGITAL MAMMOGRAPHY

For mammography, there is a greater requirement for very high resolution relative to the majority of other medical imaging. This is especially true when assessing the morphology of the margins of a mass or the morphology of faint calcifications, which may be the presenting radiological sign of DCIS. When digital imaging techniques first became available, the great importance of mammographic screening had already been demonstrated with analog techniques—a demonstration that had required multiple large trials and much scrutiny to prove efficacy (see the section on randomized, controlled trials and Table 2.11). Thus, as digital technology was developed, there were some initial concerns that digital mammography might not be as sensitive for the detection of cancers as film/screen technology. The FDA was initially going to require a postapproval screening trial for manufacturers of digital mammography equipment, and Congress earmarked $25 million to help perform this trial. Subsequently, because of testimony by experts and knowledge of the physics of digital imaging, the

FDA dropped the requirement. However, the American College of Radiology Imaging Network (ACRIN) was then able to use the earmarked funds to undertake a multi-institutional side-by-side comparison between film/screen and digital mammography, resulting in a study called the Digital Mammographic Imaging Screening Trial (DMIST).

From 2001, more than 49,500 healthy women attending screening centers were enrolled in the United States and Canada, and each underwent both a digital and a conventional screen/film mammogram on the same day, with each woman followed up for at least 10 months (17). The trial, sponsored by the National Cancer Institute, was a multi-institutional study conducted in 33 different centers in the United States and Canada. The overall data demonstrate that there is no decrease in detection of cancer using digital mammography. Moreover, in certain select subgroups—women under age 50, women with dense breasts (ACR density 3 or 4), and premenopausal or perimenopausal women—digital mammography appears to provide a 30% improvement in sensitivity over conventional film/screen mammography. It is clear that digital imaging can safely replace analog (film/screen) technology.

The major benefit of digital mammography is logistical. The precise x-ray exposure values and careful film processing required for analog film/screen mammography are no longer necessary because of the wide dynamic range and much wider latitude of digital imaging. The appearance of the processed film in the analog technique is directly related to and dependent on the exposure and processing values used; however, the digital image can be adjusted after exposure to optimize viewing. Increasingly less expensive and redundant computer servers can replace complex film libraries. Exact copies of the images can be reproduced at the same time essentially anywhere in the world. Digital images are rarely, if ever, lost in the way that film images can be misplaced.

An additional benefit of digital technology is the facility of using computer-aided detection (CAD) software to assist the interpretation of a mammogram. The use of CAD to supplement a radiologist's interpretation has been demonstrated to increase the cancer detection rate in a similar fashion to having two radiologists review a study (double reading) (18).

There has been a gradual shift to the newer technology. Digital units accounted for only 2.2% of all mammography units in 2002, increasing to 10.4% in 2005, and, by 2008, as many as 40% of mammography units in the United States were digital (19). It is likely that as analog devices need replacing, they will all be replaced by digital mammography devices. DMIST added evidence to support the fact that it is safe to change over from film/screen to digital mammography.

■ PROVING THE EFFICACY OF SCREENING TESTS

Proving efficacy for a cancer screening test is not as simple a task as one might believe. It is intuitive that a good screening test must detect cancer at a smaller size and earlier stage than the disease would otherwise present. However, since it is the metastatic spread of a cancer that is lethal in most cancers and not simply the presence of the cancer itself, it must be shown that detecting the cancer earlier actually prevents metastatic spread. If the tumor has already seeded other organs at the time of detection, then simply finding the index breast lesion earlier will have little benefit in terms of preventing death. Thus, showing the efficacy of a screening test for cancer requires proof both that undergoing screening leads to earlier detection of the disease and that this earlier detection leads to fewer deaths from the disease in the population undergoing screening. Simply using survival data (the time from the date of discovery of the cancer to the date of death) is therefore insufficient to prove efficacy. Ultimately, the definitive proof of the efficacy of a screening test comes when it can be demonstrated that when the test is introduced into the general population, the overall death rate from the cancer is decreased.

Mammography is, perhaps, the most completely studied screening test ever devised. It has fulfilled all the requirements for proving efficacy. Initial studies showed that mammography detects cancers at a smaller size and earlier stage (with less lymph node involvement) than would be seen without screening (20). In addition, large randomized, controlled trials have shown that mammographic screening significantly reduces the death rate from breast cancer in patients who have been offered the screening test (21). Finally, when mammography screening has been introduced into the general population, the overall population death rate from breast cancer declines (1–4,22).

Fundamental Biases in Analyzing Data

Screening involves the evaluation of healthy individuals. Although the goal is to reduce morbidity and mortality by finding disease earlier, false-positive results in a subset of patients inevitably occur. Being told that the test was abnormal can induce anxiety. The patient may have to take time off from work or away from family to have additional tests. Biopsies may be necessary before it can be shown that the test interpretation or result was a false alarm. In these individuals, these inconveniences and possibly unnecessary treatments would never have occurred if the screening test had not been used. In addition, although not common, there are breast cancers that are not lethal (23) or that may never become clinically relevant (24), and there are others that are metastatic and incurable even before they are detectable. Detecting the nonlethal or the already metastatic cancers by a screening test will only harm the patients, with no value for the individuals. At this time, we are unable to distinguish which lesions will benefit from early detection. Consequently, introducing a screening test into the general population must be justified by a high level of evidence that the test is indeed efficacious.

Lead-time Bias

Screening detects cancers earlier than they would otherwise be detected, which means that the length of time between detection of the disease and death from the disease is by definition increased, even if no treatment of the disease is performed in those patients screened. But this does not actually mean that true survival is extended in the screening population compared with the unscreened population. For example, consider that identical cancers begin to form in two women at the exact same time and the cancers are destined to be lethal in 10 years. If one woman is screened and her cancer is detected 2 years after it begins, she will appear to have survived 8 years from disease detection (10 years after the cancer began). If the second woman's cancer isn't detected until it is large enough to feel—say, 4 years after the cancer began—and she also dies 10 years from the time the cancer began, her survival of 6 years after detection will appear to be 2 years shorter than that of the woman whose cancer was screen detected. Comparing survival data will make it appear that the screened woman lived 2 years longer than the unscreened woman when, in fact, both died at the same time after their cancers began, and the first woman only learned of her cancer 2 years earlier, with no true benefit. Finding cancer earlier and making survival appear longer when the date of death is actually unaffected is known as lead-time bias. Lead-time bias is why merely measuring and comparing survival data—the time from diagnosis of cancer to the time of death from cancer—is not sufficient to demonstrate the efficacy of a screening test

Length Bias Sampling

The sojourn time is the time between the time a cancer can be detected by a screening test and the time it becomes evident clinically. More aggressive cancers inherently have a worse prognosis and typically a faster growth rate than less virulent lesions. Since screening exams are performed only intermittently and periodically, it is more likely that the faster-growing and more aggressive cancers (with a shorter sojourn time) will become clinically evident in the interval between screens (interval cancers). Thus screening is more likely to identify slower-growing cancers, as opposed to more virulent, inherently worse-prognosis cancers that are more likely to present as interval cancers between screening exams. This is called length bias sampling. Comparing the survival of patients with screen-detected lesions (more indolent and slower growing) with that of patients with cancers that were not detected by screening (faster-growing and more virulent) will falsely suggest that screening is beneficial because the screening will, preferentially, detect those less aggressive cancers that would have longer survival anyway.

Overdiagnosis and "Pseudodisease" Bias

Another reason we cannot rely on survival data is that there are some lesions that look like cancer to the pathologist but may never become lethal. In fact, in the absence of screening, some cancers may never become clinically evident. It is possible that some of the cancers detected by screening are these slower-growing, indolent cancers (24). Detecting these lesions can also make survival data appear to improve with no true reduction in deaths. For example, assume that, before screening was available, 75 women out of 100 diagnosed with breast cancer survived 5 years (survival at 5 years is 75/100 = 75%). If we assume that screening added nothing but indolent cancers or pseudolesions and we found 25 of these, the total number of cancers detected would be 125. If the same 25 women died, the 5-year survival would appear to improve to 80% (100/125 = 80%). Increasing the number of cancers detected may artificially make survival results appear to improve.

Screening may also lead to overtreatment. For example, DCIS is detected virtually only by mammography. There are no direct data to determine what percentage of women with DCIS will progress to invasive cancers. It may take as long as 20 years for invasion and death to occur (25). It is likely that not all cases of DCIS, if left alone, would progress to invasive and possibly lethal lesions, yet many women undergo mastectomy or lumpectomy with radiation for these lesions. Some would argue that this is a harm from screening (26). As a result, DCIS is evaluated separately when cancer statistics are reviewed. One indication of the importance of DCIS is the fact that there has recently been a decreasing incidence of invasive cancers in the United States. Some reports have, nonscientifically, suggested this decrease is due mainly to decreased use of hormones. The decrease actually began years before the reduction in hormone use, however. Therefore, it is more likely that some of the decrease is due to the removal of DCIS lesions 10 to 20 years earlier (27). Nevertheless, counting these lesions in survival data may skew the results, and this is another reason that survival data are not sufficient for proving the efficacy of screening.

Selection Bias

Individuals who volunteer for studies are usually in overall better health than people who do not volunteer. They may have longer survival as a subgroup of the population than the general population. Consequently, screening tests that are used to evaluate volunteers may falsely suggest that there is a reduction in mortality from breast cancer because these women volunteers are generally healthier at baseline. To truly identify a benefit from a screening test, the study population and the control population must be randomly chosen to avoid selection bias.

Randomized, Controlled Trials: Proof of Efficacy of a Screening Test

The only way to prove the efficacy of a screening test is through large randomized, controlled trials. As a consequence of the biases defined above, survival data alone are insufficient for proving the efficacy of a screening test. To best understand how to avoid these biases we can return to the example of the two women who develop an identical cancer at the same time and, thus, without intervention are expected to die at the same time. If early detection actually works, then the woman whose cancer was detected earlier because of screening would not have died and would have outlived the woman who was not screened. This would be direct proof for the efficacy of screening.

Obviously, it is impossible to identify women such as these with identical cancers, but the concept is the basis of randomized, controlled trials. By taking large groups of women and randomly dividing them into two groups, by the laws of probability, each woman in one group will have an identical counterpart in the other group (these trials need to be extremely large for this to be true). If the two groups were merely followed, the same number of women would die each year from breast cancer in both groups. If one group is screened, however, and if early detection actually saves lives, then there will be fewer deaths among the screened group than among the unscreened controls. If the decrease in deaths is statistically significant, then the efficacy of screening is demonstrated. The advantage of randomized, controlled trials is that they rely not on date of diagnosis but only on the date of death. Consequently, if properly performed, they eliminate all the biases described above.

■ EVIDENCE SUPPORTING MAMMOGRAPHY SCREENING

Understanding the history of the screening mammography trials is a gateway to understanding the utility of screening tests in general; it is also important as we navigate the future of breast cancer detection with different imaging modalities and perhaps even tailor screening to patients with different levels of risk. A detailed discussion of the mammography controversies is beyond the scope of this chapter, but a brief summary of each of the trials and the

issues that were raised is warranted in order to understand fully the importance of screening mammography today (Table 2.11).

The Randomized, Controlled Trials of Screening Mammography

Mammography was first used for breast evaluation in 1913 (28); however, the technique was not standardized or shown to be reproducible until the 1950s, when Robert Egan described his technique (29,30). In the 1960s, the first randomized, controlled trial to evaluate the effectiveness of screening using mammography and clinical breast examination was performed in New York (Health Insurance Plan, or HIP, Trial). The HIP Trial demonstrated a 23% statistically significant mortality benefit from earlier detection (31). Despite this proof of benefit, mammographic screening was not immediately widely accepted. There were major debates as to the feasibility and clinical effectiveness of the test, and concerns were raised over the possible harms of radiation exposure (32). Consequently, other randomized, controlled trials (31,33–38) and large-scale utilization projects have been undertaken around the world, with seven additional prospective randomized, controlled trials performed since the New York HIP trial (see Table 2.11). The individual trials—as well as numerous subsequent analyses and meta-analyses—have repeatedly documented the benefits of screening mammography. After much scrutiny, and many debates, it is now well established that screening mammography is unquestionably beneficial, with a dramatic reduction in breast cancer mortality. In fact, the overall estimated reduction in mortality that can be achieved by mammography is estimated to be as high as 50% (2,39).

In addition, following the first demonstration of a clear mortality reduction from screening in the HIP Trial, concerns were raised that it would be financially and structurally impossible to provide large-scale screening to the millions of women who might benefit in the general population. Consequently, the Breast Cancer Detection Demonstration Project was begun in 1973 to determine whether mass screening of the general population was feasible on a wide scale. This was not a randomized, controlled trial; however, it enrolled approximately 10,000 women in 27 different regions and successfully demonstrated large-scale feasibility and provided a large source of data confirming that mammography could detect many cancers at a smaller size and earlier stage than clinical breast examination (20).

The Randomized, Controlled Trials Underestimate the Benefit of Screening

What is often not understood is that the randomized, controlled trials actually underestimate the benefit of

■ Table 2.11 The randomized controlled trials of mammography screening

Year of First Entrollment and Trial Name	% Reduction in Deaths	# of Women	Length of Follow-up (years)	Age (years)	# Mammographic Views/Screening Interval (months)	% Compliance
1963 HIP[a]	23	60,995	18	40–64	2+ clinical exam/12	67
1976 Malmo I[b]	20	42, 283	19.2	45–69	2/18–24	74
1976 Malmo II[b]	49	17,793	9.1	43–49	2/18–24	75–80
1977 Swedish Two-County[c]	31	133,065	17.4–20	40–74	1 MLO /24–33	89
1979 Edinburgh[d]	21–29	44,268 (10,000 women aged 45–49 later added)	12.6	45–64	1–2+ clinical exam/24	61
1980 Canada NBSSI[e]	0	50,430	13.0	40–49	2+ clinical exam/12	100
1980 Canada NBSSII[e]	0	39,405	13.0	50–59	2+ clinical exam/12	100
1981 Stockholm[f]	21*	60,117	14.9	40–65	1/18–24	91
1982 Gothenborg[g]	20–30**	51,611	13.3	40–59	2/18	84

*not statistically significant

**dramatic 44% reduction in women aged 39 to 49

[a]HIP: Likely underestimated the true benefit of screening mammography secondary to use of conventional x-ray equipment, and old film mammography which was well below the quality available today.

[b]Malmo I/II: Women aged 45 to 49 demonstrated a dramatic 49% reduction in mortality at 10-year follow-up

[c]Swedish 2-County Trial (Kopparberg, now Dalarma, and Ostergotland Counties): The mortality reduction was almost certainly due to the fact that in the two-county trial there was a marked 25% reduction in the number of stage II cancers in the screening group relative to the control group, documenting that improved early detection leads to decreased deaths and validating the benefit of screening mammography.

[d]Edinburgh: Concerns have been raised because the randomization technique used resulted in imbalances in the socioeconomic distribution of the women in the two groups.

[e]Canada NBSSI /NBSSII: In women aged 40 to 49, there was an actual excess of breast cancer deaths among the screened women, however, these studies are among the most highly criticized and their results repeatedly questioned. All participants were volunteers, so the results are not generalizable to the entire population. The NBSS1 instructed all women in self-breast exam and included a clinical breast exam in all women prior to randomization, with unblended randomization on open lists inserting an inherent potential randomization bias for allocation. The NBSS2 included clinical breast exam in both groups and added screening mammography to the screening group. Women underwent a clinical breast examination prior to being allocated to the mammography or control groups. Women with palpable cancers, and even those with palpable axillary adenopathy (advanced cancers) were permitted in the trial and were examined prior to allotment in the control or screening group, adding a preferential bias in these women with palpable abnormalities to ensure they were placed in the screening group.

[f]Stockholm: Unfortunately, the study was terminated early before it had any statistical power. It had begun in 1981, but soon after the first screen, the Two-County Trial began showing a clear benefit and it was felt that all women in the Stockholm control group should be offered screening thus ending the trial. As a consequence of the small numbers and short-term follow-up of only two screens, the study was unable to achieve statistical significance.

[g]Gothenborg: Dramatic 44%, statistically significant reduction in breast cancer deaths in screened women ages 39 to 49.

Source: Smith R, Duffy S, Gabe R, Tabar L, Yen A, and Chen T. The randomized trials of breast cancer screening: what have we learned? *Radiol Clin North Am* 2004;42(5):793–806.

screening mammography. The randomized, controlled trials invited women to be screened. No woman was coerced into being screened, and many women who were invited declined the offer. Nevertheless, to avoid biasing the results, once random allocation was made, each woman was counted in the group to which she was assigned even if she was noncompliant. Consequently, if a woman was assigned to be screened but refused the offer and died of breast cancer, her death was still included with the screened group. A woman who was allocated to be an unscreened control but who decided on her own to get a mammogram that saved her life was still counted with the unscreened controls. Thus the mortality reductions shown in the trials underestimate the true benefit that could have been achieved if everyone invited had complied with their trial assignments (43). In addition, the sensitivity and cancer detection rate in the trials is likely lower than what can be achieved using mammography today owing to the fact that many of the trials did not screen annually, many used single-view mammography, which is known to lead to some cancers being overlooked (40), and many used techniques that one would consider below today's standards and therefore likely had lower sensitivity of detection than would be achievable today.

Controversies Surrounding the Randomized, Controlled Trials

Questions have been raised about the results of the mammography randomized, controlled trials. Some of the concerns have been valid, but others are due to a failure to understand the science behind these studies. One of the most inflammatory concerns was raised by two Danish reviewers in a meta-analysis of the trials. The authors, Gotzsche and Olsen, reviewed the randomized, controlled trials of mammography screening many years after the trials had been completed and reported. They excluded all but two trials in their final assessment—the Malmo and the Canadian NBSS1 and NBSS2 trials—and then misinterpreted the results of the Malmo trial to state that there had been no benefit of screening in that trial, with the subsequent conclusion that there was no benefit from screening mammography for anyone, regardless of age. It is outside the scope of this chapter to detail the unscientific reasoning in this meta-analysis; however, in-depth analyses of errors in adhering to scientific principles are provided in an article by Kopans (41) and another by Duffy and colleagues (42).

Nevertheless, the Gotzsche and Olsen analysis was critical to the history of mammography because it led to a reevaluation that produced a global consensus that indeed mammographic screening is efficacious. Because the media made a great deal of this review, a Global Summit on Mammographic Screening was held in Italy in 2002, where the lead biostatistician of the European Institute of Oncology and two other peer reviewers for *The Lancet* stated that they had rejected the Gotzsche and Olsen review as being scientifically flawed. The global summit concluded that the trials did, indeed, show a 30% decrease in breast cancer deaths that was attributable to screening (54).

Since the Global Summit on Mammographic Screening, at least three other major worldwide reviews have been performed and have reached the conclusion that screening mammography shows a clear benefit, including reviews by the US Preventive Task Force, the International Association

for Research in Cancer, and the National Health Council of the Netherlands.

■ INTRODUCING SCREENING INTO THE GENERAL POPULATION

The randomized, controlled trials of screening have clearly shown that early detection using mammography screening can reduce the death rate in the most rigorous of scientific studies, the randomized trials. The final piece of evidence to support general screening comes from observing what happens when mammography screening is offered to the general population. The death rate in the general population decreases with the introduction of widespread screening. For example, studying the two counties in the Swedish Two-County Trial, Tabar and colleagues (54) showed that the death rate (number of deaths per 10,000 women in the population), a statistic that is unaffected by the number of cancers detected, decreased dramatically in the entire population after the large-scale introduction of screening. Using the death rate among women prior to the institution of generalized mammography screening, the authors found that when screening was made available to all women, deaths were decreased by 63% in women aged 40 to 69 during the period 1988 to 1996 compared with prescreening data for 1968 to 1977. Over the same period, all women had access to the same improvements in therapy, but the women who chose not to participate in screening had very little change in death rate, demonstrating that the majority of the benefit in women screened was due to screening. The benefit of screening was confirmed in Sweden in a second study in 2002 evaluating the death rate in 30% of the population that demonstrated a 44% reduction in deaths among those women undergoing screening compared with the death rate during the prescreening period.

Similarly, in the United States, the death rate from breast cancer has decreased significantly since the implementation of mammographic screening, confirming a causal relationship (1). The reported incidence of breast cancer in the United States increased between 1940 and 1983, from 60 in 100,000 to 90 in 100,000. Then, suddenly, in 1984, the reported incidence of breast cancer increased dramatically, concurrent with the onset of widespread screening programs. The increase in incidence was a marker for the large-scale implementation of screening in the United States because cancers that were undetectable clinically were all of a sudden detected by mammography. As would be expected, 5 to 7 years later, breast cancer mortality decreased dramatically in the United States, in 1990, for the first time in 50 years, echoing the large-scale screening mammographic intervention that had begun in the early 1980s. Although a small portion of the mortality reduction may be attributable to improved therapy, the majority of this reduction is solely attributable to large-scale implementation of screening programs with mammography. This benefit was confirmed in studies in the Netherlands, where the death rate was slowly increasing despite improvements in therapy but began to decline in line with the introduction of mammography screening as screening centers came online (4).

■ OTHER CONTROVERSIES OVER MAMMOGRAPHY SCREENING

The challenge by Gotzsche and Olsen against the mammography trials was just one of many that have been raised against screening mammography.

Radiation Risk From Mammography

In 1976, Bailar suggested that mammograms might cause as many cancer deaths as could be avoided by early detection (2). This suggestion has proven to be a gross overestimate of the risk of radiation, but it caused great concerns that persist today. The theoretical risk from mammography is based on data collected from different groups of women with radiation exposures that were much greater than that from mammograms. These included survivors of the atomic bombs, women treated with radiation for postpartum mastitis, teenage girls with scoliosis who underwent multiple x-ray studies as teenagers, and, more recently, girls and women who underwent high doses of chest radiation for treatment of Hodgkin's lymphoma. All the radiation exposures in these populations were much larger than the level of exposure used for mammography. By statute, mammography systems must be calibrated to provide no more than 300 mrem per exposure to a breast that is 4.5 cm thick and 50% fat and 50% fibroglandular tissue.

Even at high doses, risk to the breast is likely confined to teenage women and those in their early twenties, as evidenced by women treated for Hodgkin's disease (44–46). The data clearly show that radiation risk to the breast is related to the age at exposure. The undifferentiated teenage breast (before the individual has undergone a full-term pregnancy) is highly susceptible to radiation. However, once the breast has matured (terminal differentiation has occurred), there is no evidence that radiation has any effect on the breast. If stem cells prove to be the cells that can become malignant, it would make sense that the undifferentiated breast would be more susceptible to carcinogens than the mature, differentiated breast. In fact, it is likely that for women of recommended screening age (above 39 years old), the real risk from radiation is negligible. There is no direct evidence that mammographic doses will cause any cancers among women aged 40 and over. Even assuming the smallest benefit and extrapolating

the highest risk, the risk-benefit ratio is heavily weighted toward screening (47).

Perhaps the most direct evidence we have of the safety of mammograms can be seen in US national statistics. If mammograms were causing breast cancer, then the cancer incidence in the United States should be slowly increasing relative to the onset and wide-scale utilization of screening of tens to hundreds of millions of women starting in 1985. In fact, however, after accounting for the expected initial increase in incidence due to early detection, the cancer incidence is now decreasing.

Other Risks

A more subtle issue is the psychological and inherent physical risk of false-positive tests and the subsequent unnecessary biopsies or other interventions performed for false-positive screens. It has been estimated that almost 50% of women may be called back from screening mammography for at least additional mammographic views at some point over the course of 10 consecutive annual screens (48). Although this is an overestimate, there is a theoretical risk of increased patient anxiety from this screening callback. It is of interest, and perhaps unexpected, that two studies in the literature actually demonstrate improved patient satisfaction following recalls (49,50). Only 2% or fewer of women who have been screened will be referred for biopsy (usually needle biopsy). Approximately 20% to 30% of these women will be diagnosed with breast cancer. In addition, breast biopsies are inherently a safe procedure, with very low morbidity and mortality and few long-term side effects. These false-positive risks are far outweighed by the huge benefit in mortality from undergoing screening mammography.

■ EVIDENCE SUPPORTS STARTING SCREENING PROGRAMS AT AGE 40

One of the major controversies of the past 30 years revolves around the age at which mammographic screening should begin. The reason that US guidelines chose the age 40 as a starting point for screening is based purely on the fact that the randomized, controlled trials of mammography screening, with the exception of the Gothenburg trial, which included women aged 39, did not include any younger women. At the age of 30, the probability that a woman will be diagnosed with breast cancer in the next 10 years is 0.4%; however, this jumps to 1.4% by age 40 and continues to 2.5% by age 70 (51). The chance of breast cancer in women in the United States aged 39 or younger is 1 in 228; however, jumps to 1 in 24 between the ages of 40 and 59. To have sufficient numbers of women with cancer and sufficient numbers of cancer deaths to provide statistical power in the trials, the age of 40 was chosen as the arbitrary starting point for recruiting patients.

Some analysts have suggested that there is no benefit from mammography screening prior to age 50 (52). In many European countries it has been argued that screening should not begin prior to this age. The data clearly show, however, that age 50 is nothing more than another arbitrary threshold (53). There is no direct evidence that the age of 50, or any other age, represents a true threshold for the benefit of mammography screening. There is a clear benefit from screening beginning at age 40, as has been well proven by the data. The following list summarizes some of the arguments that have been used to suggest screening should not start until 50 and presents the data demonstrating that screening is also of marked benefit to women in their forties.

- *Argument against screening before age 50:* Subgroup analyses of the mammography randomized, controlled trials show no statistically significant mortality reduction in women under age 50 in the early years (5 years after the baseline screen) following the start of the trials.
- *Facts:* The age controversy began in an effort to determine whether menopause had any influence on the screening results. Since menopausal data had not been collected in the randomized trials, age 50 was chosen as its surrogate for the subgroup analysis. The trials were designed to evaluate screening from ages 40 to 64, 45 to 65, and so on. With the exception of the Canadian trial, none of the trials was designed to permit the subgroup analysis of women aged 40 to 49 separately (54). There is insufficient statistical power to support this type of retrospective stratification; therefore, a statistically significant benefit from analyzing the deaths among these women 5 years after the start of the trials is a mathematical impossibility (54). By retrospectively evaluating women aged 40 to 49 as a separate subgroup, all statistical power was lost. Longer follow-up (more deaths and greater person-years) increases the statistical power of the trials, and the data now show a statistically significant mortality reduction from screening women aged 40 to 49 that is as high as a 44% mortality reduction among women in Gothenburg (55).
- *Argument against screening before age 50:* It has been argued that the cancer detection rate changes abruptly at age 50 and that breast cancer is not a major problem in women younger than age 50, so screening programs should offer screening only to women aged 50 and above (56,57).
- *Facts:* The cancer detection rate parallels the prior probability of cancer in the population. The

incidence of breast cancer increases steadily with increasing age, with no abrupt change at age 50 or any other age (51). Analysts have, at times, inappropriately grouped the data, comparing all women under age 50 with all women over age 50 in a dichotomous analysis. This dichotomous grouping is misleading because it makes data that change gradually with increasing age appear to change abruptly at the age selected (58). There are no ungrouped data that show that any of the parameters of screening change abruptly at age 50 or any other age. If cancer incidence is evaluated by decade age grouping, no decade of life from age 40 on accounts for more than 25% of all the cancers each year. Although cancer incidence increases steadily with increasing age, the absolute number of women diagnosed varies with the number of women in a particular age group. In 1995, for example, because of the large number of women in their forties, there were actually more women diagnosed with breast cancer in their forties than the number of women diagnosed with breast cancer who were in their fifties.

- *Argument against screening before age 50:* The theory of "age creep." It has been argued that the benefit from screening women who were in their forties when they entered the trials occurs only after they become age 50 or over (59) and therefore that screening should not start until they are age 50 or over.
- *Facts:* The theory of age creep was based on a paper by de Koning and colleagues published in 1995 (60) in which incomplete data from the randomized, controlled trials were used to make the argument. When presented with the complete data at the Consensus Development Conference in 1997, the principal investigator recanted his analysis and agreed that most of the benefit had occurred prior to women reaching age 50 (53).
- *Argument against screening before age 50:* It has been argued that women aged 40 to 49 should be screened only if they are at high risk. This argument has been proposed in the recommendations of the American College of Physicians (ACP) (61,62).
- *Facts:* The randomized, controlled trials of mammography show a clear benefit for beginning screening at age 40 for all women when the data are analyzed scientifically. Adding support for screening women in their forties are the data from Sweden. Since the introduction of mammography screening into the Swedish general population, the mortality rate has dropped by almost 50% for women in their forties, primarily due to screening. There has also been a decline in the mortality rate from breast cancer in the United States since 1990, primarily as a result of mammography screening, which includes women in

their forties. The ACP has no data to support recommending that women in their forties be screened on the basis of their individual risk for breast cancer. None of the randomized, controlled trials stratified by risk. Furthermore, screening only women at increased risk for breast cancer in this age group will miss 75% to 80% of cancer cases (63).

Currently, the ACR, the ACS, the American College of Surgeons, the American Academy of Family Practice, the American College of Obstetrics and Gynecology, and other professional societies all recommend beginning mammographic screening at age 40 in average-risk women. It may indeed be the case that owing to economic constraints, some screening programs worldwide begin at age 50. However, there are no scientific data to conclude that women aged 40 to 49 do not derive great benefit from mammographic screening. If health care programs and costs allow, two-view annual screening mammography beginning at age 40 is optimal for large-scale reduction of breast cancer deaths.

At What Age Should Screening Stop?

Although the randomized, controlled trials included women aged 70 to 74, there were, again, insufficient numbers to permit accurate subgroup analysis of these women. There is no reason to suspect that the benefit of screening would end abruptly at age 69. Two studies specifically investigating the benefits of mammography in elderly women have demonstrated that cancers detected by screening in this age group are still of lesser stage than those detected by clinical presentation alone (64,65). Currently, most sources suggest that women over age 70 can benefit from screening mammography and that it should be performed in this age group on the basis of an individual assessment of other comorbidities and health status (66).

■ ALTERNATIVE AND SUPPLEMENTARY METHODS OF SCREENING

To date, mammography is the only scientifically proven screening test to demonstrate a mortality benefit for breast cancer. However, many other modalities, from clinical exam to imaging, may be beneficial as supplements to mammography, especially in the case of high-risk patients.

Clinical Breast Examination and Breast Self-examination

Many women still find their own cancers. There have been efforts to test the efficacy of breast self-examination (BSE). The most rigorous study was performed in China and has, to date, not shown any advantage for BSE among Chinese

women (67). Multiple other studies, including a large meta-analysis of 20 observational studies and three clinical trials of women using BSE as a screening method, demonstrate that BSE is not an effective method of screening for breast cancer, likely does not reduce mortality, and instead causes a larger number of women to seek medical advice or undergo unnecessary biopsies (68).

A similar lack of demonstrated benefit exists for clinician-performed breast examination (CBE). It has been reported that in women of average risk, CBE may detect only 3% to 8% of cancers that are mammographically occult and a mere 1% to 3% of such cancers in high-risk women (69). Worse, this slight increase in sensitivity comes at the cost of more false-positive results. The only randomized, controlled study that can be invoked to support CBE as an effective screening method is the oldest mammographic screening trial, the HIP Trial. It is likely that when the control group has very large cancers, as were common in the 1960s in the HIP Trial, CBE might result in earlier detection and a decrease in deaths. However, this benefit is likely not relevant in today's population of mammographically screened women. The Edinburgh trial included CBE, but its results do not support any benefit.

We continue to recommend that women practice BSE and undergo CBE annually, but there is no definite scientific support for their use. The ACS and the US Preventive Services Task Force recommend that clinicians inform their patients of average risk that CBE may increase sensitivity and that it be performed, especially on the basis of other factors such as age or breast density, with the woman knowing that she may be subject to more false-positive results. In the high-risk population, annual or semiannual CBE is advocated by many leading medical organizations, including the American Medical Association, the ACS, the ACR, and the American College of Obstetricians and Surgeons.

Screening MRI

Recommendations for Supplemental MRI Screening and High-risk Women

There are no data to prove that screening with any test other than mammography can save lives. Although it is well established that MRI can detect unsuspected cancers in many women, the use of MRI to screen the general population has not been studied. Consequently, there is no support at the present time for widespread screening of women of average risk with gadolinium-enhanced breast MRIs.

However, women at high risk may benefit from more than annual screening mammography. The risk of developing breast cancer for a woman of average risk in the United States is one in seven over her lifetime (5), whereas women with an inherited predisposition to breast cancer, such as a known *BRCA1* or *BRCA2* gene mutation, have an estimated risk of 50% to 85% of developing breast cancer over their lifetime (83). These women have little to be offered on top of screening except for prophylactic mastectomy or chemoprevention. Recommendations are for women to be screened with annual mammography starting at age 25 years or 5 to 10 years before youngest age of diagnosis of breast cancer in the family. Women with a history of mantle radiation for pediatric malignancy, such as treatment for Hodgkin's lymphoma, because of their very high risk of developing breast cancer, are recommended to be screened by annual mammography beginning at age 25 or 8 years after receiving the radiation, whichever comes later. Screening mammography in this very high-risk population, although still useful, has been shown to have much less sensitivity than in women at average risk, detecting only about 33% of cancers, with a higher chance of nodal positivity (70,71). Many consensus panels also recommend CBE every 6 to 12 months and BSE monthly in these high-risk populations (72).

In addition, the current ACS guidelines recommend supplemental screening in the high-risk population with annual MRI. Although there is no randomized trial of MRI, multiple small studies have suggested a benefit, by detecting small, unsuspected cancers, from annual screening breast MRI as an adjunct to mammography in the population of women who are at very high risk of breast cancer (Fig. 2.4). The ACS currently recommends that women who are estimated to have a risk of more than 20% to 25% of developing breast cancer, including those women with a known significant *BRCA1* or *BRCA2* mutation or other predisposing family history, be screened with annual gadolinium-enhanced breast MRI in addition to mammography. Other high-risk women in the ACS guidelines for screening recommendations using supplemental MRI include women who are first-degree relatives of known *BRCA* mutation carriers or women with premenopausal breast cancer, women with a known cancer syndrome (e.g., *p53* mutations, Cowden's, Li-Fraumeni), and women with a history of mantle

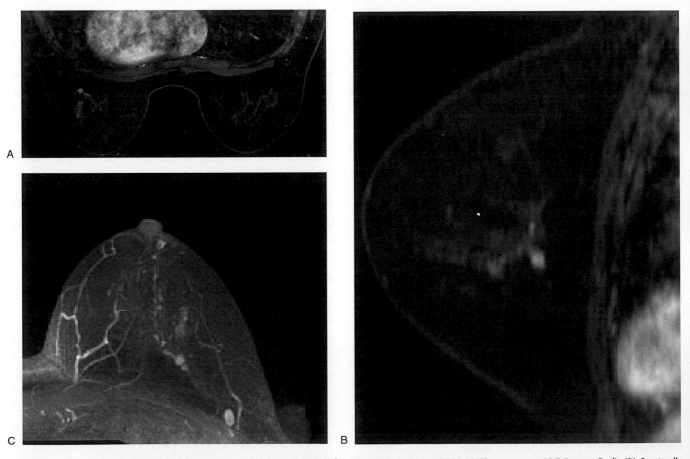

FIGURE 2.4 (A) Postcontrast axial fat suppressed Volume Imaging for Breast Assessment (VIBRANT) sequences (GE Breast Coil). (B) Sagittally reconstructed VIBRANT images of the postcontrast left breast. (C) Maximun intensity projection images of the left breast demonstrating a small 3 mm enhancing rounded focus with clumped nodular patchy enhancement extending anteriorly for approximately 1 cm. [A lymph node and mild background scattered physiologic enhancement are also noted in (C).] The tiny 3 mm enhancing focus in the left breast was new since the prior screening MRI 1 year before in a patient with a >25% risk of breast cancer on the basis of a very strong family history. There was no mammographic or sonographic correlate. Biopsy with subsequent excision yielded a 3 mm high-grade (grade 3) invasive ductal carcinoma. with low-grade DCIS extending anteriorly for 1 cm. The patient was treated successfully with breast conservation therapy.

■ **Table 2.12** Current ACS recommendations for screening women with breast MRI

Annual MRI screening recommended in addition to mammography:

BRCA1 or *BRCA2* known mutation carrier[a]
First-degree relative of a *BRCA* known mutation carrier but woman untested[a]
Lifetime risk >20–25% (as defined by statistical models, most based on family history)[a]
Chest radiation between 10 and 30 years of age (i.e., history of Hodgkin's lymphoma)[b]
Li-Fraumeni syndrome[b]
Cowden and Bannayan-Riley-Ruvalcaba syndromes[b]
First-degree relative with one of above syndromes[b]

Insufficient evidence to recommend for or against screening:

Lifetime risk of 15–20%
Prior biopsy of lobular carcinoma in situ
Prior biopsy of atypical lobular hyperplasia
Prior biopsy of atypical ductal hyperplasia
Heterogeneously dense or extremely dense breasts on mammography
Personal history of breast cancer, invasive or in situ

Recommend against MRI screening:

Women <15% lifetime risk[b]

---

[a]Based on scientific evidence from nonrandomized screening trials or observational studies.
[b]Based on expert consensus opinion.

Source: Saslow D, Boetes C, Burke W, et al. American Cancer Society guidelines for breast screening with MRI as an adjunct to mammography. *CA Cancer J Clin.* 2007;57:75–89.

radiation (e.g., for Hodgkin's lymphoma), among others (Table 2.12). Note that for women with a prior biopsy demonstrating high-risk pathology [such as lobular carcinoma in situ (LCIS), atypical lobular hyperplasia (ALH), or atypical ductal hyperplasia (ADH)] and for women with a personal history of breast cancer, the benefit of the addition of annual MRI to the screening mammogram remains indeterminate, and MRI may or may not be recommended as a supplement on an individual basis depending on other risk factors, including breast density (see Table 2.12) (73).

In all the cases where MRI screening is to be considered, it is important to remember that screening with MRI in high-risk women is recommended as a supplement to, and not a replacement for, annual mammography. Some centers prefer performing the annual MRI at the same time as the annual mammogram to aid interpretation, whereas others feel strongly that staggering the exams at 6-month intervals yields the possibility of detecting more interval cancers. Neither of these approaches has been proven more beneficial than the other at this time.

Scientific Data to Support MRI Supplemental Screening

As discussed, a randomized, controlled trial is the gold standard to prove efficacy for a screening trial. Such a trial for breast MRI, however, would be an enormous undertaking, would be extremely expensive, would require many years of follow-up data, and would require multi-institutional support. Given the difficulty of doing such a study, one has not been carried out as of yet, but it has been argued that surrogate endpoints can be used to establish the efficacy of MRI screening. No perfect one-to-one direct correlative marker has yet been demonstrated. However, the size and stage of a breast cancer at the time of diagnosis have been shown to be fairly predictive of mortality in mammographic studies (74).

It has been demonstrated that cancers detected in women undergoing screening MRI in addition to mammography are more than twice as likely to be node-negative as those cancers detected in women screened by mammography alone. These cancers detected by MRI are also smaller as a group than those detected by mammography, with more T_1 lesions (71). Multiple other studies of MRI in the high-risk population have established that the sensitivity of cancer detection increases dramatically with the addition of MRI to the mammographic protocol, from 25% to 60% sensitive with mammography alone to 86% to 100% with mammography and MRI together. Therefore, finding cancers at a smaller size and lower stage, as MRI clearly has been proven to do in high-risk women, has been used to justify recommending the use of MRI for screening high-risk women.

Screening Whole-Breast Ultrasound

A number of initial studies have shown that some mammographically occult cancers may be detected by screening ultrasound (75). In 2007, a large multi-institutional blinded trial (ACRIN 6666) evaluating more than 2600 high-risk patients demonstrated that there are indeed breast cancers that can be detected by ultrasound that are not evident on mammograms (76). Many of these cancers were small, less than 1 cm, and lymph node–negative. With the addition of whole-breast screening sonography to the mammography screening protocol, the cancer detection rate increased by 30% beyond cancers detected by mammography alone (although ultrasound did fail to detect 83% of DCIS-only cancers in this study). In a high-risk population with an elevated percentage of women with mammographically dense breasts, the sensitivity of screening was increased by approximately 25% when whole-breast sonographic screening was added to the mammographic protocol. Unfortunately, in achieving this high detection rate, screening ultrasound also resulted in a very high false-positive rate. The number of suspicious (BIRADS 4 or 5) lesions detected nearly doubled from screening mammography

(4.4%) to ultrasound alone (8.1%) and to an even more extreme 10.4% for ultrasound and mammography combined. This false-positive rate is unacceptably high. In addition, at present, bilateral whole-breast sonography is very time-consuming and likely not cost-effective. If automation of the process becomes possible with improved technology, and if the false-positive rate can be reduced, sonography for screening may become feasible. At present, however, the use of ultrasound should be confined to diagnostic evaluation for targeting areas of clinical concern or to better characterize lesions seen on mammography or MRI.

Digital Breast Tomosynthesis

The new test most likely to be introduced into the screening clinic is digital breast tomosynthesis (DBT). This is an evolution in x-ray mammography made possible by the development of digital detectors. Projection images are obtained from varying angles, and a computer synthesizes slices through the breast (limited-angle tomography). This three-dimensional image reduces the confusion caused by normal breast structures (structure noise) and decreases the false-positive rate for mammography without increasing the radiation dose to the patient over mammography. It promises to aid in the detection of cancers that are missed using conventional mammography. The technique is currently undergoing approval by the FDA and likely will be approved for at least the diagnostic setting soon with potential for investigation as a screening tool in the future.

Other Possible Screening Modalities

A number of other tests are being developed that might one day contribute to the early detection of breast cancers. Because none are yet in widespread use or have demonstrated efficacy for screening, we will only briefly mention them here.

The use of radioactive tracers with nuclear imaging for cancer detection has been evaluated for decades. Technetium-99m sestamibi concentrates in many cancers and is being evaluated as a tracer for breast-specific gamma imaging. The difficulty with this technique lies in distinguishing the signal given off by a small tumor from the background radiation signal from the intravenous injection. In addition, although the amount of radiation exposure is relatively low, it is unlikely that annual injections will be acceptable if the test is ever shown to be efficacious for screening. Furthermore, the resolution of these images is low compared with that of other modalities. The same is true for the use of positron-emission tomography using fluorodeoxyglucose. Although the technology for imaging the breast has improved, it is unlikely that this will ever be efficacious for breast cancer screening.

Other tests, including optical imaging and electrical impedance studies, are in the very early stages of development and are not ready for clinical application at this time.

■ CONCLUSION

Screening mammography is the only test currently proven to be efficacious for reducing the mortality from breast cancer. Women aged 40 and above should continue to be encouraged by their physicians to obtain annual bilateral mammograms, either digital or analog (film/screen), to reduce their chances of dying from breast cancer. Women at high risk likely may benefit from entering screening mammography at an even earlier age and from supplemental screening with additional tests such as CBE or supplemental annual MRI, although there are, as yet, no randomized, controlled studies to prove the benefit of supplemental screening. Since there is currently no safe method to prevent breast cancer in the general population, and since no universal cure is on the horizon, screening mammography, with early detection of disease, can continue to have a major impact on the reduction of breast cancer deaths.

■ REFERENCES

1. Kopans DB. Beyond randomized, controlled trials: organized mammographic screening substantially reduces breast cancer mortality. *Cancer.* 2002;94:580–581.
2. Tabar L, Vitak B, Tony HH, Yen MF, Duffy SW, Smith RA. Beyond randomized controlled trials: organized mammographic screening substantially reduces breast carcinoma mortality. *Cancer.* 2001;91:1724–1731.
3. Duffy SW, Tabar L, Chen H, et al. The impact of organized mammography service screening on breast carcinoma mortality in seven Swedish counties. *Cancer.* 2002;95:458–469.
4. Otto SJ, Fracheboud J, Looman CWN, et al. Initiation of population-based mammography screening in Dutch municipalities and effect on breast-cancer mortality: a systematic review. *Lancet.* 2003;361:411–417.
5. Jemal A, Tiwari RC, Murray T, et al. Cancer statistics, 2004. *CA Cancer J Clin.* 2004;54:8–29.
6. Feig SA. Effect of service screening mammography on population mortality from breast carcinoma. *Cancer.* 2002;95:451–457.
7. Smith RA, Saslow D, Sawyer KA, et al. American Cancer Society guidelines for breast cancer screening: update 2003. *CA Cancer J Clin.* 2003;53:141–169.
8. Burke W, Daly M, Garber J, et al. Recommendations for follow-up care of individuals with an inherited predisposition to cancer. II. BRCA1 and BRCA2. Cancer Genetics Studies Consortium. *JAMA.* 1997;277:997–1003.
9. Blanks RG, Moss SM, Wallis MG. Use of two view mammography compared with one view in the detection of small invasive cancers: further results from the National Health Service breast screening programme. *J Med Screen.* 1997;4(2):98–101.
10. Feig SA. Increased benefit from shorter screening mammography intervals for women ages 40–49 years. *Cancer.* 1997;80:2035–2039.
11. DuBard CA, Schmid D, Yow, A, Rogers AB, Lawrence WW. Recommendation for and receipt of cancer screenings among

Medicaid recipients 50 years and older. *Arch Intern Med.* 2008; 168(18):2014–2021.

12. Oeffinger KC, Gord JS, Moskowitz CS, et al. Breast cancer surveillance practices among women previously treated with chest radiation for a childhood cancer. *JAMA.* 2009;301(4):404–414.

13. http://www.fda.gov/CDRH/MAMMOGRAPHY/frmamcom2. html#s90011

14. Jackson VP, Hendrick RE, Feig SA, Kopans DB. Imaging of the radiographically dense breast. *Radiology.* 1993;188:297–301.

15. Boyd NF, Dite GS, Stone J, et al. Heritability of mammographic density, a risk factor for breast cancer. *N Engl J Med.* 2002; 347(12):886–894.

16. Kopans DB. Basic physics and doubts about relationship between mammographically determined tissue density and breast cancer risk. *Radiology.* 2008;246:348–353.

17. Pisano ED, Gatsonis C, Hendrick E, et al. Diagnostic performance of digital versus film mammography for breast-cancer screening. *N Engl J Med.* 2005;353(17):1773–1783.

18. Gromet M. Comparison of computer-aided detection to double reading of screening mammograms: review of 231,221 mammograms. *Am J Roentgenol.* 2008;190:854–859.

19. Rao VM, Levin DC, Parker L, Frangos A. Recent trends in mammography utilization in the Medicare population: is there a cause for concern? *J Am Coll Radiol.* 2008;5(5):652–656.

20. Baker LH. Breast Cancer Detection Demonstration Project: five-year summary report. *CA Cancer J Clin.* 1982;32(4):194–225.

21. Duffy SW, Smith RA, Gabe R, Tabár L, Yen AM, Chen TH. Screening for breast cancer. *Surg Oncol Clin N Am.* 2005;14: 671–697.

22. American Cancer Society. Cancer statistics 2008 presentation. Available at http://www.cancer.org/docroot/PRO/content/ PRO_1_1_Cancer_Statistics_2008_Presentation.asp

23. Nielsen M, Jensen J, Andersen J. Precancerous and cancerous breast lesions during lifetime and at autopsy: a study of 83 women. *Cancer.* 1984;54:612–615.

24. Zackrisson S, Andersson I, Janzon L, Manjer J, Garne JP. Rate of over-diagnosis of breast cancer 15 years after end of Malmö mammographic screening trial: follow-up study. *Br Med J.* 2006;332:689–692.

25. Page DL, Dupont WD, Rogers LW, Jenson RA, Schuyler PA. Continued local recurrence of carcinoma 15–25 years after a diagnosis of low grade ductal carcinoma in situ of the breast treated only by biopsy. *Cancer.* 1995;76:1197–1200.

26. Ernster VL, Barclay J, Kerliikowske K, Grady D, Henderson C. Incidence of and treatment for ductal carcinoma in situ of the breast. *JAMA.* 1996;275:913–918.

27. Cady B, Chung MA, Michaelson JS. A decline in breast cancer incidence. *N Engl J Med.* 2007;357:511.

28. Gold RH, Bassett LW, Widoff BE. Radiologic history exhibit: highlights from the history of mammography. *Radiographics.* 1990;10:1111–1131.

29. Egan RL. Experience with mammography in a tumor institution: evaluation of 1,000 studies. *Radiology.* 1960;75:894–900.

30. Clark RL, Copeland MM, Egan RL, et al. Reproducibility of the technic of mammography (Egan) for cancer of the breast. *Am J Surg.* 1965;109:127–133.

31. Shapiro S, Venet W, Strax P, Venet L. *Periodic Screening for Breast Cancer: The Health Insurance Plan Project and Its Sequelae, 1963–1986.* Baltimore, MD: Johns Hopkins University Press; 1988.

32. Bailar, JC. Mammography: a contrary view. *Ann Intern Med.* 1976;84:77–84.

33. Tabár L, Fagerberg CJ, Gad A, et al. Reduction in mortality from breast cancer after mass screening with mammography: randomised trial from the Breast Cancer Screening Working Group of the Swedish National Board of Health and Welfare. *Lancet.* 1985;1(8433):829–832.

34. Alexander FE, Anderson TJ, Forrest APM, et al. 14 Years of follow-up from the Edinburgh randomised trial of breast-cancer screening. *Lancet.* 2000;353:1903–1908.

35. Bjurstam N, Bjorneld L, Warwick J, et al. The Gothenburg breast screening trial. *Cancer.* 2003;97(10):2387–2396.

36. Frisell J, Eklund G, Hellström L, Glas U, Somell A. The Stockholm breast cancer screening trial: 5-year results and stage at discovery. *Breast Cancer Res Treat.* 1989;13:79–87.

37. Miller AB, Baines CJ, To T, Wall C. Canadian National Breast Screening Study: 1. Breast cancer detection and death rates among women aged 40–49. *Can Med Assoc J.* 1992;147;1459–1476.

38. Miller AB, Baines CJ, To T, Wall C. Canadian National Breast Screening Study: 2. Breast cancer detection and death rates among women aged 50–59. *Can Med Assoc J.* 1992;147;1477–1594.

39. Feig S. Estimation of currently attainable benefit from mammographic screening of women aged 40–49 years. *Cancer.* 1995;75: 2412–2419.

40. Blanks RG, Bennett RL, Patnick J, Cush S, Davison C, Moss SM. The effect of changing from one to two views at incident (subsequent) screens in the NHS breast screening programme in England: impact on cancer detection and recall rates. *Clin Radiol.* 2005;60:674–80.

41. Kopans DB. The most recent breast cancer screening controversy about whether mammographic screening benefits women at any age: nonsense and nonscience. *Am J Roentgenol.* 2003; 180:21–26.

42. Duffy SW. Interpretation of the breast screening trials: a commentary on the recent paper by Gotzsche and Olsen. *Breast.* 2001; 10:209–212.

43. Jackson VP. Screening mammography: controversies and headlines. *Radiology.* 2002;225:323–326.

44. Janjan NA, Wilson JF, Gillin M, et al. Mammary carcinoma developing after radiotherapy and chemotherapy for Hodgkin's disease. *Cancer.* 1988;61:252–254.

45. Dershaw D, Yahalom J, Petrek JA. Breast carcinoma in women previously treated for Hodgkin's disease: mammographic evaluation. *Radiology.* 1992;184:421–423.

46. Bhatia S, Robison LL, Oberlin O, et al. Breast cancer and other second neoplasms after childhood Hodgkin's disease. *N Engl J Med.* 1996;334:745–751.

47. Mettler FA, Upton AC, Kelsey CA, Rosenberg RD, Linver MN. Benefits versus risks from mammography: a critical assessment. *Cancer.* 1996;77:903–909.

48. Elmore JG, Barton MB, Moceri VM, Polk S, Arena PJ, Fletcher SW. Ten-year risk of false positive screening mammograms and clinical breast examinations. *New Engl J Med.* 1998;338: 1089–1096.

49. Tyndel S, Austoker J, Henderson BJ, et al. What is the psychological impact of mammographic screening on younger women with a family history of breast cancer? Findings from a prospective cohort study by the PIMMS Management Group. *J Clin Oncol.* 2007;25:3823–3830.

50. Currence BV, Pisano ED, Earp JA, et al. Does biopsy, aspiration or six-month follow-up of a false-positive mammogram reduce future screening or have large psychosocial effects? *Acad Radiol.* 2003;10:1257–1266.

51. Collaborative Group on Hormonal Factors in Breast Cancer. Familial breast cancer: collaborative reanalysis of individual data from 52 epidemiological studies including 58,209 women with breast cancer and 101,986 women without the disease. *Lancet.* 2001;358:1389–1399.

52. Fletcher SW, Black W, Harris R, Rimer BK, Shapiro S. Report of the International Workshop on Screening for Breast Cancer. *J Natl Cancer Inst.* 1993;85:1644–1656.

53. Kopans DB. Bias in the medical journals: a commentary. *Am J Roentgenol.* 2005;185:176–182.

54. Kopans DB, Halpern E, Hulka CA. Statistical power in breast cancer screening trials and mortality reduction among women 40–49 with particular emphasis on the national breast screening study of Canada. *Cancer.* 1994;74:1196–1203.

55. Hendrick RE, Smith RA, Rutledge JH, Smart CR. Benefit of screening mammography in women ages 40–49: a new meta-analysis

of randomized controlled trials. *Monogr Natl Cancer Inst.* 1997;22:87–92.

56. Kerlikowske K, Grady D, Barclay J, Sickles EA, Eaton A, Ernster V. Positive predictive value of screening mammography by age and family history of breast cancer. *JAMA.* 1993;270:2444–2450.

57. Sox H. Screening mammography in women younger than 50 years of age. *Ann Inter Med.* 1995;122:550–552.

58. Kopans DB, Moore RH, McCarthy KA, et al. Biasing the interpretation of mammography screening data by age grouping: nothing changes abruptly at age 50. *Breast J.* 1998;4:139–145.

59. Fletcher SW. Breast cancer screening among women in their forties: an overview of the issues. *J Natl Cancer Inst Monogr.* 1997; 22:5–9.

60. de Koning HJ, Boer R, Warmerdam PG, Beemsterboer PMM, van der Maas PJ. Quantitative interpretation of age-specific mortality reductions from the Swedish breast cancer-screening trials. *J Natl Cancer Inst.* 1995;87:1217–1223.

61. Efficacy Assessment Subcommittee of the American College of Physicians. Screening mammography for women 40 to 49 years of age: a clinical practice guideline from the American College of Physicians. *Ann Int Med.* 2007:146;511–515.

62. Kopans DB. Screening mammography for women age 40 to 49 years. *Ann Intern Med.* 2007;147:740–741.

63. Seidman H, Stellman SD, Mushinski MH. A different perspective on breast cancer risk factors: some implications of nonattributable risk. *Cancer.* 1982;32(5):301–313.

64. Badgwell BD, Giordano SH, Duan ZZ, et al. Mammography before diagnosis among women age 80 years and older with breast cancer. *J Clin Oncol.* 2008;26:2482–2488.

65. Smith-Bindman R, Kerliklowske K, Gebretsadik T, Newman J. Is screening mammography effective in elderly women? *Ann J Med.* 2000;108:112–119.

66. Costanza ME, ed. Breast cancer screening in older women. *J Gerontol.* 1992;47(special issue):1–152.

67. Thomas DB, Gao DL, Ray RM, et al. Randomized trial of breast self-examination in Shanghai: final results. *J Natl Cancer Inst.* 2002;94:1445–1457.

68. Hackshaw AK, Paul EA. Breast self-examination and death from breast cancer: a meta-analysis. *Br J Cancer.* 2003;88: 1047–1053.

69. Oestreicher N, Lehman C, Seger D, Buist DSM, White E. The incremental contribution of clinical breast examination to invasive cancer detection in a mammography screening program. *Am J Roentgenol.* 2005;185:428–432.

70. Brekelmans CT, Seynaeve C, Bartels CC, et al. Effectiveness of breast cancer surveillance in BRCA1/2 gene mutation carriers and women with high familial risk. *J Clin Oncol.* 2001;19: 924–930.

71. Kriege MMA, Brekelmans CTM, Coetes C, et al. Efficacy of MRI and mammography for breast-cancer screening in women with a familial or genetic predisposition. *N Engl J Med.* 2004;351: 427–437.

72. Robson M, Offit K. Management of an inherited predisposition to breast cancer. *N Engl J Med.* 2007;357:154–162.

73. Saslow D, Boetes C, Burke W, et al. American Cancer Society guidelines for breast screening with MRI as an adjunct to mammography. *CA Cancer J Clin.* 2007;57:75–89.

74. Carter CL, Allen C, Henson DE. Relation of tumor size, lymph node status, and survival in 24,740 breast cancer cases. *Cancer.* 1989;63:181–187.

75. Kolb TM, Lichy J, Newhouse JH. Comparison of the performance of screening mammography, physical examination, and breast US and evaluation of factors that influence them: an analysis of 27,825 patient evaluations. *Radiology* 2002;225:165–175.

76. Berg WA, Blume JD, Cormack JB, et al. Combined screening with ultrasound and mammography vs mammography alone in women at elevated risk of breast cancer. *JAMA.* 2008;299(18): 2151–2163.

Intake of New Patients for Multidisciplinary Clinics

MARTHA LAKE

GWENDOLYN MITCHELL

The initial diagnosis of breast cancer is an overwhelming experience for virtually all patients. It signifies a life-threatening situation to which most individuals have had little exposure. This lack of knowledge compounds what is often a debilitating sense of loss of control and resulting lack of direction. With proper preparation, the initial office visit not only provides patients with an assessment of the best course of treatment but also allows them to regain their composure for the difficult days ahead.

■ LIMITATIONS OF THE STANDARD APPROACH

In most practice settings, a newly diagnosed breast cancer patient is first seen by a single physician in a private office setting. Patients may be asked bring their pathology slides and imaging studies to their appointment. The physician or their office staff can only then begin to obtain pathology and radiology review of materials, and results are not available for some time. Many decisions about treatment cannot be made until these results are available, resulting in the potential for delays and fragmentation of care. Because little information is available prior to the appointment, the patient may not even be seeing the appropriate provider. At the very least, the patient is likely to require multiple appointments on separate days before a treatment plan can be made.

■ THE MULTIDISCIPLINARY APPROACH

Most patients with breast cancer require consultation with a surgical oncologist, radiation oncologist, and medical oncologist, and many will receive treatment from each of these specialists. For patients with early-stage disease, the first decision to be made is whether they will have a lumpectomy or mastectomy. This decision requires input from a surgeon and a radiation oncologist, usually with input from breast pathology and breast imaging to assess the feasibility of breast preservation and plan the extent of surgery. The patient may also require genetic testing before deciding between lumpectomy and bilateral mastectomy. She may wish to consider fertility issues.

If the cancer is more advanced, the initial decision may be whether surgery or chemotherapy will come first. Pathology results and imaging findings will be important in making this decision.

A multidisciplinary approach makes it possible to streamline decision making and shorten the time from diagnosis to finalization of a treatment plan. Treating physicians, support services, and consultants are brought together in a structured way to discuss an individual patient's issues and make consensus recommendations, with each specialty's expertise brought to bear. In addition, economies of scale can result from sharing costs of office expenses for clinical and research activities, making more services available than would be possible in a single practitioner's office.

The Multidisciplinary Team

Core members of the multidisciplinary team include the access nurse (sometimes known as nurse coordinator or nurse navigator), administrative coordinator, and dedicated breast oncology physicians specializing in the areas of surgical oncology, radiation oncology, and medical oncology. Other team members are made available to patients depending on their particular needs and circumstances. These team members include social workers, genetic counselors, nurse researchers, plastic surgeons, nutritionists, physical therapists, psychiatrists, interpreters, and chaplains.

Administrative Coordinator

The multidisciplinary administrative coordinator will receive the initial call identifying a patient with a new diagnosis of breast cancer. The administrative coordinator

■ **Table 3.1** Multidisciplinary clinical information needed prior to initial appointment

Information to be faxed
1. Pathology reports
2. Mammography, ultrasound, and breast MRI reports
3. Reports of CT scans, bone scans, and other imaging studies
4. Operative reports
5. Laboratory results

Materials to be sent in advance of visit
1. Pathology glass slides—to arrive 48–72 h prior to appointment for internal review

Imaging studies to be brought to appointment (hardcopy or disk)
1. Mammograms, most recent and last 3 years
2. Breast ultrasounds
3. CT scans, bone scans, MRI, and chest x-ray images

■ **Table 3.2** Initial appointment guidelines for multidisciplinary patients by diagnosis

Ductal carcinoma in situ (DCIS)
1. Core or open biopsy diagnosis—surgery and radiation oncology
2. Surgery completed, margins clear—radiation and medical oncology, postoperative check by surgery

Invasive carcinoma
1. Core or open biopsy diagnosis—surgery and radiation oncology
2. Core or open biopsy diagnosis, large tumor size or locally advanced—surgery and radiation oncology, medical oncology available for consideration of neoadjuvant chemotherapy
3. Surgery and axillary staging completed—medical and radiation oncology, postoperative check by surgery
4. Metastatic disease—medical oncology

Hereditary breast/ovarian cancer (BRCA1/2)
Patients to refer for cancer genetics consultation at initial visit:
• Breast cancer under age 40
• Ovarian cancer at any age *and* another relative with breast or ovarian cancer
• Breast cancer under age 50 *and* another relative with breast cancer
• Three relatives with breast cancer at any age
• More than one family member under age 50 with breast or ovarian cancer at any age plus Jewish ancestry

Fertility concerns
• Experienced specialists are made available to provide consultation and treatment for those facing issues with fertility

works closely with the patient to obtain all relevant pathology slides, films, and reports. Pathology slides are received 48 to 72 hours prior to the scheduled appointment in order for advance pathology review (Table 3.1).

Access Nurse

Prior to the multidisciplinary appointment, the access nurse has the opportunity to review all outside information to determine which caregivers a patient should see at the initial visit (Table 3.2). The access nurse then contacts each new patient by telephone prior to the visit. Communicating with patients in their own environment decreases anxiety tremendously and eliminates many fears. Patients are given an opportunity to tell their story, a medical history is obtained, and an overview of the upcoming appointment is provided to the patient (Figure 3.1).

During this conversation, the access nurse has the opportunity to identify additional needs (e.g., genetic testing and additional imaging studies) and to gain insight into the patient's individual circumstances. The patient is encouraged to write down questions for each physician and to bring someone along to the office visit. The patient is left with a direct contact name and telephone number to call in case of additional questions prior to the visit.

The role of the access nurse is multidimensional. The nurse not only performs the intake of new patients but has the opportunity to provide education and clarify misconceptions. Most important, the nurse provides emotional support to patients who may be unprepared for the reality of a breast cancer diagnosis. A newly diagnosed patient often has little or no idea how to cope with this new phase of life. The nurse's assessment of each patient is critical in helping to acquire the resources needed during care.

The nurse develops a short but meaningful relationship with every patient. Every patient, whether through anger, humor, strength of character, or apathy, gives insight not only into the individual situation but also into our human character. The knowledge, understanding, and compassion the nurse extends to patients reflects the philosophy of the entire program.

The Multidisciplinary Visit

The multidisciplinary visit is tailored to meet the individual patient's needs according to disease stage, workup to date, health status, and other personal needs. Appointments are generally divided into preoperative visits, for patients with a biopsy showing cancer who have not started treatment, and postoperative visits, for patients who have completed surgical staging. Each category of visit will require different specialty input (see Table 3.2), with appointments arranged accordingly by the access nurse.

Patients who have had only an initial core needle or surgical biopsy will require consultation to make initial

TELEPHONE INTAKE FORM

Name: _____   Appt Date: _____

MR#: _____   Age: _____

Initial Onset:

    Chief Complaint: _____

    Date: _____

Treatment Summary:

Procedure: _____   R   L   Date:

    _____   R   L   Date:

Risk Factors:

    Oral Contraceptives: Y ☐   N ☐

    Hormone Replacement Therapy: Y ☐   N ☐

    Menarche: _____   Gravida: _____   Para: _____

    Abortion: _____   Miscarriage: _____   Age 1st Pregnancy: _____

    Menopause: Y ☐ N ☐   LMP: _____

    Alcohol: Y ☐ N ☐   No. Drinks/Wk: _____

    Smoking: Y ☐ N ☐   PPD: _____ Pk-yrs: _____

    Prior Breast Bx: Y ☐ N ☐

Medical Problems: _____

_____

Surgical Problems: _____

_____

Medications: _____ _____ _____ _____

    _____ _____ _____ _____

Allergies: _____

Family Cancer History: *(Record breast and ovarian first)* _____

_____

_____

Social History: _____

_____

Occupation: _____

Additional Concerns: _____

_____

_____

Bx, biopsy; LMP, last menstrual period; Pk-yrs, pack-years; PPD, packs per day.

FIGURE 3.1

decisions as to whether their surgery will be breast conservation or mastectomy. If their tumor is large or locally advanced, consultations address whether surgery or systemic therapy will come first. Patients who have completed their surgery will require consultation aimed at finalizing radiation and systemic therapy decisions.

Additional consultations and imaging studies required can be scheduled in advance by the access nurse or can be arranged following the multidisciplinary visit.

After each patient at the multidisciplinary session has been examined, the physicians meet to discuss each patient and review pathology and radiology materials. Ideally, pathology slides are presented by the pathologist and radiology materials are reviewed with a breast imaging radiologist. Eligibility for participation in clinical trials is reviewed. A consensus on treatment options is reached among the physicians and presented to the patient.

In our program, an educational session is provided for the patients attending each multidisciplinary clinic during the time that the physicians' working conference takes place. This educational session includes presentations by a nurse, social worker, and research assistant. Basic information on breast cancer is provided, and patients are informed about resources available within the cancer center and the community. General information about clinical trials is given, including information about specimen and data collection studies and the consent process for these studies. A packet of written educational materials is also distributed at this time.

Patient Satisfaction/Program Evaluation

It is important for a multidisciplinary program to work to continually improve the quality of care and to measure patient satisfaction. Some of the information frequently collected in a quality measures survey should include assessment of patient experience and satisfaction with the following measures:

- *Access:* the wait time between calling and the first scheduled appointment
- *Waits and delays:* Are patients kept informed regarding wait times in the check-in area and exam room?

- *Telephone:* ease of reaching office staff and courtesy and helpfulness of staff
- *Phlebotomy:* wait time and courtesy of the staff
- *Education and information resources:* access, relevance, and usefulness of educational material and workshops
- *Psychosocial issues:* culturally sensitive care for patient and families

Survey results are valuable in helping identify areas for improvement and, in areas where satisfaction is high, validate the worth of services provided in the multidisciplinary session.

Our own experience with patient surveys obtained following multidisciplinary sessions has shown us that these sessions are a significant step in planning a patient's course of care. In particular, breast cancer patients place a high value on the ease of making appointments and on receiving courtesy and compassion from staff. Patients tell us how grateful they are to have an opportunity to actively participate in decision making. They highly value knowing that the nurse they have connected with on the phone will be supporting and will advocate for them during their visit and throughout the decision-making process.

■ CONCLUSIONS

The central goal of a current, state-of-the-art breast cancer program is to deliver patient-focused care that ensures the best possible quality of life during and following treatment. A multidisciplinary approach is key in achieving these goals.

4 Multidisciplinary Issues for Newly Diagnosed Patients

Biopsy Techniques

ELIZABETH A. RAFFERTY

For many years, the standard of care for diagnosing breast pathology was surgical excision (with or without preoperative needle localization). More recently, however, techniques of percutaneous breast biopsy have evolved that offer less invasive options for the diagnosis of breast pathology. Percutaneous sampling offers several advantages. It is expeditious (often being performed on the same day that the lesion is identified) and less invasive than surgical biopsy while maintaining very high rates of accuracy. The percutaneous route of sampling produces little or no scarring and has very few complications. When used appropriately, percutaneous biopsy also offers significant cost savings over excisional biopsy. But perhaps most important is that the ability to make an accurate diagnosis of a breast lesion percutaneously reduces the number of subsequent operations for the patient. If a concordant benign diagnosis is obtained, no further evaluation is needed, and the patient is spared a surgery. If a malignant diagnosis is obtained, appropriate delineation of the extent of disease can be made, and a definitive surgical procedure can be undertaken, including assessment of the axilla if an invasive process is found.

■ METHODS OF PERCUTANEOUS BIOPSY

Preprocedural Evaluation

A complete evaluation of all breast lesions should be performed prior to contemplating biopsy; this is particularly true of cases referred from outside your facility. Be particularly wary of patients referred for biopsy of lesions "seen only on one view"; in these cases, diagnostic evaluation has often been incomplete, and biopsy may in fact be unnecessary. Review all relevant imaging (including imaging of the contralateral breast), and perform any additional imaging that may be required to define the apparent radiological extent of disease; this will enable formulation of a comprehensive biopsy plan that will yield maximal information for treatment planning.

Fine-Needle Aspiration

The use of fine-gauge (20 to 23) needle aspiration for diagnosing malignancy in palpable breast masses has been described for more than 30 years (1). While the convenience of the technique cannot be disputed, its reliability has been recognized to be variable, and its diagnostic accuracy is imperfect. In an analysis of 10,197 patients, Grant and colleagues reported sensitivities of fine-needle aspiration biopsy of palpable breast lesions ranging from 53% to 99% (2). Similar results have been described when fine-needle aspiration techniques are employed to assess nonpalpable primary breast lesions under imaging guidance (3).

Particularly problematic is the high rate of inadequate samples seen when fine-needle aspiration techniques are employed, with insufficient material for diagnosis reported in 15% to 35% of procedures (2–4). Further histological investigation of lesions yielding insufficient diagnostic results on fine-needle aspiration biopsy is necessary, and the operator should not be falsely reassured of a benign process from an inadequate sample. The number of insufficient samples can be decreased and the overall accuracy of fine-needle aspiration biopsy can be maximized by having a trained cytopathologist present at the time of lesion sampling to enable immediate assessment of the adequacy of the specimen (4); however, this is not always possible. Widespread availability of core needle biopsy techniques that have demonstrated superior diagnostic yield and greater reproducibility call into question the role of fine-needle aspiration biopsy in the evaluation of primary breast lesions.

Stereotactic Core Needle Biopsy

Technical Considerations

The principle of stereotaxis allows the three-dimensional location of an object to be precisely predicted from two-dimensional images; this concept is used in localizing lesions for stereotactic breast biopsy. Because the technique employs x-ray imaging of the breast for targeting, a lesion must be visible mammographically to enable stereotactic biopsy. Biopsy can be accomplished either on a dedicated prone table or though use of an upright unit.

With either technique, the breast is positioned such that the lesion of interest is visible within a fenestrated compression paddle affording a limited field of view. Visualization of the lesion is confirmed with a scout image (Figure 4.1). Subsequently, the x-ray tube is moved so that images are acquired 15 degrees off the perpendicular in both the positive and negative directions (the stereotactic paired images) to yield a pair of images seen at a 30-degree differential (Figure 4.2). The patient remains stationary, with her breast in compression, during this process. Stereotactic biopsy is based on the principle of parallax. The targeted lesion will appear to shift from its original location (as demonstrated on the scout image) to a different location on each of the stereotactic paired images. The degree of this apparent shift (the parallax shift) is related to the depth of the lesion within the breast. If the location of a fixed reference point on the stereotactic platform is known, the stereotactic unit can mathematically calculate the distance into the breast using the degree of parallax shift and thus direct the biopsy needle to the target lesion for sampling. It is the operator who must identify the lesion

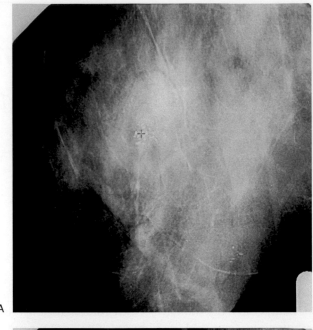

A

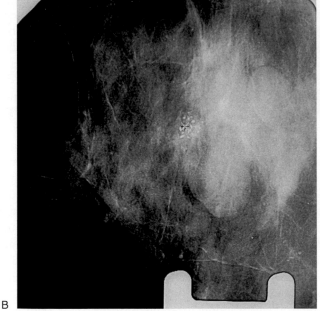

B

FIGURE 4.2 A and B: Calcifications are identified and targeted on the paired stereotactic images. Pathology showed ductal carcinoma in situ.

of interest on each of the stereotactic paired images, and the accuracy of the technique is predicated on the correct identification of the same unique point in space on each of the paired images. Failure to identify the same unique aspect of the lesion on each of the paired images will result in an inaccurate depth calculation and failure to retrieve the desired target.

Fine-Needle Aspiration

Initial stereotactic experiences successfully employed fine-needle aspiration techniques to sample lesions on the

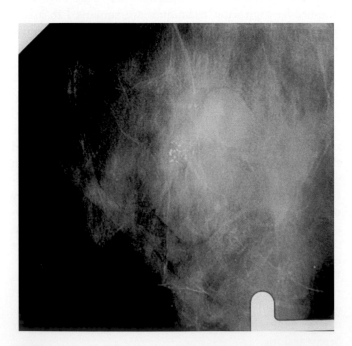

FIGURE 4.1 Calcifications are centered on the stereotactic scout image.

stereotactic platform (5). While this approach did allow the diagnosis of malignancy, it was recognized that sampling error leading to false-negative results, specimens of insufficient diagnostic quality, and underestimation of disease limited the usefulness of the technique (6–8).

Large-Core Automated Sampling

Application of core needle sampling techniques using an automated biopsy device on the stereotactic platform ushered in the era of histological rather than cytological evaluation of breast lesions. Core biopsy material allows for more confident diagnosis of benign lesions as well as more comprehensive characterization of malignant lesions—in particular the ability to distinguish in situ from invasive disease (9,10). Parker and colleagues reported on a series of 102 patients undergoing 14-gauge core needle biopsy under stereotactic guidance immediately followed by needle localization and surgical excision of mammographically suspicious lesions (10). Pathological agreement of a benign or malignant diagnosis was achieved in 96% of cases. Furthermore, all core needle samples were deemed sufficient for histological analysis, overcoming the major obstacle of insufficient cytological material inherent in fine-needle aspiration biopsy.

Directional Vacuum-assisted Biopsy Sampling

While the issue of nondiagnostic sampling was effectively addressed by the adoption of the 14-gauge automated biopsy device, significant underestimation of disease stage remained, with 50% of atypical ductal hyperplasia found at stereotactic biopsy upgraded to ductal carcinoma in situ (DCIS) or invasive carcinoma at subsequent surgical excision (11,12). Introduction of the directional vacuum-assisted biopsy (DVAB) device in 1996 provided the ability to more thoroughly sample mammographically suspicious lesions, particularly calcifications (13). The device is inserted once and then serially rotated to enable sampling of different areas of the lesion and an overall retrieval of substantially larger quantities of tissue. The more complete sampling afforded by vacuum-assisted biopsy has resulted in a significant decrease in underestimation of disease. Underestimation of disease when using 14- and 11-gauge DVAB devices has been reported at 18% to 39% and 10% to 25%, respectively (14–17). Interestingly, the introduction of even larger-gauge DVAB instruments has not resulted in any further reduction in upgrade rates (18,19), thereby underscoring the continued need for surgical re-excision of all atypical ductal hyperplasia diagnosed at core needle biopsy.

Clinical Considerations

One of the fundamental benefits of percutaneous breast biopsy over open surgical biopsy in the evaluation of suspicious breast lesions is the ability to spare a woman unnecessary surgeries. Liberman and colleagues demonstrated that in women with calcifications highly suggestive of malignancy [Breast Imaging Reporting and Data System (BIRADS) category 5], the utilization of stereotactic core needle biopsy for diagnosis significantly reduced the total number of operations performed; the likelihood of a woman undergoing a single operation was 68.5% when undergoing stereotactic biopsy for diagnosis versus 38.0% when undergoing surgical excision for diagnosis (20). Moreover, use of an 11-gauge DVAB device rather than a 14-gauge instrument was significantly more likely to result in sparing of a surgical procedure (76.6% versus 38.1%) while reducing the cost of diagnosis by 22.2%.

Specimen radiography plays a critical role in stereotactic biopsy, particularly when calcifications are being targeted (Figure 4.3). Failure to retrieve calcifications in the stereotactic specimen has been associated with a high rate of underestimation of malignancy (21). Use of an 11-gauge DVAB device results in calcification retrieval in 95% of cases. Failure to retrieve calcifications is more likely to occur with targets spanning less than 5 mm, calcifications that are amorphous in shape, and when the biopsy device is fired outside the breast and manually advanced to the lesion (16). At biopsy, if the operator suspects that all or most of the targeted lesion has been removed, it is advisable to place a tissue marker at the site of biopsy to facilitate localization of the biopsy cavity for excision should the pathological results require it. Immediate postbiopsy mammography is also important and allows the operator to confirm that the lesion of interest has been successfully sampled and that the tissue marker has deployed accurately. Correlation of the histological diagnosis with the imaging findings is critical to the success of any percutaneous biopsy procedure.

Stereotactic core needle biopsy represents an important advance in evaluating mammographically evident

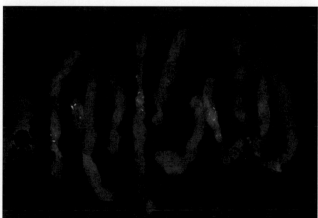

FIGURE 4.3 Specimen radiography of stereotactic core biopsy samples demonstrates calcifications.

breast lesions. The evolution of technology has resulted in a highly accurate procedure that can provide expeditious diagnosis at a lower cost, sparing the patient unnecessary surgeries and facilitating surgical planning. Important factors in ensuring success include the use of a DVAB device that is 11-gauge or larger, accurate targeting on the stereotactic paired imaging, performance of specimen radiography to ensure adequate target retrieval, and meticulous radiological-pathological correlation.

Ultrasound-Guided Core Needle Biopsy

Technical Considerations

In general, ultrasound guidance is selected for interventions in which the lesion is visible by ultrasound because this approach is readily available, does not employ ionizing radiation, and is generally more comfortable for both the patient and the operator. In addition, sonography offers the operator the advantage of real-time visualization of the needle as it advances into and samples the lesion. Cyst aspiration, abscess drainage, fine-needle aspiration biopsy, needle localization, and core needle biopsy all can be accomplished using sonographic guidance. Orientation of the needle parallel to the chest wall is recommended to ensure that the chest wall is not transgressed and to improve visualization of the needle through superior sound reflection (Figure 4.4).

Clinical Considerations

Masses fulfilling the sonographic criteria of a simple cyst do not require intervention unless symptomatic. Cysts containing low-level internal echoes can have their cystic nature confirmed through sonographically guided cyst aspiration. Cyst aspirates yielding bloody fluid should

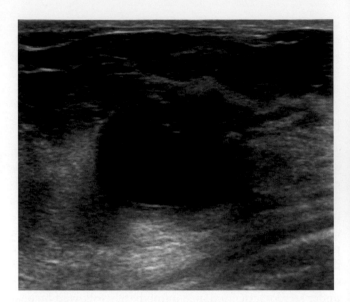

FIGURE 4.5 Complex cystic mass with thick wall. Pathology showed papillary carcinoma.

be sent for cytological analysis; nonbloody aspirates can be safely discarded (22,23). In contrast, in a series published by Berg and colleagues, sonographically evaluated masses demonstrating a thick wall (Figure 4.5), thick septations, mural nodularity, or a combination of cystic and solid components were shown to be malignant 23% of the time at biopsy and should be evaluated with core biopsy (24).

Solid masses that are sonographically visible are appropriately managed with core needle biopsy (25,26). In a series of 1352 lesions undergoing core biopsy with a 14-gauge automated device under sonographic guidance, a false-negative rate of 1.6% (11 of 671 malignant lesions) was reported (27). As with stereotactic core needle biopsy, meticulous attention to technique as well as radiological-pathological correlation is critical in minimizing false-negative results.

Technology has also been developed to allow DVAB under sonographic guidance using a handheld device (28). On the stereotactic platform, the transition from large-core automated biopsy to DVAB devices was accompanied by increased accuracy and a reduction in underestimation of disease (14,16,17); however, under ultrasound guidance, the use of DVAB devices has not shown a diagnostic advantage (29). The differential performance of the vacuum-assisted method under the two modalities may be attributable to lesion selection; stereotactic core biopsy is used primarily in the evaluation of indeterminate and suspicious microcalcifications. Calcified lesions have been shown to be more accurately sampled using vacuum-assisted techniques (16,30), suggesting that these lesions have more inherent heterogeneity than masses and would perhaps be optimally addressed with the excision of a larger volume of contiguous tissue.

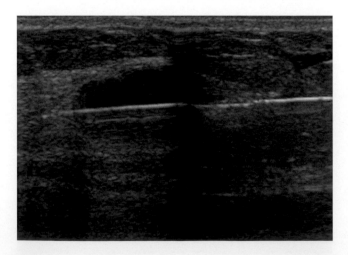

FIGURE 4.4 Postfire image of ultrasound-guided core needle biopsy shows biopsy needle traversing the lesion and positioned parallel to the chest wall.

MRI-Guided Core Needle Biopsy

Intermodality Correlation

In the past several years, MRI has assumed an increasingly important role in the evaluation of breast disease for both diagnostic and screening applications, and the growing utilization of the modality has mandated the ability to biopsy findings seen only on MRI. Because access to the magnet to perform MRI-guided intervention is relatively limited and expensive, an attempt to find a sonographic correlate for suspicious findings observed at MRI is reasonable, yet few studies have addressed the ability to reliably find sonographic correlates for lesions initially diagnosed on MRI. LaTrenta and colleagues identified an ultrasound correlate for 23% of suspicious lesions identified on MRI (31). Notably, the likelihood of malignancy in MRI-detected lesions demonstrating a sonographic correlate was significantly greater than in those failing to demonstrate such a correlate (43% versus 14%); however, the rate of diagnosis of malignancy in lesions seen only on MRI was sufficiently high as to require the ability to perform MRI-guided intervention (Figures 4.6 and 4.7).

Clinical Performance

MRI-guided biopsy can be accomplished using a dedicated breast coil and a grid system specifically designed

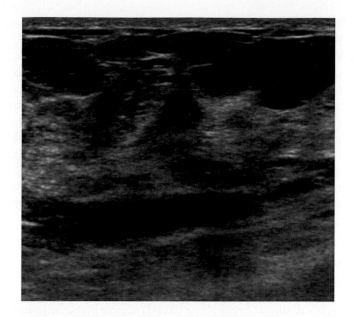

FIGURE 4.7 Second-look ultrasound is able to demonstrate a correlate for the MRI finding, allowing biopsy under ultrasound guidance. Pathology showed invasive ductal carcinoma.

for intervention. With an MRI-compatible coaxial system, multiple core biopsies can be obtained using a 9-gauge MRI-compatible DVAB device (32,33). A tissue marker can be placed at the site of biopsy, thus obviating the need to return to the magnet should further intervention be required. With this system, the yield of malignancy on MRI-guided biopsy has been reported to be 25% to 26% (32,34).

Unlike percutaneous biopsy performed under sonographic or stereotactic guidance, confirmation of target retrieval on MRI-guided breast biopsy is challenging. Lesion enhancement, integral to targeting and sampling during the procedure, is transient and seen only in vivo. Accordingly, the operator must use particular care when assessing lesion histology and imaging concordance. In a series of 342 lesions undergoing MRI-guided biopsy, Lee and colleagues found 7% of the pathology results to be discordant with the imaging findings (35), a rate higher than that reported with either ultrasound- or stereotactic-guided biopsy (36). Moreover, at surgical excision, malignancy was diagnosed in 30% of the discordant lesions (35). These data highlight the need for meticulous and skeptical radiological-pathological correlation with this modality.

■ MANAGEMENT CONSIDERATIONS IN PERCUTANEOUS BIOPSY

Radiological-Pathological Correlation

A critical aspect of any percutaneous core needle biopsy is correlation of the pathological data with the imaging.

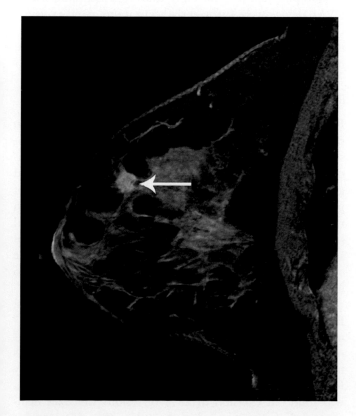

FIGURE 4.6 Enhancing lesion (arrow) identified on gadolinium-enhanced MRI.

In particular, the operator must ascertain: (a) whether the lesion of concern was accurately and adequately sampled, (b) whether the pathology and imaging findings are concordant (in agreement with the preprocedure expectation based on the radiological findings) or discordant (*not* in agreement with the preprocedure expectation based on the radiological findings), (c) whether the histology suggests the possibility of an adjacent higher-stage lesion, and (d) whether the histological diagnosis is one that warrants additional evaluation on its own merit. Any lesion yielding a histological diagnosis that is not concordant with the imaging findings must be rebiopsied or surgically removed.

Lesions Warranting Special Consideration

Atypical Ductal Hyperplasia

Atypical ductal hyperplasia (ADH) is a proliferative lesion of the breast that shares some, but not all, of the cytological features of DCIS and can be seen in proximity to both in situ and invasive malignancy (37). Identification of ADH is more common when core needle biopsy is performed in the evaluation of microcalcifications rather than masses (38). ADH is present in only 1.7% of sonographically guided breast biopsies (39). Despite the relative rarity of ADH on sonographic core biopsy, excision of these lesions yielded malignancy in 44% of cases. Because of this association, ADH seen on core biopsy requires surgical excision to exclude adjacent malignancy regardless of the nature of the target, the type of biopsy device employed, or the modality used for image guidance.

Lobular Neoplasia

The significance and optimal management of lobular neoplasia incidentally diagnosed on percutaneous core needle biopsy have generated substantial debate. The term *lobular neoplasia* describes the spectrum of histological changes ranging from atypical lobular hyperplasia to lobular carcinoma in situ (LCIS). The identification of lobular neoplasia at biopsy is recognized to represent a risk factor for the subsequent development of breast cancer (40); however, its potential role as a precursor to invasive carcinoma is controversial.

Lobular neoplasia is diagnosed in only 0.9% to 1.2% of core needle biopsies (41,42). Although the pleomorphic form of LCIS may present with mammographically suspicious calcifications (43), most lobular neoplasia is not associated with imaging findings.

Several studies have noted a significant incidence of malignancy when lobular neoplasia diagnosed at percutaneous core biopsy is excised, with upgrade rates of 17% to 23% reported (42,44,45). Several reasons have been postulated to explain this association: The targeted lesion was missed at the time of biopsy; the targeted lesion was accurately sampled, and both the lobular neoplasia and the subsequently diagnosed malignancy are incidental; the targeted lesion was initially misdiagnosed as lobular neoplasia but was, in fact, DCIS; or the lobular neoplasia is a nonobligate precursor of invasive carcinoma and should be treated similarly to ADH (45).

Papillary Lesions

Papillary lesions of the breast comprise a histologically diverse group of lesions ranging from solitary intraductal papilloma to papillary carcinoma. Individual lesions can also demonstrate heterogeneity, complicating definitive histological diagnosis and introducing the potential for underestimation of disease with core needle sampling. Single-institution series have been small and have generated conflicting recommendations regarding the need for re-excision (46,47).

More recently, Mercado and colleagues noted an upgrade rate of 26% to either ADH or DCIS on excision of benign papillary lesions (48). Rizzo and colleagues reviewed 142 cases of benign papillary lesions diagnosed at core needle biopsy and identified an upgrade rate of almost 25% (14.0% to ADH and 10.5% to DCIS) at subsequent surgical excision (49). In an analysis of 103 papillary lesions diagnosed as benign by histology and concordant with the imaging findings, 17% were upgraded to malignancy or high-risk lesion at excision (50). Neither sonographic features nor more thorough sampling with a DVAB device were sufficiently accurate to avoid excision. Given these results, excision of all papillary lesions diagnosed at core needle biopsy would seem prudent to avoid missing a malignant diagnosis.

Radial Scars

Radial scars are complex, proliferative lesions that can mimic carcinoma on imaging studies as well as microscopically (51,52). Pathologically, they consist of a central fibroelastic core that is associated with entrapped glandular elements demonstrating varying degrees of proliferation. The heterogeneous nature of the lesion raises concern for underestimation of disease when radial scar is diagnosed at percutaneous core biopsy; results of surgical excision from relatively small studies add to the confusion, with yields of malignancy ranging from 0% to 40% (53–55).

In a review of the data gathered from 11 institutions, Brenner and colleagues evaluated the outcome of 157 mammographically detected lesions that resulted in a diagnosis of radial scar on core needle biopsy (56). All lesions had undergone surgical excision or demonstrated stability for at least two years of imaging follow-up. Carcinoma was found at excision in 28% of lesions that had demonstrated atypia at core biopsy and in 4% of lesions not showing evidence of atypia at core biopsy. Interestingly, underestimation occurred in 9% of lesions biopsied with a large-core automated device, but in 0% of lesions sampled with a vacuum-assisted device. The number of core specimens retrieved also affected outcome, with an upgrade rate of 8% occurring when fewer than 12 specimens were obtained and an upgrade rate of 0% resulting from biopsies yielding 12 or more core samples. The authors suggest that these data allow a subset of radial scars diagnosed at core needle biopsy to forgo excision; however, given the conflicting data, this recommendation requires validation, and continued excision of radial scars diagnosed at core biopsy remains a prudent approach.

■ SURGICAL BIOPSY

Indications for Surgical Biopsy

Because it is expeditious, minimally invasive, cost-effective, and highly accurate, core biopsy is generally preferred to surgical biopsy in the histological assessment of suspicious breast lesions. However, technical challenges such as insufficient breast thickness or faint calcifications may preclude successful percutaneous biopsy. Complex cystic and solid lesions may also require surgical excision to ensure adequate sampling. When patient comorbidities are considered or there is a clinical need to minimize any interruption of anticoagulation, surgical biopsy may also be preferred. Clinically suspicious lesions lacking an imaging correlate will also require surgical biopsy. Finally, core needle biopsies yielding nonconcordant histological results or demonstrating atypia or specific histologies such as papillary lesions and radial scars should be surgically excised.

Needle Localization and Surgical Excision

Prior to the advent of mammography, the vast majority of breast biopsies was performed for diagnosis of a palpable breast mass. As mammographic screening became more prevalent, an increasing number of clinically occult lesions were detected by mammography and required evaluation. Preoperative placement of a guidewire immediately adjacent to the lesion under imaging guidance enables the surgeon to excise the abnormality in a minimal volume of tissue and can be accomplished under mammographic, sonographic, or MRI guidance.

Specimen radiography is essential to ensure that the area of concern is contained within the surgical sample. If the target is not within the specimen, limited additional excision is reasonable if the likely location of the lesion can be ascertained. Otherwise, the procedure should be terminated and repeat imaging should be undertaken after a few weeks when the patient can tolerate mammographic compression and repeat localization and excision.

Surgical Biopsy Considerations

Incision placement for every surgical biopsy must take into account the possibility that malignancy may be present and that mastectomy ultimately may be required. Excessive tunneling should be avoided, and whenever possible, incisions should be placed so as not to preclude skin-sparing mastectomy.

Specimen orientation is essential for all diagnostic breast biopsies to permit the pathologist to specify which margins are positive or close if malignancy is identified. Such orientation allows selective re-excision of involved margins rather than a global re-excision of the entire cavity. Specimen orientation may be achieved with two or more marking sutures followed by six-color inking of the specimen to uniquely identify superior, inferior, medial, lateral, anterior, and deep aspects of the specimen.

■ SUMMARY

The introduction of techniques for percutaneous breast biopsy has transformed the way that breast pathology is diagnosed. Offering expeditious, accurate, and cost-effective diagnosis, these techniques have gained widespread acceptance by both patients and practitioners. Critical to success is a thorough evaluation of the patient's preprocedural imaging to permit development of a comprehensive plan for biopsy. Familiarity with the full scope of modalities available for imaging guidance as well as the array of equipment and instruments available for intervention ensures the optimal approach to each lesion. The importance of meticulous radiological-pathological correlation cannot be overstated; rigorous attention to the concordance or discordance of histological results with imaging findings allows sampling error to be minimized and underestimation of disease to be avoided.

■ MULTIDISCIPLINARY CONSIDERATIONS

- Core biopsy should be the first diagnostic approach whenever possible, but collaboration between radiologist and surgeon in selecting the biopsy technique for an individual patient ensures optimal outcome.
- Meticulous radiological-pathological correlation of core biopsy results is essential to ensure accurate diagnosis.

■ REFERENCES

1. Kern WH. The diagnosis of breast cancer by fine-needle aspiration smears. *JAMA*. 1979;241:1125–1127.

2. Grant CS, Goellner JR, Welch JS, Martin JK. Fine-needle aspiration of the breast. *Mayo Clin Proc.* 1986;61:377–381.

3. Evans WP, Cade SH. Needle localization and fine-needle aspiration biopsy of nonpalpable breast lesions with use of standard and stereotactic equipment. *Radiology.* 1989;173:53–56.

4. Pisano ED, Fajardo LL, Caudry DJ, et al. Fine-needle aspiration biopsy of nonpalpable breast lesions in a multicenter clinical trial: results from the Radiologic Diagnostic Oncology Group V. *Radiology.* 2001;219:785–792.

5. Lofgren M, Andersson I, Lindholm K. Stereotactic fine-needle aspiration for cytologic diagnosis of nonpalpable breast lesions. *AJR Am J Roentgenol.* 1990;154:1191–1195.

6. Azavedo E, Svane G, Auer G. Stereotaxic fine-needle biopsy in 2,594 mammographically detected non-palpable lesions. *Lancet.* 1989;1:1033–1036.

7. Dowlatshahi K, Gent HJ, Schmidt R, et al. Nonpalpable breast tumors: diagnosis with stereotaxic localization and fine-needle aspiration. *Radiology.* 1989;170:427–433.

8. Ciatto S, Del Turco MR, Bravetti P. Non-palpable breast lesion: stereotaxic fine-needle aspiration cytology. *Radiology.* 1989;173:57–59.

9. Parker SH, Lovin JD, Jobe WE, et al. Stereotactic breast biopsy with a biopsy gun. *Radiology.* 1990;176:741–747.

10. Parker SH, Lovin JD, Jobe WE, et al. Non-palpable breast lesions: stereotactic automated large core biopsies. *Radiology.* 1991;180:403–407.

11. Jackman RJ, Nowels KW, Shepard MJ, et al. Stereotaxic large-core needle biopsy of 450 breast lesions with surgical correlation in lesions with cancer or atypical hyperplasia. *Radiology.* 1994;193:91–95.

12. Liberman L, Cohen MA, Dershaw DD, et al. Atypical ductal hyperplasia diagnosed at stereotaxic core biopsy of breast lesions: an indication for surgical biopsy. *AJR Am J Roentgenol.* 1995;164:1111–1113.

13. Burbank F, Parker SH, Fogarty TJ. Stereotactic breast biopsy: improved tissue harvesting with the Mammotome. *Am Surg.* 1996;62:738–744.

14. Jackman RJ, Burbank F, Parker SH, et al. Atypical ductal hyperplasia diagnosed at stereotactic breast biopsy: improved reliability with a 14-gauge, directional, vacuum-assisted biopsy. *Radiology.* 1997;204:485–488.

15. Darling ML, Smith DN, Lester SC, et al. Atypical ductal hyperplasia and ductal carcinoma in situ as revealed by large-core needle breast biopsy: results of surgical excision. *AJR Am J Roentgenol.* 2000;175:1341–1346.

16. Liberman L, Smolkin JH, Dershaw DD, et al. Calcification retrieval at stereotactic, 11-gauge, directional, vacuum-assisted breast biopsy. *Radiology.* 1998;208:251–260.

17. Brem RF, Behrndt VS, Sanow L, Gatewood OMB. Atypical ductal hyperplasia: histologic underestimation of carcinoma in tissue harvested from impalpable breast lesions using 11-gauge stereotactically guided directional vacuum-assisted biopsy. *AJR Am J Roentgenol.* 1999;172:1405–1407.

18. Eby PR, Ochsner JE, DeMartini WB, et al. Frequency and upgrade rates of atypical ductal hyperplasia diagnosed at stereotactic vacuum-assisted breast biopsy: 9- versus 11-gauge. *AJR Am J Roentgenol.* 2009;192:229–234.

19. Brem RF, Schoonians JM, Goodman SN, et al. Nonpalpable breast cancer: percutaneous diagnosis with 11- and 8-gauge stereotactic vacuum-assisted biopsy devices. *Radiology.* 2001;219:793–796.

20. Liberman L, Gougoutas, CA, Zakowski MF, et al. Calcifications highly suggestive of malignancy: comparison of breast biopsy methods. *AJR Am J Roentgenol.* 2001;177:165–172.

21. Dershaw DD, Morris EA, Liberman L, Abramson AF. Nondiagnostic stereotaxic core breast biopsy: results of rebiopsy. *Radiology.* 1996;198:323–325.

22. Smith DN, Kaelin CM, Korbin CD, et al. Impalpable breast cysts: utility of cytologic examination of fluid obtained with radiologically guided aspiration. *Radiology.* 1997;204:149–151.

23. Ciatto S, Cariaggi P, Bulgaresi P. The value of routine cytologic examination of breast cyst fluids. *Acta Cytol.* 1987;31:301–304.

24. Berg WA, Campassi CI, Ioffe OB. Cystic lesions of the breast: sonographic-pathologic correlation. *Radiology.* 2003;227:183–191.

25. Parker SH, Jobe WE, Dennis MD, et al. US-guided automated large-core breast biopsy. *Radiology.* 1993;187:507–511.

26. Liberman L, Feng TL, Dershaw DD, et al. Ultrasound-guided core breast biopsy: utility and cost-effectiveness. *Radiology.* 1998; 208:717–723.

27. Schueller G, Jaromi S, Ponhold L, et al. US-guided 14-gauge core-needle breast biopsy: results of a validation study in 1352 cases. *Radiology.* 2008;248:406–413.

28. Parker SH, Klaus AJ, McWey PJ, et al. Sonographically guided directional vacuum-assisted breast biopsy using a handheld device. *AJR Am J Roentgenol.* 2001;177:405–408.

29. Philpotts LE, Hooley RJ, Lee CH. Comparison of automated versus vacuum-assisted biopsy methods for sonographically guided core biopsy of the breast. *AJR Am J Roentgenol.* 2003;180:347–351.

30. Meyer JE, Smith DN, DiPiro PJ, et al. Stereotactic breast biopsy of clustered microcalcifications with a directional, vacuum-assisted device. *Radiology.* 1997; 204:575–576.

31. LaTrenta LR, Menell JH, Morris EA, et al. Breast lesions detected with MR imaging: utility and histopathologic importance of identification with US. *Radiology.* 2003;227:856–861.

32. Liberman L, Bracero N, Morris E, et al. MRI-guided 9-gauge vacuum-assisted breast biopsy: initial clinical experience. *AJR Am J Roentgenol.* 2005;185:183–193.

33. Orel SG, Rosen M, Mies C, Schnall MD. MR-imaging guided 9-gauge vacuum-assisted core-needle breast biopsy: initial experience. *Radiology.* 2006;238:54–61.

34. Han BK, Schnall MD, Orel SG, Rosen M. Outcome of MRI-guided breast biopsy. *AJR Am J Roentgenol.* 2008;191:1798–1804.

35. Lee JM, Kaplan JB, Murray MP, et al. Imaging-histologic discordance at MRI-guided 9-gauge vacuum-assisted breast biopsy. *AJR Am J Roentgenol.* 2007;189:852–859.

36. Liberman L, Drotman MB, Morris EA, et al. Imaging-histologic discordance at percutaneous breast biopsy. *Cancer.* 2000;89: 2538–2546.

37. Sneige N, Fornage BD, Saleh G. Ultrasound-guided fine needle aspiration of non-palpable breast lesions: cytologic and histologic findings. *Am J Clin Pathol.* 1994;102:98–101.

38. Liberman L, Dershaw DD, Glassman JR, et al. Analysis of cancers not diagnosed at stereotactic core breast biopsy. *Radiology.* 1997;203:151–157.

39. Jang M, Cho N, Moon WK, et al. Underestimation of atypical ductal hyperplasia at sonographically guided core biopsy of the breast. *AJR Am J Roentgenol.* 2008;191:1347–1351.

40. Chuba PJ, Hamre MR, Yap J, et al. Bilateral risk for subsequent breast cancer after lobular carcinoma-in-situ: analysis of surveillance, epidemiologic, and end results data. *J Clin Oncol.* 2005;23:5534–5541.

41. Liberman L, Sama M, Susnik B, et al. Lobular carcinoma in situ at percutaneous breast biopsy: surgical biopsy findings. *AJR Am J Roentgenol.* 1999;173:291–299.

42. Brem RF, Lechner MC, Jackman RJ, et al. Lobular neoplasia at percutaneous breast biopsy: variables associated with carcinoma at surgical excision. *AJR Am J Roentgenol.* 2008;190:637–641.

43. Georgian-Smith D, Lawton TJ. Calcifications of lobular carcinoma in situ of the breast: radiologic-pathologic correlation. *AJR Am J Roentgenol.* 2001;176:1255–1259.

44. Foster MC, Helvie MA, Gregory NE, et al. Lobular carcinoma in situ or atypical lobular hyperplasia at core-needle biopsy: is excisional biopsy necessary? *Radiology.* 2004;231:813–819.

45. Cohen MA. Cancer upgrades at excisional biopsy after diagnosis of atypical lobular hyperplasia or lobular carcinoma in situ at core-needle biopsy: some reasons why. *Radiology.* 2004;231:617–621.

46. Rubin E, Dempsey PJ, Pile NS, et al. Needle-localization biopsy of the breast: impact of a selective core needle biopsy program on yield. *Radiology.* 1995;195:627–631.

47. Liberman L, Bracero N, Vuolo M, et al. Percutaneous large-core biopsy of papillary breast lesions. *AJR Am J Roentgenol.* 1999;172:331–337.

48. Mercado CL, Hamele-Bena D, Oken SM, et al. Papillary lesions of the breast at percutaneous core-needle biopsy. *Radiology.* 2006;238:801–808.

49. Rizzo M, Lund MJ, Oprea G, et al. Surgical follow-up and clinical presentation of 142 breast papillary lesions diagnosed by ultrasound-guided core-needle biopsy. *Ann Surg Oncol.* 2008; 15:1040–1047.

50. Shin HJ, Kim HH, Kim SM, et al. Papillary lesions of the breast diagnosed at percutaneous sonographically guided biopsy: comparison of sonographic features and biopsy methods. *AJR Am J Roentgenol.* 2008;190:630–636.

51. Cohen MA, Sferlazza SJ. Role of sonography in evaluation of radial scars of the breast. *AJR Am J Roentgenol.* 2000;174:1075–1078.

52. Kennedy M, Masterson AV, Kerin M, et al. Pathology and clinical relevance of radial scars: a review. *J Clin Pathol.* 2003; 56:721–724.

53. Philpotts LA, Shaheen NA, Jain KS, et al. Uncommon high-risk lesions of the breast diagnosed at stereotactic core-needle biopsy: clinical importance. *Radiology.* 2000;216:831–837.

54. Jackman RJ, Nowels KW, Rodriguez-Soto J, et al. Stereotactic, automated large-core needle biopsy of non-palpable breast lesions: false-negative and histologic underestimation rates after long-term follow-up. *Radiology.* 1999;210:799–805.

55. Lopez-Medina A, Cintora E, Mugica B, et al. Radial scars diagnosed at stereotactic core-needle biopsy: surgical biopsy findings. *Eur Radiol* 2006;16:1803–1810.

56. Brenner RJ, Jackman RJ, Parker SH, et al. Percutaneous core needle biopsy of radial scars of the breast: when is excision necessary? *AJR Am J Roentgenol.* 2002;179:1179–1184.

Surgical Pathology

ELENA F. BRACHTEL

The surgical pathological findings for breast specimens—both for cancer and for benign changes—determine the subsequent treatment course for a patient. Although most entities in breast pathology are well defined, there is considerable variation in the way specimens are handled and findings are reported. Diagnostic terminology also remains problematic in some areas (1–4). The information to allow accurate staging must be provided in the pathology report (5). Pertinent information (such as tumor size, histological grade, distance to margins, lymph nodes) is often listed in a tabular format (Table 4.1). Ancillary tests such as hormone receptor and HER-2 studies or gene expression profiling may be integrated or added to the reports (6,7). This chapter will highlight topics important for multidisciplinary breast cancer care.

■ Table 4.1 Summary of pathological tumor characteristics

PATHOLOGY REPORT	EXAMPLE
PATIENT INFORMATION	Name Date of birth Age Medical record number
COMMUNICATING PHYSICIANS	Surgeon Medical oncologist Radiation oncologist Pathologist
SPECIMENS SUBMITTED (parts listed separately with exact localization; completed by surgeon)	A - Left Axillary Sentinel Lymph Node B - Left Breast Excision C - Left Breast Final Margin Superior Hemisphere D - Left Breast Final Margin Inferior Hemisphere
FINAL DIAGNOSIS (listed for each specimen part; completed by pathologist)	**LYMPH NODE (LEFT AXILLARY SENTINEL)** THERE IS NO EVIDENCE OF MALIGNANCY IN ONE LYMPH NODE (0/1). Keratin-positive tumor cells are not identified on three AE 1.3/Cam 5.2 immunostained levels. The frozen section diagnosis is confirmed.
FINAL DIAGNOSIS	**BREAST (LEFT), EXCISION:** 1. INVASIVE DUCTAL CARCINOMA. 2. DUCTAL CARCINOMA IN-SITU, SOLID AND CRIBRIFORM TYPE, WITH CALCIFICATIONS. 3. LOBULAR NEOPLASIA (LOBULAR CARCINOMA IN SITU). 4. HEALING BIOPSY SITE.
TUMOR TABLE	TUMOR SIZE: 1.5 x 1 x 1 cm (gross measurement) GRADE: 2. LYMPHATIC VESSEL INVASION: Not identified. BLOOD VESSEL INVASION: Not identified. MARGIN OF INVASIVE CARCINOMA: The distances to all margins measure 0.2 cm or greater. LOCATION OF DUCTAL CARCINOMA IN SITU: Within the region of the mass, few foci. GRADE OF DUCTAL CARCINOMA IN SITU: 1 MARGIN OF DUCTAL CARCINOMA IN SITU: Ductal carcinoma in-situ extends to less than 0.1 cm from the superior margin one focus. STAINS FOR RECEPTORS: Requested on block B1.

Continued

■ **Table 4.1** Summary of pathological tumor characteristics *(Continued)*

PATHOLOGY REPORT	EXAMPLE
NOTE	Foci of ductal carcinoma in situ are surrounded by myoepithelial cells as demonstrated by immunohistochemical stains for p63, calponin and smooth-muscle myosin. Lobular neoplasia cells are negative for E-cadherin.
FINAL DIAGNOSIS	BREAST (LEFT, FINAL MARGIN SUPERIOR HEMISPHERE), EXCISION: THERE IS NO EVIDENCE OF MALIGNANCY.
FINAL DIAGNOSIS	BREAST (LEFT, FINAL MARGIN INFERIOR HEMISPHERE), EXCISION: THERE IS NO EVIDENCE OF MALIGNANCY.
FROZEN SECTION DIAGNOSIS	LYMPH NODE (LEFT AXILLARY "SENTINEL"): NO TUMOR SEEN. AWAIT PERMANENTS.
GROSS DESCRIPTION (listed for each specimen part; completed by pathologist)	LYMPH NODE (LEFT AXILLARY "SENTINEL") Received fresh in the frozen section lab, labeled "Name", Medical record number "#" and "left axillary sentinel lymph node", is a 2 x 2 x 1 cm fibroadipose tissue that contains a 1.3 x 1 x 0.5 cm pink rubbery lymph node, which is bisected and entirely frozen as FX#1, now thawed and submitted as A1. The remainder of the adipose tissue in A2.
GROSS DESCRIPTION	BREAST (LEFT), EXCISION: Received fresh, labeled "Name", Medical record number "#" and "left breast excision", is a 5 x 4 x 3.5 cm portion of breast tissue with a localization wire in place and accompanied by a specimen radiograph. A long suture indicates lateral, a short suture superior, as designated by the surgeon. The specimen is inked as follows: anterior—blue, posterior—black, superior—green, inferior—yellow. The specimen and serially sectioned along the long axis from medial to lateral to reveal a poorly defined firm, white mass of 1.5 x 1 x 1 cm, which comes to within 0.2 cm from the superior, 0.3 cm from the posterior, 1 cm from anterior and inferior margins, 1.5 from the lateral and 2 cm from the medial margin. Medially adjacent to the mass is a 0.3 x 0.3 x 0.2 cm hemorrhagic cavity, grossly consistent with prior biopsy site. The remainder of the breast parenchyma is grossly unremarkable. Representative sections are submitted as follows: B1–B4: Mass and biopsy site, entirely submitted, with closest margins. B5: Grossly unremarkable breast parenchyma, away from the mass. B6: Medial margin, en face. B7: Lateral margin, en face.
GROSS DESCRIPTION	BREAST (LEFT, FINAL MARGIN SUPERIOR HEMISPHERE), EXCISION: Received fresh, labeled "Name", Medical record number "#" and "left breast final margin superior hemisphere", is a 3.5 x 3 x 1 cm unoriented breast tissue. The specimen is serially sectioned to reveal grossly unremarkable fibroadipose tissue and entirely submitted as C1–C8.
GROSS DESCRIPTION	BREAST (LEFT, FINAL MARGIN INFERIOR HEMISPHERE), EXCISION: Received fresh, labeled "Name", Medical record number "#" and "left breast final margin inferior hemisphere", is a 3 x 2.5 x 1 cm unoriented breast tissue. The specimen is serially sectioned to reveal grossly unremarkable fibroadipose tissue and entirely submitted as D1–D6.

■ SPECIMEN TYPES, ORIENTATION, AND GROSS EXAMINATION

Core Biopsy

Core biopsies of the breast are commonly performed to obtain tissue diagnosis of breast lesions and show high concordance with histopathological findings on excision (8,9).

Core biopsies may be obtained with various techniques using ultrasound or stereotactic mammographic guidance and are increasingly performed for MRI-enhancing lesions (10). For calcifications, specimen radiographs are performed to demonstrate the presence of calcifications in the tissue, and correlation of radiographic with histopathological findings is required (11–13).

Excision

Excisions include specimens that may also be labeled "excisional biopsy," "lumpectomy," or "partial mastectomy." Formalin fixation makes tissue firm; therefore it is preferred for the gross evaluation of a specimen in its intact, fresh, unfixed state, to better appreciate changes in color and texture of the tissue (Fig. 4.8). The surface of unoriented excisions is inked in one color, the specimen is sectioned, and sections are submitted for histological evaluation either in a representative fashion or in their entirety, depending on the size of the specimen and the diagnostic question. Breast excisions may be oriented by the surgeon with sutures (e.g., with a long suture for the lateral aspect and a short suture for the superior aspect of a specimen). These are then inked with multiple colors, either by the surgeon in the operating room or by the pathologist during initial gross examination of the specimen (Fig. 4.9). The color designation for each margin needs to be documented in the gross description. Specimen radiographs may reveal mass lesions, calcifications, or metal clips. The presence of a healing biopsy site or metal clips is documented during gross examination. Re-excisions after a prior excision

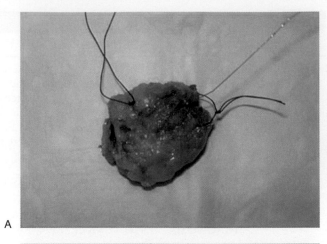

A

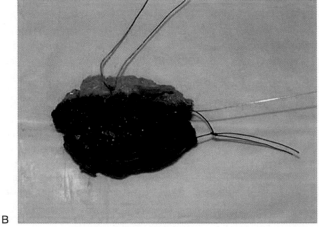

B

FIGURE 4.9 Example of a breast excision specimen oriented by a long suture (lateral) and a short suture (superior) by the surgeon (A). The localizing wire can move or fall out and should not be used for orientation. In this example, the anterior surface is inked blue; the superior surface, yellow; the inferior surface, green. The posterior surface is not visible in this view. Lateral and medial margins show a confluence of all four colors and are submitted separately (B).

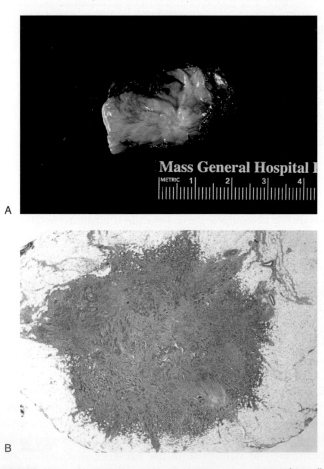

Mass General Hospital

A

B

FIGURE 4.8 An invasive carcinoma appears as a tan-white, ill-defined mass in this gross photograph (A) and histologically (B).

with positive or close margins generally follow the same workup as excisions (14).

Mastectomy

Mastectomy specimens are designated on the basis of the extent of skin and lymph node tissue included. A modified radical mastectomy specimen consists of the breast parenchyma with adipose tissue containing axillary lymph nodes in the upper-outer quadrant, the so-called axillary tail. A simple or total mastectomy specimen may contain a few lymph nodes but does not include a formal axillary lymph node dissection. The appearance of a mastectomy specimen depends on the surgical technique: the conventional, skin-sacrificing mastectomy specimen shows a large skin ellipse, which makes up most of the anterior surface and includes the nipple and areola. A skin-sparing mastectomy consists of breast tissue with only nipple and areola skin included. A nipple-sparing mastectomy specimen consists of breast tissue with no skin taken. Histological sampling is dependent on the lesion and the purpose of the mastectomy: a therapeutic, tumor-bearing mastectomy specimen requires adequate sampling of the tumor in relation to margins. Correlation with preoperative radiographic images is helpful to localize multifocal breast cancers. Representative sections of grossly unremarkable breast parenchyma are performed on a prophylactic mastectomy specimen in the absence of distinct lesions (14).

Margin Evaluation

Margin evaluation is an essential part of the gross description of each breast excision or mastectomy specimen. Each mass lesion is grossly described in its spatial relationship to the margins. Specimen orientation is critical to reduce the volume of tissue removed during breast-conserving surgery. A specimen without orientation can provide only distance from tumor to the closest margin, without information as to which margin is close or positive, making it necessary to re-excise all margins if any one is positive. An oriented excision on the other hand provides the distance from a mass to six possible margins (anterior, posterior/deep, inferior, superior, medial, and lateral), allowing selective re-excision of only those margins that are close or positive.

Margins can be sampled radially (i.e., perpendicular to the mass) or en face (Fig. 4.10) (15,16). Additional

shaved margins of the excision cavity may be submitted as separate specimens. On microscopic examination, the nature of the malignant tumor [invasive carcinoma or ductal carcinoma in situ (DCIS)] and distance to the closest margin are defined. In perpendicular (radial) sections, the distance between tumor and respective inked margins is measured, while en face margins are considered positive or negative. Close margins often include a distance measurement for the tumor in relation to margins ranging from less than 0.1 to 0.2 cm. The details of reporting the distance between tumor and margins are variable, and ultimately the surgeon decides whether the surgical clearance is considered sufficient. Relation to margins is not usually given for lobular neoplasia [lobular carcinoma in situ (LCIS)] in its typical form (17).

■ HISTOPATHOLOGICAL EXAMPLES

Invasive Carcinoma

Tumor Grade and Size

The histological tumor grade for invasive breast carcinoma ranges from well differentiated (grade 1, low grade), to moderately differentiated (grade 2, intermediate grade), to poorly differentiated (grade 3, high grade) (Fig. 4.11) (2,3). In a commonly used grading scheme for

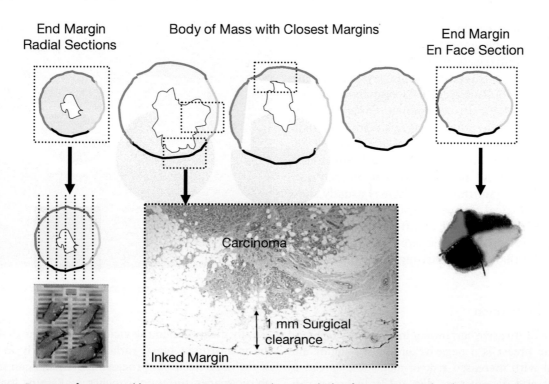

FIGURE 4.10 Diagram of an oriented breast excision specimen with mass, inked surface margins, and end margins. Radial margins are often taken if the mass is close to the margin and allow microscopic measurements of the distance between tumor and inked margin (surgical clearance). En face margins include a section of the surface tissue, which is submitted "face down" into the cassette for histological evaluation.

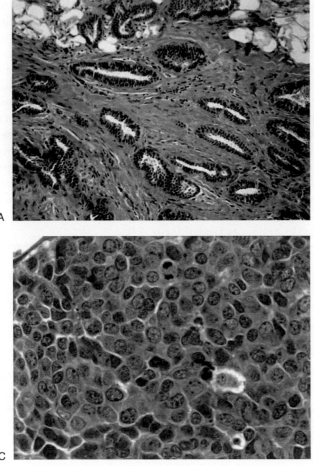

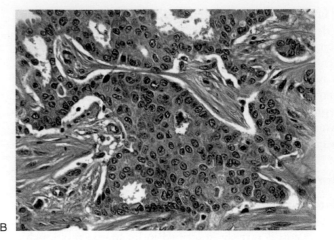

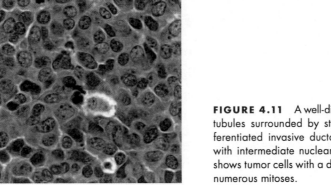

FIGURE 4.11 A well-differentiated invasive ductal carcinoma (A) shows tubules surrounded by stroma (tubular carcinoma). A moderately differentiated invasive ductal carcinoma (B) shows no tubule formation, with intermediate nuclear pleomorphism. A high-grade carcinoma (C) shows tumor cells with a diffuse growth pattern, pleomorphic nuclei, and numerous mitoses.

invasive carcinoma, the histological features of tubule formation, nuclear pleomorphism, and mitotic rate are assessed and summarized as a cumulative score (18). DCIS also follows a three-tier grading system in most classifications (19). Tumor size is usually measured grossly, with histological confirmation. For small carcinomas or those that do not present as a distinct, grossly recognizable mass, microscopic measurements of the greatest tumor extent on any slide are used. For tumors that consist of multiple nodules, the size of each nodule is given. While multifocal carcinomas usually show similar morphological features throughout, heterogeneity and variations in histological differentiation are possible. Microinvasive carcinomas are small invasive foci (usually smaller than 0.1 cm) arising in the background of DCIS (20).

Lymphovascular Invasion

The presence of invasive carcinoma in lymphatic or blood vessels in the breast is a negative prognostic factor and is associated with increased risk of metastatic spread to lymph nodes and distant sites (Fig. 4.12). In breast cancer, lymphatic tumor emboli are more frequently observed than invasion of blood vessels. Lymph vessel invasion is

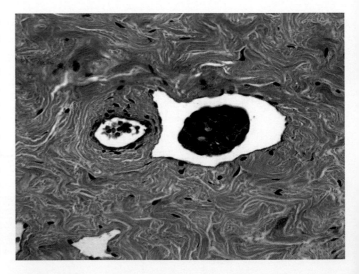

FIGURE 4.12 Invasive carcinoma in a lymphatic vessel.

usually diagnosed in the vicinity of or some distance from the main tumor mass, rather than directly in the center of the mass itself. As processing artifacts can mimic lymphatic spaces, immunohistochemical stains for lymphatic or blood vessels may be helpful for identifying true lymphovascular invasion (1,21,22).

Invasive Carcinoma of Ductal or Lobular Type

The vast majority of invasive breast cancers are ductal carcinomas. These are characterized by mostly cohesive groups of tumor cells that grow in glandlike formations or sheets with various grades of histological differentiation (see Fig. 4.11). Invasive lobular carcinoma is characterized by small dyshesive tumor cells that infiltrate in a single-file pattern, often surrounded by a dense stromal reaction. The traditional nomenclature (ductal vs lobular type) reflects not the anatomical structure of origin (duct vs lobule) but rather the different growth pattern and morphology of tumor cells. Most invasive lobular carcinomas (classic type) are well to moderately differentiated, but a subset of high-grade lobular carcinomas, pleomorphic lobular carcinoma, is now recognized. The loss of cellular cohesion is associated with the absence of the adhesion molecule E-cadherin, which can be demonstrated by immunohistochemistry (Fig. 4.13). Lobular carcinomas often present as ill-defined densities rather than distinct mass lesions and may show a somewhat different metastatic pattern

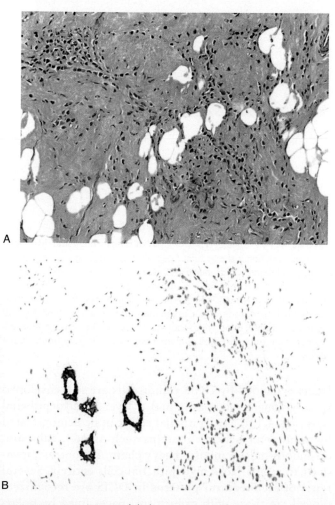

FIGURE 4.13 Invasive lobular carcinoma shows small, dyshesive tumor cells infiltrating the tissue in a single-file pattern (A). The lobular type tumor cells are negative for E-cadherin by immunostain; few remaining normal ducts are positive (B).

from invasive ductal carcinomas. Occasionally, tumors show features of both ductal and lobular differentiation and cannot be unequivocally categorized (1–3,23).

Special Types of Invasive Carcinoma

There are numerous special types of invasive breast carcinoma (Fig. 4.14). Although many are rare, the recognition of their peculiar morphological features is helpful and may be clinically relevant (2,3). Mucinous or colloid carcinoma of the breast has abundant extracellular mucin, which grossly produces a gelatinous appearance and in which groups or strips of carcinoma cells are suspended. Colloid carcinoma is often admixed with conventional invasive ductal carcinoma; pure colloid carcinomas tend to have a more favorable prognosis (24). Micropapillary carcinomas are composed of papillary clusters without fibrovascular cores and are associated with a high rate of metastasis (25). Carcinomas with neuroendocrine features occur mostly in older women; these tumor cells often show a spindled appearance and are positive for neuroendocrine markers such as chromogranin and synaptophysin (26). Metaplastic carcinomas comprise a heterogeneous group that includes matrix-producing malignancies and those with squamous or spindle cell differentiation, ranging from low to high grade (27,28). Intracystic papillary carcinomas appear well circumscribed and surrounded by a fibrous capsule but often show foci of invasion, and their cyst walls generally lack myoepithelial cells (29). Tubular carcinomas are mostly well differentiated and composed of glands that are lined by a one-cell layer of cancer cells (see Fig. 4.11A).

Tumor Characterization After Neoadjuvant Chemotherapy

Locally advanced breast cancers may be treated by chemotherapy prior to definitive surgical excision. Preoperative chemotherapy can lead to clinical shrinking of the tumor mass and permit more conservative surgery in selected cases. The tumor response to the preoperative chemotherapeutic agents may range from complete to partial to absent when pathological response is assessed after the tumor is excised (Fig. 4.15). Several schemas have been proposed to assess and classify the histological response observed after preoperative treatment (30–32).

Distant Metastases

When distant metastases are detected in liver, bone, lung, pleural space, or other sites, tissue is often obtained for diagnosis (Fig. 4.16). Depending on the clinical scenario, cytological rather than histological evaluation may be indicated, particularly for tumor sites where only fine-needle aspiration biopsy is feasible. It is helpful to compare the morphology of the metastatic deposit with that of the

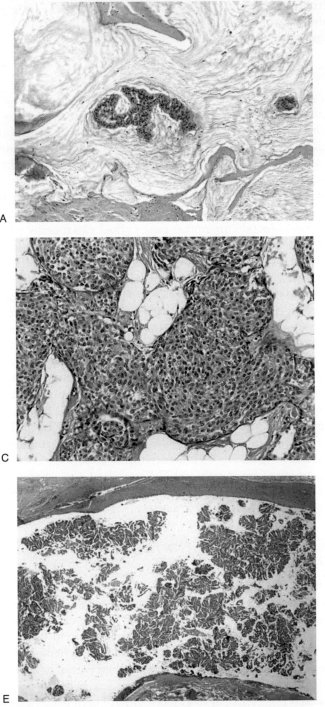

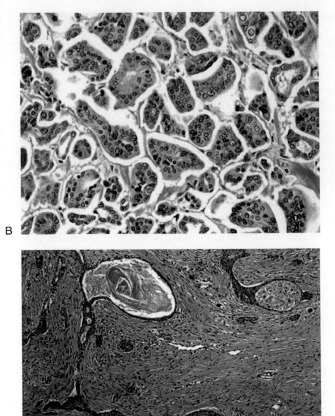

FIGURE 4.14 Special types of invasive breast carcinoma. Mucinous or colloid carcinoma shows tumor cells that appear suspended in pools of abundant extracellular mucin (A). Invasive micropapillary carcinoma shows clusters of tumor cells surrounded by clear spaces (B). Tumor cells of an invasive carcinoma with neuroendocrine features appear spindled (C). Low-grade adenosquamous carcinoma has glandular and squamous differentiation with focal keratinization (D). Intracystic papillary carcinoma appears well circumscribed with papillary fronds in the center (E).

primary tumor. Although most metastases morphologically resemble the original primary, variations due to tumor heterogeneity are possible; hormone receptor and HER-2 studies may be used diagnostically on the metastatic lesion to confirm its origin from the prior primary lesion and to assess sensitivity to therapeutic agents (33,34).

Ductal Carcinoma In Situ

DCIS tumor cells are confined within preexisting ducts and are considered a precursor of invasive carcinoma.

Ducts expanded by DCIS tumor cells are still enveloped by a basement membrane and a layer of myoepithelial cells (Fig. 4.17). Myoepithelial cells can be demonstrated by immunohistochemical stains such as p63, calponin, or smooth-muscle myosin heavy chain. In contrast, invasive carcinoma lacks myoepithelial cells entirely. Several types of architectural patterns in DCIS are recognized; typical are those with cribriform spaces lined by polarized glandular cells (previously compared to "Roman arches") or solid DCISs with comedonecrosis, among others (2,35).

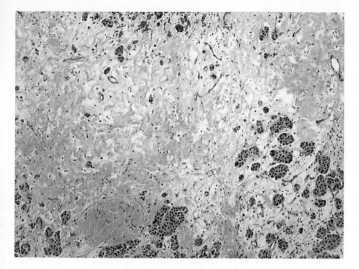

FIGURE 4.15 Breast cancer treated by neoadjuvant chemotherapy. Few cell clusters are present in a tumor bed of loose fibrous tissue.

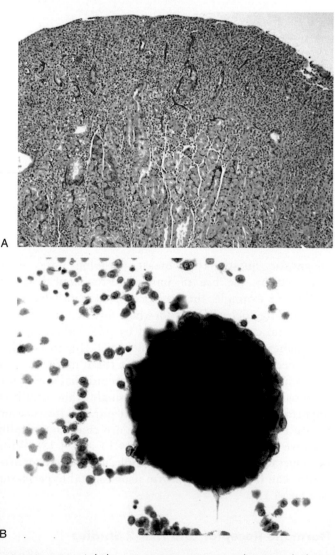

FIGURE 4.16 Lobular carcinoma metastatic to the stomach shows tumor cells infiltrating between gastric glands (A). Cytology shows metastatic ductal carcinoma in pleural fluid (B).

Low-grade Precursor Lesions

Low grade precursor lesions [lobular neoplasia, atypical ductal hyperplasia (ADH), and flat epithelial atypia (FEA)] are associated with an increased risk of breast cancer (Fig. 4.18). Lobular neoplasia, variably referred to as atypical lobular hyperplasia (ALH) or LCIS includes the often multifocal and patchy intraductal proliferation of tumor cells of lobular type, which are characteristically negative for E-cadherin by immunohistochemistry (36,37). Long-term studies have found the presence of lobular neoplasia and ADH to be an indicator of a higher risk for developing breast cancer in either breast rather than an obligatory precursor (17,38). ADH is an intraductal proliferation with cytological atypia but falls short of producing definitive architectural or cytological abnormalities seen in DCIS. Often those ducts appear enlarged and are lined by a thickened layer of ductal epithelial cells with mildly atypical elongated nuclei. Nuclear pseudostratification may produce the impression of "piled-up" ductal epithelium. FEA is a related entity that encompasses abnormal ductal cells that appear in a multilayered but flat epithelium without definitive architectural abnormalities such as the Roman arches of DCIS (39,40).

Benign Findings

A wide variety of breast proliferations and architectural alterations is benign but can mimic malignant lesions radiographically, grossly, and microscopically. Microcalcifications or masses may be detected by screening mammograms, and tissue diagnosis is often necessary to distinguish benign changes from those found in DCIS or invasive carcinoma (1,13). Fibrocystic changes are very frequent in the breast and show cysts lined by apocrine metaplasia or ducts filled by usual ductal hyperplasia (Fig. 4.19). A radial scar, for example, can appear radiographically as a spiculated breast mass, and tissue diagnosis usually is necessary to differentiate this benign lesion from breast cancer (41). Sclerosing adenosis is a benign proliferation of glands that undergo a fibrous scarring reaction and may harbor microcalcifications. Pseudoangiomatous stromal hyperplasia may cause a mass lesion (1,42).

Fibroepithelial Lesions: Fibroadenoma, Phyllodes Tumor

Fibroadenomas are the most common benign breast neoplasms and are characterized by an epithelial component surrounded by an increased amount of stromal tissue, producing a characteristic architectural pattern of compressed, interconnecting ducts (Fig. 4.20). Phyllodes tumors are biphasic breast tumors that contain both epithelial and stromal elements with potentially malignant behavior. They are typically characterized by

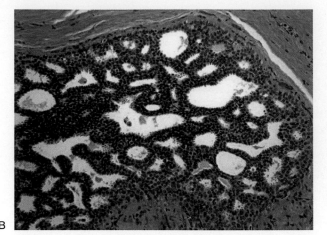

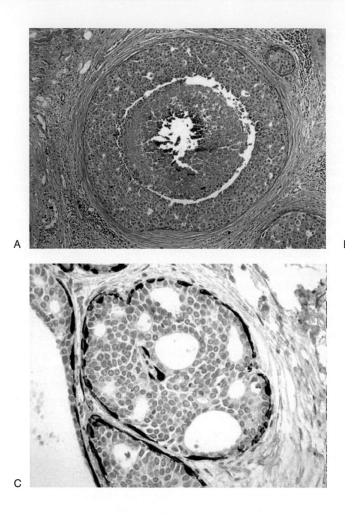

FIGURE 4.17 Ductal carcinoma in situ with central comedonecrosis and calcifications (A), and cribriform pattern (B). Ductal carcinoma in situ is enveloped by myoepithelial cells (C, calponin immunostain).

leaflike fronds in cystic spaces (hence the traditional term "cystosarcoma phyllodes"). They range from low-grade to high-grade tumors; some show stromal overgrowth or frankly sarcomatous appearance with heterologous elements (1,43).

Axillary Lymph Nodes

Pathological assessment of axillary lymph nodes is an important component of breast cancer staging (5). Mapping and excision of sentinel lymph nodes is now widely employed in breast cancer staging and minimizes the side effects of a complete axillary dissection. Sentinel lymph nodes are evaluated in a histologically detailed way to find not only macrometastases (>0.2 cm) but also micrometastases (<0.2 cm), or isolated tumor cells that may be apparent only with immunohistochemical cytokeratin stains (Fig. 4.21). If a sentinel node shows tumor deposits on histological assessment, completion axillary dissection is generally performed. Intraoperative frozen section or cytological evaluation may be done at the discretion of the treating team to permit completion axillary dissection during the same operative procedure (14,44–46).

■ IMMUNOHISTOCHEMISTRY IN BREAST PATHOLOGY

Diagnostic questions in breast pathology are often answered by the use of immunohistochemical stains (1,47). For example, the presence of myoepithelial cells surrounding foci of DCIS (or their absence in invasive carcinoma) can be demonstrated by p63, calponin, and myosin heavy chain stains (see Fig. 4.17). Due to overlapping specificity profiles of many of these markers, it is recommended to use a panel of myoepithelial stains for diagnosis rather than relying on a single stain, and it is important to be aware of potential pitfalls. Invasive or in situ tumor cells of lobular type are characteristically negative for E-cadherin (see Figs. 4.13 and 4.18). With intraductal proliferations, high-molecular-weight cytokeratins can be useful to confirm usual ductal hyperplasia (see Fig. 4.19).

Hormone Receptor and HER-2 Studies

The hormone receptor and HER-2 profiles of breast cancers have prognostic importance and determine treatment approach. Estrogen and progesterone receptor studies

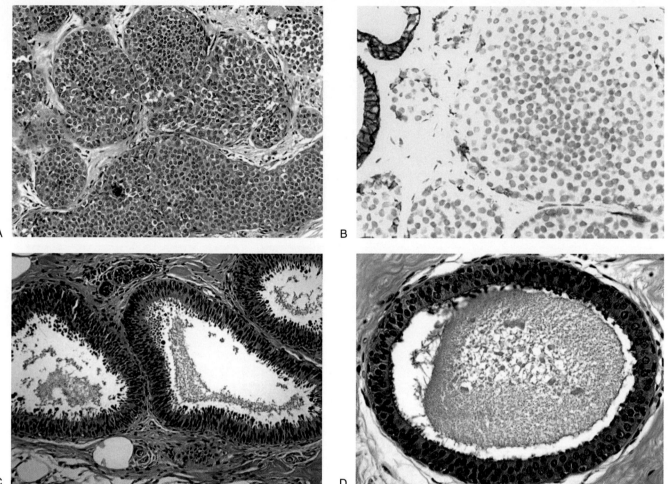

FIGURE 4.18 Lobular neoplasia (lobular carcinoma in situ, LCIS) shows expanded lobules and ducts, filled with small, dyshesive cells (A). The lobular neoplasia cells are negative for E-cadherin by immunostain (B). Atypical ductal hyperplasia is present in enlarged ducts lined by pseudostratified "piled-up" cells (C). Flat epithelial atypia is present in a duct lined by cuboidal cells with enlarged, round nuclei (D).

are routinely performed by immunohistochemistry on formalin-fixed, paraffin-embedded tissue with semiquantitative scoring of positive nuclei (6,48). HER-2 amplification may be determined by visualization of the protein by immunohistochemistry or amplification of the *HER-2* gene by in situ hybridization methods (7). Fluorescent in situ hybridization uses a fluorescent pigment attached to the gene probe (Fig. 4.22).

Intraoperative Consultations and Frozen Sections

The extent of intraoperative gross evaluation of breast specimens and frozen sections depends on institutional experience, expertise, and preference. Most breast masses now receive a tissue diagnosis by core biopsy or fine-needle aspiration, which allows for advance planning of surgical strategy in conjunction with imaging findings (8,10). In general, breast tissue is not routinely submitted for frozen section, and margin evaluation is generally deferred to permanent sections. However,

institutional preferences in this regard vary (14). Sentinel lymph nodes are often submitted for frozen section at the discretion of the surgeon if the operative procedure is to be modified on the basis of frozen section results (44,49). The remainder of the frozen tissue is then thawed and fixed in formalin for permanent sections. Some institutions employ touch-preps or imprint cytology rather than frozen sections for margin and sentinel node evaluation (50–54).

■ QUALITY ASSURANCE AND CONTROL IN BREAST PATHOLOGY

Surgical pathology reports provide the link between imaging, surgery, and further therapeutic interventions. Appropriate communication of pathological findings is the single most important component of surgical pathology practice and the basis for multidisciplinary patient care (55,56). Consistent reporting is necessary. While

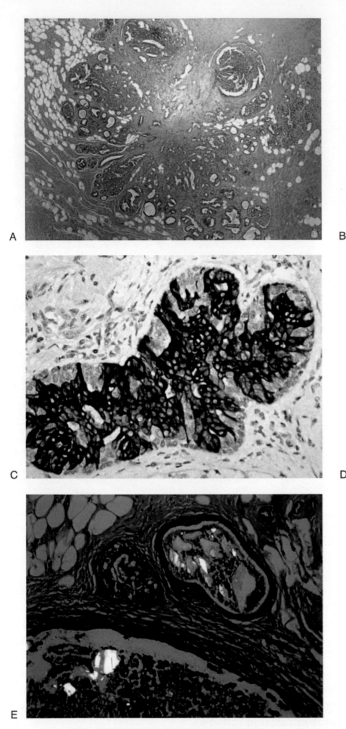

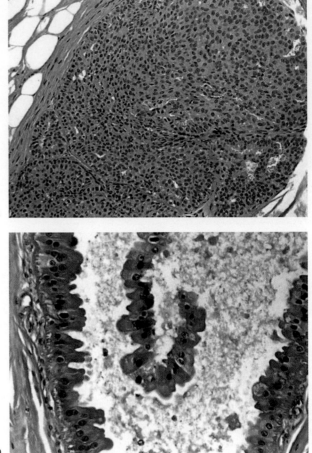

FIGURE 4.19 Benign breast lesions. A radial scar is a benign breast lesion characterized by elastotic material in the center surrounded by intraductal proliferations and cysts in the periphery (A). Usual ductal hyperplasia shows small nuclei in a syncytial pattern, slitlike spaces, and streaming pattern without polarization filling ducts (B). Usual ductal hyperplasia often is positive for high-molecular-weight cytokeratin by immunohistochemistry (C). Apocrine cysts are part of the spectrum of fibrocystic changes (D) and may contain calcium oxalate crystals that appear birefringent when viewed with polarized light (E).

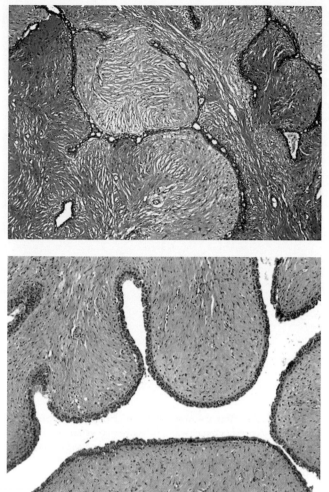

A

B

FIGURE 4.20 Fibroadenomas are benign breast neoplasms with a stromal and compressed epithelial component (A). Fronds of a low-grade phyllodes tumor are shown (B).

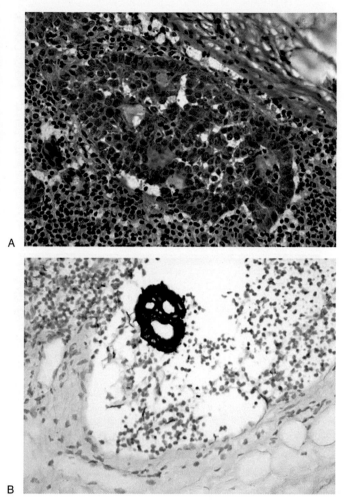

A

B

FIGURE 4.21 Micrometastasis in a sentinel lymph node (A). A deeper tissue section shows a cluster of cytokeratin-positive cells (B).

many histopathological entities in breast pathology are diagnostically straightforward, others are not (1). For this purpose, slide conferences and seminars are important to discuss interesting and controversial cases, enhance sub-specialty expertise, minimize errors, and support continued learning.

■ MULTIDISCIPLINARY CONSIDERATIONS

- Specimen orientation by the surgeon is essential for correct pathological reporting.
- Clinical information needs to be provided to the pathologist.
- There should be agreement about margin assessment: how close is close?
- Results should correlate between surgeons and pathologists: are results concordant?
- Consensus is required among pathologists about unusual pathological findings.

■ REFERENCES

1. Koerner FC. *Diagnostic Problems in Breast Pathology.* Philadelphia: Saunders Elsevier; 2009.
2. Rosen PP. *Rosen's Breast Pathology.* 3rd ed. Philadelphia, PA: Lippincott Williams & Wilkins; 2008.
3. Tavassoli FA, Devilee P. *Tumours of the Breast, Tumours of the Breast and Female Genital Organs. World Health Organization Classification of Tumours.* Lyon: IARC Press; 2003.
4. O'Malley FP, Pinder SE. Breast pathology. In Goldblum JR, ed. *Foundations in diagnostic pathology.* Philadelphia: Churchill Livingstone Elsevier; 2006.
5. Greene F, Page DL, Fleming I. *American Joint Committee on Cancer Staging Manual.* New York: Springer; 2002:223–239.
6. Badve SS, Baehner FL, Gray RP, et al. Estrogen- and progester-one-receptor status in ECOG 2197: comparison of immunohis-tochemistry by local and central laboratories and quantitative reverse transcription polymerase chain reaction by central laboratory. *J Clin Oncol.* 2008;26:2473–2481.
7. Wolff AC, Hammond ME, Schwartz JN, et al. American Society of Clinical Oncology/College of American Pathologists guideline recommendations for human epidermal growth factor receptor 2 testing in breast cancer. *J Clin Oncol.* 2007;25:118–145.
8. Burge CN, Chang HR, Apple SK. Do the histologic features and results of breast cancer biomarker studies differ between core biopsy and surgical excision specimens? *Breast.* 2006;15:167–172.

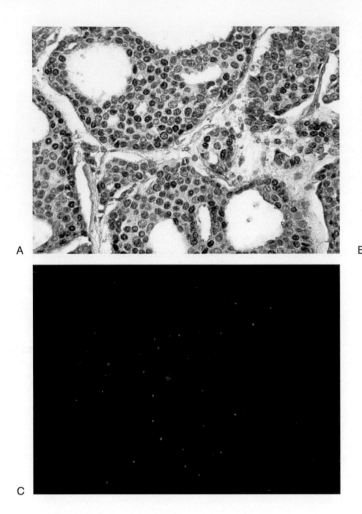

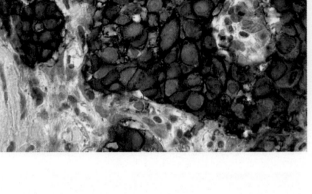

FIGURE 4.22 This invasive ductal carcinoma is estrogen receptor positive (A). A breast cancer with strong overexpression of HER-2 protein is shown (B). HER-2 fluorescent in situ hybridization shows amplification of the *HER-2* gene (red signals) when compared with the green signals of the chromosome 17 centromere (C).

9. Richter-Ehrenstein C, Mueller S, Noske A, et al. Diagnostic accuracy and prognostic value of core biopsy in the management of breast cancer: a series of 542 patients. *Int J Surg Pathol.* 2009;17:323.

10. Hazard HW, Hansen NM. Image-guided procedures for breast masses. *Adv Surg.* 2007;41:257–272.

11. Margolin FR, Kaufman L, Jacobs RP, et al. Stereotactic core breast biopsy of malignant calcifications: diagnostic yield of cores with and cores without calcifications on specimen radiographs. *Radiology.* 2004;233:251–254.

12. Liu X, Inciardi M, Bradley JP, et al. Microcalcifications of the breast: size matters! a mammographic-histologic correlation study. *Pathologica.* 2007;99:5–10.

13. Tse GM, Tan PH, Cheung HS, et al. Intermediate to highly suspicious calcification in breast lesions: a radio-pathologic correlation. *Breast Cancer Res Treat.* 2008;110:1–7.

14. Rosen PP: Pathologic examination of breast and lymph node specimens. Rosen's Breast Pathology. 3rd ed. Philadelphia, PA: Lippincott, Williams & Wilkins; 2008:1034–1102.

15. Wright MJ, Park J, Fey JV, et al. Perpendicular inked versus tangential shaved margins in breast-conserving surgery: does the method matter? *J Am Coll Surg.* 2007;204:541–549.

16. Guidi AJ, Connolly JL, Harris JR, et al. The relationship between shaved margin and inked margin status in breast excision specimens. *Cancer.* 1997;79:1568–1573.

17. Rosen PP, Kosloff C, Lieberman PH, et al. Lobular carcinoma in situ of the breast. Detailed analysis of 99 patients with average follow-up of 24 years. *Am J Surg Pathol.* 1978;2:225–251.

18. Robbins P, Pinder S, de Klerk N, et al. Histological grading of breast carcinomas: a study of interobserver agreement. *Hum Pathol.* 1995;26:873–879.

19. Silverstein MJ, Poller DN, Waisman JR, et al. Prognostic classification of breast ductal carcinoma-in-situ. *Lancet.* 1995;345:1154–1157.

20. Silver SA, Tavassoli FA. Mammary ductal carcinoma in situ with microinvasion. *Cancer.* 1998;82:2382–2390.

21. Rosen PP. Invasive duct carcinoma: assessment of prognosis, morphologic prognostic markers, and tumor growth rate. *Rosen's Breast Pathology.* Philadelphia, PA: Lippincott, Williams & Wilkins; 2008:358–404.

22. Mohammed RA, Martin SG, Gill MS, et al. Improved methods of detection of lymphovascular invasion demonstrate that it is the predominant method of vascular invasion in breast cancer and has important clinical consequences. *Am J Surg Pathol.* 2007;31:1825–1833.

23. Hanby AM, Hughes TA. In situ and invasive lobular neoplasia of the breast. *Histopathology.* 2008;52:58–66.

24. Barkley CR, Ligibel JA, Wong JS, et al. Mucinous breast carcinoma: a large contemporary series. *Am J Surg.* 2008;196:549–551.

25. Marchio C, Iravani M, Natrajan R, et al. Genomic and immunophenotypical characterization of pure micropapillary carcinomas of the breast. *J Pathol.* 2008;215:398–410.

26. Rovera F, Masciocchi P, Coglitore A, et al. Neuroendocrine carcinomas of the breast. *Int J Surg.* 2008;6(suppl 1):S113–S115.

27. Tse GM, Tan PH, Putti TC, et al. Metaplastic carcinoma of the breast: a clinicopathological review. *J Clin Pathol.* 2006;59:1079–1083.

28. Ho BC, Tan HW, Lee VK, et al. Preoperative and intraoperative diagnosis of low-grade adenosquamous carcinoma of the breast: potential diagnostic pitfalls. *Histopathology.* 2006;49:603–611.

29. Collins LC, Carlo VP, Hwang H, et al. Intracystic papillary carcinomas of the breast: a reevaluation using a panel of myoepithelial cell markers. *Am J Surg Pathol.* 2006;30:1002–1007.

30. Pinder SE, Provenzano E, Earl H, et al. Laboratory handling and histology reporting of breast specimens from patients who have received neoadjuvant chemotherapy. *Histopathology.* 2007;50: 409–417.

31. Ogston KN, Miller ID, Payne S, et al. A new histological grading system to assess response of breast cancers to primary chemotherapy: prognostic significance and survival. *Breast.* 2003; 12:320–327.

32. Symmans WF, Peintinger F, Hatzis C, et al. Measurement of residual breast cancer burden to predict survival after neoadjuvant chemotherapy. *J Clin Oncol.* 2007;25:4414–4422.

33. Gong Y, Booser DJ, Sneige N. Comparison of HER-2 status determined by fluorescence in situ hybridization in primary and metastatic breast carcinoma. *Cancer.* 2005;103:1763–1769.

34. Gomez-Fernandez C, Daneshbod Y, Nassiri M, et al. Immunohistochemically determined estrogen receptor phenotype remains stable in recurrent and metastatic breast cancer. *Am J Clin Pathol.* 2008;130:879–882.

35. Lester SC, Bose S, Chen YY, et al. Protocol for the examination of specimens from patients with ductal carcinoma in situ of the breast. *Arch Pathol Lab Med.* 2009;133:15–25.

36. Mastracci TL, Tjan S, Bane AL, et al. E-cadherin alterations in atypical lobular hyperplasia and lobular carcinoma in situ of the breast. *Mod Pathol.* 2005;18:741–751.

37. Koerner F, Maluf H. Uncommon morphologic patterns of lobular neoplasia. *Ann Diagn Pathol.* 1999;3:249–259.

38. Collins LC, Baer HJ, Tamimi RM, et al. Magnitude and laterality of breast cancer risk according to histologic type of atypical hyperplasia: results from the Nurses' Health Study. *Cancer.* 2007;109:180–187.

39. Lerwill MF. Flat epithelial atypia of the breast. *Arch Pathol Lab Med.* 2008;132:615–621.

40. Collins LC, Achacoso NA, Nekhlyudov L, et al. Clinical and pathologic features of ductal carcinoma in situ associated with the presence of flat epithelial atypia: an analysis of 543 patients. *Mod Pathol.* 2007;20:1149–1155.

41. Farshid G, Rush G. Assessment of 142 stellate lesions with imaging features suggestive of radial scar discovered during population-based screening for breast cancer. *Am J Surg Pathol.* 2004;28:1626–1631.

42. Rabban JT, Sgroi DC. Sclerosing lesions of the breast. *Semin Diagn Pathol.* 2004;21:42–47.

43. Lerwill MF. Biphasic lesions of the breast. *Semin Diagn Pathol.* 2004;21:48–56.

44. Schwartz GF, Krill LS, Palazzo JP, et al. Value of intraoperative examination of axillary sentinel nodes in carcinoma of the breast. *J Am Coll Surg.* 2008;207:758–762.

45. Alkuwari E, Auger M. Accuracy of fine-needle aspiration cytology of axillary lymph nodes in breast cancer patients: a study of 115 cases with cytologic-histologic correlation. *Cancer.* 2008; 114:89–93.

46. Turner RR, Weaver DL, Cserni G, et al. Nodal stage classification for breast carcinoma: improving interobserver reproducibility through standardized histologic criteria and image-based training. *J Clin Oncol.* 2008;26:258–263.

47. Lerwill MF. Current practical applications of diagnostic immunohistochemistry in breast pathology. *Am J Surg Pathol.* 2004;28: 1076–1091.

48. Harvey JM, Clark GM, Osborne CK, et al. Estrogen receptor status by immunohistochemistry is superior to the ligand-binding assay for predicting response to adjuvant endocrine therapy in breast cancer. *J Clin Oncol.* 1999;17:1474–1481.

49. McLaughlin SA, Ochoa-Frongia LM, Patil SM, et al. Influence of frozen-section analysis of sentinel lymph node and lumpectomy margin status on reoperation rates in patients undergoing breast-conservation therapy. *J Am Coll Surg.* 2008;206:76–82.

50. Bakhshandeh M, Tutuncuoglu SO, Fischer G, et al. Use of imprint cytology for assessment of surgical margins in lumpectomy specimens of breast cancer patients. *Diagn Cytopathol.* 2007;35:656–659.

51. Creager AJ, Geisinger KR, Shiver SA, et al. Intraoperative evaluation of sentinel lymph nodes for metastatic breast carcinoma by imprint cytology. *Mod Pathol.* 2002;15:1140–1147.

52. Forbes RC, Pitchford C, Simpson JF, et al. Selective use of intraoperative touch prep analysis of sentinel nodes in breast cancer. *Am Surg.* 2005;71:955–960, discussion 961–962.

53. Klimberg VS, Westbrook KC, Korourian S. Use of touch preps for diagnosis and evaluation of surgical margins in breast cancer. *Ann Surg Oncol.* 1998;5:220–226.

54. Vanderveen KA, Ramsamooj R, Bold RJ. A prospective, blinded trial of touch prep analysis versus frozen section for intraoperative evaluation of sentinel lymph nodes in breast cancer. *Ann Surg Oncol.* 2008;15:2006–2011.

55. Newman EA, Guest AB, Helvie MA, et al. Changes in surgical management resulting from case review at a breast cancer multidisciplinary tumor board. *Cancer.* 2006;107:2346–2351.

56. Onerheim R, Racette P, Jacques A, et al. Improving the quality of surgical pathology reports for breast cancer: a centralized audit with feedback. *Arch Pathol Lab Med.* 2008;132:1428–1431.

Multidisciplinary Approach to Breast Cancer

JERRY YOUNGER

■ MASSACHUSETTS GENERAL HOSPITAL BREAST CANCER MULTIDISCIPLINARY PROGRAM

Multidisciplinary care is a familiar concept for oncologists. Clinics attended by medical, surgical, and radiation oncologists have been a part of most cancer programs for many years. As the treatments for cancer have become more sophisticated, multidisciplinary diagnostic and treatment planning requires a more comprehensive, integrated program with other specialists available.

The Massachusetts General Hospital (MGH) multidisciplinary breast cancer program was initiated in 1995 to address the care of breast cancer patients in a large general hospital. The program was developed to answer several needs for the overall cancer program at MGH. New information and new treatments for patients with breast cancer are rapidly advancing. It is difficult for each individual caring for a patient with breast cancer to maintain the knowledge base, skills, and experience to provide complex evaluations and treatments for breast cancer patients, and easy access to consultation is required. For example, our breast cancer program, like many others, encounters patients who want to have children after chemotherapy or who are pregnant at the time of breast cancer diagnosis. Skilled reproductive medicine consultation, which must be available as a part of the initial treatment planning program, is required to lay out the options and deliver care. Reconstructive surgery needs to be planned prior to initial surgery and may affect how radiation can be administered.

A multidisciplinary breast cancer clinic was the first component of the breast cancer program developed at our institution. The primary purpose of the clinic was to integrate the clinical care of patients with a new diagnosis of breast cancer so that they would be able to see a team of breast cancer specialists who could evaluate and plan care for them without their having to make multiple office visits. The initial clinic scheduled patients with a new primary diagnosis of breast cancer so that breast cancer surgeons, medical oncologists, radiation oncologists, breast imaging radiologists, and breast pathologists saw patients together one or two afternoons per week. The clinic was held in the office of a breast cancer surgeon, and the other team members came to the clinic, although their offices and support staff were not located in the clinic. This provided a venue for patients to be seen for consultation by multiple physicians in one location and enhanced communication between the physicians. This system did not provide truly integrated care for the patient, nor did it provide a sense of full participation in an integrated care program for the physicians and staff.

As the clinical program grew, we were able to obtain space in the cancer center clinics. Primary offices became available for the main physician and nurse participants in the program. Clinical space and support were available for all participants to see all of their patients with breast cancer within the clinic. Nurses, nurse practitioners, and clinical support staff were also located in the clinic. Social workers and genetic counselors were available to come to the clinic, although their offices were not located there. Many but not all patients with a new diagnosis of breast cancer were seen in the clinic for their initial and follow-up care. Radiation and chemotherapy were easily accessible nearby. Intake nurses developed a method for contacting patients in advance of their appointment to provide information and to ascertain data required for a full consultation (pathology review, prior treatments and procedures, x-rays, and so on).

As the MGH Cancer Center grew, coverage of all aspects of cancer care increased. Major components, including a large medical oncology fellowship program, clinical and basic research, electronic records, clinical genetics, and pharmacology, have required and offered new opportunities for program development.

The current breast cancer program is located within a large cancer center outpatient clinic. Most patients with breast cancer seen at MGH see their physicians and nurses in the breast cancer clinic. Some physicians have an office in the breast cancer center, and some have offices outside the center but come to the center to see patients. Clinical support for these activities is provided. Clinical genetics, chemotherapy, radiation, acute care, radiology, social services, and a resource room are conveniently located together. All clinical support (scheduling, clinical assistants, billing, and so on) is provided and is supervised by a practice manager.

With the complexities inherent in digital mammography, ultrasound, and MRI and the need for localization technology, breast imaging is not located in the breast cancer center, and patients who are coming in for diagnostic studies such as mammograms and biopsies prior to the diagnosis of breast cancer are seen in clinical space designed for this purpose.

Multidisciplinary clinic sessions are held four afternoons per week. Patients can be referred by their physician or can be self-referred. Prior to the initial consultation, patients are contacted by an intake nurse to explain the multidisciplinary process, to obtain history and necessary clinical information, and to arrange receipt of any x-rays and pathology specimens required for the consultation. Each session is attended by a surgeon, a medical oncologist, and a radiation oncologist specializing in breast cancer. During a clinic, patients may be seen by all three specialties or the visit may be confined to a specific specialist or combination of specialists, depending on the need. All patients evaluated in the clinic are discussed at a conference, and x-rays, pathology slides, and information are reviewed the same day as the clinic. The conference is attended by the oncologists assigned to the clinic session, as well as nurses, trainees (medical oncology fellows, radiation oncology residents, and surgery fellows), breast pathologists, and clinical research staff. Appropriate referrals for genetics, plastic surgery, and reproductive medicine are made. In some cases, genetics consultations can be completed at the time of the initial visit.

The program expressly focuses on the initial care of the patient with a new diagnosis of breast cancer and the provision of continued integrated care throughout the course of breast cancer diagnosis. The program aims to facilitate as much as possible and ease the decision-making process for the patient. Long-term follow-up is provided, although the emphasis is on initial management. Many components of the program can be used to provide care for the patient with advanced disease, especially since many of the medical personnel are the same.

■ IMPORTANT ISSUES FOR CARE INTEGRATION

One important requirement in the development of an integrated breast cancer care program is that all participants are invested in the program. It is essential that the care providers are adequately supported to provide the best care for the patient, that they are confident of the care provided by the group, and that they feel comfortable in suggesting ideas for change and new programs. At our institution we have encouraged investment by providing a center with examination space and workspace, providing clinical support staff, and providing administrative needs for all the participants in the program.

Collocation of clinical workspace enhances communication. Working in a centralized clinical facility encourages understanding the problems and concerns of other participants. Problem solving and group interaction are improved. Respect for colleagues and integrated care develop in this environment.

An easily accessible record used by all the providers is essential. MGH has developed over the years an electronic medical record with diagnostic information, medical notes, order entry (including complex chemotherapy algorithms), procedures, referrals, medication, allergies, treatment regimens, and clinical trials integrated into one convenient source. The importance of integrated information technology in a large multidisciplinary clinical and research program cannot be overemphasized.

It is important to have the cooperation of colleagues from radiology and pathology. The participation of these specialties in multidisciplinary clinical conferences provides a much better understanding of diagnostic issues.

In addition to clinic time, development of conference structure allows open and frequent discussion among the entire group. We have a weekly tumor board and weekly didactic conference.

Projects and initiatives that have attracted both philanthropic and federal and private funding have grown out of staff discussions and suggestions. Examples of new program development are: lymphedema care, an annual memorial service in support of the families of patients treated for breast cancer in our program, and the HOPES (helping our patients through education and support) program, which has been in operation for over a decade. The HOPES program provides free wellness services, plus education and support workshops for patients with cancer, their families, and their friends. Examples of educational topics are

- Chemotherapy
- Radiation therapy
- Clinical trials
- Cancer pain management
- The interpretation of blood counts
- Nutrition
- Fatigue

Complementary or integrative services include

- Acupuncture
- Exercise
- Expressive arts (art and writing)
- Gentle yoga
- Healing harp music
- Humor therapy
- Massage therapy
- Music therapy
- Qigong
- Reflexology
- Relaxation methods

■ PATIENTS' PERSPECTIVE

The multidisciplinary clinic is popular with patients and has steadily grown since it was initiated. The clinic provides "one-stop shopping" for the new patient dealing with the diagnosis of breast cancer. There are many confusing options for treatment, which require expert advice and education. This forum represents one time when the patient can hear a discussion of her individual problem and receive a consultation from the medical providers who will be involved in her care. Different options for treatment can be discussed from various perspectives.

Studies indicate that few patients want to have autonomy in making decisions about treatment, especially early treatment. Most prefer shared informed decision making, especially when there is good communication and trust with the involved physicians. Patient satisfaction scores for our multidisciplinary program demonstrate excellent satisfaction for the multidisciplinary clinic experience.

The clinic requires a significant time commitment for the patient. In order for information to be reviewed by multiple physicians and treatment recommendations to be communicated to the patient, patients may be in the clinic for several hours. A significant amount of information is given and multiple decisions are made during this time. Some patients can be overwhelmed by the process at a time when they feel particularly vulnerable. Thus it is important to prepare patients for the potential of a longer and more complex initial visit prior to the actual day.

■ PHYSICIANS' PERSPECTIVE

The program provides an efficient way to see new patients. Opinions from different specialties can be immediately discussed, avoiding the need to contact colleagues unnecessarily, saving time, and improving understanding. Referral information, such as pathology and x-ray reports, risk factors, and medications, is provided at the time of consultation. Treatment scheduling needs such as surgery, chemotherapy, and radiation can be anticipated.

Upfront discussion among the specialties enhances confidence in the care plan. Because all the providers are involved in the initial discussion and planning, it is unlikely that a decision about treatment will need to be changed. For example, a decision about needing neoadjuvant chemotherapy can be made at the time of the initial consultation.

New treatment options can be discussed and treatment patterns can evolve. Interstaff teaching occurs during the conference. Clinical trials and eligibility are discussed in real time, and research staff are available to help.

For the pathologist and radiologist, however, the clinic is less efficient. Their input and review is nonetheless invaluable to a full consultation and to treatment planning. It is recognized that all specialists may sacrifice a slight degree of efficiency for a significantly improved patient experience and an improvement in communication and, hopefully, outcomes. The exact cost of this experience is not certain.

■ MEDICAL EDUCATION PERSPECTIVE

Oncology fellows, residents, nurses, and students participate in the multidisciplinary clinics. A conference to discuss all patients seen during the multidisciplinary clinic occurs during each clinic. The history, pathology, x-rays, and treatment plans are reviewed during this conference. Medical staff, fellows, and residents present the cases for each of the patients they have seen. During this conference a treatment plan is formulated, with the healthcare providers for the patient involved in the discussion. Trainees are expected to defend their opinions about treatment options and provide information to patients after the conference. Although not every patient is seen by the entire team, the conference provides a format for participants to hear about all patients seen in the clinic that day.

A tumor board meets once a week to review those cases seen in the multidisciplinary clinic that the staff wish to present. The tumor board provides a forum for discussion of patients with difficult issues that the attending physician wishes to discuss. National guidelines for care are discussed in the context of MGH practices. The tumor board provides an opportunity for all of the specialty care teams throughout the program to meet and discuss common practices and concerns and is an important way to disseminate new information and discuss best practices. It is also an opportunity for trainees to present a discussion, for care policy development, and for staff and student education. The tumor board is open to all staff in the breast cancer center. A separate didactic conference with guest and in-house speakers occurs weekly.

New staff education occurs in a supportive way. Medical staff with various levels of experience participate in all aspects of the program. The model of physicians working alongside nurse practitioners and physician assistants provides a supportive and supervised learning experience. Care policies are informally developed. Peer review has not been formally incorporated but occurs in a supportive, interactive way.

Fellows, residents, medical students, nurses, and research assistants can be exposed to multiple patient issues in a confined time period in the multidisciplinary clinics. There is also exposure to multiple senior staff and practice support personnel communicating with other physicians and patients.

■ RESEARCH PERSPECTIVES

The multidisciplinary clinics were created primarily to enhance clinical care. During multidisciplinary sessions, however, patients are reviewed for clinical trial eligibility. Trials are discussed, and appropriate participation is encouraged. New trial development and research issues are discussed in other forums, but it is commonplace for ideas for trial development to originate in the multidisciplinary conferences and tumor board sessions. Thus, multidisciplinary care can act as a powerful catalyst for the research program.

■ INTEGRATION OF NEW SERVICES

The multidisciplinary concept has encouraged new programs because needs are defined and the staff become interested in developing programs to meet those needs. Examples of new programs are lymphedema diagnosis and treatment, physical therapy, exercise, yoga, acupuncture, and therapeutic massage. Our institution has a large and active genetics program, which is now fully integrated into the multidisciplinary system.

In summary, the multidisciplinary process is a venue that serves to bring better care to our patients. The particulars of any individual program reside with many of the local resources. We are fortunate to practice in a large general hospital that provides significant resources for the care of the cancer patient through the cancer center. Support from multiple specialties, physical therapy, nursing, and administration are essential components. There

is a large medical education program, including fellows, residents, medical students, and nursing programs, that provides a challenging environment for learning. The institution is highly involved in clinical and basic research, and all of these factors serve to stimulate growth and expertise of the participating staff.

■ SUMMARY

- Institutional commitment is vital to provide high-quality multidisciplinary care to patients with breast cancer.
- Components of a successful program include all the cancer specialties working in an interdisciplinary fashion.
- Facilitation of one-stop care for patients far outweighs the time investment individual specialists may need to make to participate in a multidisciplinary program.
- Cancer programs highlighting breast cancer treatment should consider multidisciplinary programs as the standard of care, particularly when patients require knowledge related to reconstruction, genetics, and reproductive issues.

Diagnosis and Initial Evaluation

ELIZABETH A. GUANCIAL

STEVEN J. ISAKOFF

The importance of the multidisciplinary approach to the care of a patient with breast cancer is most readily apparent during the initial evaluation following diagnosis. This is an opportunity for medical, surgical, and radiation oncologists to integrate their treatment modalities and act as oncologists first and technical specialists second. Benefits of this system include: thorough review of primary data by pathologists and radiologists, interaction between specialties to shorten time from diagnosis to intervention, coordination of multiple stages of treatment, and ultimately improved communication between the medical team, patient, and caregivers. This chapter will review components of the evaluation of newly diagnosed patients with invasive breast cancer, including relevant history, physical exam, laboratory studies, and imaging; the role of staging; and multidisciplinary issues to consider in the selection of treatment. The evaluation of patients with proliferative lesions and pre-invasive carcinomas is discussed in Chapters 5 and 6 and will not be covered in this section.

DIAGNOSIS

The advent of large-scale screening efforts in the United States has led to decreasing mortality from breast cancer and lower stage at diagnosis in screened populations. The data supporting the utility of screening mammograms are described in detail in Chapter 2. Nevertheless, it is important to emphasize that many experts attribute roughly half the approximately 3% per year decrease in breast cancer mortality since 1990 to increasing rates of mammographic screening. The diagnosis of invasive breast cancer is most commonly based on obtaining an adequate biopsy of the region of concern in the breast. Less commonly, symptoms of systemic disease may prompt patients to seek medical attention, and upon evaluation a primary breast cancer is identified.

Staging

Following the initial diagnosis, further staging is based on the TNM system established by the American Joint Committee of Cancer and updated in 2002 (Table 4.2) (1). The goal of staging is to provide prognostic information and guide therapy selection by grouping TNM classifications

with a similar prognosis together. The sixth edition of the TNM system incorporates the increased use of immunohistochemical (IHC) testing and amends the prior TNM staging system. Specific revisions include defining the size of micrometastases (between 0.2 and 2.0 mm) detected in regional lymph nodes, as distinguished from isolated tumor cells detected via IHC or hematoxylin and eosin (H&E) staining, thus providing more detailed cytological information. It is advised that H&E staining follow IHC identification of lesions, designated by (i +) for "immunohistochemical," to confirm malignant characteristics. The designation (mol +), for "molecular," is applied to lesions that are histologically negative by H&E staining but positive by reverse transcriptase/polymerase chain reaction in order to aid in data collection. The seventh edition of the staging system will go into effect January 1, 2010.

Patients are grouped according to the number of positive axillary lymph nodes, one of the most powerful prognostic indicators for survival. The presence of infraclavicular lymph nodes (N3 nodes) is now categorized with metastases in 10 or more axillary lymph nodes to reflect the similarly poor prognosis. Metastasis to supraclavicular lymph nodes was changed from classification as a distant metastasis (M1) to an advanced regional lymph node metastasis (N3) to avoid undertreatment of this group of patients. Finally, metastasis to the internal mammary (IM) nodes is classified according to the method of detection, with clinically apparent nodes having a worse prognosis than clinically occult microscopically involved nodes. Involvement of IM nodes portends a worse prognosis when axillary nodes are involved than when they are unaffected.

In addition to histological diagnosis, biopsy specimens are subjected to molecular characterization. Estrogen receptor and progesterone receptor should be assessed in primary invasive breast tumors and metastatic lesions in order to identify patients who may benefit from endocrine therapies and for prognostic information. HER-2 expression, amplification, or both should be measured to guide the selection of HER-2-directed therapy. However, measurement of circulating extracellular domain of HER-2 has no clinical utility at this time.

INITIAL EVALUATION

History, Physical Exam, and Laboratory Studies

Following the diagnosis of invasive breast cancer, the initial assessment should include an evaluation for local and

■ **Table 4.2** Staging based on the American Joint Committee on Cancer TNM system, 2002

Primary tumor (T)

Tx	Primary tumor cannot be assessed
T0	No evidence of primary tumor
Tis	Carcinoma in situ
Tis (DCIS)	Ductal carcinoma in situ
Tis (LCIS)	Lobular carcinoma in situ
Tis (Paget's)	Paget's disease[a] of the nipple with no tumor
T1	Tumor ≤2 cm in greatest dimension
T1mic	Microinvasion ≤0.1 cm in greatest dimension
T1a	Tumor >0.1 cm but ≤0.5 cm in greatest dimension
T1b	Tumor >0.5 cm but ≤1 cm in greatest dimension
T1c	Tumor >1 cm but ≤2 cm in greatest dimension
T2	Tumor >2 cm but ≤5 cm in greatest dimension
T3	Tumor >5 cm in greatest dimension
T4	Tumor of any size with direct extension to (a) chest wall or (b) skin, only as described below
T4a	Extension to chest wall, not including pectoralis muscle
T4b	Edema (including peau d'orange) or ulceration of the skin of the breast, or satellite skin nodules confined to the same breast
T4c	Both T4a and T4b
T4d	Inflammatory carcinoma

Regional lymph nodes (N)

Clinical

Nx	Regional lymph nodes cannot be assessed (e.g., previously removed)
N0	No regional lymph node metastasis
N1	Metastasis in movable ipsilateral axillary lymph node(s)
N2	Metastases in ipsilateral axillary lymph nodes fixed or matted, or in clinically apparent[b] ipsilateral internal mammary nodes in the absence of clinically evident axillary lymph node metastasis
N2a	Metastasis in ipsilateral axillary lymph nodes fixed to one another (matted) or to other structures
N2b	Metastasis only in clinically apparent[b] ipsilateral internal mammary nodes and in the absence of clinically evident axillary lymph node metastasis
N3	Metastasis in ipsilateral infraclavicular lymph node(s), or in clinically apparent[b] ipsilateral internal mammary lymph node(s) and in the presence of clinically evident axillary lymph node metastasis; or metastasis in ipsilateral supraclavicular lymph node(s) with or without axillary or internal mammary lymph node involvement
N3a	Metastasis in ipsilateral infraclavicular lymph node(s) and axillary lymph node(s)
N3b	Metastasis in ipsilateral internal mammary lymph node(s) and axillary lymph node(s)
N3c	Metastasis in ipsilateral supraclavicular lymph node(s)

Pathological (pN)[c]

pNx	Regional lymph nodes cannot be assessed (e.g., previously removed, or not removed for pathological study)
pN0	No regional lymph node metastasis histologically, no additional examination for isolated tumor cells[d]
pN0(i –)	No regional lymph node metastasis histologically, negative IHC
pN0(i +)	No regional lymph node metastasis histologically, positive IHC, no IHC cluster >0.2 mm
pN0(mol –)	No regional lymph node metastasis histologically, negative molecular findings (RT-PCR)
pN0(mol +)	No regional lymph node metastasis histologically, positive molecular findings (RT-PCR)
pN1	Metastasis in 1–3 axillary lymph nodes, or in internal mammary nodes with microscopic disease detected by sentinel lymph node dissection but not clinically apparent[e]
pN1mi	Micrometastasis (>0.2 mm, none >2.0 mm)
pN1a	Metastasis in 1–3 axillary lymph nodes
pN1b	Metastasis in internal mammary nodes with microscopic disease detected by sentinel lymph node dissection but not clinically apparent[e]
pN1c	Metastasis in 1–3 axillary lymph nodes and in internal mammary lymph nodes with microscopic disease detected by sentinel lymph node dissection but not clinically apparent[e] (if associated with >3 positive axillary lymph nodes, the internal mammary nodes are classified as pN3b to reflect increased tumor burden)
pN2	Metastasis in 4–9 axillary lymph nodes, or in clinically apparent[b] internal mammary lymph nodes in the absence of axillary lymph node metastasis
pN2a	Metastasis in 4–9 axillary lymph nodes (at least 1 tumor deposit >2.0 mm)
pN2b	Metastasis in clinically apparent[b] internal mammary lymph nodes in the absence of axillary lymph node metastasis

Continued

■ **Table 4.2**   Staging based on the American Joint Committee on Cancer TNM system, 2002 *(Continued)*

pN3	Metastasis in ≥10 axillary lymph nodes, or in infraclavicular lymph nodes, or in clinically apparent[b] ipsilateral internal mammary lymph nodes in the presence of ≥1 positive axillary lymph nodes; or in >3 axillary lymph nodes with clinically negative microscopic metastasis in internal mammary lymph nodes; or in ipsilateral supraclavicular lymph nodes
pN3a	Metastasis in ≥10 axillary lymph nodes (at least 1 tumor deposit >2.0 mm), or metastasis to the infraclavicular lymph nodes
pN3b	Metastasis in clinically apparent[b] ipsilateral internal mammary lymph nodes in the presence of ≥1 positive axillary lymph nodes; or in >3 axillary lymph nodes and in internal mammary lymph nodes with microscopic disease detected by sentinel lymph node dissection but not clinically apparent[e]
pN3c	Metastasis in ipsilateral supraclavicular lymph nodes

Distant metastasis (M)

Mx	Distant metastasis cannot be assessed
M0	No distant metastasis
M1	Distant metastasis

Stage Grouping

Stage 0	Tis	N0	M0
Stage 1	T1[f]	N0	M0
Stage 2A	T0	N1	M0
	T1[f]	N1	M0
	T2	N0	M0
Stage 2B	T2	N1	M0
	T3	N0	M0
Stage 3A	T0	N2	M0
	T1[f]	N2	M0
	T2	N2	M0
	T3	N1	M0
	T3	N2	M0
Stage 3B	T4	N0	M0
	T4	N1	M0
	T4	N2	M0
Stage 3C	Any T	N3	M0
Stage 4	Any T	Any N	M1

Abbreviations: IHC, immunohistochemistry; RTPCR, reverse transcriptase/polymerase chain reaction.

[a]Paget's disease associated with a tumor is classified according to the size of the tumor.

[b]Clinically apparent is defined as detected by imaging studies (excluding lymphoscintigraphy) or by clinical examination or grossly visible pathologically.

[c]Classification is based on axillary lymph node dissection with or without sentinel lymph node dissection. Classification based solely on sentinel lymph node dissection without subsequent axillary lymph node dissection is designated (sn) for "sentinel node"—e.g., pN0(i +)(sn).

[d]Isolated tumor cells are defined as single tumor cells or small cell clusters ≤0.2 mm, usually detected only by immunohistochemical or molecular methods but which may be verified on hematoxylin and eosin stains. Isolated tumor cells do not usually show evidence of metastatic activity (e.g., proliferation or stromal reaction).

[e]Not clinically apparent is defined as not detected by imaging studies (excluding lymphoscintigraphy) or by clinical examination.

[f]T1 includes T1mic.

Note: Definitions for classifying the primary tumor (T) are the same for clinical and pathological classification. If the measurement is made by physical examination, the examiner will use major headings (T1, T2, or T3). If other measurements, such as mammographic or pathological measurements, are used, the subsets of T1 can be used. Tumors should be measured to the nearest 0.1 cm increment.

Source: Used with the permission of the American Joint Committee on Cancer (AJCC), Chicago, Illinois. The original source for this material is the *AJCC Cancer Staging Manual*, Sixth Edition (2002), published by Springer Science and Business Media LLC, www.springerlink.com.

systemic disease through a complete history, a review of systems, and a physical exam. Signs and symptoms specific to the breast include pain, palpable masses, unilateral discharge, peau d'orange skin changes (seen with inflammatory breast cancer), nipple crusting (suggestive of Paget's disease) or inversion, and other skin changes.

Additional symptoms of bone pain, shortness of breath, jaundice, fatigue, weight loss, and visceral or neurological complaints are also elicited. Within the context of a complete physical exam, special focus on several areas may identify findings that warrant further evaluation. The breast and nipple should be carefully examined for the above findings; careful palpation of axillary lymph nodes as well as supraclavicular and infraclavicular nodes may identify the presence of regional lymph nodes, which has prognostic implications. Abnormal abdominal findings may suggest possible involvement of the liver or peritoneum. Pain with palpation in the skeletal system may indicate sites of bone metastases and, together with the history, may require further imaging. Careful neurological exam for evidence of central nervous system involvement is particularly important for subtypes of breast cancer with high rates of brain metastases, such as hormone receptor–negative or HER-2+ breast cancer.

The history should review known risk factors for breast cancer through a detailed reproductive history (age at menarche, age at first pregnancy, menopausal status); personal history of breast biopsies, breast cancer, or other cancers, including ovarian; and family history with *BRCA* status if known. In the multidisciplinary setting, such information may contribute to decision making regarding contralateral prophylactic breast surgery. Detailed review of the medical history focuses on conditions that may impact breast cancer chemotherapy, endocrine therapy, or radiation therapy. For example, cardiomyopathy may limit the ability to deliver anthracycline-based therapy, as will risk factors such as hypertension and uncontrolled diabetes mellitus. Connective tissue disorders and rheumatologic disorders may alter the therapeutic window of radiation therapy. A history of osteoporosis or thromboembolic disease may affect selection of hormonal therapy. Medications should be reviewed, including careful attention to herbal supplements, to determine potential drug interactions with treatments. History of hormone replacement therapy should be sought and agents discontinued if the disease is hormone receptor–positive. Recently, the impact of agents that inhibit cytochrome P450 2D6 (CYP2D6) has been recognized. Agents such as the selective-serotonin reuptake inhibitor antidepressants fluoxetine and paroxetine, as well as bupropion and diphenhydramine, are now recognized as impairing the metabolism of tamoxifen to its active metabolite endoxifen and should be avoided wherever possible in patients treated with tamoxifen (2).

Laboratory studies upon initial evaluation are intended to screen for organ dysfunction that may impact treatment, as well as to elicit evidence of systemic disease. Studies include general chemistries, complete blood count, liver function tests, and alkaline phosphatase (a surrogate for osteoblast activity). The American Society of Clinical Oncology 2007 guidelines evaluating the clinical utility of tumor markers in the diagnosis and management of breast cancer concluded that there is no established role for measurement of serum tumor markers (CA 15-3, CA 27.29, or carcinoembryonic antigen) in the initial diagnosis and staging of early-stage breast cancer (3). Similarly, there is no role for evaluating markers of proliferation, such as DNA content or S phase, by flow cytometry. The panel

also highlighted the lack of data to support testing for circulating tumor cells or bone marrow biopsy to assess for micrometastases at the time of diagnosis. Tumor markers may play a role in monitoring patients with metastatic breast cancer receiving therapy by providing supplementary information to assess response to therapy or to monitor for disease recurrence.

Initial evaluation should include an assessment of modifiable lifestyle factors, including diet and exercise. Recently, vitamin D levels have been suggested to impact breast cancer risk (4). In the prospective Nurses' Health Study, patients in the highest quintile for plasma 25(OH) vitamin D had a 27% reduction in the relative risk of developing breast cancer compared with the lowest quintile (5). In a retrospective case-control study, the lowest quartile of 25(OH) vitamin D had a fivefold increase in risk of breast cancer compared with the highest quartile (6). While no studies to date have evaluated the impact of vitamin D on risk of recurrence after a diagnosis of breast cancer, a goal of normal vitamin D levels is reasonable. Importantly, many patients will go on to receive adjuvant aromatase inhibitor therapy, for which calcium and vitamin D supplementation are recommended to reduce the risk of bone loss.

The relationship between dietary fat intake and breast cancer is a controversial issue, with inconsistent associations observed in epidemiologic studies. The Women's Intervention Nutrition Study (WINS) was the first large-scale, multicenter, randomized trial, and it assigned more than 2,400 women who had undergone breast cancer resection to a dietary intervention to reduce or control fat intake. The results demonstrated improved relapse-free survival in the intervention group compared with controls, with a hazard ratio of relapse events of 0.76, thus supporting the reduction of fat intake to improve clinical outcomes in this population (7). Interestingly, in exploratory analyses, hormone receptor–negative patients had a greater reduction in recurrence risk than hormone receptor–positive patients. The impact of physical activity on survival among women with breast cancer has been difficult to evaluate. The Nurses' Health Study found that women who engaged in the highest level of activity compared with the lowest had a 26% to 40% lower risk of an adverse outcome (including death or recurrence). Furthermore, these benefits were greatest among women with hormone-responsive tumors (8). Despite the difficulty in assessing the impact of diet and exercise on breast cancer outcomes, emerging data suggest it is reasonable to assess these issues at the initial diagnosis and encourage lifestyle choices that include a healthy diet and physical activity.

Gene expression profiling is a technological advancement developed within the past 10 years that generates a molecular signature when applied to tumor tissue; it has the potential for multiple clinical applications for breast cancer. Through multiparameter gene expression analysis, patient-specific information generates personalized estimates of disease recurrence and informs the selection of therapy. At this time, Onco*type* DX and the MammaPrint test are the only commercially available assays, and both are currently undergoing further evaluation in prospective phase III trials. Details of these molecular pathological tests are described in Chapter 16. Adjuvant!Online is a clinically based risk assessment tool made publically available on the Internet to help predict the risk of recurrence of breast cancer and death from breast cancer as well as the benefit of endocrine therapy or chemotherapy. It is a useful tool to supplement but not substitute for clinical decision making in the multidisciplinary clinic.

Genetic testing is not necessary for all patients diagnosed with breast cancer, but *BRCA* mutation testing is advised on the following criteria, which are supported by the Preventative Services Task Force (9) and discussed in more detail in Chapter 2. Characteristics that suggest a higher risk of familial cancer syndromes and warrant referral to a genetic counselor include age <40 at diagnosis, Ashkenazi Jewish heritage, a first-degree relative diagnosed with breast cancer before the age of 50, two or more first- or second-degree relatives with a history of breast cancer, a personal history or first- or second-degree relative with history of bilateral breast cancer, a male relative with a history of breast cancer, and a personal or first- or second-degree relative with a history of ovarian cancer. In the multidisciplinary setting, testing prior to definitive surgery may influence patient choice of mastectomy or lesser surgery. For example, patients who had breast-conserving surgery ultimately may elect to undergo a mastectomy with or without a prophylactic contralateral mastectomy and may forgo subsequent radiation therapy. Therefore, in the multidisciplinary setting, evaluation for genetic risk and referral for appropriate testing are necessary for the patient and all collaborating members of the team to develop an informed management plan.

Initial Imaging Studies of the Breast

Breast imaging plays a key role in the initial diagnosis and management of breast cancer and is discussed in detail Chapter 2. Once a breast cancer is identified, bilateral mammography helps identify multifocal or multicentric disease as part of surgical planning. Multifocal disease refers to sites of disease in the same quadrant, usually along the same duct. Multicentric disease refers to multiple areas within different quadrants, likely involving multiple ducts.

Ultrasound may be employed to further evaluate palpable breast masses and aid in interventional procedures. It is capable of distinguishing between cystic and solid masses, and ultrasound guidance allows for aspiration of complex cysts. For patients receiving neoadjuvant chemotherapy, ultrasound may be used to localize the primary tumor with radio-opaque clips so that the tumor location can later be identified in cases of clinical and radiographic response to therapy.

The role of breast magnetic resonance imaging (MRI) as a screening tool is still evolving, but it is increasingly being used in the preoperative setting and has important implications for the multidisciplinary approach to breast cancer. MRI is used preoperatively to assess the extent of breast tumors, occasionally to rule out chest wall involvement, and to screen for unsuspected disease in the ipsilateral and contralateral breasts. This imaging modality detects additional unsuspected ipsilateral breast disease in 6% to 34% of women with breast cancer (10) and unsuspected contralateral tumors in 3% to 5% of cases (11). However, the clinical implications of these findings remain controversial, and no study to date has shown a survival advantage for patients evaluated with this modality. Importantly, use of presurgical MRI has been shown to delay time to treatment by up to three weeks and may contribute to increasing rates of mastectomy (12,13). MRI has a lower specificity than mammography, resulting in an increased number of breast biopsies for benign lesions. Thus its use in the general population should be carefully restricted. At the current time, MRI in the newly diagnosed patient may be useful for all suspected risk gene carriers, for patients with suboptimal imaging or where imaging has raised additional questions, or on a case-by-case basis where clinical judgment may be altered by the procedure. Patients must be informed of the risks and benefits of MRI imaging as health outcomes remain uncertain.

Once a breast tumor has been identified and localized by imaging, tissue is obtained for pathological review and histological diagnosis. Minimally invasive percutaneous image-guided or palpation-guided procedures are preferred over surgical biopsy because they provide a diagnosis before surgery and thus minimize the number of surgical procedures required. For example, if a patient is known to have clinically positive ipsilateral lymph nodes based on ultrasound evaluation and percutaneous fine-needle aspiration (FNA) before surgery, a full axillary dissection will be planned.

Alternatively, a preoperative diagnosis of invasive carcinoma enables the surgeon to prepare for a procedure that includes sentinel lymph node biopsy or axillary dissection as well as primary tumor resection. In addition, diagnosis by needle biopsy before surgery allows for multidisciplinary consideration of neoadjuvant therapy and evaluation of response to therapy.

FNA biopsy of breast lesions can be rapidly performed at the time of diagnostic imaging, and results may be available the same day, depending upon the institution. This technique is preferred over core needle biopsy (CNB) for masses in technically difficult areas, such as those near breast implants or the pectoralis muscle, and for patients who are therapeutically anticoagulated because it carries a lower risk of bleeding. IHC can often be obtained if enough material is collected to make a cell block. The FNA procedure cannot distinguish between in situ and invasive carcinoma because it destroys the surrounding tissue architecture. Another limitation is its rate of false negatives and nondiagnostic samples, which reflects lack of operator experience (14). CNB has the advantage of obtaining a histological rather than cytological diagnosis and has a lower rate of false negative results, thus making it the procedure of choice. For nonpalpable lesions, such as calcifications, stereotactic core biopsy is employed. The target site is identified between two digital mammographic images, and a vacuum-assisted biopsy needle samples from the vicinity of the lesion. Titanium clips may be placed in the area after sampling in order to locate the site in the event that surgery is later required.

Imaging to Evaluate for Metastatic Disease

According to the National Comprehensive Cancer Network clinical practice guidelines, evaluation for metastatic breast cancer is guided by symptoms and abnormal physical findings. Radionucleotide bone scan is indicated in patients who have an elevated alkaline phosphatase concentration or localized bone symptoms. Abdominal or pelvic computed tomography (CT), ultrasound, or MRI is utilized for abnormal liver function tests, abdominal complaints, or abnormalities detected on exam. Brain MRI (or CT if MRI is not readily available) is recommended for neurological complaints or abnormalities detected on physical exam. Chest imaging is indicated in early-stage breast cancer if pulmonary symptoms are present or for patients with stage 3A and above. The initial evaluation of patients presenting with stage 4 breast cancer or recurrent disease should include complete staging studies with chest and abdominal imaging and bone scan.

Positron-emission tomography (PET) scans are not recommended in the initial diagnosis or staging of asymptomatic patients because of the high rate of false positives. Furthermore, some studies suggest that tumors under 1 cm and those of lobular histology may have reduced uptake of 18-fluorodeoxyglucose, leading to false negatives. The role of PET in stage 3 disease or in women with multiple positive axillary lymph nodes is unclear. Integrated PET/CT scanning provides greater spatial resolution than PET alone and may be useful in evaluation of the mediastinum and internal mammary lymph nodes. This modality can be an alternative to CT imaging of the chest, abdomen, and pelvis with bone scan, but it is generally discouraged except in cases where other staging studies are equivocal.

Further Evaluation for Risks of Treatment

Evaluation of left ventricular ejection fraction (LVEF) provides baseline information for patients considering treatment with an anthracycline-based chemotherapy regimen or trastuzumab, both of which are associated with cardiotoxicity. In general, doxorubicin should not be administered to women with a reduced LVEF because of cardiotoxicity risk, which increases with increased cumulative dose. LVEF can be assessed with a transthoracic echocardiogram or a multiple-gated acquisition (MUGA) scan, although debate exists as to whether a MUGA scan is warranted for patients identified as low risk for cardiac disease given how infrequently such information changes treatment plans (15). While anthracycline cardiotoxicity may be permanent, limited follow-up to date indicates that congestive heart failure secondary to trastuzumab is reversible. Radiation therapy of the left chest wall is also associated with a small risk of cardiovascular toxicity, but the increased rate of cardiovascular events is generally outweighed by the reduction in risk of breast cancer recurrence for most patients. In addition, modern CT planning has substantially reduced the risk of cardiac toxicity from radiation administered in the adjuvant setting.

Other long-term risks of breast cancer treatment include osteoporosis secondary to aromatase inhibitors (AIs) or early menopause. Patients receiving AI therapy should have baseline measurement of bone mineral density. In this population, osteoporosis or osteopenia is treated according to standard management with calcium and vitamin D supplementation and consideration of bisphosphonates if indicated. Adequate history of dental health should be obtained to assess for risk of osteonecrosis of the jaw. Increased risk of venous thromboembolic events is associated with tamoxifen use, and risk factors for thrombosis should be assessed during the initial evaluation. Tamoxifen is generally contraindicated in patients with a history of thromboembolic events, such as pulmonary emboli, deep venous thrombosis, and embolic stroke. However, screening is not recommended in patients without a personal history of hypercoagulability given the relatively small increase in absolute risk (16).

Fertility preservation is a pressing issue for women who desire to become pregnant following treatment of their breast cancer and plays a prominent role in the selection and timing of therapy for this demographic. Approximately 25% of women diagnosed with breast cancer are premenopausal. Given the trend toward increasing maternal age at first pregnancy, a significant number of women face the potential of infertility from chemotherapy. The most commonly used adjuvant chemotherapy regimens include gonadotoxic agents such as cyclophosphamide, doxorubicin, and possibly paclitaxel, which cause follicle loss through apoptosis and ultimately result in premature ovarian failure (17). Animal data suggest that taxanes also cause ovarian toxicity. Factors that determine the likelihood of infertility include patient age and the type and cumulative dose of cytotoxic agents.

Currently, options for assisted reproductive technologies include the established technique of embryo cryopreservation following in vitro fertilization (IVF) and more experimental approaches such as oocyte and ovarian cryopreservation. Pregnancy rates with frozen oocytes are significantly lower than with unfrozen oocytes. As a result, this procedure is most commonly performed in single women who choose not to proceed with IVF with donor sperm. Cryopreservation of ovarian tissue is still an investigational protocol since transplantation of this tissue carries a theoretical risk of reseeding cancer cells. Studies demonstrate that in addition to standard methods of ovulatory induction, tamoxifen and AIs can safely be used to induce ovulation in patients with breast cancer (18). Both embryo and oocyte cryopreservation require approximately 2 weeks of ovarian stimulation, beginning with the onset of the patient's menstrual cycle, and it is advised that this occur prior to initiation of chemotherapy in order to avoid the risk of fertilization or harvesting of a damaged oocyte. Therefore, it is imperative that patients be educated on the risks of infertility from proposed chemotherapy regimens and referred to fertility centers immediately after diagnosis in order to avoid delays in cancer treatment. The multidisciplinary evaluation of premenopausal women with breast cancer should always include an assessment of the patient's desire for fertility preservation. This will foster efficient coordination with the reproductive endocrinology team to minimize delays in treatment owing to embryo or oocyte cryopreservation.

Clinical Trials Assessment

Clinical trials are an integral component of the armamentarium against breast cancer and are responsible for the many advances that have been made in recent years in both the early-stage and advanced breast cancer setting. The multidisciplinary setting is the ideal environment for consideration of trial participation for patients as it affords the opportunity to bring together primary caregivers with research staff to discuss issues of eligibility and candidacy for trials. In particular, certain types of trials, such as preoperative therapy, are greatly facilitated by the multidisciplinary input at the initial evaluation. The multidisciplinary approach to clinical trials is described in Chapter 16. Many organizations, including the National Comprehensive Cancer Network, advocate for enrollment in a clinical trial for all eligible patients. While data suggest that outcomes of patients on trial are similar to those of patients not on trial, the benefits of participation in a clinical trial for an individual patient may include: multidisciplinary care by members of the research team, close monitoring of disease response or recurrence and potential side effects, and access to the latest advances

in treatment methods and therapeutic agents up to years before they are widely available. Furthermore, patients have the opportunity to make an invaluable contribution to the field of oncology that benefits other patients as a direct result of the knowledge gained from clinical trials. Therefore, assessment for clinical trial participation should be included in the multidisciplinary initial evaluation of all patients.

■ CONCLUSIONS

A newly diagnosed woman with breast cancer faces a number of life-altering options that require careful thought and evaluation before proceeding with a treatment plan. The initial evaluation by multidisciplinary teams offers patients an approach to care that centers on the coordination of data collection, review, and synthesis in order to provide patients with timely access to the most appropriate therapies. Recent guidelines for the diagnosis and evaluation of breast cancer incorporate advances in imaging modalities, laboratory techniques, and gene expression profiling that, together with the promise of new therapies, will translate into improved outcomes for patients with breast cancer.

■ SUMMARY

- The goal of staging using the TNM system is to provide prognostic information and guide the initial evaluation and treatment selection.
- Molecular characterization of estrogen receptor, progesterone receptor, and HER-2 status is required to aid in prognostication and treatment selection.
- Initial evaluation of the newly diagnosed breast cancer patient includes: history, physical exam, chemistries, complete blood count, liver function tests, diagnostic mammography, and pathological review of biopsies.
- No established role exists during the initial evaluation for measurement of tumor markers, markers of proliferation, circulating tumor cells, or bone marrow biopsy.
- Genomic profiling of tumors is a recent advancement that may aid in treatment selection in certain patients.
- Appropriate patients should be referred for genetic counseling.
- The role of MRI in newly diagnosed patients is evolving. MRI may detect additional ipsilateral or contralateral abnormalities, but this may account for increasing rates of mastectomy and delays in treatment and has not been shown to improve long-term outcomes in this group.

- Imaging to evaluate for advanced disease is guided by symptoms or based on abnormal findings on physical exam or laboratory studies in stage 1 or 2. Chest and abdominal imaging should be considered in stage 3 disease. PET scans are not recommended in staging operable breast cancer.
- Fertility preservation should be discussed prior to treatment, with appropriate referral to fertility specialists if indicated.
- The initial multidisciplinary evaluation should include consideration of clinical trial participation.

■ REFERENCES

1. Greene FL, Page DL, Fleming ID, et al. *AJCC Cancer Staging Manual*, 6th ed. New York: Springer; 2002:255–282.
2. Goetz MP, Kamal A, Ames MM. Tamoxifen pharmacogenomics: the role of CYP2D6 as a predictor of drug response. *Clin Pharmacol Ther*. 2008;83(1):160–166.
3. Harris L, Fritsche H, Mennel R, et al. American society of clinical oncology 2007 update of recommendations for the use of tumor markers in breast cancer. *J Clin Oncol*. 2007;25(33):5287–5312.
4. Bertone-Johnson ER. Vitamin D and breast cancer. *Ann Epidemiol*. 2009;19(7):462-467.
5. Bertone-Johnson ER, Chen WY, Holick MF, et al. Plasma 25-hydroxyvitamin D and 1,25-dihydroxyvitamin D and risk of breast cancer. *Cancer Epidemiol Biomarkers Prev*. 2005;14(8): 1991–1997.
6. Lowe LC, Guy M, Mansi JL, et al. Plasma 25-hydroxy vitamin D concentrations, vitamin D receptor genotype and breast cancer risk in a UK Caucasian population. *Eur J Cancer*. 2005;41(8): 1164–1169.
7. Chlebowski RT, Blackburn GL, Thomson CA, et al. Dietary fat reduction and breast cancer outcome: interim efficacy results from the Women's Intervention Nutrition Study. *J Natl Cancer Inst*. 2006;98(24):1767–1776.
8. Holmes MD, Chen WY, Feskanich D, Kroenke CH, Colditz GA. Physical activity and survival after breast cancer diagnosis. *JAMA*. 2005;293(20):2479–2486.
9. U.S. Preventive Services Task Force (USPSTF). Genetic risk assessment and BRCA mutation testing for breast and ovarian cancer susceptibility: recommendation statement. *Ann Intern Med*. 2005;143(5):355–361.
10. Liberman L, Morris EA, Dershaw DD, Abramson AF, Tan LK. MR imaging of the ipsilateral breast in women with percutaneously proven breast cancer. *AJR Am J Roentgenol*. 2003;180(4):901–910.
11. Lehman CD, Gatsonis C, Kuhl CK, et al. MRI evaluation of the contralateral breast in women with recently diagnosed breast cancer. *N Engl J Med*. 2007;356(13):1295–1303.
12. Bleicher RJ, Ciocca RM, Egleston BL, et al. The influence of routine pretreatment MRI on time to treatment, mastectomy rate, and positive margins. *Breast Cancer Symp*. 2008. Abstract 227.
13. Katipamula R, Hoskin TL, Boughey JC, et al. Trends in mastectomy rates at the Mayo Clinic Rochester: effect of surgical year and preoperative MRI. *J Clin Oncol*. 2008;26(suppl.). Abstract 509.
14. Pisano ED, Fajardo LL, Caudry DJ, et al. Fine-needle aspiration biopsy of nonpalpable breast lesions in a multicenter clinical trial: results from the radiologic diagnostic oncology group V. *Radiology*. 2001;219(3):785–792.
15. Sabel MS, Levine EG, Hurd T, et al. Is MUGA scan necessary in patients with low-risk breast cancer before doxorubicin-based adjuvant therapy? Multiple gated acquisition. *Am J Clin Oncol*. 2001;24(4):425–428.
16. Hayes DF. Clinical practice. Follow-up of patients with early breast cancer. *N Engl J Med*. 2007;356(24):2505–2513.
17. Sonmezer M, Oktay K. Fertility preservation in young women undergoing breast cancer therapy. *Oncologist*. 2006;11(5): 422–434.
18. Oktay K, Buyuk E, Libertella N, Akar M, Rosenwaks Z. Fertility preservation in breast cancer patients: a prospective controlled comparison of ovarian stimulation with tamoxifen and letrozole for embryo cryopreservation. *J Clin Oncol*. 2005;23(19): 4347–4353.

Fertility and Pregnancy Considerations

KATHRYN J. RUDDY

ANN H. PARTRIDGE

Young women with newly diagnosed breast cancer are often concerned about how treatment will affect their fertility and the safety of any future pregnancy (1,2). Although many studies suggest that pregnancy after treatment for early-stage breast cancer does not adversely affect a woman's risk of breast cancer recurrence or survival, breast cancer treatment does often compromise a woman's fertility. At the time of diagnosis and in follow-up, premenopausal breast cancer patients should receive adequate information about risks to their future child-bearing potential and available options for fertility preservation (1). Figure 4.23 details an algorithm for considering fertility issues in women with newly diagnosed breast cancer. Because treatment of early-stage breast cancer is usually not a medical emergency, delaying systemic therapy for the time needed to pursue fertility preservation options is often reasonable. However, because many breast cancers are hormonally responsive, breast cancer patients and their healthcare providers may be uniquely apprehensive about the impact of fertility preservation techniques and future pregnancies on prognosis. In order to avoid excessive delays in treatment, all women interested in fertility preservation should be counseled regarding infertility risks and safety of pregnancy after breast cancer, and they should be promptly referred to a fertility specialist for consideration of reproductive technologies prior to treatment when appropriate.

■ SAFETY OF PREGNANCY AFTER BREAST CANCER

Research suggests that 5% to 15% of young women with breast cancer will go on to become pregnant (2–4). The current literature suggests that pregnancy after breast cancer does not increase a woman's risk of recurrence of or death from breast cancer. Large studies have shown that women who become pregnant after early-stage breast cancer are no more likely to experience recurrence than those who do not (4–16). In several, pregnancy appeared even to be associated with a *lower* rate of recurrence of breast cancer. For example, Ives and colleagues performed a population-based study of pregnancy after breast cancer using the Western Australia data linkage system and medical record review to identify women who were diagnosed with breast cancer under age 45 between 1982 and 2000 (4). These authors reported that 123 of 2,539 (5%) became pregnant in follow-up, and these women had better breast cancer outcomes than those who did not have a subsequent pregnancy after breast cancer. This apparent beneficial effect of pregnancy may reflect a "healthy mother bias" in that only the healthiest women attempt and are able to become pregnant after cancer treatment (6). However, it is also possible that there is a biological effect by which pregnancy protects against breast cancer recurrence. Because of the inherent limitations of the studies, some physicians and patients remain concerned that pregnancy-related hormones may stimulate growth of dormant breast cancer cells and worsen breast cancer outcomes (8). This is a challenging issue to study because it would be unethical and impractical to randomize

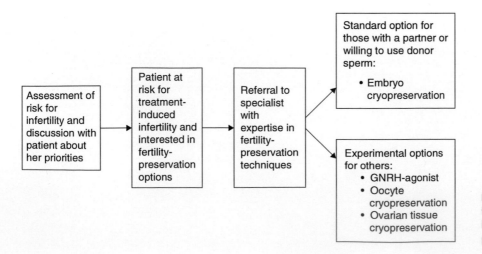

FIGURE 4.23 Algorithm for considering fertility issues in women with newly diagnosed breast cancer. (Adapted from Ref. 1, with permission.)

women to pregnancy after breast cancer, although ongoing prospective studies may add to current knowledge. At present, providers should assist breast cancer patients to make decisions about subsequent pregnancy based on the current data, which suggest safety, while considering of the patient's preferences, values, and underlying risk of recurrence.

■ IMPACT OF TREATMENT ON FERTILITY AND TIMING OF PREGNANCY

Breast cancer treatment can impair fertility in several ways. First, optimal hormonal therapy for hormone receptor–positive breast cancer generally requires that a woman delay pregnancy for 5 or more years. During this period, a woman's fertility declines with age. At approximately age 37, the rate of decline increases significantly in most women. Although tamoxifen, ovarian suppression, and aromatase inhibitors do not directly damage the ovaries, a woman who begins treatment at age 35 may have greater difficulty conceiving when hormonal therapy is complete at age 40. Some women, particularly those with low-risk tumors, may choose to forgo some or all of their hormonal therapy, giving up some reduction of risk of recurrence, in an effort to pursue a pregnancy at an earlier age.

Those who do choose to receive hormonal therapy must be aware of the teratogenicity of tamoxifen, which due to the drug's long half-life, may persist for some time after one has stopped taking the drug. Because it may take 6 to 8 weeks for tamoxifen metabolites to be cleared from the bloodstream, most women should plan to wait at least 3 months after stopping tamoxifen before attempting to conceive (17). In contrast, there is no evidence that ovarian suppression using a gonadotropin-releasing hormone agonist, GnRH-a, is teratogenic. Also, aromatase inhibitors (given in conjunction with GnRH-a as a nonstandard hormonal therapy for breast cancer in premenopausal women) do not appear to be teratogenic on the basis of exposure of embryos to aromatase inhibitors as part of infertility treatments, but there are limited data in this regard (18). The increasingly frequent consideration of bisphosphonates for prevention of bone loss and possibly recurrence for early-stage, premenopausal breast cancer patients is problematic for the patient considering future pregnancy. The long biological half-life of these agents, coupled with a lack of safety data in pregnancy, should contraindicate their use in women considering future pregnancy.

Even for women not treated with hormonal therapy (e.g., hormone receptor–negative breast cancer), a delay before conception is often recommended. Owing to the risk of treatments harming a developing fetus, it is recommended that women wait at least several months after completion of radiation therapy or chemotherapy before attempting conception. In fact, because the rate of recurrence is highest during the first 2 to 3 years, particularly for hormone receptor–negative cancers, women have traditionally been advised to wait at least 2 years after diagnosis with early-stage breast cancer before conceiving a child. However, there is no evidence to suggest that earlier pregnancy is detrimental to prognosis. Thus a shorter delay before pregnancy may be reasonable for some women.

The second major way in which breast cancer treatment can impair fertility is via direct damage to the ovaries by chemotherapy. Most studies have used chemotherapy-related amenorrhea (CRA) as a surrogate for menopause and associated infertility. However, women who experience CRA may still be fertile and therefore premenopausal, and many will resume menses after a period of amenorrhea following treatment. Furthermore, women who continue to menstruate after treatment may still have impaired fertility. Risk of CRA increases with increasing patient age and with greater cumulative dose of alkylating agents (19–21). In one study, the likelihood of menstruation 6 months after a variety of different chemotherapeutic regimens for breast cancer was 85% in those aged below 35 years, 61% in those aged 35 to 40 years, and less than 25% in those aged above 40 years (20). Alkylating agents such as cyclophosphamide are particularly gonadotoxic because they are not cell-cycle specific, so they may damage cells that are not actively dividing, including oocytes and the estrogen-producing granulosa cells and pregranulosa cells of primordial follicles (22). Other cytotoxic agents may have additional substantial effect on ovarian function. Table 4.3 details estimated rates of amenorrhea after standard adjuvant breast cancer regimens. Rates vary widely from study to study, due in part to differences in the definitions of menopause and lengths of follow-up. In general, anthracyclines are thought to be less gonadotoxic than alkylating agents. Taxanes have become commonly prescribed drugs in the treatment of early-stage breast cancer in recent years, but data regarding their gonadotoxicity are mixed. Most recent studies suggest limited if any increase in CRA with the addition of paclitaxel (23–28). Radiation and surgery for early-breast cancer therapy do not impact future fertility.

Even among women who resume menses after chemotherapy, premature ovarian failure may occur. A retrospective evaluation of long-term follow-up of women treated on International Breast Cancer Study Group (IBCSG) trials V and VI showed that 227 women who remained premenopausal after six cycles of adjuvant CMF (cyclophosphamide, methotrexate, 5-fluorouracil) with oral cyclophosphamide had high rates of menopause at 5 years, even in younger age cohorts (29). In this study, a patient who was 30 years old at diagnosis and who was

■ **Table 4.3** Risk of chemotherapy-related amenorrhea with common treatment regimens

| Regimen | Percentage With CRA (Varies by Study) | | | |
	Results From Studies (Including All Ages)	Age <40 yrs	Age >40 yrs	References
None		<5	20–25	21
Tamoxifen	14	16	74	59,60
AC	53	13–44	81	20,60–62
AC-T or AC-D	13–74	9–61	65–85	20,25,27,60,63–65
AC-TH		14	67	60
CMF	43–82	33–40	76–81	21,20,59,61,66,67
CEF or FEC or ddFEC or FAC	51–77	39–62	75–100	59,65–68
TX/AC	67–90			65

AC, doxorubicin and cyclophosphamide; AC-D, AC and docetaxel; AC-T, AC and paclitaxel; AC-TH, AC followed by paclitaxel and a year of trastuzumab; CAF, cyclophosphamide, doxorubicin, 5-fluorouracil; CEF, cyclophosphamide, epirubicin, 5-fluorouracil; CMF, cyclophosphamide, methotrexate, 5-fluorouracil; CRA, chemotherapy-related amenorrhea; dd, dose dense; FAC, 5-fluorouracil, doxorubicin, cyclophosphamide; TX/AC, docetaxel and capecitabine (TX) as neoadjuvant therapy and then adjuvant AC or AC as neoadjuvant therapy followed by adjuvant TX.

Sources: Adapted from Refs. 57 and 58, with permission.

menstruating after six cycles of oral CMF had a 37% risk of menopause at age 35 and an 84% risk at age 40, much higher than would be expected at those ages.

■ **PREDICTING FUTURE FERTILITY**

Given the limitations of using CRA to reflect fertility and menopausal status, there is interest in developing more accurate markers of fertility and menopause for use before and after breast cancer treatment in order to assist women in their family-planning decisions. For example, if fertility markers were low at the time of diagnosis, a woman who highly valued an opportunity to have a biological child might decide to undergo embryo cryopreservation before chemotherapy or might forgo chemotherapy if the projected absolute reduction in risk of recurrence were small. She might also opt to cut hormonal therapy short in order to attempt conception before further natural waning of fertility occurred. Alternatively, she might choose to forgo having a biological child in the future and seek other routes of parenthood sooner if the likelihood of future pregnancy were low. Improved information would be of great value in managing expectations for these patients.

Several markers of ovarian reserve have been studied extensively in noncancer patients undergoing fertility treatments. Serum hormone levels in the early follicular phase

of a menstrual cycle (days 2 to 4) are predictive of success with fertility treatment. In general, even if periods are absent, levels of follicle-stimulating hormone (FSH) less than 20 mIU/mL, luteinizing hormone (LH) less than 20 mIU/mL, and estradiol (E2) greater than 20 pg/mL suggest that ovulation is possible. Other potential markers of ovarian reserve include serum inhibin levels, serum anti-mullerian hormone (AMH), and measurements of antral follicle count (AFC) and ovarian volume by transvaginal ultrasound. Higher inhibin levels (30,31), AMH (32), and AFC (33) during the early follicular phase of the menstrual cycle correlate with fertility in the general population of women seeking care at infertility clinics. There have been early studies in breast cancer survivors suggesting that these measures may add information regarding fertility after treatment, although further research is warranted (23,27,34,35). For breast cancer survivors interested in their fertility, these measures of ovarian reserve ideally can be done before women begin adjuvant hormonal therapy because hormonal treatment may affect these values without actually changing fertility. One caveat for using these measures in women who have received breast cancer treatment is that some women who appear to be postmenopausal and infertile by these hormonal levels for months or years after chemotherapy may later experience an "ovarian awakening" and premenopausal hormone levels may return.

■ OPTIONS FOR FERTILITY PRESERVATION

For women at significant risk of future infertility, several strategies have been explored for fertility preservation. Embryo cryopreservation is the standard method for the protection of fertility in the breast cancer patient population. A premenopausal patient who has a partner or wants to use donor sperm can freeze embryos before breast cancer treatment in order to plan pregnancy using in vitro fertilization (IVF) after cancer treatment is completed. The delay required to harvest the oocytes before additional breast cancer treatment is generally between 2 and 6 weeks, depending on when in the menstrual cycle a woman presents to a reproductive specialist. Later, pregnancy rates of approximately 20% to 30% per transfer of two to three embryos to the woman herself or to a surrogate can be expected, according to studies in patients without cancer (36,37). The success rate of this technique may be slightly lower in cancer patients due to fewer high-quality oocytes (38). The ovarian stimulation required for creation of embryos does result in high estradiol levels (10 times higher than in the normal menstrual cycle) and carries a theoretical risk of promoting cancer cell growth. In order to avoid this potential risk, tamoxifen and aromatase inhibitor ovarian stimulation protocols have been developed (39–41). In a small study comparing early-stage breast cancer patients who received prechemotherapy ovarian stimulation for IVF with tamoxifen alone, tamoxifen plus FSH, or letrozole plus FSH, Oktay and colleagues found that embryo yield was highest in the letrozole plus FSH group, which had the lowest peak estradiol levels (42). In a subsequent study, these investigators compared short-term breast cancer recurrence rates in survivors who did not undergo IVF to rates in patients who underwent letrozole plus FSH stimulation; they found that rates were similar in the two groups (41). At the present time, there is no evidence that any fertility preservation technique increases risk of recurrence in breast cancer survivors; however, this research is in its infancy and future research is warranted.

Other methods of fertility preservation are more experimental and have been less successful to date. Data from preclinical studies suggest that GnRH-a could reduce the ovarian damage caused by chemotherapy by halting ovarian cycling and perhaps by inhibiting ovarian cell death directly (43–45). However, results of clinical studies of GnRH-a have been mixed in women with breast cancer as well as other cancers (3,46–52). In the coming years, the effects of GnRH-a should be clarified by larger ongoing prospective, randomized trials. A study being conducted by the Southwestern Oncology Group (www.cancer.gov/clinicaltrials/SWOG-S0230) randomizes women with hormone receptor–negative early-stage breast cancer to receive or not receive goserelin during chemotherapy.

Trials by the Anglo Celtic Cooperative Oncology Group in the United Kingdom (www.isdscotland.org/isd/1663.html) and by the Gruppo Italiano Mamella in Italy are of similar design, but they also include women with hormone receptor–positive disease.

Oocyte cryopreservation and ovarian tissue cryopreservation are experimental options offered in some centers to patients who do not have a partner and do not wish to create embryos using a sperm donor. Success rates with oocyte cryopreservation are only approximately 1.6% live births per frozen oocyte, three to four times lower than standard embryo cryopreservation because oocytes are more vulnerable to damage during the freezing process than are embryos (53). Concerns about hormonal stimulation of breast tissue are similar to those in embryo cryopreservation. Ovarian tissue cryopreservation theoretically could preserve hundreds of primordial follicles without any need for ovarian stimulation or treatment delay, as menstrual phase is irrelevant when a piece of ovarian tissue is stored, and tissue can be re-implanted either orthotopically (for natural conception) or heterotopically (for ease). However, it has proven difficult to mature these follicles into oocytes that are ready for fertilization, and there are concerns that cancer cells residing in the ovarian tissue could be reintroduced during re-implantation (54–56). Furthermore, ischemia-reperfusion injury may occur. Currently, neither oocyte cryopreservation nor ovarian cryopreservation is ready for widespread use.

■ CONCLUSION

Although pregnancy after breast cancer does not appear to increase risk of breast cancer recurrence or decrease survival, breast cancer treatments can impair a woman's ability to conceive in the future. Early identification of women who will benefit from meeting with a fertility specialist allows patients to decide whether they wish to pursue oocyte retrieval with embryo cryopreservation or other fertility technologies with minimal delay to their treatment. Discussions regarding the safety of future pregnancies and options for fertility preservation should be tailored to each patient's individual priorities and risk for recurrence and infertility. References that physicians may provide to patients to help inform them of their risks and their options include websites such as www.plwc.org, www.BreastCancer.Org/fertility_pregnancy_adoption.html, and www.fertilityandcancerproject.org, and www.fertilehope.org. Additional research is needed to improve measurement of ovarian function before and after breast cancer treatment so that women can understand their fertility potential and fertility-focused interventions can be targeted appropriately. Furthermore, more data are needed regarding the impact of newer chemotherapy regimens on ovarian function so that this risk of treatment can be considered adequately when choosing treatment regimens.

■ KEY POINTS

- Treatment for breast cancer can impair fertility by allowing natural waning of ovarian function over time as well as by directly damaging the ovaries.
- Early in the course of care, oncologists should discuss the potential for infertility and the available data regarding the apparent safety of future pregnancies with women of childbearing age who are diagnosed with breast cancer.
- Prompt referral to specialists in reproductive technologies allows women who desire embryo preservation or other fertility preservation to minimize delay in oncologic treatment and maximize options for fertility preservation strategies.

■ REFERENCES

1. Lee SJ, Schover LR, Partridge AH, et al. American Society of Clinical Oncology recommendations on fertility preservation in cancer patients. *J Clin Oncol.* 2006;24:2917–2931.
2. Partridge AH, Gelber S, Peppercorn J, et al. Web-based survey of fertility issues in young women with breast cancer. *J Clin Oncol.* 2004;22:4174–4183.
3. Fox KR, Scialla J, Moore H. Preventing chemotherapy-related amenorrhea using leuprolide during adjuvant chemotherapy for early-stage breast cancer [abstract 50]. *Proc Am Soc Clin Oncol.* 2003;22:13.
4. Ives A, Saunders C, Bulsara M, et al. Pregnancy after breast cancer: population based study. *BMJ* 2007;334:194.
5. Kroman N, Wohlfahrt J, Andersen KW, et al. Time since childbirth and prognosis in primary breast cancer: population based study. *BMJ* 1997;315:851–855.
6. Sankila R, Heinavaara S, Hakulinen T. Survival of breast cancer patients after subsequent term pregnancy: "healthy mother effect". *Am J Obstet Gynecol.* 1994;170:818–823.
7. von Schoultz E, Johansson H, Wilking N, et al. Influence of prior and subsequent pregnancy on breast cancer prognosis. *J Clin Oncol.* 1995;13:430–434.
8. Petrek JA. Pregnancy safety after breast cancer. *Cancer.* 1994; 74:528–531.
9. Gemignani ML, Petrek JA. Pregnancy after breast cancer. *Cancer Control.* 1999;6:272–276.
10. Velentgas P, Daling JR, Malone KE, et al. Pregnancy after breast carcinoma: outcomes and influence on mortality. *Cancer.* 1999;85:2424–2432.
11. Dow KH, Harris JR, Roy C. Pregnancy after breast-conserving surgery and radiation therapy for breast cancer. *J Natl Cancer Inst Monogr.* 1994;16:131–137.
12. Higgins S, Haffty BG. Pregnancy and lactation after breast-conserving therapy for early-stage breast cancer. *Cancer.* 1994; 73:2175–2180.
13. Gelber S, Coates AS, Goldhirsch A, et al. Effect of pregnancy on overall survival after the diagnosis of early-stage breast cancer. *J Clin Oncol.* 2001;19:1671–1675.
14. Upponi SS, Ahmad F, Whitaker IS, et al. Pregnancy after breast cancer. *Eur J Cancer.* 2003;39:736–741.
15. Mueller BA, Simon MS, Deapen D, et al. Childbearing and survival after breast carcinoma in young women. *Cancer.* 2003; 98:1131–1140.
16. Blakely LJ, Buzdar AU, Lozada JA, et al. Effects of pregnancy after treatment for breast carcinoma on survival and risk of recurrence. *Cancer.* 100:465–469.
17. Guerrieri-Gonzaga A, Baglietto L, Johansson H, et al. Correlation between tamoxifen elimination and biomarker recovery in a primary prevention trial. *Cancer Epidemiol Biomarkers Prev.* 2001;10:967–970.
18. Tulandi T, Martin J, Al-Fadhli R, et al. Congenital malformations among 911 newborns conceived after infertility treatment with letrozole or clomiphene citrate. *Fertil Steril.* 2006;85:1761–1765.
19. Walshe JM, Denduluri N, Swain SM. Amenorrhea in premenopausal women after adjuvant chemotherapy for breast cancer. *J Clin Oncol.* 2006;24:5769–5779.
20. Petrek JA, Naughton MJ, Case LD, et al. Incidence, time course, and determinants of menstrual bleeding after breast cancer treatment: a prospective study. *J Clin Oncol.* 2006;24:1045–1051.
21. Goldhirsch A, Gelber RD, Castiglione M. The magnitude of endocrine effects of adjuvant chemotherapy for premenopausal breast cancer patients. The International Breast Cancer Study Group. *Ann Oncol.* 1990;1:183–188.
22. Falcone T, Attaran M, Bedaiwy MA, et al. Ovarian function preservation in the cancer patient. *Fertil Steril.* 2004;81:243–257.
23. Anderson RA, Themmen AP, Al-Qahtani A, et al. The effects of chemotherapy and long-term gonadotrophin suppression on the ovarian reserve in premenopausal women with breast cancer. *Hum Reprod.* 2006;21:2583–2592.
24. Kramer R, Tham YL, Sexton K, et al. Chemotherapy-induced amenorrhea is increased in patients treated with adjuvant doxorubicin and cyclophosphamide (AC) followed by a taxane (T). *J Clin Oncol.* 2005;23:651.
25. Fornier MN, Modi S, Panageas KS, et al. Incidence of chemotherapy-induced, long-term amenorrhea in patients with breast carcinoma age 40 years and younger after adjuvant anthracycline and taxane. *Cancer.* 2005;104:1575–1579.
26. Abusief ME, Missmer SA, Ginsburg ES, et al. Chemotherapy-related amenorrhea in women with early breast cancer: the effect of paclitaxel or dose density. *J Clin Oncol.* 2006;24:10506.
27. Reh A, Oktem O, Oktay K. Impact of breast cancer chemotherapy on ovarian reserve: a prospective observational analysis by menstrual history and ovarian reserve markers. *Fertil Steril.* 2008;90:1635–1639.
28. Minisini AM, Menis J, Valent F, et al. Determinants of recovery from amenorrhea in premenopausal breast cancer patients receiving adjuvant chemotherapy in the taxane era. *Anticancer Drugs.* 2009;20(6):503–507.
29. Partridge A, Gelber S, Gelber RD, et al. Age of menopause among women who remain premenopausal following treatment for early breast cancer: long-term results from International Breast Cancer Study Group Trials V and VI. *Eur J Cancer.* 2007;43:1646–1653.
30. Blumenfeld Z, Ritter M, Shen-Orr Z, et al. Inhibin A concentrations in the sera of young women during and after chemotherapy for lymphoma: correlation with ovarian toxicity. *Am J Reprod Immunol.* 1998;39:33–40.
31. Blumenfeld Z. Preservation of fertility and ovarian function and minimalization of chemotherapy associated gonadotoxicity and premature ovarian failure: the role of inhibin-A and -B as markers. *Mol Cell Endocrinol.* 2002;187:93–105.
32. van Rooij IA, Broekmans FJ, te Velde ER, et al. Serum anti-Mullerian hormone levels: a novel measure of ovarian reserve. *Hum Reprod.* 2002;17:3065–3071.
33. Scheffer GJ, Broekmans FJ, Looman CW, et al. The number of antral follicles in normal women with proven fertility is the best reflection of reproductive age. *Hum Reprod.* 2003;18:700–706.
34. Lutchman Singh K, Muttukrishna S, Stein RC, et al. Predictors of ovarian reserve in young women with breast cancer. *Br J Cancer.* 2007;96:1808–1816.

35. Partridge AH, Ruddy KJ, Gelber S, et al. Ovarian reserve in women who remain premenopausal after chemotherapy for early-stage breast cancer. *Fertil Steril.* Epub ahead of print.

36. Richter KS, Shipley SK, McVearry I, et al. Cryopreserved embryo transfers suggest that endometrial receptivity may contribute to reduced success rates of later developing embryos. *Fertil Steril.* 2006;86:862–866.

37. Mocanu EV, Cottell E, Waite K, et al. Frozen-thawed transfer cycles: are they comparable with fresh? *Ir Med J.* 2008;101:181–184.

38. Pal L, Leykin L, Schifren JL, et al. Malignancy may adversely influence the quality and behaviour of oocytes. *Hum Reprod.* 1998;13:1837–1840.

39. Oktay K, Buyuk E, Davis O, et al. Fertility preservation in breast cancer patients: IVF and embryo cryopreservation after ovarian stimulation with tamoxifen. *Hum Reprod.* 2003;18:90–95.

40. Mitwally MF, Casper RF. Single-dose administration of an aromatase inhibitor for ovarian stimulation. *Fertil Steril.* 2005;83: 229–231.

41. Azim AA, Costantini-Ferrando M, Oktay K. Safety of fertility preservation by ovarian stimulation with letrozole and gonadotropins in patients with breast cancer: a prospective controlled study. *J Clin Oncol.* 2008;26:2630–2635.

42. Oktay K, Buyuk E, Libertella N, et al. Fertility preservation in breast cancer patients: a prospective controlled comparison of ovarian stimulation with tamoxifen and letrozole for embryo cryopreservation. *J Clin Oncol.* 2005;23:4347–4353.

43. Ataya K, Rao LV, Lawrence E, et al. Luteinizing hormone-releasing hormone agonist inhibits cyclophosphamide-induced ovarian follicular depletion in rhesus monkeys. *Biol Reprod.* 1995; 52:365–372.

44. Letterie GS. Anovulation in the prevention of cytotoxic-induced follicular attrition and ovarian failure. *Hum Reprod.* 2004;19:831–837.

45. Grundker C, Emons G. Role of gonadotropin-releasing hormone (GnRH) in ovarian cancer. *Reprod Biol Endocrinol.* 2003;1:65.

46. Waxman JH, Ahmed R, Smith D, et al. Failure to preserve fertility in patients with Hodgkin's disease. *Cancer Chemother Pharmacol.* 1987;19:159–162.

47. Dann EJ, Epelbaum R, Avivi I, et al. Fertility and ovarian function are preserved in women treated with an intensified regimen of cyclophosphamide, adriamycin, vincristine and prednisone (Mega-CHOP) for non-Hodgkin lymphoma. *Hum Reprod.* 2005;20:2247–2249.

48. Blumenfeld Z, Eckman A. Preservation of fertility and ovarian function and minimization of chemotherapy-induced gonadotoxicity in young women by GnRH-a. *J Natl Cancer Inst Monogr.* 2005;40–43.

49. Pereyra Pacheco B, Mendez Ribas JM, Milone G, et al. Use of GnRH analogs for functional protection of the ovary and preservation of fertility during cancer treatment in adolescents: a preliminary report. *Gynecol Oncol.* 2001;81:391–397.

50. Recchia F, Sica G, De Filippis S, et al. Goserelin as ovarian protection in the adjuvant treatment of premenopausal breast cancer: a phase II pilot study. *Anticancer Drugs.* 2002;13:417–424.

51. Badawy A, Elnashar A, El-Ashry M, et al. Gonadotropin-releasing hormone agonists for prevention of chemotherapy-induced ovarian damage: prospective randomized study. *Fertil Steril.* 2009;91:694–697.

52. Ismail-Khan R, Minton S, Cox C, et al. Preservation of ovarian function in young women treated with neoadjuvant chemotherapy for breast cancer: a randomized trial using the GnRH agonist (triptorelin) during chemotherapy, American Society of Clinical Oncology Annual Meeting, *J Clin Oncol.* 2008;26(Suppl.). Abstract 524.

53. Lee JK, Grace KA, Taylor AJ. Effect of a pharmacy care program on medication adherence and persistence, blood pressure, and low-density lipoprotein cholesterol: a randomized controlled trial. *JAMA.* 2006;296:2563–2571.

54. Kim SS, Radford J, Harris M, et al. Ovarian tissue harvested from lymphoma patients to preserve fertility may be safe for autotransplantation. *Hum Reprod.* 2001;16:2056–2060.

55. Donnez J, Dolmans MM, Demylle D, et al. Restoration of ovarian function after orthotopic (intraovarian and periovarian) transplantation of cryopreserved ovarian tissue in a woman treated by bone marrow transplantation for sickle cell anaemia: case report. *Hum Reprod.* 2006;21:183–188.

56. Donnez J, Dolmans MM, Demylle D, et al. Livebirth after orthotopic transplantation of cryopreserved ovarian tissue. *Lancet.* 2004;364:1405–1410.

57. Partridge AH, Ruddy KJ. Fertility and adjuvant treatment in young women with breast cancer. *Breast.* 2007;16(suppl 2): S175–S181.

58. Maltaris T, Weigel M, Mueller A, et al. Cancer and fertility preservation: fertility preservation in breast cancer patients. *Breast Cancer Res.* 2008;10:206.

59. Goodwin PJ, Ennis M, Pritchard KI, et al. Risk of menopause during the first year after breast cancer diagnosis. *J Clin Oncol.* 1999;17:2365–2370.

60. Abusief ME, Missmer SA, Ginsburg ES, et al. The effects of paclitaxel, dose density and trastuzumab on treatment-related amenorrhea in premenopausal women with breast cancer. *Cancer.* In press.

61. Bines J, Oleske DM, Cobleigh MA. Ovarian function in premenopausal women treated with adjuvant chemotherapy for breast cancer. *J Clin Oncol.* 1996;14:1718–1729.

62. Burstein HJ, Winer EP. Primary care for survivors of breast cancer. *N Engl J Med.* 2000;343:1086–1094.

63. Tham YL, Sexton K, Weiss H, et al. The rates of chemotherapy-induced amenorrhea in patients treated with adjuvant doxorubicin and cyclophosphamide followed by a taxane. *Am J Clin Oncol.* 2007;30:126–132.

64. Martin M, Pienkowski T, Mackey J, et al. Adjuvant docetaxel for node-positive breast cancer. *N Engl J Med.* 2005;352: 2302–2313.

65. Han HS, Ro J, Lee KS, et al. Analysis of chemotherapy-induced amenorrhea rates by three different anthracycline and taxane containing regimens for early breast cancer. *Breast Cancer Res Treat.* 2009;115:335–342.

66. Levine MN, Bramwell VH, Pritchard KI, et al. Randomized trial of intensive cyclophosphamide, epirubicin, and fluorouracil chemotherapy compared with cyclophosphamide, methotrexate, and fluorouracil in premenopausal women with node-positive breast cancer. National Cancer Institute of Canada Clinical Trials Group. *J Clin Oncol.* 1998;16:2651–2658.

67. Parulekar WR, Day AG, Ottaway JA, et al. Incidence and prognostic impact of amenorrhea during adjuvant therapy in high-risk premenopausal breast cancer: analysis of a National Cancer Institute of Canada Clinical Trials Group Study—NCIC CTG MA.5. *J Clin Oncol.* 2005;23:6002–6008.

68. Venturini M, Del Mastro L, Aitini E, et al. Dose-dense adjuvant chemotherapy in early breast cancer patients: results from a randomized trial. *J Natl Cancer Inst.* 2005;97:1724–1733.

5 Medical and Surgical Management of Atypical Hyperplasia and Lobular Carcinoma in situ

PRAKASH K. PANDALAI

VERÓNICA C. MARICIANI

MELINDA F. LERWILL

CONSTANCE A. ROCHE

KEVIN S. HUGHES

In addition to malignancy, the breast is the site of numerous benign diseases. More than 50% of women will develop some form of benign breast disease in their lifetime (1,2). The relationship between these benign conditions and the development of malignant disease has been a topic of controversy (3,4). Currently, the best characterized high-risk lesions are atypical ductal hyperplasia (ADH), atypical lobular hyperplasia (ALH), and lobular carcinoma in situ (LCIS). The major objectives of this chapter are to define these premalignant lesions, to describe their histological features, to describe the risk of invasive breast cancer they confer, to discuss associated factors that may increase this risk, and to outline our approach to the clinical management of patients with these conditions.

■ ATYPICAL DUCTAL HYPERPLASIA AND ATYPICAL LOBULAR HYPERPLASIA

Incidence

The widespread acceptance of screening mammography has increased the frequency of breast biopsies, most of which yield benign findings (5–7). Benign breast disease is a known risk factor for subsequent development of breast cancer. Early studies indicate an incidence of breast cancer from 1.4 to 2.7 times greater in women with histologically confirmed benign breast disease than in the general population. Among women with biopsy-confirmed benign disease, those with atypical hyperplasia have the highest breast cancer rate. In most studies, ADH and ALH have been combined into a single atypical hyperplasia category to strengthen the statistical power of the analysis because

both are relatively uncommon lesions. However, combining these two histologically distinct patterns of atypical hyperplasia into a single group potentially obscures important differences between them. The biological meaning of atypical hyperplastic lesions is controversial primarily because their natural history is unclear. A central issue is whether these atypical lesions are markers of general breast cancer risk or are precursor lesions.

In the classic series reported by Dupont and Page in 1985, 69.7% of 10,366 benign lesions examined could be classified as nonproliferative, 26.7% as proliferative lesions with hyperplasia, and 3.6% as atypical lesions (8). In the Mayo Clinic's series, the incidence of atypical hyperplasia was 3.7% in a cohort of 9,087 women with benign breast disease, as determined by open surgical biopsy (9). Among women who have a breast biopsy because of a palpable mass, atypical hyperplasia is seen in approximately 2% to 4% of cases (8,10). In contrast, atypical hyperplasia was identified in 12% to 17% of biopsies performed because of the presence of mammographic microcalcifications (11,12).

The overall incidence of atypical hyperplasia was roughly 3.7% in the series by Dupont and Page, with 2.1% classified as ADH and 1.6% as ALH (8). In a nested case-control study of participants in the Nurses' Health Study, the incidence of ADH was 7.3%, and the incidence of ALH was 3.8% (13). In another large retrospective study by Worsham, the incidence of ADH was 4% and that of ALH was 1% (14).

Risk of Breast Cancer

Two factors must be considered in assessing the risk of breast cancer associated with ADH and ALH: first, a number of studies report their results with ADH and ALH combined into a single category in order to improve statistical power; second, histological criteria used for classification of biopsy specimens are not always the same, which can result in differences among results from different series. Dupont and Page examined more than 10,000 biopsy specimens from two decades (8). Follow-up of these patients was more than 90% and averaged 17.5 years. Proliferative disease was noted in 1,925 women.

In women without atypia, a relative risk of 1.9 was seen, whereas the 232 women with atypical hyperplasia carried a fourfold increased risk of breast cancer, and the 39 women with both atypical hyperplasia and a positive family history of breast cancer carried a ninefold increased risk for subsequent breast cancer. A subgroup analysis later found that for women with ADH, the relative risk of subsequent cancer was increased 4.3-fold and, for those with ALH, 4.2-fold compared with the general population. Furthermore, of the 12% of women with ADH who went on to develop invasive cancer, 56% developed disease on the same side as the high-risk disease. The average interval from diagnosis of ADH until diagnosis of invasive cancer was 8.2 years. For women with ALH, 12.6% went on to develop invasive cancer, 69% in the same breast as the previous disease, and at an average of 11.9 years following diagnosis. This study confirmed that women with ADH and ALH carried a significantly greater risk of developing breast cancer than the general population and that follow-up was needed for more than a decade following excision (4).

The Nurses' Health Study reported a relative risk of 3.7 among women with atypical hyperplasia versus women with nonproliferative disease (15). Five-year follow-up including subtype analysis confirmed a relative risk for development of breast cancer of 3.4 for any atypical hyperplasia: 2.4 for ADH and 5.3 for ALH. The difference between these relative risks was of borderline statistical significance (16). A recent update of this cohort confirmed the relative risk of breast cancer of 4.0 for atypical hyperplasia; the relative risk for ADH was 3.9, lower than the relative risk of 5.49 seen with ALH (17). Among the small subset of women who had benign biopsies that showed both ADH and ALH, the relative risk of breast cancer was 6.94, although there were only 15 patients in

this subgroup. Although the risk of future breast cancer among women with ADH in this study was lower than the risk reported for women with ADH by Page and colleagues, these risk estimates are within the 95% confidence intervals of each other (Tables 5.1 and 5.2).

Variables Associated With Risk

Many factors have been studied that may change the magnitude of breast cancer risk in patients with ADH and ALH. The association of family history of breast cancer and the age at which the benign disease is diagnosed has been well investigated. Dupont and Page (4,8) demonstrated that patients with first-degree relatives with a history of breast cancer had a risk in the same range as women with lobular carcinoma in situ and 11 times higher (8.9) than patients with nonproliferative disease and no family history of breast cancer. In the same series, the relative risk specific for ADH was 3.2 when the family history was negative and 9.7 when it was positive. When a diagnosis of ALH and a positive family history are paired, there is an eightfold increased risk compared with the general population. This suggests a twofold additional risk when both an atypical lesion and a positive family history are present.

Family history alone was an independent risk factor for subsequent breast cancer in the Mayo Clinic series (18), with no additive elevation in risk of breast cancer based on the histology of the benign biopsy combined with a positive family history. In women with a strong family history of breast cancer, even nonproliferative findings were associated with a risk ratio of 1.62. In this series, women with atypia were at significantly increased risk, but family history did not significantly modify the atypia-associated risk.

■ Table 5.1 Relative risk of breast cancer defined by histological criteria of benign breast proliferative disease

Authors	Design	Nonproliferative	Proliferative Without Atypia	Atypical Hyperplasia
Dupont and Page (Ref. 8)	Retrospective	1	1.9	5.3
Marshall et al. (Ref. 16)	Case-control	1	1.6	3.9
Dupont et al. (Ref. 19)	Case-control	1	1.3	4.3

■ Table 5.2 Relative risk of breast cancer defined by histological criteria of benign breast disease

Authors	Atypical Hyperplasia	Atypical Ductal Hyperplasia	Atypical Lobular Hyperplasia
Page et al. (Ref. 4)	5.3	4.7	5.8
Marshall et al. (Ref. 16)	3.4	2.4	5.3

The Breast Cancer Detection Demonstration Project showed similar frequencies of breast cancer in women with atypia combined with a family history (6.1%) compared with those with atypia alone (4.9%) (19). Recent data from the Nurses' Health Study confirm the finding that a family history of breast cancer in a first-degree relative does not further increase risk in women with atypical hyperplasia (13). To explain these findings it has been postulated that atypical hyperplasia is a phenotype reflecting increased risk and that this phenotype derives from both inherited risk and lifetime exposures. Thus the histological presence of atypia could already reflect the increased breast cancer risk inherent in a positive family history. It is important to note that these studies contained a relatively small number of women who had the combination of atypical hyperplasia and a positive family history of breast cancer.

The association between age and menopausal status and breast cancer risk has been well characterized. London and colleagues demonstrated that the risk of breast cancer among women with atypical hyperplasia was higher among premenopausal women than among postmenopausal women (15). The relatively small number of patients in this study precluded a definitive association between menopause and breast cancer risk, but the variation in the relative risk with menopausal status was greater than that observed for age alone. The age at diagnosis of benign breast disease appears to modify the risk related to the histological appearance of benign breast disease. The presence of atypia in women under 45 years of age conveyed twice the risk observed among women over 55 years of age (6.99 and 3.37, respectively) (18). The Breast Cancer Detection and Demonstration Project showed that the risk of breast cancer among premenopausal women with atypia was elevated by a factor of 12.0, as compared with 3.3 among postmenopausal women with atypia (19). An alternate explanation of the effect of age on relative risk is that atypical hyperplasia produces almost the same absolute risk regardless of age. If so, the lower population risk of younger women and the higher population risk of older women would cause the relative risk of atypical hyperplasia to vary with age.

In the most recent report of the Mayo cohort, increasing risk was seen with greater numbers of foci of atypia: Relative risk (RR) = 2.33 with a single focus, 5.26 for two foci, and 7.97 for three or more foci (9). Risk was dramatically increased in the small group of women (n = 38) with both calcifications and three or more foci of atypia. If confirmed, this could reflect the identification of a new histological variable that appears to stratify risk in women with atypia: multifocality. In the highest-risk subgroup of women with three or more foci and histological calcifications, the cumulative incidence exceeded 50% over 25 years. This level of risk approaches that reported for carriers of *BRCA* mutations. It is postulated that a more widespread distribution of atypical foci within breast tissue signals a field defect that predisposes a woman to malignancy.

Time Course

It is debated whether there is any variation of risk related to the time elapsed since benign breast biopsy. According to Page and colleagues, the time between diagnosis of ADH and invasive carcinoma averaged 8.2 years and varied widely (4,8). Eight of these 18 women developed carcinoma within 5 years of biopsy, and a total of 14 had developed invasive disease within 10 years of biopsy. These patterns suggest that the breast cancer risk is greatest in the first 10 years after the benign breast biopsy.

Conversely, in the Nurses' Health Study, breast cancer risk remained elevated over time (16). The relative risk of breast cancer within 10 years after a benign breast biopsy was 3.31, whereas the risk of developing breast cancer more than 10 years after benign biopsy was 5.15. ALH was strongly associated with the development of breast cancer within 10 years [odds ratio (OR) = 5.57] compared with ADH (OR = 2.4). In contrast, the risk of breast cancer more than 10 years after the benign breast biopsy was similar for women with ALH (OR = 5.8) and women with ADH (OR = 4.82). Risk of breast cancer was fairly constant over time for women with ALH but increased over time for women with ADH, although this difference was not statistically significant. In the Mayo Clinic cohort the median time from the original biopsy to the diagnosis of breast cancer was 10.7 years, and the excess risk persisted for at least 25 years after the initial biopsy (9).

Laterality

The laterality of subsequent breast cancer in relation to the initial benign breast disease has been a subject of interest. Page and colleagues documented that 68% of subsequent breast cancers were found in the ipsilateral breast, while 24% were seen in the contralateral breast (4). Women with atypical hyperplasia in whom breast cancer developed within 10 years after the initial biopsy were 2.5 times more likely to have the cancer in the same breast as the original atypical hyperplasia (9). Studies examining laterality have demonstrated that only about half of the invasive breast cancers arise in the same breast in which atypical hyperplasia was previously diagnosed. In a case-control study, Collins and colleagues demonstrated that the site of invasive breast cancer was ipsilateral in 50% to 56% of women with ADH and in 58% to 69% of women with ALH (17). The consistency of these data suggests that breast cancer risk associated with atypical hyperplasia is bilateral. It has been considered indirect evidence that atypical lesions are risk markers rather than direct precursors of malignancy. Breast cancers occurring in the first 10 years after diagnosis of atypia may be more likely to occur in the ipsilateral breast, and a recent study of gene expression profiling identified remarkably similar alterations in gene expression among ADH, ductal carcinoma in situ (DCIS), and invasive cancers found in the same specimen, supporting the role of atypical hyperplasia as a precursor lesion (20), although these results remain inconclusive (Figures 5.1 and 5.2).

Surgical Management of ADH and ALH

Large-core needle biopsy of the breast has become a widely accepted alternative to open surgical biopsy for

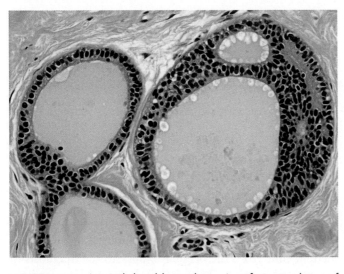

FIGURE 5.1 Atypical ductal hyperplasia. A uniform population of ductal cells with hyperchromatic nuclei has replaced the normal epithelium of these small ducts. There is focal cellular stratification and early cribriform space formation (right). Although low-grade cytological atypia is present, the degree of architectural atypia and the extent of duct involvement are limited. Thus the overall features fall short of a diagnosis of ductal carcinoma in situ.

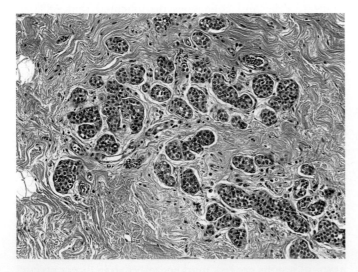

FIGURE 5.2 Atypical lobular hyperplasia. A monomorphic population of small, round cells demonstrates only minimal filling of the terminal duct lobular unit.

the initial diagnosis of suspicious abnormalities visible on mammography. The incidence of atypical hyperplasia is 2% to 11% of cases when percutaneous needle biopsy is performed for suspicious breast imaging findings (21–25). Because ADH and DCIS have been shown to be pathologically similar and often coexist, it is accepted that a diagnosis of ADH after image-guided core biopsy of a breast lesion may underestimate the presence of DCIS or invasive carcinoma (21–25). When the initial histopathological diagnosis of ADH is made and subsequent surgical excision reveals either DCIS or invasive carcinoma, the lesion is considered "upgraded." The reported rates of upgrade for ADH lesions is discussed on page 88. Following the diagnosis of ADH on percutaneous needle sampling, surgical excision should be performed to exclude the presence of noninvasive or invasive breast cancer.

■ LOBULAR CARCINOMA IN SITU

LCIS, first described by Foote and Stewart in 1941, was initially believed to be a premalignant lesion that would inevitably progress to invasive lobular carcinoma, and ipsilateral mastectomy was uniformly recommended (26). Long term follow-up of these patients demonstrated that many developed carcinoma in the contralateral breast, suggesting that LCIS was a marker of overall risk rather than a direct precursor. It is now understood that about 20% to 30% of women with LCIS will develop breast cancer, most commonly invasive ductal carcinoma. LCIS has been extensively characterized, and its management has undergone considerable evolution. Given the current understanding of the natural history of LCIS, surveillance, with the possible addition of chemoprevention, has become the accepted practice.

Incidence

The true incidence of LCIS in the general population is uncertain. Autopsy studies suggest an incidence of 0.5% to 3% (27,28). In the premammography era, LCIS predominated over its noninvasive counterpart, DCIS, by as much as 3:1 (29,30); however, this has changed dramatically with the widespread use of screening mammography since the early 1980s, with DCIS now predominating 5:1 over LCIS (31). LCIS is now found in 1.1% to 1.6% of all breast biopsies (31,32). It should be noted that LCIS is seldom associated with a mass lesion and does not seem to produce calcifications, and hence it is usually an incidental finding. This explains why its incidence has not markedly increased with widespread mammography, as has the incidence of DCIS. The mean age at diagnosis is 44 to 47 years (27,33,34).

Risk of Breast Cancer

LCIS is considered a high-risk lesion, conferring a risk of developing invasive breast cancer of about 1% to 2% per year, with a lifetime risk of 30% to 40% (34,35). This represents an eightfold to tenfold increased risk of invasive breast cancer compared with the general population. The earliest report of subsequent cancer risk after a diagnosis of LCIS was by Hutter and Foote in 1969 (36). This series demonstrated development of breast cancer in 15 of 46 (33%) women with LCIS. In subsequent studies, breast cancer was found to occur in the contralateral breast in 9.3% and in the ipsilateral breast in 15% of patients with previously diagnosed LCIS (33,37). These early reports were criticized for their small sample size and lack of uniform histopathological classification. In 1978, Haagensen published the largest series at the time, consisting of 211 patients (34). This study was unique in that standard criteria were applied in distinguishing LCIS lesions. It was also seminal in that Haagensen chose to observe LCIS rather than perform bilateral mastectomy, which had been the standard approach. Of the 211 patients, 36 (17%) developed invasive cancer over 15 years of follow-up. Of the subsequent cancers that were diagnosed, 20 were ipsilateral and 19 contralateral to the original LCIS diagnosis. This study concluded that LCIS predisposed women to a significant degree of subsequent carcinoma, that the interval of this development was fairly long, and that the risk was bilateral. It suggested that bilateral mastectomy was unjustified.

In 1991 Page and colleagues confirmed an absolute risk of breast cancer of 17% following a diagnosis of LCIS over a follow-up period of 15 years (38). The authors reviewed more than 10,000 biopsies performed over 10 years and identified 49 cases of LCIS using strict criteria, an incidence of 0.5%. This study demonstrated an eightfold increased risk of subsequent cancer within 15 years of LCIS diagnosis compared with the general population. Among women with LCIS, 45% were under the age of 45. Contrary to the notion that LCIS was not associated with mammographic findings, this study found that 33% of women with LCIS had microcalcifications identified histologically, versus only 10% in the control group. The risk of malignancy was again noted to be bilateral in this study population, and family history was not a significant additive risk factor. While the number of women who ultimately developed invasive cancers was small, the authors note that their criteria for defining LCIS were stricter than those in any previous study and that previous studies with higher rates of malignancy included a more heterogeneous population of patients. Of the 10 women who developed invasive breast cancer, 9 had cancer of the lobular subtype, in stark contrast to previous studies suggesting that invasive ductal cancer was the predominant form of cancer associated with LCIS.

Variables Associated With Risk

Time Course

The relationship between risk and time was first reported in 1991 by Page and Kidd (38). Using a novel time-dependent hazard model they documented that women with LCIS have a relative risk of 10.8 for development of invasive breast cancer during the first 15 years after biopsy. This study showed that for those women who remain free of disease for 15 years, the relative risk after this time is reduced to 4.2, but the numbers of patients in this study was small and this reduction in risk has not been confirmed by other studies.

Laterality

Women with LCIS are at increased risk of developing breast cancer in either breast. Numerous studies have shown that LCIS is itself commonly bilateral and multicentric (37). More than 50% of women with LCIS have multicentric disease in the ipsilateral breast, and up to 30% have involvement of the contralateral breast (39,40). Cancer was noted in the contralateral breast in 9.3% and in the ipsilateral breast in 15% of patients with previously diagnosed LCIS (34,37). In a meta-analysis of 228 women diagnosed with LCIS that was treated with observation after excision, 15.1% went on to develop invasive breast cancer in the ipsilateral breast and 9.3% in the contralateral breast (37). Rates of breast cancer in the contralateral breast were three times higher in women with LCIS than in the general population (41). Recent literature confirms the finding that the ipsilateral breast is still at three times greater risk for malignancy in women with LCIS (16,42).

Surgical Management of LCIS

It is generally accepted that LCIS diagnosed on excisional biopsy does not warrant further surgical treatment. Wide surgical excision with histologically negative margins is not advocated, because LCIS is multicentric and bilateral in 23% to 35% of women (39). Continued surveillance is mandatory, and chemoprevention in these high-risk women may be beneficial.

In the past, prophylactic bilateral mastectomy played a role in the surgical management of LCIS. In the original description of LCIS in 1941, Foote and Stewart suggested that their observations of bilateral disease and bilateral subsequent risk of malignancy made surgical excision of both breasts the ideal prevention strategy (27). This was the prevailing dogma for the next several years. In 1978, however, Haagensen challenged this concept by reporting that while women with LCIS certainly were at higher risk than the general population, the majority do not go on to develop breast cancer (35). He concluded that "we do not recommend mastectomy for lobular neoplasia, but only systematic follow-up by palpation." In that same year

Rosen published another large series of 99 patients with LCIS and drew the opposite conclusion, suggesting that "follow-up without further surgery should be considered an investigative procedure" (40). Both these studies were reported in the era before screening mammography, when the ability to find early cancer was limited, and the mortality from breast cancer was high. With the advent of effective screening, the use of bilateral mastectomy for this disease has become uncommon, if not rare, and surveillance with clinical breast examination every 6 to 12 months and annual mammography has become standard. Bradley and colleagues published a meta-analysis that included 389 women who underwent local excision and surveillance and were followed for a mean of 10.9 years (52). Invasive cancer was seen in 16.4% of these women, who were then treated with mastectomy, and the cancer-related mortality was 2.8%, not statistically different from that in a cohort of 391 women who underwent mastectomy initially. This confirms the efficacy of surveillance in women with LCIS (Figures 5.3–5.5).

■ MANAGEMENT OF ATYPICAL HYPERPLASIA AND LCIS FOUND ON CORE BIOPSY

It is important to note that estimates of breast cancer risk are based on the follow-up of patients in whom ADH was identified in excisional biopsy specimens. When ADH is encountered in core needle biopsy specimens taken because of a mammographic abnormality, the major concern is whether the histological finding of ADH in the core biopsy is completely representative of the target lesion. This concern is due to the recognition that in many cases

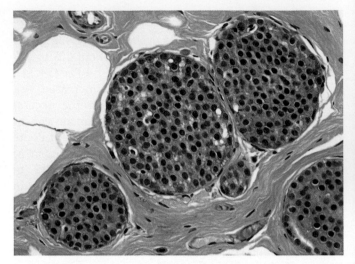

FIGURE 5.4 Typical cytological features of lobular carcinoma in situ. The lobular carcinoma cells are cytologically uniform, with relatively small nuclei and limited amounts of eosinophilic cytoplasm.

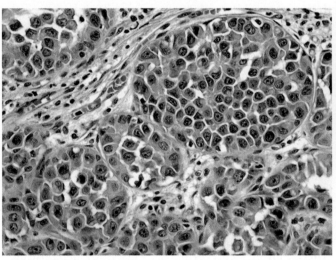

FIGURE 5.5 Pleomorphic lobular carcinoma in situ. In contrast to classic lobular carcinoma in situ, the cells of pleomorphic lobular carcinoma in situ have larger, more atypical nuclei with coarser chromatin and prominent nucleoli.

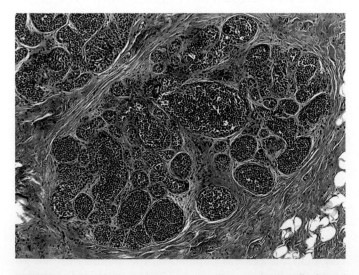

FIGURE 5.3 Lobular carcinoma in situ. The neoplastic cells distend more than 50% of the acini in the terminal duct lobular units. The loosely cohesive lobular carcinoma cells have a solid growth pattern.

there are foci of ADH adjacent to DCIS. Making the distinction between ADH and low-grade DCIS is sometimes challenging in surgical biopsy specimens. It can be even more difficult on the limited tissue sample obtained during core biopsy. Studies using the automated biopsy gun method and 14-gauge needles have shown that ADH on core biopsy may prove to be frank carcinoma if additional tissue is obtained, with carcinoma found in up to 50% of cases when surgical excision is performed, with about two-thirds being DCIS. Data from series using larger-gauge and vacuum-assisted core biopsies have shown a lower rate of underdiagnosis of carcinoma among patients with ADH on core biopsy, presumably the result of more extensive tissue sampling and the greater likelihood of complete removal of the radiologically targeted lesions. The risk of underdiagnosis with 11-gauge vacuum-assisted biopsy devices has been reported to be about 15% to 19% in different series. Other factors related to the likelihood of underdiagnosis of malignancy include the extent to which the mammographic lesion has been sampled and the nature of the mammographic lesion being targeted. Carcinoma was found at excision in 30% of those in whom the targeted lesion was microcalcifications, compared with 5% of those in whom the target lesion was a mass (21).

Ely and colleagues assessed the risk of carcinoma based on the number of foci of ADH present in the surgical excision (43). None of the 24 cases in which ADH involved two or fewer foci had carcinoma on excision. In contrast, of the 15 cases with four or more foci of ADH on core biopsy, 13 (86.7%) had carcinoma on excision (12 DCIS and 1 invasive carcinoma). When LCIS is seen on biopsy, concurrent invasive lobular carcinoma is found 5% to 16% of the time (44).

■ CHEMOPREVENTION FOR HIGH-RISK LESIONS

The role of estrogen in the development of breast cancer has long been recognized. Selective estrogen receptor modulators (SERMs) that antagonize estrogen receptors in some tissues and mimic their action in other tissues play a key role in chemoprevention strategies. The National Surgical Adjuvant Breast and Bowel Project (NSABP P-1) evaluated the use of tamoxifen for the prevention of breast cancer in 13,175 women considered at high risk (45). Inclusion criteria were strict, and high risk was defined as age >60 years or between 35 and 59 years of age with a 5-year Gail model–predicted risk of 1.66% or a history of LCIS. These high-risk women were randomized to receive 20 mg of tamoxifen or placebo daily for 5 years. This study demonstrated a 49% risk reduction in invasive breast cancer and a 50% risk reduction in noninvasive breast cancer overall. Subgroup analysis of the 6.3% of women with LCIS showed a 56% risk reduction in breast cancer development. These results also demonstrated the risk of subsequent breast cancer in women with LCIS to be 12.9 per 1,000 women, which is a 5-year breast cancer rate of 6.5%. Subgroup analysis of the 8.8% of women with atypical hyperplasia showed an 86% risk reduction in breast cancer development.

Recent evidence suggests a similar risk reduction with raloxifene. The NSABP P-2 study randomized more than 19,000 women with a 5-year Gail model–predicted risk of 1.66% who were at least 35 years old and postmenopausal to receive either tamoxifen or raloxifene, a second-generation SERM (46). Although there was no difference in effect between tamoxifen and raloxifene on the incidence of invasive breast cancer, tamoxifen was superior to raloxifene in the reduction of carcinoma in situ (DCIS and LCIS cases combined). In subgroup analyses of women with LCIS or atypical hyperplasia, tamoxifen and raloxifene were equivalent for risk reduction.

Aromatase inhibitors have been shown to decrease the risk of contralateral breast cancer in women treated for primary breast cancer (47–50). Data from several adjuvant trials has led to two large trials studying the use of aromatase inhibitors for prevention, one using anastrozole and the other exemestane. The International Breast Cancer Intervention Study (IBIS)-II trial is comparing anastrozole to placebo in 6,000 postmenopausal women at increased risk of breast cancer. The NCIC trial is comparing 5 years of exemestane versus placebo in 3,000 postmenopausal women at increased risk. Eligibility in both studies includes: (a) a Gail score >1.66, (b) age >60 years, (c) prior ADH or ALH, and (d) DCIS treated with mastectomy (51).

■ SUMMARY OF ADH AND ALH

ADH and ALH are benign breast lesions that confer an increased risk of subsequent breast cancer four times that of the normal population. Lesions that demonstrate all the qualitative features of DCIS but fail to meet the size criterion are classified as ADH. ADH is present in 5% to 17% of breast biopsies performed for calcifications and less frequently in biopsies performed for mammographic densities or palpable masses. ALH is a cellular proliferation identical to LCIS, with involvement of less than 50% of the lobule. ALH is an incidental finding present in fewer than 5% of biopsies performed for any reason. It is accepted that the risk of subsequent breast cancer among women with atypical hyperplasia is between 3.7 and 5.3 times that of the general population. For women diagnosed with ADH on biopsy, the risk of developing breast cancer is roughly four times that of the general population. Women with ALH carry a fivefold elevation for subsequent breast cancer compared with the general population. For women with ADH or ALH and a family history of breast cancer in a first-degree relative, there is a risk of subsequent breast cancer (ninefold increase) that is twice as high as that of women with ADH/ALH alone (fourfold increase). It is unclear whether high-risk lesions developing in women with a family history represent transmitted genetic aberrations or represent a larger field defect within breast tissue. The relationship between these high-risk lesions and family history remains to be elucidated. The risk for subsequent breast cancer continues for up to 20 years following the diagnosis of ADH or ALH, although the highest risk occurs within the first decade after diagnosis. These women are at greatest risk for the development of invasive ductal carcinoma.

ADH or ALH diagnosed on core needle biopsy mandates surgical excision to rule out adjacent noninvasive or invasive breast cancer, which is demonstrated on 15% to 60% of specimens following surgical excision. Negative surgical margins are not required on excisional biopsies for ADH and ALH. Following treatment, continued surveillance with monthly self breast exams, clinical breast exams every 6 to 12 months, and annual mammography is the standard of care. Large randomized trials have shown a benefit of chemoprevention with either tamoxifen or raloxifene. The administration of tamoxifen increases the risk of endometrial cancer, and both agents increase the risk of thromboembolic events, factors that must be assessed in relation to potential gains in breast cancer risk reduction.

■ SUMMARY OF LCIS

LCIS is an incidental finding on breast biopsy performed for other indications. LCIS is found in approximately 1.5% of all biopsies performed. LCIS is typically diagnosed in premenopausal women and is multicentric and bilateral in 30% to 50% of women. LCIS confers a risk of breast cancer up to 10 times that of the general population, with a 1% to 2% annual risk that persists for the patient's lifetime. Both breasts are at risk for either invasive ductal or invasive lobular carcinoma. While invasive ductal cancer predominates in this population, the incidence of invasive lobular cancer is higher in these women than in the general population. LCIS diagnosed on excisional biopsy does not warrant further surgery; however, LCIS seen on core needle biopsy currently is followed by excision to rule out an undiagnosed invasive component. Excision with negative margins is not necessary for pure LCIS. Following treatment, continued surveillance with monthly self breast exams, clinical breast exams every 6 to 12 months, and annual mammography is the standard of care. Large randomized trials have shown a significant benefit to chemoprevention with either tamoxifen or raloxifene in these high-risk women. The administration of tamoxifen increases the risk of endometrial cancer, and both agents increase the risk of thromboembolic events, factors that must be assessed in relation to potential gains in breast cancer risk reduction.

■ REFERENCES

1. Kalache A. Risk factors for breast cancer: a tabular summary of the epidemiological literature. *Br J Surg.* 1981;68(11):797–799.
2. Wellings SR, Jensen HM, Marcum RG. An atlas of subgross pathology of the human breast with special reference to possible precancerous lesions. *J Natl Cancer Inst.* 1975;55(2):231–273.
3. Black MM, Asire AJ. Palpable axillary lymph nodes in cancer of the breast. Structural and biologic considerations. *Cancer.* 1969;23(2):251–259.
4. Page DL, et al. Atypical hyperplastic lesions of the female breast. A long-term follow-up study. *Cancer.* 1985;55(11):2698–2708.
5. Choucair RJ, et al. Biopsy of nonpalpable breast lesions. *Am J Surg.* 1988;156(6):453–456.
6. Schwartz GF, Feig SA, Patchefsky AS. Significance and staging of nonpalpable carcinomas of the breast. *Surg Gynecol Obstet.* 1988;166(1):6–10.
7. Thompson WR, et al. Mammographic localization and biopsy of nonpalpable breast lesions. A 5-year study. *Arch Surg.* 1991;126(6):730–733; discussion 733–734.
8. Dupont WD, Page DL. Risk factors for breast cancer in women with proliferative breast disease. *N Engl J Med.* 1985;312(3):146–151.
9. Degnim AC, et al. Stratification of breast cancer risk in women with atypia: a Mayo cohort study. *J Clin Oncol.* 2007;25(19):2671–2677.
10. Schnitt SJ, Morrow M. Lobular carcinoma in situ: current concepts and controversies. *Semin Diagn Pathol.* 1999;16(3):209–223.
11. Owings DV, Hann L, Schnitt SJ. How thoroughly should needle localization breast biopsies be sampled for microscopic examination? A prospective mammographic/pathologic correlative study. *Am J Surg Pathol.* 1990;14(6):578–583.
12. Rubin E, et al. Proliferative disease and atypia in biopsies performed for nonpalpable lesions detected mammographically. *Cancer.* 1988;61(10):2077–2082.
13. Collins LC, et al. The influence of family history on breast cancer risk in women with biopsy-confirmed benign breast disease: results from the Nurses' Health Study. *Cancer.* 2006;107(6):1240–1247.
14. Worsham MJ, et al. Breast cancer incidence in a cohort of women with benign breast disease from a multiethnic, primary health care population. *Breast J.* 2007;13(2):115–121.
15. London SJ, et al. A prospective study of benign breast disease and the risk of breast cancer. *JAMA.* 1992;267(7):941–944.
16. Marshall LM, et al. Risk of breast cancer associated with atypical hyperplasia of lobular and ductal types. *Cancer Epidemiol Biomarkers Prev.* 1997;6(5):297–301.
17. Collins LC, et al. Magnitude and laterality of breast cancer risk according to histologic type of atypical hyperplasia: results from the Nurses' Health Study. *Cancer.* 2007;109(2):180–187.
18. Hartmann LC, et al. Benign breast disease and the risk of breast cancer. *N Engl J Med.* 2005;353(3):229–237.
19. Dupont WD, et al. Breast cancer risk associated with proliferative breast disease and atypical hyperplasia. *Cancer.* 1993;71(4):1258–1265.
20. Ma XJ, et al. Gene expression profiles of human breast cancer progression. *Proc Natl Acad Sci U S A.* 2003;100(10):5974–5979.
21. Darling ML, et al. Atypical ductal hyperplasia and ductal carcinoma in situ as revealed by large-core needle breast biopsy: results of surgical excision. *AJR Am J Roentgenol.* 2000;175(5):1341–1346.
22. Jackman RJ, et al. Stereotaxic large-core needle biopsy of 450 nonpalpable breast lesions with surgical correlation in lesions with cancer or atypical hyperplasia. *Radiology.* 1994;193(1):91–95.
23. Liberman L, et al. Atypical ductal hyperplasia diagnosed at stereotaxic core biopsy of breast lesions: an indication for surgical biopsy. *AJR Am J Roentgenol.* 1995;164(5):1111–1113.
24. Liberman L, et al. Analysis of cancers not diagnosed at stereotactic core breast biopsy. *Radiology.* 1997;203(1):151–157.
25. Tocino I, Garcia BM, Carter D. Surgical biopsy findings in patients with atypical hyperplasia diagnosed by stereotaxic core needle biopsy. *Ann Surg Oncol.* 1996;3(5):483–488.
26. Hutter RV. Classics in Oncology. Lobular carcinoma in situ by Foote and Stewart. *CA Cancer J Clin.* 1982;32(4):232–237.
27. Page DL and Dupont WD. Proliferative breast disease: diagnosis and implications. *Science.* 1991;253(5022):915–916.

28. Li CI, et al. Risk of invasive breast carcinoma among women diagnosed with ductal carcinoma in situ and lobular carcinoma in situ, 1988–2001. *Cancer.* 2006;106(10):2104–2112.

29. Rosner D, et al. Noninvasive breast carcinoma: results of a national survey by the American College of Surgeons. *Ann Surg.* 1980; 192(2):139–147.

30. Frykberg ER, et al. Lobular carcinoma in situ of the breast. *Surg Gynecol Obstet.* 1987;164(3):285–301.

31. Frykberg ER. Lobular carcinoma in situ of the breast. *Breast J.* 1999;5(5):296–303.

32. Bland KI, et al. The National Cancer Data Base 10-year survey of breast carcinoma treatment at hospitals in the United States. *Cancer.* 1998;83(6):1262–1273.

33. Wheeler JE, et al. Lobular carcinoma in situ of the breast. Long-term followup. *Cancer.* 1974;34(3):554–563.

34. Haagensen CD, et al. Lobular neoplasia (so-called lobular carcinoma in situ) of the breast. *Cancer.* 1978;42(2):737–769.

35. Anderson JA. Invasive breast carcinoma with lobular involvement. Frequency and location of lobular carcinoma in situ. *Acta Pathol Microbiol Scand [A].* 1974;82(6):719–729.

36. Hutter RV, Foote FW. Lobular carcinoma in situ. Long-term follow-up. *Cancer.* 1969;24(5):1081–1085.

37. Anderson JA. Multicentric and bilateral appearance of lobular carcinoma in situ of the breast. *Acta Pathol Microbiol Scand [A].* 1974;82(6):730–734.

38. Page DL, et al. Lobular neoplasia of the breast: higher risk for subsequent invasive cancer predicted by more extensive disease. *Hum Pathol.* 1991;22(12):1232–1239.

39. Urban JA. Bilaterality of cancer of the breast. Biopsy of the opposite breast. *Cancer.* 1967;20(11):1867–1870.

40. Rosen PP, et al. Lobular carcinoma in situ of the breast. Detailed analysis of 99 patients with average follow-up of 24 years. *Am J Surg Pathol.* 1978;2(3):225–251.

41. Haagensen CD, Lane N, Bodian C. Coexisting lobular neoplasia and carcinoma of the breast. *Cancer.* 1983;51(8):1468–1482.

42. Page DL, et al. Atypical lobular hyperplasia as a unilateral predictor of breast cancer risk: a retrospective cohort study. *Lancet.* 2003;361(9352):125–129.

43. Ely KA, et al. Core biopsy of the breast with atypical ductal hyperplasia: a probabilistic approach to reporting. *Am J Surg Pathol.* 2001;25(8):1017–1021.

44. Hutter RV. The management of patients with lobular carcinoma in situ of the breast. *Cancer.* 1984;53(3 Suppl):798–802.

45. Fisher B, et al. Tamoxifen for prevention of breast cancer: report of the National Surgical Adjuvant Breast and Bowel Project P-1 Study. *J Natl Cancer Inst.* 1998;90(18):1371–1388.

46. Vogel VG, et al. Effects of tamoxifen vs raloxifene on the risk of developing invasive breast cancer and other disease outcomes: the NSABP Study of Tamoxifen and Raloxifene (STAR) P-2 trial. *JAMA.* 2006;295(23):2727–2741.

47. Howell A, et al. Results of the ATAC (arimidex, tamoxifen, alone or in combination) trial after completion of 5 years' adjuvant treatment for breast cancer. *Lancet.* 2005;365(9453):60–62.

48. Boccardo F, et al. Switching to anastrozole versus continued tamoxifen treatment of early breast cancer: preliminary results of the Italian Tamoxifen Anastrozole Trial. *J Clin Oncol.* 2005; 23(22):5138–5147.

49. Coates AS, et al. Five years of letrozole compared with tamoxifen as initial adjuvant therapy for postmenopausal women with endocrine-responsive early breast cancer: update of study BIG 1-98. *J Clin Oncol.* 2007;25(5):486–492.

50. Goss PE, et al. A randomized trial of letrozole in postmenopausal women after five years of tamoxifen therapy for early-stage breast cancer. *N Engl J Med.* 2003;349(19):1793–1802.

51. Cuzick J. Chemoprevention of breast cancer. *Breast Cancer.* 2008;15(1):10–16.

52. Bradley SJ, Weaner DW, Bowman DL. Alternatives in surgical management of in situ breast cancer. A meta-analysis of outcome. *American Surgeon.* 1990;56(7):428–432.

6 Multidisciplinary Approach in the Treatment of Ductal Carcinoma in situ

Surgical Management of DCIS

MICHELLE SPECHT

■ INCIDENCE AND NATURAL HISTORY

Ductal carcinoma in situ (DCIS) accounts for approximately 20% of breast cancers identified in the United States (1,2), up from 5% of cancers in the early 1980s, largely owing to increasing use of screening mammography (3).

Histologically, DCIS is characterized by a proliferation of malignant epithelial cells that fill the lumen of the ducts without invasion through the basement membrane. DCIS is thought to be a nonobligate precursor to invasive breast cancer. It is postulated that up to 47% to 86% of patients with DCIS will not progress to invasive breast cancer even after 30 years of follow-up (4–7). In one cohort of patients with low-grade DCIS treated with excisional biopsy alone, only 39% of patients progressed to ipsilateral invasive cancer at 30 years of follow-up (8). Currently, information regarding factors that predict progression to invasion is limited, and therefore treatment of DCIS is predicated on treating all DCIS as if it has the potential to progress to invasive breast cancer.

■ DIAGNOSIS OF DCIS

DCIS may be detected by screening mammography, clinical breast exam, or screening breast magnetic resonance imaging (MRI). More than 90% of DCIS is found via mammography, most commonly as microcalcifications (9,10). About 10% of DCIS is mammographically occult and presents as a palpable mass, as nipple discharge (11), or on MRI. Recent reports demonstrate that MRI has a sensitivity for detection of DCIS ranging from 88% to 92% (12,13).

Historically, open surgical biopsy using wire localization was the only method to sample suspicious microcalcifications. Today, management guidelines recommend tissue sampling of suspicious mammographic lesions via stereotactic guided vacuum-assisted biopsy rather than open surgical biopsy, whenever possible. Stereotactic core needle biopsy provides an accurate, minimally invasive method of tissue acquisition. Core biopsy is immediately followed by placement of a radioopaque clip at the site of biopsy that is easily detected on subsequent breast imaging and allows localization of the site for further excision if malignancy is found. Interestingly, a review of the Surveillance, Epidemiology and End Results (SEER) database between 1991 and 1999 demonstrated a percutaneous needle biopsy rate of 24%, with a majority of surgeons continuing to use open surgical biopsy, although use of percutaneous biopsy did increase over time (14). A recent single-institution review demonstrated a percutaneous biopsy rate of 40% for mammographically suspicious lesions in 2007 (15).

■ SURGICAL TREATMENT OPTIONS FOR DCIS

For many years, DCIS was treated primarily with modified radical mastectomy, which resulted in very low rates of local or distant recurrence. A meta-analysis of 21 studies including 1,574 patients with DCIS treated with mastectomy demonstrated a local recurrence rate of only 1.4% (16). When data from trials comparing mastectomy to breast conservation in patients with invasive breast cancer demonstrated low rates of local recurrences and equivalent survival (17), nonrandomized trials were initiated to evaluate the safety of breast conservation in patients with DCIS (18–20). These nonrandomized trials revealed local recurrence rates of 11% to 13% at 10 years after wide excision with radiation therapy for DCIS. Randomized trials of wide excision with or without radiation for DCIS showed ipsilateral local recurrence rates of 22% to 31.7% without radiation and 7% to 16% with radiation therapy (21–24). Approximately 30% to 35% of patients with DCIS are treated with mastectomy today (25).

■ PREOPERATIVE PLANNING: LUMPECTOMY VERSUS MASTECTOMY

Multiple factors impact the decision for lumpectomy or mastectomy in DCIS and may require input from breast imaging, surgical oncology, radiation oncology, plastic surgery, and medical oncology specialists, as well as from the patient. A multidisciplinary clinic is an excellent way to inform the patient of her options and develop a treatment plan.

Prior to lumpectomy, it is important to obtain a detailed imaging evaluation. Magnification views of the affected breast are performed to rule out multicentric disease and help delineate the extent of the mammographic abnormality. If there is no evidence of multicentric disease, which would warrant a mastectomy, the extent of calcifications associated with biopsy-proven DCIS should be mapped. Unfortunately, the extent of the calcifications may underestimate the pathological size of the lesion (13), and even with excision of all suspicious microcalcifications, DCIS may be found at the margins.

MRI has shown high sensitivity for detection of DCIS (12,13) and is used increasingly to assess the extent of DCIS prior to surgery. However, it has been shown that breast MRI may overestimate the extent of DCIS (13). To date, there are no prospective data evaluating the ability of MRI to improve local failure rates after breast conservation therapy in DCIS. In a retrospective review of a cohort of 756 women treated with breast conservation for early-stage invasive breast cancer or DCIS, Solin and colleagues did not find any reduction in local recurrence in women evaluated with breast MRI prior to definitive surgery (26). At this time, selective use of MRI is favored for patients diagnosed with DCIS where necessary to determine multicentricity and extent of disease and to screen the contralateral breast.

Once it has been determined that a DCIS lesion is amenable to breast conservation, developing a plan for optimal localization in collaboration with the breast imaging team is critical. If the volume of disease is small, a single-wire needle localization procedure may be performed. If calcifications are extensive or in an eccentric shape, multiple-wire bracketed lumpectomy has been shown to increase breast conservation rates and decrease re-excision rates (27). MRI-guided localization with a bracketed wire technique may help in defining the extent of small invasive breast cancers for excision but may also overestimate the volume of DCIS lesions and therefore lead to excision of excess normal breast tissue (13).

■ OPTIMIZING LUMPECTOMY MARGINS

In order to minimize risk of local recurrence, margins on a lumpectomy for DCIS must be free of tumor. There is,

however, no consensus on what defines a clear margin, with recommendations ranging from at least 1 mm to at least 10 mm.

There is no consensus as to the optimum margin width for DCIS when wide excision and radiation therapy are used. A meta-analysis of 4,660 DCIS patients demonstrated that the likelihood of an ipsilateral breast recurrence was significantly decreased when margins were 2 mm or wider compared with patients whose margins were less than 2 mm. In addition, there was no significant difference in local recurrence in patients with a 2 mm margin compared with a 5 mm or greater clear margin. Therefore, the authors concluded that a clear margin of 2 mm was appropriate for DCIS patients treated with lumpectomy and radiation therapy (28).

It has been suggested that radiation may be omitted for select DCIS lesions that are excised with a sufficiently wide margin. Silverstein and colleagues reported that wide excision alone of DCIS with a margin of at least 10 mm resulted in a local recurrence rate of 6% at 53 months of follow-up (29). This retrospective, nonrandomized analysis is unique in its low rate of local recurrence after wide excision without radiation. A single-arm prospective trial of 158 patients who underwent wide excision without radiation for grade 1 or 2 DCIS measuring 2.5 cm or less, with at least 1 cm clear margins, failed to confirm low local recurrence rate when radiation was omitted. Patients in this trial had a 2.4% annual rate of ipsilateral breast recurrence, with an actuarial recurrence rate of 12% at 5 years (30). Finally, a prospective trial following 580 grade 1 or 2 DCIS lesions measuring 2.5 cm or less and 102 patients with high-grade DCIS measuring 1 cm or less excised with at least 3 mm of clear margin reported 5-year ipsilateral recurrence rates of 6.8% and 14.8%, respectively (31). Further follow-up in these large trials will help to define appropriate margin width and select patients who may be candidates for wide excision alone.

Limitations of currently available preoperative breast imaging modalities prevent accurate assessment of the actual histopathological extent of DCIS preoperatively. As a result, approximately 50% of lumpectomies for DCIS will have close or positive margins (32–34). Since such a large fraction of DCIS patients will require re-excision, the initial lumpectomy must be performed in a manner that facilitates margin assessment and potential re-excision.

Accurate assessment of margins requires specimen orientation at the time of excision with placement of sutures to orient the lumpectomy or with intraoperative application of multicolor inks by the surgeon. By orienting the specimen, the pathologist can then report which margins are close or positive with DCIS. A targeted, rather than global, re-excision of the involved margin(s) as a second procedure may then be performed. This selective re-excision can decrease the overall volume of tissue excised and yield a better cosmetic result.

An intraoperative specimen radiograph is performed to confirm complete excision of the mammographic abnormality and may also aid in attaining clear margins. Identification of calcifications extending to the margin of the lumpectomy specimen indicates the need for additional excision of that margin at the time of surgery.

Some authors have advocated routinely re-excising the cavity at the time of initial lumpectomy by obtaining additional oriented shaved margins to decrease risk of positive margins (32–34). The use of shaved margins may decrease the likelihood of a falsely positive margin that results from seepage of the ink into cracks in the lumpectomy specimen or inadvertent removal of friable tissue at the edge of the lumpectomy specimen. Some centers have adopted intraoperative frozen section of margins for patients undergoing wide excision for breast cancer, and this has decreased the need for a second operation in patients with invasive breast cancer and to a lesser extent for patients with DCIS (35).

If the margin of the initial lumpectomy is positive for DCIS, then the decision must be made as to whether to proceed with a re-excision or convert to mastectomy. Factors that influence this decision include: the likelihood of a successful re-excision, the ability to maintain a good cosmetic result after removal of additional tissue, and patient preference. Re-excision is usually performed within 4 to 6 weeks of the initial lumpectomy to ensure that a seroma cavity is still present but to allow some of the initial tissue edema to resolve. A postexcision mammogram to look for residual calcifications is performed 3 to 6 weeks after surgery and prior to re-excision at some centers. Needle localization of the residual calcifications at the time of re-excision may increase the chance of obtaining clear margins.

select patients may be considered for wide excision without radiation.

Some patients with DCIS may begin their surgical treatment with lumpectomy but ultimately be treated with mastectomy when multiple re-excisions demonstrate residual DCIS and clear margins cannot be obtained. There is no specific limit to the number of re-excisions that may be performed before a recommendation for mastectomy is made. Rather, it is a decision that is based on the total volume of tissue excised in relationship to the overall volume of the breast, the cosmetic result obtained, and the patient's desire for breast conservation.

A family history of breast cancer may play a role in the decision to opt for mastectomy. Patients who are diagnosed with DCIS in the context of a positive gene mutation for *BRCA1* or *BRCA2* have a 40% likelihood of a contralateral breast cancer at 10 years (36). Therefore, some patients with a *BRCA* mutation may choose to treat their DCIS with bilateral mastectomies in order to decrease the likelihood of a second breast cancer.

Patient preference is a strong predictor of choice in local treatment. Overall survival for patients with DCIS is greater than 97% (20). Consequently, the greatest risks associated with DCIS are local recurrence or development of a new primary breast cancer. In patients with DCIS who do not have a risk gene mutation, the risk of a second breast cancer is estimated to be about 1% per year. Some women may opt to treat their DCIS with bilateral mastectomy in order to avoid this risk of a second cancer. However, it is important to ensure that these patients completely understand DCIS, including their risk of local recurrence and their extremely low risk of a systemic recurrence. In a longitudinal cohort study of women diagnosed with DCIS, researchers demonstrated that more than 50% of women overestimated the risk of subsequent breast cancer (37).

■ MASTECTOMY FOR DCIS

Total mastectomy is indicated for patients with multicentric DCIS, for those with diffuse microcalcifications that occupy a large proportion of the breast, for patients with a contraindication to radiation therapy, for positive margins after re-excision, and for patient preference. Multicentric DCIS is defined as DCIS that occupies sites in more than one quadrant of the breast. Stereotactic core biopsy of separate areas of mammographic abnormality may be performed to prove multicentricity. Radiation therapy after lumpectomy is contraindicated in a patient with active collagen vascular disease (such as scleroderma or systemic lupus) or a patient with previous therapeutic radiation to the breast or chest (e.g., mantle irradiation for Hodgkin's disease) or in a pregnant patient. The majority of these patients will undergo mastectomy due to their inability to receive radiation after lumpectomy, although

■ SKIN-SPARING MASTECTOMY

Skin-sparing mastectomy is a procedure in which only the nipple and areola skin are removed, leaving all remaining skin for use in the reconstruction. Breast tissue including the nipple-areola complex is excised through a circumareolar incision, with or without a lateral extension of the incision for exposure. The incidence of local recurrence after skin-sparing mastectomy is similar to that seen with standard total mastectomy (38). Preservation of the skin allows optimal immediate reconstruction with either implant or autologous tissue. Nipple and areola reconstruction is performed as a second procedure. Studies have demonstrated a high level of patient satisfaction with skin-sparing mastectomy and immediate reconstruction (39). Risks of skin-sparing mastectomy include infection, bleeding, necrosis of the skin flaps, and close or positive margins.

■ NIPPLE-SPARING MASTECTOMY

Nipple-sparing mastectomy spares all breast skin and retains the skin of the nipple-areola complex. Preservation of the nipple-areola complex provides improved cosmesis but is associated with loss of nipple sensation. This operation is presumed to be safe in patients with DCIS that does not extend into the nipple-areola complex. Between 8% and 30% of patients undergoing mastectomy for treatment of their breast cancer have been shown to have tumor involvement of the nipple-areola complex (40–42). Patients considering nipple-sparing mastectomy should be screened for involvement of the nipple-areola complex with preoperative mammography with magnification of the subareola area to rule out microcalcifications extending to the nipple. Some centers advocate the use of breast MRI to select patients for nipple-sparing mastectomy (43). Frozen section analysis of a disk of duct tissue just underneath the areola can be performed intraoperatively. Evidence of malignancy in the tissue just under the nipple would warrant conversion to a skin-sparing, nipple-sacrificing mastectomy. Ongoing trials are investigating intraoperative radiation therapy of the nipple-areola complex following excision of the breast tissue to decrease the likelihood of a local recurrence (44). Immediate reconstruction may be performed with either immediate implant reconstruction or autologous tissue.

Complications of nipple-sparing mastectomy include infection, bleeding, necrosis of the skin flaps, and potential nipple loss owing to necrosis. In one series, smokers had the highest nipple-areola complex necrosis rate, at 60%, compared with approximately 20% in nonsmokers (43).

■ SENTINEL LYMPH NODE BIOPSY FOR DCIS

Pure DCIS is believed to have no metastatic potential, and therefore surgical staging of the axilla is not indicated. However, a 1% to 2% disease-specific mortality is reported for patients with DCIS (45), and when modified mastectomy was routinely performed for DCIS, 1% to 2% of patients were found to have positive axillary nodes.

At present, sentinel lymph node biopsy is used selectively in patients with DCIS. Some patients initially diagnosed with DCIS will be upstaged to invasive cancer at definitive surgical excision. The frequency of such upstaging depends on the method of initial diagnostic biopsy and clinicopathological features of the DCIS (Table 6.1).

■ Table 6.1 Predictors of invasion on final pathology after biopsy showing ductal carcinoma in situ (DCIS)

Young age (<55 yrs)

Palpable DCIS

Mammographic density

Large lesion size (>4 cm)

Paget's disease of the nipple

Patients undergoing mastectomy (owing to lesion size)

High-grade DCIS

DCIS, ductal carcinoma in situ.

Because of the risk of invasive carcinoma on final pathological analysis, sentinel lymph node biopsy is recommended when mastectomy is performed for DCIS because mapping is not possible after mastectomy has been performed. Sentinel node biopsy may be used selectively for patients undergoing lumpectomy for DCIS because the option of sentinel node biopsy remains viable if invasive tumor is identified (46). Sentinel node biopsy is considered during lumpectomy for DCIS with microinvasion or with areas suspicious for microinvasion, although some authors have suggested that this is not always necessary (47). Prior to surgery, the surgeon and the patient should discuss whether to proceed with sentinel lymph node biopsy at the time of initial lumpectomy or, alternatively, at a second operation only if invasive tumor is found.

■ MULTIDISCIPLINARY CONSIDERATIONS

- Collaboration between the breast surgeon and the breast imaging team is essential for diagnosis, identifying the extent of disease, and preoperative localization for lumpectomy.
- Collaboration between the breast surgeon and the breast pathologist is essential for diagnosis, selecting patients with microinvasion for sentinel lymph node biopsy, and assessing margins of the surgical specimen.
- Collaboration between the breast surgeon and plastic surgeon is essential for patients needing mastectomy.
- Collaboration with pathologists and translational researchers to identify predictors of progression to invasion is important to identify novel treatments for patients with DCIS.

■ REFERENCES

1. Ernster VL, Ballard-Barbash R, Barlow WE, et al. Detection of ductal carcinoma in situ in women undergoing screening mammography. *J Natl Cancer Inst.* 2002;94:1546–1554.

2. Jemal A, Murray T, Ward E, et al. Cancer statistics, 2005. *CA Cancer J Clin.* 2005;55:10–30.

3. Rosener D, Bedwani RN, Vana J, et al Noninvasive breast carcinoma: results of a national survey by the American College of Surgeons. *Ann Surg.* 1980;192:139–147.

4. Rosen PP, Braun DW Jr, Kinne DE. The clinical significance of preinvasive breast carcinoma. *Cancer.* 1980;46(4 suppl):919–925.

5. Page DL, Dupont WD, Rogers LW, et al. Intraductal carcinoma of the breast: follow up after biopsy only. *Cancer.*1982;49:751–758.

6. Eusebi V, Feudale E, Foschini MP, et al. Long term follow up of in situ carcinoma of the breast. *Semin Diagn Pathol.* 1994;11:223–235.

7. Collins LC, Tamimi RM, Baer HJ, et. al. Outcome of patients with ductal carcinoma in situ untreated after diagnostic biopsy: results from the Nurses' Health Study. *Cancer.* 2005;103:1778–1784.

8. Sanders ME, Schuyler PA, Dupont WD, Page DL. The natural history of low-grade ductal carcinoma in situ of the breast in women treated by biopsy only revealed over 30 years of longitudinal follow-up. *Cancer.* 2005;103:2481–2484.

9. Barreau B, De Mascarel I, Feuga C, et al. Mammography of ductal carcinoma in situ of the breast: review of 909 cases with radiographic-pathologic correlations. *Eur J Radiol.* 2005;54:55–61.

10. Holland R, Hendriks JH. Microcalcifications associated with ductal carcinoma in situ: mammographic-pathologic correlation. *Semin Diagn Pathol.* 1994;11:181–192.

11. Ikeda DM, Andersson I. Ductal carcinoma in situ: atypical mammographic appearances. *Radiology.* 1989;172:661–666.

12. Kuhl CK, Schrading S, Bieling HB, et al. MRI for diagnosis of pure ductal carcinoma in situ: a prospective observational study. *Lancet.* 2007;370:485–492.

13. Schouten van der Velden AP, Boetes C, Bult P, et al. The value of magnetic resonance imaging in diagnosis and size assessment of in situ and small invasive breast carcinoma. *Am J Surg.* 2006;192:172–178.

14. Friese CR, Nevill BA, Edge SB, Hassett MJ, Earle CC. Breast biopsy patterns and outcomes in Surveillance, Epidemiology and End Results-Medicare data. *Cancer.* 2009;115:716–724.

15. Clarke-Pearson, Jacobson AF, Boolbol SK, et al. Quality assurance initiative at one institution for minimally invasive breast biopsy as the initial diagnostic technique. *J Am Coll Surg.* 2009;208:75–78.

16. Boyages J, Delaney G, Taylor R. Predictors of local recurrence after treatment of ductal carcinoma in situ: a meta-analysis. *Cancer.* 1999;85:616–628.

17. Fisher B, Anderson S, Bryant J, et al. Twenty year follow up of a randomized trial comparing total mastectomy, lumpectomy, and lumpectomy plus irradiation therapy for the treatment of invasive breast cancer. *New Engl J Med.* 2002;347(16):1233–1241.

18. Mirza NQ, Vlastos G, Meric F, et al. Ductal carcinoma-in-situ: long term results of breast-conserving therapy. *Ann Surg Oncol.* 2000;7:656–664.

19. Rodrigues N, Carter D, Dillon D, et al. Correlation of clinical and pathologic features with outcome in patients with ductal carcinoma in situ of the breast treated with breast-conserving surgery and radiotherapy. *Int J Radiot Oncol Biol Phys.* 2002;54:1331–1335.

20. Vargas C, Kestin L, Go N, et al. Factors associated with local recurrence and cause-specific survival in patients with ductal carcinoma in situ of the breast treated with breast-conserving therapy or mastectomy. *In J Radiat Oncol Biol Phys.* 2005;63:1514–1521.

21. Fisher B, Land S, Mamounas E, et al. Prevention of invasive breast cancer in women with ductal carcinoma in situ: an update of the National Surgical Adjuvant Breast and Bowel Project experience. *Semin Oncol.* 2001;28:400–418.

22. Bijker N, Meijnen P, Peterse JL, et al. Breast-conserving treatment with or without radiotherapy in ductal carcinoma-in-situ: ten year results of European Organisation for Research and Treatment of Cancer randomised phase III trial 10853—a study by the EORTC Breast Cancer Cooperative Group and EORTC radiotherapy Group. *J Clin Oncol.* 2006;24:3381–3387.

23. Houghton J, George WD, Cuzick J, et al. Radiotherapy and tamoxifen in women with completely excised ductal carcinoma in situ of the breast in the UK, Australia, and New Zealand: randomised controlled trial. *Lancet.* 2003;362:95–102.

24. Emdin SO, Granstrand B, Ringberg A, et al. SweDCIS: radiotherapy after sector resection for ductal carcinoma in situ of the breast. Results of a randomised trial in a population offered mammography screening. *Acta Oncol.* 2006;45:536–543.

25. Rakovitch E, Pignol JP, Chartier C, et al. The management of ductal carcinoma in situ of the breast: a screened population based analysis. *Breast Cancer Res Treat.* 2007;101:335–347.

26. Solin LJ, Orel SG, Hwang WT, Harris EE, Schnall MD. Relationship of breast magnetic resonance imaging to outcome after breast-conservation treatment with radiation for women with early-stage invasive breast carcinoma or ductal carcinoma in situ. *J Clin Oncol.* 2008;26:386–391.

27. Kirstein LJ, Rafferty E, Specht MC, et al. Outcomes of multiple wire localization for larger breast cancers: when can mastectomy be avoided? *J Am Coll Surg.* 2008;207:342–346.

28. Dunne C, Burke JP, Morrow M, Kell MR. Effect of margin status on local recurrence after breast conservation and radiation therapy for ductal carcinoma in situ. *J Clin Oncol.* 2009;27:1615–1620.

29. Silverstein MJ, Lagios MD, Groshen S, et al. The influence of margin width on local control of ductal carcinoma in situ of the breast. *New Engl J Med.* 1993;340:1455–1461.

30. Wong JS, Kaelin CM, Troyan SL, et al. Prospective study of side excision alone for ductal carcinoma in situ of the breast. *J Clin Oncol.* 2006;24:1031–1036.

31. Hughes L, Wang M, Page D, et al. Five year results of intergroup study E5194: local excision alone (without radiation treatment) for selected patients with ductal in situ. *Breast Cancer Res Treat.* 2006;100(suppl):S15.

32. Jacobson AF, Asad, J, Boolbol SK, Osborne MP, Boachie-Adjei, K, Felman SM. Do additional shaved margins at the time of lumpectomy eliminate the need for re-excision? *Am J Surg.* 2008;196:556–558.

33. Cao D, Lin C, Woo SH, et al. Separate cavity margin sampling at the time of initial breast lumpectomy significantly reduces the need for re-excision. *Am J Surg Pathol.* 2005;29:1625–1632.

34. Huston T, Pigalarga R, Osborne M. Tousimis E. The influence of additional surgical margins on the total specimen volume excised and the re-operative rate after breast-conserving surgery. *Am J Surg.* 2006;192:509–512.

35. Cabioglu N, Hunt KK, Sahin AA, et al. Role for intraoperative margin assessment in patients undergoing breast-conserving surgery. *Ann Surg Oncol.* 2007;14:1458–1471.

36. Metcalfe K, Lynch HT, Ghadirian P, et al. Contralateral breast cancer in BRCA 1 and BRCA 2 mutation carriers. *J Clin Oncol.* 2004;22:2328–2335.

37. Partridge A, Adloff K, Blood E, et al. Risk perceptions and psychosocial outcomes of women with ductal carcinoma in situ: longitudinal results from a cohort study. *J Natl Cancer Inst.* 2008;100:243–251.

38. Carlson GW, Page A, Johnson E, et al. Local recurrence of ductal carcinoma in situ after skin-sparing mastectomy. *J Am Coll Surg.* 2007;204:1074–1080.

39. Salhab M, Al Sarakbi W, Joseph A, et al. Skin-sparing mastectomy and immediate breast reconstruction: patient satisfaction and clinical outcomes. *Int J Clin Oncol.* 2006;11:51–54.

40. Lagios MD, Gates EA, Westdahl PR, Richards V, Alpert BS. A guide to the frequency of nipple involvement in breast cancer: a study of 149 consecutive mastectomies using a serial

subgross and correlated radiographic technique. *Am J Surg.* 1979;138:135–140.

41. Morimoto T, Komaki K, Inui K, et al. Involvement of nipple and areola in early breast cancer. *Cancer.* 1985;55:2459–2463.

42. Rusby JE, Brachtel EF, Othus M, et al. Development and validation of a model predictive of occult nipple involvement in women undergoing mastectomy. *Br J Surg.* 2008;95:1356–1361.

43. Wijayanayagam A, Kumar AS, Foster RD, Esserman LJ. Optimizing the total skin-sparing mastectomy. *Arch Surg.* 2008;143:38–45.

44. Petit JY, Veronesi U, Orecchia R, et al. Nipple-sparing mastectomy in association with intra operative radiation therapy (ELIOT): a new type of mastectomy for breast cancer treatment. *Breast Cancer Res Treat.* 2006;96:47–51.

45. Ernster VL, Barclay J, Kerlikowske K, et al. Mortality among women with ductal carcinoma in situ of the breast in the population based surveillance, epidemiology, and end results program. *Arch Intern Med.* 2000;160:953–958.

46. Wong SL, Edwards MJ, Chao C, et al. The effect of prior breast biopsy method and concurrent definitive breast procedure on success and accuracy of sentinel lymph node biopsy. *Ann Surg Oncol.* 2002;9:272–277.

47. Murphy CD, Jones JL, Javid SH, et al. Do sentinel lymph node micrometastases predict recurrence risk in patients with ductal carcinoma in situ and patients with ductal carcinoma in situ with microinvasion? *Am J Surg.* 2008;196:566–568.

Radiation Treatment of DCIS

MARGARITA RACSA

ARIEL E. HIRSCH

SHANNON M. MACDONALD

Ductal carcinoma in situ (DCIS), or intraductal carcinoma, is characterized by the proliferation of malignant epithelial cells within the confines of the mammary ducts. Although DCIS is included under the umbrella of breast cancer, by strict definition DCIS is noninvasive. The primary concern in patients diagnosed with DCIS is the potential for progression from DCIS to invasive disease. Interestingly, while most invasive carcinomas arise from DCIS, not all patients with DCIS go on to develop invasive breast cancer (1,2). However, in the absence of a means for identifying which patients will develop invasive breast cancer, the local management of patients with DCIS is very similar to that of patients with early invasive breast cancer. As will be discussed, the evolution of treatment options for DCIS closely followed that of treatments for early invasive breast cancer—with breast-conserving surgery (BCS) followed by radiation therapy emerging as a safe and effective alternative to mastectomy, which historically had been the gold standard.

■ EPIDEMIOLOGY AND RISK FACTORS

Prior to the advent of screening mammography, DCIS was a relatively rare diagnosis, comprising less than 5% of all breast cancers, the majority of which were detected clinically as a palpable mass (3). According to recent estimates, DCIS accounts for approximately 20% of all breast malignancies, most of which are identified mammographically (4). In 2008, an estimated 67,770 women were diagnosed with DCIS in the United States (5). The risk factors for developing DCIS are similar to those for invasive cancer and include increasing age, family history of breast cancer, early menarche, late menopause, advanced gestational age, nulliparity, prior breast biopsy, hormonal therapy, and *BRCA1* and *BRCA2* mutations (6).

■ PATHOLOGY

Breast carcinomas are described as either "in situ" or "invasive" carcinomas. In the former case, tumor cells are confined to the ducts or lobules and show no evidence of invasion into the surrounding stroma. In the latter case, there is evidence of invasion into the stroma, with the potential of tumor cells to metastasize. The in situ carcinomas can be further described as either DCIS or lobular carcinoma in situ (LCIS), each with distinct clinical and pathological features. DCIS is predominantly located in the ducts, typically presents as a mammographic abnormality, is unifocal, and has a higher risk of invasive cancers, which tend to occur in the ipsilateral breast. In contrast, LCIS most commonly occurs in the lobules, is infrequently visible on a mammogram, is multifocal, and has a lower risk of invasive cancers, which tend to occur in the ipsilateral or contralateral breast. LCIS is considered a marker for increased risk of developing invasive carcinoma (7).

The pathological classification of DCIS is determined by the architectural pattern (comedo, cribriform, micropapillary, papillary, and solid), nuclear grade (low, intermediate, or high), and the presence or absence of necrosis (8). While no single classification scheme has been widely adopted (9,10), the College of American Pathologists recommends the following be included in the surgical pathology report: the type and size of the specimen (partial or total breast), the type of surgery performed, the type of lymph node sampling performed (if any), specimen laterality, tumor location within the breast, the size and extent of DCIS, the histological type, architectural patterns, nuclear grade, necrosis, surgical margins, lymph nodes, pathological staging (pTNM), hormone receptor status, microcalcifications, and clinical history (11). The evaluation of surgical margins is of paramount importance and is discussed later in this chapter.

Finally, in cases where an occult microinvasive tumor is found, with a focus less than 1 mm, the tumor is staged as microinvasive breast cancer (T1mic) (12). Microinvasive tumors are more likely to occur in patients who present with palpable masses or nipple discharge, large DCIS lesions (measuring greater than 2.5 cm), or lesions with high-grade DCIS or comedonecrosis (13–15).

■ CLINICAL PRESENTATION AND MAMMOGRAPHY

Prior to the widespread use of screening mammography, DCIS was an unusual clinical finding and was detected by a palpable mass or nipple discharge, particularly when associated with an underlying invasive lesion. However, at present, less than 10% of patients with DCIS will present with a palpable mass independent of microcalcifications (16).

The incidence of DCIS has risen owing to the increased use of mammography, and up to 30% of mammographically detected breast cancers contain DCIS (17). A full 90% of DCIS cases are identified on mammography as suspicious microcalcifications, which can vary from pleomorphic to clustered to linear in distribution (18). Characterization of the microcalcifications with regard to number, morphology, distribution, and size is critical, particularly as many benign conditions can contain microcalcifications as well (16). As mammography can underestimate the pathological extent of DCIS, even with additional magnification views, and as sonography does not play a role in the evaluation of microcalcifications, there is interest in breast magnetic resonance imaging (MRI) as an emerging technology in the pre-irradiation evaluation of DCIS patients, particularly in those patients who are candidates for partial breast irradiation (PBI) protocols (19). Contrast-enhanced breast MRI can provide excellent anatomical and extent-of-tumor information with a high sensitivity. Breast MRI, however, has a low specificity in the detection of DCIS, and there are a high number of false negative findings. It may be most helpful in the diagnosis of DCIS lesions that lack calcifications or necrosis (20). Figure 6.1 shows a lesion representing DCIS that was detected by MRI.

■ MANAGEMENT

Patients with DCIS have several options, including mastectomy or breast conserving surgery followed by radiation therapy, with hormonal therapy as indicated. Although the diagnosis of DCIS was much less common in the premammography era, mastectomy was considered the standard of care for decades until the development of breast-sparing surgical techniques. It is interesting to note that BCS followed by radiation therapy evolved in the setting of invasive breast cancer. Multiple prospective randomized trials comparing mastectomy with breast-conserving therapy (BCT) for patients with invasive disease showed no difference in survival (21–24). Moreover, the addition of whole breast radiation therapy following BCS further improved local control and allowed for rates comparable to mastectomy, establishing radiation therapy as an integral component of BCT (21–24). BCS without radiation resulted in unacceptable rates of local recurrence in these studies and, therefore, was not considered an acceptable alternative for patients with invasive breast cancer. There are no randomized, controlled trials comparing mastectomy with BCT for DCIS, and it is unlikely that these trials will ever be performed. The management of DCIS with BCS was extrapolated from such trials for invasive cancer and is considered acceptable on the basis of the earlier stage of disease at the time of detection. It does seem logical that patients with

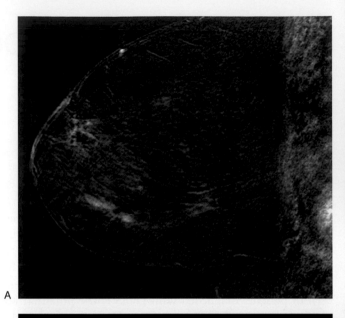

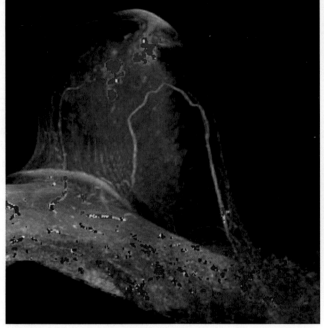

FIGURE 6.1 (A) Magnetic resonance imaging (MRI)–detected ductal carcinoma in situ (DCIS). Subtracted sagittal MRI image of the left breast performed in a patient with biopsy-proven DCIS of the left breast (*superior arrow*). Inferior arrow showing a new region of abnormality that was not detectable by mammogram or ultrasound. Biopsy by MRI guidance revealed a second separate lesion of DCIS. (Courtesy of Phoebe Freer, MD.) (B) maximum intensity projection (MIP) image of the left breast with CADstream kinetics color mapping showing the two areas of enhancement in the left breast: the subareolar area representing the known malignancy (DCIS) and the more central, six o'clock area representing the new suspicious area (later shown to represent a second area of DCIS). (Courtesy of Phoebe Freer, MD.)

a lesser stage of disease should be spared a more extensive surgery. It is, however, important to keep in mind that the major goal of therapy for DCIS is to prevent a local recurrence, especially an invasive local recurrence.

For extensive or multicentric DCIS or for cases for which negative margins cannot be achieved with reasonable cosmesis, mastectomy is still recommended.

Mastectomy

The rates of local control with mastectomy are excellent, at approximately 98% in most series (25,26). Although mastectomy may be considered overtreatment for most cases of DCIS, it does provide the best rates of local control, and in cases of multicentric disease or findings of calcifications that are too widespread to be removed with reasonable cosmesis, it is considered the most desirable option. Total (or simple) mastectomy is the surgical procedure indicated for patients with DCIS and involves removal of the entire breast, with preservation of the pectoralis muscles and axillary lymph nodes. Sentinel lymph node biopsy (SLNB) is not routinely performed for patients with DCIS but should be considered in patients with extensive disease or when there is a suspicion of invasive disease. Some published series report that more than 20% of patients with DCIS will have findings of invasive disease in the surgical specimen (27–29). These patients will require some form of axillary staging. If mastectomy is being performed, many surgeons prefer to perform a SLNB at the time of mastectomy rather than lose this option and be forced to perform a full axillary dissection if invasive disease is found in the mastectomy specimen (30). Radiation therapy is not generally indicated in patients with DCIS who have undergone a mastectomy owing to historically low recurrence rates. However, a recent publication suggests a subset of patients with close margins, particularly when combined with high-grade disease and young age, may have unacceptably high rates of local recurrence (31). Another small series suggests that when isolated local relapses do occur following mastectomy for DCIS, resection followed by radiation results in high rates of cure (32).

For patients in whom radiation therapy is contraindicated, mastectomy is recommended. Several other relative contraindications to BCT exist. Absolute and relative contraindications for BCT are listed in Table 6.2.

BCS and the Role of Radiation Therapy

There are no prospective randomized trials comparing mastectomy with BCS and radiation therapy in patients diagnosed with DCIS. As the long-term follow-up data from early invasive breast cancer comparing mastectomy and excision followed by radiation matured, investigators became more confident that BCT was a reasonable treatment option for women with invasive breast cancer. It seemed logical to offer BCT to women with a lesser stage of disease, and this ultimately evolved as a standard option for DCIS without ever being tested in a phase III randomized setting. Many did question, however, whether there

■ Table 6.2 Absolute and relative contraindications for breast-conserving therapy with radiation

Absolute:
- Prior radiation therapy to the breast or chest wall
- Radiation therapy during pregnancy
- Diffuse suspicious or malignant appearing microcalcifications
- Widespread disease that cannot be incorporated by local excision through a single incision that achieves negative margins with a satisfactory cosmetic result.
- Positive pathologic margin

Relative:
- Active connective tissue disease involving the skin (especially scleroderma and lupus)
- Tumors >5 cm (category 2B)
- Focally positive margin
- Women ≤35 y or premenopausal women with a known BRCA 1/2 mutation:
  — May have an increased risk of ipsilateral breast recurrence or contralateral breast cancer with breast conserving therapy
  — Prophylactic bilateral mastectomy for risk reduction may be considered.

Source: National Comprehensive Cancer Network Clinical Practice Guidelines in Oncology: Breast Cancer, vol.1, 2009.

was a benefit to adding radiation in patients with DCIS. Three prospectively randomized trials compared BCS alone with BCS followed by radiation therapy for patients with DCIS (33–35). Given the long natural history of DCIS, it is important to review the long-term results of these studies (36,37).

The National Surgical Adjuvant Breast and Bowel Project (NSABP) B-17 study randomized 813 women with DCIS to BCS alone or BCS followed by whole breast radiation therapy (50 Gy in 25 fractions) (34,37). Of note is the fact that in this study a negative margin was defined as no tumor cells touching the inked margin. At a median follow-up of 12 years, there was a decrease in the risk of local recurrence with the addition of radiation when compared with BCS alone (31.7% versus 15.7%). Specifically, the risk of recurrence was decreased from 16.8% to 7.7% in patients who recurred with invasive disease and from 14.6% to 8% in patients who recurred with DCIS. Notably, there was no difference in overall survival between the two groups.

The European Organisation for Research and Treatment of Cancer (EORTC) 10853 trial randomized 1,010 women with DCIS who underwent BCS to no further treatment or BCS followed by whole breast radiation therapy (50 Gy in 25 fractions) (33,36). Surgical margins were considered negative if they measured greater than 1 mm.

With a median follow-up of 10.5 years, the EORTC 10853 trial confirmed the results that BCS followed by radiation decreased the risk of local recurrence compared with BCS alone (26% versus 15%). Again, there was no difference in overall survival between the two arms.

Finally, the United Kingdom Coordinating Committee on Cancer Research (UKCCCR) conducted a trial that randomized women using a 2 × 2 factorial design to BCS or BCS followed by radiation therapy (50 Gy in 25 fractions) (35). This study also investigated the role of tamoxifen in decreasing the risk of ipsilateral and contralateral disease. The trial included four arms: BCS alone, BCS and radiation therapy, BCS and tamoxifen, and BCS with radiation therapy and tamoxifen. A margin was considered positive if it "extended to the margin of the specimen." At a median follow-up of 4.5 years, there was a decrease in the rate of local recurrence with the addition of radiation therapy (14% versus 6%).

The results of these three trials show an improvement in local control with the addition of radiation therapy in patients undergoing BCS and establish radiation therapy as a critical component of BCT. The results of these trials are summarized in Table 6.3. Of note is the fact that in all these trials, radiation therapy was administered to the whole breast to 50 Gy without a boost to the tumor bed. While a subsequent trial demonstrated a further reduction in local recurrence in invasive breast cancer with an additional dose of 16 Gy to the tumor bed (38), an additional boost to the tumor bed is sometimes administered but has not been universally employed in patients with DCIS.

As yet, no clinical or pathological subgroup of patients has been definitively identified that does not benefit from radiation therapy. Arguably, the magnitude of benefit differs among patients; however, in view of the above findings, all patients undergoing BCS for DCIS should be considered for radiation therapy.

Omission of Radiation Therapy

Despite three prospective trials demonstrating improved local control, there remains substantial controversy regarding whether all patients should be treated with radiation therapy. Silverstein and colleagues developed the Van Nuys Prognostic Index (VPNI) in 1995 to predict the risk of local recurrence following BCS using different clinical and pathological features (39). In a retrospective study of 333 patients three factors were used in the initial analysis: tumor size, margin width, and pathological classification. Each predictor was assigned a score of one (favorable) to three (unfavorable), with the sum of these three factors used to calculate a cumulative score. Patients were grouped into three categories on the basis of their cumulative scores. At 8 years of follow-up among patients with a VPNI score of 3 to 4, there was no statistically significant difference in local recurrence-free survival with the addition of radiation. In contrast, patients with VPNI scores of 5 to 7 and 8 to 9 received a statistically significant recurrence-free survival benefit, with the greatest relative benefit in patients with scores of 8 to 9, when radiation therapy was given after BCS.

In an update to their analysis, age was added to the VPNI scoring system, which is shown in Table 6.4. Their findings were similar to those reported earlier (40). There was no statistically significant benefit in local recurrence-free survival with radiation therapy in patients with a low score (VPNI scores of 4, 5, or 6). Patients with intermediate scores (VPNI scores of 7, 8, or 9) or high scores (VPNI scores of 10, 11, or 12) showed a statistically significant benefit in local recurrence-free survival.

In a subsequent analysis of 469 patients, margin status was determined to be the most important predictor of local recurrence in patients treated with BCS alone (41). Among patients with a margin width of 10 mm or more, there was no benefit with radiation therapy [relative risk (RR) 1.14, $P = 0.92$]. In contrast, in patients with a margin width of less than 1 mm, there was a statistically significant benefit with radiation therapy (RR 2.54, $P = 0.01$). Patients with margins between 1 and 9 mm did not derive a statistically significant benefit with radiation therapy (RR 1.49, $P = 0.24$). Moreover, at 8 years, among patients with a margin of less than 1 mm, the rate of local recurrence was decreased from 58% to 30%.

■ **Table 6.3** Randomized trials of breast-conserving therapy with or without radiation								
			LR (%)			OS (%)		
Trial	Number of Patients	Follow-up (years)	BCS	BCS + RT	*P*	BCS	BCS + RT	*P*
NSABP B-17	813	12	31.7	15.7	<0.00005	86	87	0.8
EORTC 10853	1,010	10.5	26	15	<0.0001	95	95	0.53
UKCCCR	1,030	4.5	14	6	<0.0001	NR	NR	

BCS, breast-conserving surgery; EORTC, European Organisation for Research and Treatment of Cancer; LR, local recurrence; NSABP, National Surgical Adjuvant Breast and Bowel Project; NR, not recorded; OS, overall survival; RT, radiation thereapy; UKCCCR, United Kingdom Coordinating Committee on Cancer Research.

Table 6.4	Van Nuys Prognostic Index for ductal carcinoma in situ		
Size	Margin	Pathological Classification	Age (yrs)
1 = ≤15 mm	1 = ≥10 mm	1 = Non–high-grade lesion without comedonecrosis	1 = ≥60
2 = 16–40 mm	2 = 1–9 mm	2 = Non–high-grade lesion with comedonecrosis	2 = 40–60
3 = ≥41 mm	3 = <1 mm (involved or close)	3 = All high-grade lesions, with or without necrosis	3 = ≤40

Source: Ref. 76.

The aforementioned data are derived from retrospective studies and suffer from the biases of such. Unfortunately, attempts to replicate these results in a prospective manner have been unsuccessful. Wong and colleagues conducted a prospective, single-arm study in which patients with low-grade DCIS (grade 1 or 2), small tumors (mammographic extent less than or equal to 2.5 cm), and margins greater than or equal to 1 cm or a negative re-excision for close margins were treated with BCS alone (40). Radiation therapy was omitted, and patients were followed closely with mammographic follow-up of the involved breast every 6 months and annual mammograms for the uninvolved breast. The trial was stopped early because the number of local recurrences reached the predetermined study cessation rules. At a median follow-up of 40 months, the rate of local recurrence as the first site of treatment failure was 2.4%, which corresponded to a 5-year rate of 12%. In light of these findings, additional studies are needed to better identify the favorable subset of patients with DCIS who may not require radiation therapy after BCS.

Currently, there are no published data from large cooperative group or randomized, controlled trials attempting to omit radiation for patients with DCIS considered to have a lower risk of recurrence. The Eastern Cooperative Oncology Group trial (ECOG 5194) has accrued approximately 1,000 patients with favorable risk factors to a single-arm trial of excision alone for DCIS (42). This trial has closed, but results have not yet to be reported in manuscript form. The Radiation Therapy Oncology Group and Cancer and Leukemia Group (RTOG 9804/ CALGB 49801) attempted to accrue patients to a phase III randomized trial of excision alone compared with excision followed by radiation. Unfortunately, this trial closed owing to poor accrual.

■ IMPORTANCE OF SURGICAL MARGINS FOR DCIS

Data from randomized trials as well as large retrospective reviews have indicated that margins are among the most important risk factors for local recurrence (41,43–45). Despite widespread agreement that DCIS should be excised without tumor present on the edge of the specimen, the desired amount of normal breast tissue surrounding the DCIS is unknown. Distribution of DCIS in the pathological specimen varies from a single area of disease to multiple foci of disease separated by several millimeters, although most gaps are 1 mm or less (46). Careful pathological evaluation to detect all areas of involvement is of paramount importance in this disease. A study of surgical re-excision published by Neuschatz and colleagues provides information on the likelihood of residual DCIS following excision based on the width of margins (47). For patients with extensively positive, moderately positive, and focally positive margins, the likelihood of residual disease was 85%, 68%, and 30%, respectively. For patients with margins of 0 to 1 mm, 1 to 2 mm, and more than 2 mm, the risk of residual disease was 41%, 31%, and 0%, respectively ($P = 0.001$). A review of 455 patients with DCIS treated with surgery alone examined multiple risk factors and found margin status to be the single most important predictor of local recurrence (48). After adjustments for other examined risk factors, the authors found the risk of local recurrence to be 5.39 times greater for patients with margins of less than 1 cm than for those with margins of 1 cm or more. The probability of local recurrence-free survival at 8 years was 49%, 58%, and 39% for patients with margins of 1.0 to 1.9 mm, 0.1 to 0.9 mm, and 0 mm, respectively (48). While data on the required margin width in the setting of radiation therapy are even more scarce, it is clear that obtaining a rim of normal tissue is important in achieving a high likelihood of local control and margins of 2 mm or more are generally preferred (49).

In addition to pathological evaluation, verification that calcifications are completely removed by surgery is necessary to evaluate complete removal of DCIS. This is generally accomplished by thorough review of a specimen radiograph, making certain that all of the suspicious microcalcifications are identified. In addition, following lumpectomy, pre-irradiation mammography is an important tool in assessing residual microcalcifications in the breast and is especially useful in patients with DCIS (50).

■ RADIATION TECHNIQUES USED FOR WHOLE BREAST RADIATION THERAPY

Patients are most commonly placed in the supine position, with the arms above the head, and a breast board is used for immobilization. Prior to simulation it is useful to identify the clinical boundaries of the targeted breast volume with radio-opaque markers at midsternum (medially), midaxillary line (laterally), 1 to 2 cm below the inframammary line (caudad), and the base of the clavicular heads (cephalad). Another option is to place a wire around the mound of clinical breast tissue. Note that these borders can be modified depending on the location of the tumor bed. The simulation can be done using a conventional fluoroscopic simulator or, more commonly, using a computed tomography (CT) simulator. Tangential beams are used to include the targeted clinical breast volume and are angled to minimize the divergence of the beam into the lung and heart (left-sided tumors). The collimator can also be rotated to cover the breast and further minimize lung and heart exposure (left-sided tumors). Care must be taken to cover the tumor bed adequately within the radiation field. Different techniques including wedges, compensators or intensity-modulated radiation therapy may be used to optimize dose homogeneity within the breast if CT planning is used. Finally, while beam energies of 4 to 6 MV are typically used, mixed beams or beams with higher energies can be used to ensure sufficient coverage.

Prone Position

While most patients in the United States and Europe are treated in the supine position, several institutions are advocating the use of treatment in the prone position. Formenti and colleagues reported the feasibility of treatment in the prone position for patients with early-stage breast cancer and, more recently, patients with DCIS in an attempt to optimally spare heart and lung while reducing inframammary fold skin reaction (51). While patients with large, pendulous breasts are considered to benefit most from treatment in the prone position, early results from a prospective trial from New York University (NYU) suggest women with both small and large breasts may benefit from treatment in the prone position. The trial, which recently closed, included both patients with early invasive breast cancer and patients with noninvasive breast cancer, and imaged patients in both the prone and supine positions for breast radiotherapy to characterize specifically which patients are best suited for each position (52). The better position was selected on the basis of inclusion of the whole index breast, maximal heart sparing, and maximal lung sparing. The prone position was chosen more often on the basis of these criteria.

Using the prone technique, patients are simulated in the prone position with both arms about the head using a dedicated breast mattress that allows the index breast

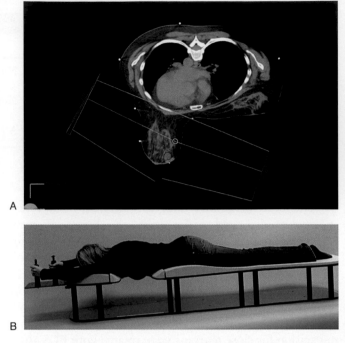

FIGURE 6.2 (A) External beam radiation therapy in the prone position. Field arrangement for prone breast treatment. Lumpectomy cavity contoured in red. Tangent treatment fields (LPO, left posterior oblique; RPO, right posterior oblique). (B) Dedicated treatment board for the treatment of breast cancer in the prone position. (Courtesy of Orbital Therapy.)

to fall freely through an opening. There are now several commercially available boards for prone positioning. It is important to ensure patient comfort and reproducibility when using the prone position. An example of prone positioning is shown in Figure 6.2.

■ DOSE AND FRACTIONATION

The most common fractionation used in patients with DCIS is 50 Gy at 2 Gy per fraction; the same fractionation scheme was used in the NSABP B-17, EORTC, and UKCCCR studies.

Hypofractionation

In recent years, there has been a strong interest in delivering a higher dose per fraction, resulting in fewer fractions (hypofractionation), in patients with early invasive breast cancer (51,53,54). The Whelan study prospectively randomized patients to receive whole breast irradiation to 50 Gy in 25 fractions or 42.5 Gy in 16 fractions (53). At a median follow-up of 12 years, there was no difference in local control, overall survival, or acute or late side effects between the two groups (55). The role of hypofractionation in patients with DCIS has not been studied extensively. Preliminary results from NYU demonstrated the feasibility of treating patients with DCIS with hypofractionation in a phase I/II trial (56). Specifically, the whole breast was treated to a total dose of 42 Gy (2.8 Gy per fraction in 15 fractions) following BCS. Overall, radiation therapy was well tolerated, with modest acute toxicity and late toxicity. At a median follow-up of 36 months, no ipsilateral or contralateral breast recurrences were reported.

Radiation Boost

A boost, or additional dose to the tumor bed, is commonly given in patients with early invasive breast cancer following whole breast irradiation. Two prospective, randomized trials have shown a small but statistically significant benefit in local control for patients with invasive breast cancer (57,58). The larger of these two trials, EORTC 22881-10882, randomized 5,318 patients to receive whole breast radiation therapy to 50 Gy followed by a 16 Gy boost or observation. At a median follow-up of 10.8 years, the cumulative incidence of local recurrence was 6.2% and 10.2% for the boost and observation groups, respectively ($P < 0.0001$), for women in all age groups (38). There was no difference in overall survival. Limited data are available on the benefit of a boost for patients with DCIS, with mixed results. A radiation boost is generally given at the discretion of the treating physician and may be based on additional risk factors (59–62). The recently opened French multicentric randomized trial will attempt to answer this question for patients with DCIS in the setting of a phase III randomized study (59). Patients in this trial will be randomized to 50 Gy whole breast irradiation or 50 Gy whole breast irradiation followed by a 16 Gy boost.

■ ACCELERATED PARTIAL BREAST IRRADIATION FOR DCIS

Accelerated partial breast irradiation (APBI) is currently under investigation for patients with both invasive and noninvasive breast cancer. The rationale for partial breast irradiation in DCIS is that the pattern of recurrence following BCS with or without radiation therapy is similar to that of invasive breast cancer: the majority (75%) of recurrences occur within or adjacent to the tumor bed (54). Moreover, only a minority of DCIS cases (8%) have satellite lesions more than 1 cm from the original tumor (47). Finally, a prospective phase I/II study at the Ochsner Clinic that included both patients with DCIS and patients with early-stage breast cancer delivered APBI with either low-dose brachytherapy delivering 45 Gy over 4 days or high-dose radiation delivery of 32 Gy in eight fractions over 4 days. This study showed rates of local control in patients treated with APBI using brachytherapy to be comparable to those in patients treated with whole

breast standard fractionation external beam radiation therapy (63). The potential benefits of partial breast irradiation include delivery of a higher radiation dose to the postoperative tumor bed, with a theoretical increase in local control, a shorter overall treatment time (typically 5–10 days), and decreased toxicity to ipsilateral heart and lung and the contralateral breast. The counterargument is that whole breast radiation therapy decreases the risk of both noninvasive and invasive disease outside the postoperative tumor bed.

To test this hypothesis a phase III prospective randomized trial is being conducted comparing partial breast irradiation with conventional whole breast irradiation for women with stage 0, 1, and 2 breast cancer. The schema for NSABP B-39/RTOG 0413 is shown in Figure 6.3. Several PBI techniques are allowed in the protocol, including interstitial brachytherapy, intracavitary balloon catheter (MammoSite), and three-dimensional conformal external beam radiation therapy.

■ SIDE EFFECTS OF WHOLE BREAST RADIATION THERAPY

There are generally two kinds of side effects from radiation therapy: acute and late side effects. Acute side effects are defined as those that occur within 90 days of a course of radiation therapy, and late side effects are defined as those that occur thereafter. The most common acute side effect is treatment-related fatigue, which can vary in severity from patient to patient. Most patients who receive breast irradiation experience mild fatigue. Other common acute effects include skin reaction in the treatment portal, including dryness, erythema, and occasionally pruritus and tenderness. Skin breakdown, particularly in the inframammary fold or axilla, occurs in up to 30% of patients, and new skin forms over the desquamated area within a week or two (64). The skin can remain hyperpigmented for a number of months after completion of radiation therapy but returns to normal thereafter (65). The most troubling late side effects are damage to the heart and lung as well as the risk of developing second malignancies (66). CT planning as well as the use of IMRT shaping has been shown to minimize dose to the heart and thereby reduce the risk of long-term cardiac damage (67). With current techniques, routine monitoring for heart and lung toxicity is not recommended (65).

■ HORMONAL THERAPY

Early trials examining the use of tamoxifen for patients with invasive breast cancer demonstrated a decrease in the risk of ipsilateral and contralateral invasive and

NSABP B-39/RTOG 0413 SCHEMA

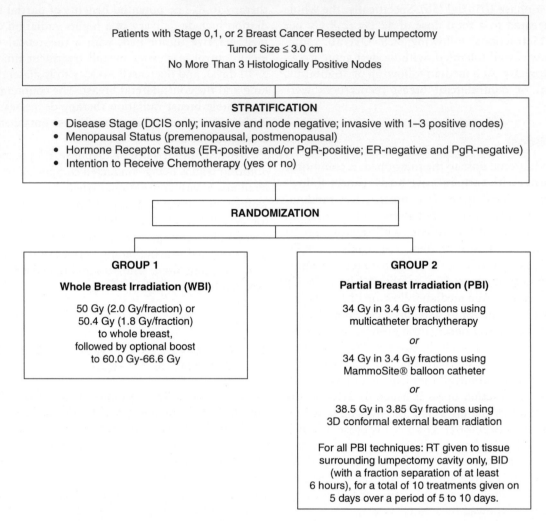

Patients with Stage 0,1, or 2 Breast Cancer Resected by Lumpectomy
Tumor Size ≤ 3.0 cm
No More Than 3 Histologically Positive Nodes

STRATIFICATION
- Disease Stage (DCIS only; invasive and node negative; invasive with 1–3 positive nodes)
- Menopausal Status (premenopausal, postmenopausal)
- Hormone Receptor Status (ER-positive and/or PgR-positive; ER-negative and PgR-negative)
- Intention to Receive Chemotherapy (yes or no)

RANDOMIZATION

GROUP 1

Whole Breast Irradiation (WBI)

50 Gy (2.0 Gy/fraction) or
50.4 Gy (1.8 Gy/fraction)
to whole breast,
followed by optional boost
to 60.0 Gy-66.6 Gy

GROUP 2

Partial Breast Irradiation (PBI)

34 Gy in 3.4 Gy fractions using
multicatheter brachytherapy

or

34 Gy in 3.4 Gy fractions using
MammoSite® balloon catheter

or

38.5 Gy in 3.85 Gy fractions using
3D conformal external beam radiation

For all PBI techniques: RT given to tissue
surrounding lumpectomy cavity only, BID
(with a fraction separation of at least
6 hours), for a total of 10 treatments given on
5 days over a period of 5 to 10 days.

FIGURE 6.3   Schema for a randomized phase 3 study of conventional whole breast irradiation (WBI) compared with partial breast irradiation (PBI) for women with stage 0, 1, or 2 breast cancer (National Surgical Adjuvant Breast and Bowel Project (NSABP) B-39/RTOB 0413.)

noninvasive breast cancers (68,69). In addition, these patients derived a small but statistically significant benefit in overall survival. Two prospective trials sought to determine whether patients with DCIS derived a similar benefit from the addition of tamoxifen following BCS and radiation.

The NSABP B-24 study randomized 1,804 patients with DCIS who underwent BCS and radiation therapy to tamoxifen (20 mg daily) or placebo for 5 years (70). At a median follow-up of 74 months, the women in the tamoxifen group had fewer breast cancer events at 5 years than those on placebo (8.2% and 13.4%, respectively). At 5 years, the cumulative incidence of invasive cancer events in the tamoxifen and placebo groups was 4.1% and 7.2%, respectively ($P = 0.004$). Interestingly, the reduction in noninvasive events from 6.2% to 4.2% in patients treated with tamoxifen was not statistically significant ($P = 0.08$). Younger women (age <50 years) and

histological findings of comedonecrosis were associated with higher rates of ipsilateral breast recurrence. There was no difference in survival between the two groups (97%) at 5 years. Figure 6.4 demonstrates the benefit that radiation and tamoxifen provide for the prevention of local recurrences.

As discussed previously, the UKCCCR conducted a trial that randomized women using a 2 × 2 factorial design that included four arms: BCS alone, BCS and radiation therapy, BCS and tamoxifen, and BCS with radiation therapy and tamoxifen (35). In contrast to NSABP B-24, at a median follow-up of 52.6 months, there was no statistically significant decrease in ipsilateral or contralateral invasive breast cancer events in patients who received tamoxifen whether or not radiation therapy was given. Of note is the fact that tamoxifen did decrease the ipsilateral recurrence of noninvasive disease [hazard ratio (HR) 0.68; $P = 0.03$].

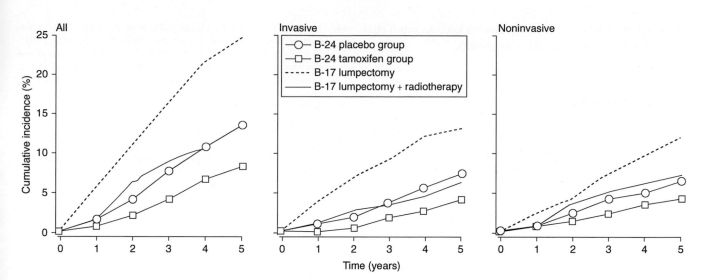

FIGURE 6.4 Data from National Surgical Adjuvant Breast and Bowel Project (NSABP) 24 (placebo versus tamoxifen) and NSABP 17 (lumpectomy alone versus lumpectomy plus radiation). The data show the cumulative incidence of all, invasive, and noninvasive recurrences. (Adapted from Ref. 70).

Although NSABP-24 did not stratify patients according to their receptor status, a subset analysis of 628 patients by Allred and colleagues demonstrated that the benefit of tamoxifen is most likely limited to estrogen receptor–positive (ER+) patients (71). Among ER+ patients, there was a decrease in the relative risk of breast cancer recurrence. In contrast, there was no decrease in the relative risk of recurrence in ER– patients. Thus information on receptor status is important in determining which patients will derive the most benefit from treatment with tamoxifen.

While the sequencing of tamoxifen and radiation therapy in DCIS has not been studied, it has been studied extensively in patients with early-stage invasive breast cancer (72–74). The issue of sequencing is of particular concern because preclinical data suggested that administering tamoxifen prior to or concurrently with radiation therapy may lead to radioresistance, resulting in a possible decrease in local control. These three independent retrospective studies reached the same conclusion: Whether tamoxifen was administered concurrently (with radiation therapy) or sequentially (after radiation therapy), there was no statistically significant difference in local control.

The role of aromatase inhibitors in patients with DCIS is still under investigation. NSABP B-35 is a prospective, randomized trial comparing tamoxifen and anastrozole in postmenopausal women in patients with DCIS. The study has completed accrual; however, the results have not yet been reported in manuscript form. A second trial, the International Breast Cancer Intervention Study (IBIS-II), is also being conducted in the United Kingdom (75). More details on the role of hormonal therapy in the treatment of DCIS are presented elsewhere in this book.

■ THE VALUE OF THE MULTIDISCIPLINARY APPROACH FOR THE MANAGEMENT OF DCIS

DCIS is a disease that carries minimal risk of systemic spread but a substantial risk of local recurrence in the form of DCIS or invasive disease. Management is aimed at decreasing this risk of local recurrence using multiple modalities. Surgical management is based on the extent of disease and patient preference, and the choice of proceeding with mastectomy or BCT almost always affects the need for irradiation. Tamoxifen may be recommended to further reduce the risk of recurrence, but this may also depend on the patient's choices regarding local management in addition to consideration of past medical and family history and the risks/benefit profile of tamoxifen for an individual. A multidisciplinary approach allows for optimal management for patients with DCIS. By providing clear options and consensus recommendations, this approach facilitates a patient's decision-making process and increases confidence in the choices she makes.

■ CONCLUSION

DCIS is a noninvasive tumor that has the potential to transform into invasive breast carcinoma. Management options are targeted at decreasing the risk of local recurrence of both invasive and noninvasive disease. BCS followed by radiation therapy has emerged as an alternative to mastectomy with comparable rates of long-term local control and is currently considered the standard of care. Given that no clinical or pathological subgroup of patients has been identified who do not benefit from radiation therapy, all patients undergoing BCS for DCIS should be considered for radiation therapy. It is important to keep in mind that survival is excellent with either approach.

■ KEY POINTS

- Treatment options for patients with DCIS include mastectomy or breast-sparing surgery followed by radiation therapy, with hormonal therapy as indicated.
- Radiation therapy should be given to the whole breast using tangential fields that maximize coverage of the breast and tumor bed while minimizing exposure of ipsilateral lung and heart (left-sided tumors).
- The standard dose to the whole breast is 50 Gy delivered in fractions of 2 Gy daily, with or without a boost of approximately 10 Gy to the tumor bed.
- While multiple prospective randomized trials have demonstrated the effectiveness of hypofractionation in invasive breast cancer, hypofractionation in DCIS is still under investigation.

■ REFERENCES

1. Page DL, Dupont WD, Rogers LW, Jensen RA, Schuyler PA. Continued local recurrence of carcinoma 15-25 years after a diagnosis of low grade ductal carcinoma in situ of the breast treated only by biopsy. *Cancer.* 1995;76(7):1197–1200.

2. Rosen PP, Braun DW Jr, Kinne DE. The clinical significance of pre-invasive breast carcinoma. *Cancer.* 1980;46(4 suppl):919–925.

3. Rosner D, Bedwani RN, Vana J, Baker HW, Murphy GP. Noninvasive breast carcinoma: results of a National Survey by the American College of Surgeons. *Ann Surg.* 1980;192(2):139–147.

4. Jemal A, Siegel R, Ward E, Murray T, Xu J, Thun MJ. Cancer statistics, 2007. *CA Cancer J Clin.* 2007;57(1):43–66.

5. American Cancer Society. *Cancer Facts and Figures 2008.* Atlanta: G.A.C.S; 2008.

6. Kerlikowske K, Barclay J, Grady D, Sickles EA, Ernster V. Comparison of risk factors for ductal carcinoma in situ and invasive breast cancer. *J Natl Cancer Inst.* 1997;89(1):76–82.

7. Chuba PJ, Hamre MR, Yap J, et al. Bilateral risk for subsequent breast cancer after lobular carcinoma-in-situ: analysis of surveillance, epidemiology, and end results data. *J Clin Oncol.* 2005;23(24):5534–5541.

8. Morrow M, Schnitt SJ, Harris JR. Ductal carcinoma in situ. In: Harris JR, Lippman ME, Morrow M, Hellman S (Eds), *Diseases of the Breast.* Philadelphia, PA: Lippincott-Raven; 1995.

9. Lagios MD, Margolin FR, Westdahl PR, Rose MR. Mammographically detected duct carcinoma in situ: frequency of local recurrence following tylectomy and prognostic effect of nuclear grade on local recurrence. *Cancer.* 1989;63(4):618–624.

10. Silverstein MJ, Poller DN, Waisman JR, et al. Prognostic classification of breast ductal carcinoma-in-situ. *Lancet.* 1995; 345(8958):1154–1157.

11. Members of the Cancer Committee, C.o.A.P. *Protocol for the Examination of Specimens from Patients with Ductal Carcinoma in Situ (DCIS) of the Breast.* www.cap.org/apps/docs/committees/cancer/cancer_protocols/2009/dcis09.doc2009.

12. Schwartz GF, Patchefsky AS, Finklestein SD, et al. Nonpalpable in situ ductal carcinoma of the breast: predictors of multicentricity and microinvasion and implications for treatment. *Arch Surg.* 1989;124(1):29–32.

13. Greene FL, Page DL, Fleming ID, Fritz A, Balch CM. *AJCC Cancer Staging Manual.* 6th ed. New York, NY: Springer; 2002.

14. Patchefsky AS, Schwartz GF, Finkelstein SD, et al. Heterogeneity of intraductal carcinoma of the breast. *Cancer.* 1989;63(4):731–741.

15. Gump FE, Jicha DL, Ozello L. Ductal carcinoma in situ (DCIS): a revised concept. *Surgery.* 1987;102(5):790–795.

16. Winchester DP, Jeske JM, Goldschmidt RA. The diagnosis and management of ductal carcinoma in-situ of the breast. *CA Cancer J Clin.* 2000;50(3):184–200.

17. Maass N, Alkasi O, Bauer M, et al. Actual management of ductal carcinoma in situ of the breast. *Arch Gynecol Obstet.* Epub ahead of print.

18. Dershaw DD, Abramson A, Kinne DW. Ductal carcinoma in situ: mammographic findings and clinical implications. *Radiology.* 1989;170(2):411–415.

19. Tendulkar RD, Chellman-Jeffers M, Rybicki LA, et al. Preoperative breast magnetic resonance imaging in early breast cancer: implications for partial breast irradiation. *Cancer.* 2009;115: 1621–1630.

20. Kuhl CK, Schrading S, Bieling HB, et al. MRI for diagnosis of pure ductal carcinoma in situ: a prospective observational study. *Lancet.* 2007;370(9586):485–492.

21. Veronesi U, Cascinelli N, Mariani L, et al. Twenty-year follow-up of a randomized study comparing breast-conserving surgery with radical mastectomy for early breast cancer. *New Engl J Med.* 2002;347(16):1227–1232.

22. Arriagada R, Lê MG, Rochard F, Contesso G. Conservative treatment versus mastectomy in early breast cancer: patterns of failure with 15 years of follow-up data. Institut Gustave-Roussy Breast Cancer Group. *J Clin Oncol.* 1996;14(5):1558–1564.

23. Fisher B, Anderson S, Bryant J, et al. Twenty-year follow-up of a randomized trial comparing total mastectomy, lumpectomy, and lumpectomy plus irradiation for the treatment of invasive breast cancer. *New Engl J Med.* 2002;347(16):1233–1241.

24. Goh BK, Yong WS. Eighteen-year results in the treatment of early breast carcinoma with mastectomy versus breast conservation therapy. *Cancer.* 2003;98(4):697–702.

25. Silverstein MJ, Barth A, Poller DN, et al. Ten-year results comparing mastectomy to excision and radiation therapy for ductal carcinoma in situ of the breast. *Eur J Cancer.* 1995;31A(9): 1425–1427.

26. Cutuli B, Cohen-Solal-Le Nir C, De Lafontan B, et al. Ductal carcinoma in situ of the breast results of conservative and radical treatments in 716 patients. *Eur J Cancer.* 2001;37(18):2365–2372.

27. Tunon-de-Lara C, Giard S, Buttarelli M, et al. Sentinel node procedure is warranted in ductal carcinoma in situ with high risk of occult invasive carcinoma and microinvasive carcinoma treated by mastectomy. *Breast J.* 2008;14(2):135–140.

28. Boughey JC, Khakpour N, Meric-Bernstam F, et al. Selective use of sentinel lymph node surgery during prophylactic mastectomy. *Cancer.* 2006;107(7):1440–1447.

29. Tan JC, McCready DR, Easson AM, Leong WL. Role of sentinel lymph node biopsy in ductal carcinoma-in-situ treated by mastectomy. *Ann Surg Oncol.* 2007;14(2):638–645.

30. Dominguez FJ, Golshan M, Black DM, et al. Sentinel node biopsy is important in mastectomy for ductal carcinoma in situ. *Ann Surg Oncol.* 2008;15(1):268–273.

31. Rashtian A, Iganej S, Amy Liu IL, Natarajan S. Close or positive margins after mastectomy for DCIS: pattern of relapse and potential indications for radiotherapy. *Int J Radiat Oncol Biol Phys.* 2008;72(4):1016–1020.

32. Kim JH, Tavassoli F, Haffty BG. Chest wall relapse after mastectomy for ductal carcinoma in situ: a report of 10 cases with a review of the literature. *Cancer J.* 2006;12(2):92–101.

33. Julien JP, Bijker N, Fentiman IS, et al. Radiotherapy in breast-conserving treatment for ductal carcinoma in situ: first results of the EORTC randomised phase III trial 10853. EORTC Breast Cancer Cooperative Group and EORTC Radiotherapy Group. *Lancet.* 2000;355(9203):528–533.

34. Fisher B, Dignam J, Wolmark N, et al. Lumpectomy and radiation therapy for the treatment of intraductal breast cancer: findings from National Surgical Adjuvant Breast and Bowel Project B-17. *J Clin Oncol.* 1998;441–452.

35. Houghton J, George WD, Cuzick J, et al. Radiotherapy and tamoxifen in women with completely excised ductal carcinoma in situ of the breast in the UK, Australia, and New Zealand: randomized controlled trial. *Lancet.* 2003;362(9378):95–102.

36. Bijker N, Meijnen P, Peterse JL, et al. Breast-conserving treatment with or without radiotherapy in ductal carcinoma-in-situ: ten-year results of European Organisation for Research and Treatment of Cancer randomized phase III trial 10853—a study by the EORTC Breast Cancer Cooperative Group and EORTC Radiotherapy Group. *J Clin Oncol.* 2006;24(21):3381–3387.

37. Fisher B, Land S, Mamounas E, Dignam J, Fisher ER, Wolmark N. Prevention of invasive breast cancer in women with ductal carcinoma in situ: an update of the national surgical adjuvant breast and bowel project experience. *Semin Oncol.* 2001;28:400–418.

38. Bartelink H, Horiot JC, Poortmans PM, et al. Impact of a higher radiation dose on local control and survival in breast-conserving therapy of early breast cancer: 10-year results of the randomized boost versus no boost EORTC 22881-10882 trial. *J Clin Oncol.* 2007;25(22):3259–3265.

39. Silverstein MJ, Lagios MD, Craig PH, et al. A prognostic index for ductal carcinoma in situ of the breast. *Cancer.* 1996; 77(11):2267–2274.

40. Wong JS, Kaelin CM, Troyan SL, et al. Prospective study of wide excision alone for ductal carcinoma in situ of the breast. *J Clin Oncol.* 2006;24(7):1031–1036.

41. Silverstein MJ, Lagios MD, Groshen S, et al. The influence of margin width on local control of ductal carcinoma in situ of the breast. *New Engl J Med.* 1999;340(19):1455–1461.

42. Leonard GD, Swain SM. Ductal carcinoma in situ, complexities and challenges. *J Natl Cancer Inst.* 2004;96(12):906–920.

43. Boyages J, Delaney G, Taylor R. Predictors of local recurrence after treatment of ductal carcinoma in situ: a meta-analysis. *Cancer.* 1999;85(3):616–628.

44. Fisher ER, Costantino J, Fisher B, et al. Pathologic findings from the National Surgical Adjuvant Breast Project (NSABP) Protocol B-17. Intraductal carcinoma (ductal carcinoma in situ). The National Surgical Adjuvant Breast and Bowel Project Collaborating Investigators. *Cancer.* 1995;75(6):1310–1319.

45. Bijker N, Peterse JL, Duchateau L, et al. Risk factors for recurrence and metastasis after breast-conserving therapy for ductal carcinoma-in-situ: analysis of European Organization for Research and Treatment of Cancer Trial 10853. *J Clin Oncol.* 2001;19(8):2263–2271.

46. Faverly DR, Burgers L, Bult P, Holland R, et al. Three dimensional imaging of mammary ductal carcinoma in situ: clinical implications. *Semin Diagn Pathol.* 1994;11(3):193–198.

47. Neuschatz AC, DiPetrillo T, Steinhoff M, et al. The value of breast lumpectomy margin assessment as a predictor of residual tumor burden in ductal carcinoma in situ of the breast. *Cancer.* 2002;94(7):1917–1924.

48. MacDonald HR, Silverstein MJ, Mabry H, et al. Local control in ductal carcinoma in situ treated by excision alone: incremental benefit of larger margins. *Am J Surg.* 2005;190(4):521–525.

49. Neuschatz AC, DiPetrillo T, Safaii H, Lowther D, Landa M, Wazer DE. Margin width as a determinant of local control with and without radiation therapy for ductal carcinoma in situ (DCIS) of the breast. *Int J Cancer.* 2001;96(suppl.):97–104.

50. Liu J, Slanetz P, Ozonoff A, Hirsch A. The value of post-excision pre-irradiation mammography in the treatment of breast cancer patients undergoing breast conservation therapy. *Int J Radiat Oncol Biol Phys.* 2008;72(suppl. 1):S187–S188.

51. Formenti SC, Gidea-Addeo D, Goldberg JD, et al. Phase I-II trial of prone accelerated intensity modulated radiation therapy to the breast to optimally spare normal tissue. *J Clin Oncol.* 2007;25:2236–2242.

52. Formenti S, Parhar PK, Goldberg JD, et al. Prospective trial of individual optimal positioning (prone versus supine) for whole breast radiotherapy: Results of the first 168 patients [Abstract]. *Int J Radiat Oncol Biol Phys.* 2007;69(suppl. 1): S74.

53. Whelan T, MacKenzie R, Julian J, et al. Randomized trial of breast irradiation schedules after lumpectomy for women with lymph node-negative breast cancer. *J Natl Cancer Inst.* 2002; 94(15):1143–1150.

54. Fisher ER, Dignam J, Tan-Chiu E, et al. Pathologic findings from the National Surgical Adjuvant Breast Project (NSABP) eight-year update of Protocol B-17: intraductal carcinoma. *Cancer.* 1999;86(3):429–438.

55. Whelan T, Pignol JP, Julian J, et al. Long-term results of a randomized trial of accelerated hypofractionated whole breast irradiation following breast-conserving surgery (abstract). Data presented at the 30th annual San Antonio Breast Cancer Symposium, San Antonio, TX, December 13th, 2007. (Abstract available online at www.abstracts2view.com/sabcs/; accessed January 3, 2008).

56. Constantine C, Parhar P, Lymberis S, et al. Feasibility of accelerated whole-breast radiation in the treatment of patients with ductal carcinoma in situ of the breast. *Clin Breast Cancer.* 2008; 8(3):269–274.

57. Romestaing P, Lehingue Y, Carrie C, et al. Role of a 10-Gy boost in the conservative treatment of early breast cancer: results of a randomized clinical trial in Lyon, France. *J Clin Oncol.* 1997; 15(3):963–968.

58. Bartelink H, Horiot JC, Poortmans P, et al. Recurrence rates after treatment of breast cancer with standard radiotherapy with or without additional radiation. *New Engl J Med.* 2001; 345(19):1378–1387.

59. Azria D, Auvray H, Barillot I, et al. [Ductal carcinoma in situ: role of the boost]. *Cancer Radiother.* 2008;12(6–7):571–576.

60. Omlin A, Amichetti M, Azria D, et al. Boost radiotherapy in young women with ductal carcinoma in situ: a multicentre, retrospective study of the Rare Cancer Network. *Lancet Oncol.* 2006;7(8):652–656.

61. Wong JS. Is radiotherapy boost needed in young patients with ductal carcinoma-in-situ? *Lancet Oncol.* 2006;7(8):615–617.

62. Yerushalmi R, Sulkes A, Mishaeli M, et al. Radiation treatment for ductal carcinoma in situ (DCIS): is a boost to the tumor bed necessary? *Neoplasma.* 2006;53(6):507–510.

63. King TA, Bolton JS, Kuske RR, Fuhrman GM, Scroggins TG, Jiang XZ. Long-term results of wide-field brachytherapy as the sole method of radiation therapy after segmental mastectomy for T(is,1,2) breast cancer. *Am J Surg.* 2000;180(4): 299–304.

64. Pignol JP, Olivotto I, Rakovitch E. A multicenter randomized trial of breast intensity-modulated radiation therapy to reduce acute radiation dermatitis. *J Clin Oncol.* 2008;26(13):2085–2092.

65. Buchholz TA. Radiation therapy for early-stage breast cancer after breast-conserving surgery. *New Engl J Med.* 2009;360(1): 63–70.

66. Clarke M, Collins R, Darby S, et al. Effects of radiotherapy and of differences in the extent of surgery for early breast cancer on local recurrence and 15-year survival: an overview of the randomised trials. *Lancet.* 2005;366(9503):2087–2106.

67. Borghero YO, Salehpour M, McNeese MD. Multileaf field-in-field forward-planned intensity-modulated dose compensation for whole-breast irradiation is associated with reduced contralateral breast dose: a phantom model comparison. *Radiother Oncol.* 2007;82(3):324–328.

68. Fisher B, Jeong JH, Dignam J, et al. Findings from recent National Surgical Adjuvant Breast and Bowel Project adjuvant studies in stage I breast cancer. *J Natl Cancer Inst Monogr.* 2001;(30):62–66.

69. Fisher B, Bryant J, Dignam JJ. Tamoxifen, radiation therapy, or both for prevention of ipsilateral breast tumor recurrence after lumpectomy in women with invasive breast cancers of one centimeter or less. *J Clin Oncol.* 2002;20(20):4141–4149.

70. Fisher B, Dignam J, Wolmark N, et al. Tamoxifen in treatment of intraductal breast cancer: National Surgical Adjuvant Breast and Bowel Project B-24 randomised, controlled trial. *Lancet*. 1999;353(9169):1993–2000.

71. Allred D, Bryant J, Land S, et al. Estrogen receptor expression as a predictor of the effectiveness of tamoxifen in the treatment of DCIS: findings from NSABP protocol B-24 [Abstract]. *Breast Cancer Res Treat*. 2002;76:S36.

72. Harris EE, Christensen VJ, Hwang WT, Fox K, Solin LJ. Impact of concurrent versus sequential tamoxifen with radiation therapy in early-stage breast cancer patients undergoing breast conservation treatment. *J Clin Oncol*. 2005;23:11–16.

73. Pierce LJ, Hutchins LF, Green SR, et al. Sequencing of tamoxifen and radiotherapy after breast-conserving surgery in early-stage breast cancer. *J Clin Oncol*. 2005;23(1):24–29.

74. Ahn PH, Vu HT, Lannin D, et al. Sequence of radiotherapy with tamoxifen in conservatively managed breast cancer does not affect local relapse rates. *J Clin Oncol*. 2005;23:10.

75. Cuzick J. Aromatase inhibitors in prevention—data from the ATAC (arimidex, tamoxifen alone or in combination) trial and the design of IBIS-II (the second International Breast Cancer Intervention Study). *Recent Results Cancer Res*. 2003;163: 96–103.

76. Silverstein MJ. The University of Southern California/Van Nuys Prognostic Index. In: Silverstein MJ, Recht A, Lagios MD, eds. *Ductal Carcinoma in Situ of the Breast*, Philadelphia, PA: Lippincott, Williams & Wilkins; 2002:465.

Medical Oncology Treatment of DCIS

JANET E. MURPHY

BEVERLY MOY

Ductal carcinoma in situ (DCIS) is a noninvasive cancerous lesion of the breast. It represents the clonal proliferation of malignant ductal cells that accumulate within but do not invade the basement membrane of mammary ductolobular units, and the architecture of the duct is preserved. Virtually all invasive carcinomas begin as in situ tumors, though not all DCIS progresses to invasive cancer (1). Approximately 62,000 new cases of DCIS are detected annually in the United States—a number that has increased significantly in the past two decades, in part as a result of widespread use of mammography for early detection (2). Screening guidelines in the United States have evolved to now recommend annual mammography for women over age 40 (American Cancer Society and National Cancer Institute guidelines), though this has not been universally implemented (3). In DCIS, there are three major concerns that invite multidisciplinary input: risk of development of DCIS, risk of invasive carcinoma progressing from DCIS, and risk of recurrence of DCIS after excision and local management. The risk factors for development of DCIS are the same as those for invasive carcinoma. They include a positive family history, prior history of breast biopsy, nulliparity, advanced gestational age, and *BRCA1* and *BRCA2* mutations and occur at the same frequency as with invasive cancer (as nearly all invasive cancers arise from in situ carcinomas, DCIS may represent lead-time bias and early detection of these lesions) (4,5).

DCIS encompasses a broad range of histopathological lesions of the breast with a wide spectrum of invasive potential. The categorization of these cancers takes into account the nuclear grade of the cells, the pattern of growth (solid, micropapillary, papillary, cribriform), and the absence or presence of comedonecrosis. Several classification schemes have been proposed for DCIS based on the histopathology of the tumor. The Lagios criteria divide tumors into low-grade, intermediate-grade, and high-grade; the Van Nuys classification divides histopathology into non-high-grade without necrosis, non-high-grade with necrosis, and high-grade; and the European system divides DCIS into well-differentiated, intermediately differentiated, and poorly differentiated subtypes (6,7). The risk of invasiveness of DCIS is correlated with the tumor grade, the tumor size, the patient's age, and the clearing of margins after surgery (8). High-grade tumors with comedonecrosis have the highest potential for invasiveness.

Our understanding of the natural history of DCIS without treatment comes from data collected from women who underwent a breast biopsy that revealed low-grade DCIS but who were not treated medically or surgically. On average, it is estimated that one third of women will progress to invasive carcinoma, with a variable latency period of between 6 and 20 years. In one small series, 11 of 28 women developed invasive carcinoma in the same breast and quadrant from which their low-grade DCIS biopsy was taken. Seven were diagnosed within 10 years of the DCIS biopsy, one was diagnosed within 12 years of the DCIS biopsy, and the remaining three invasive carcinomas were diagnosed over a period of 23 to 42 years (9).

With the advent of widespread mammography, detection of DCIS increased 10-fold (10). Early treatment consisted of mastectomy, which conferred nearly 100% local control and survival (11). However, as discussed in detail above, treatment of DCIS has evolved to include breast-conserving therapy (BCT). For most patients, mastectomy is considered unnecessary—with the exception of patients who have a field defect and widespread DCIS (larger than 5 cm). There are data from large surgical series that mastectomy lowers the risk of local or regional recurrence compared with BCT (12), but overall survival is excellent regardless—better, in fact, than age-matched all-cause mortality (13). With BCT, the majority of patients remain disease-free in long-term follow-up. However, half of all recurrences that do happen present as invasive carcinoma. Since patients are screened actively, those who recur will still have 90% survival rates. Nonetheless, for a small number of women, an invasive recurrence after primary treatment of DCIS will involve systemic treatment considerations that otherwise would have been avoided by mastectomy.

The risk of recurrence is encapsulated by the Van Nuys criteria, which calculate a recurrence score based on lesion size, adequacy of resection, age, and histological grade (from the Van Nuys classification system of non-high-grade, with or without necrosis, versus high-grade lesions). Of these features, local recurrence of DCIS is most closely correlated with completeness of resection and surgical margin width (14). Tumor grade and histological subtype play a lesser, but important, role in predicting DCIS recurrence risk after BCT. High-grade lesions, especially those exhibiting comedonecrosis, are most likely to recur (in addition to the risk they confer for invasiveness) after BCT that achieves negative margins (15).

The natural history of well-excised DCIS remains controversial and has been studied by the Eastern Cooperative Oncology Group, which selected patients by side and grade considerations (E5194) for follow-up after excision alone. This study will provide important long-term data and tissue that can be used to identify predictors of recurrence. As discussed in detail above, adjuvant radiation therapy (RT) has become the standard of care after BCT, reducing risk of local recurrence in the ipsilateral breast by approximately 50%. Several positive radiation clinical trials drive this standard, including the National Surgical Adjuvant Breast and Bowel Project (NSABP) B-17 trial, the European Organization for Research and Treatment of Cancer (EORTC) 10853 trial, and the United Kingdom, Australia, and New Zealand (UK/ANZ) trial. The UK/ANZ trial will be discussed in detail here because it also randomized patients to medical treatment in its 2 × 2 study design.

■ ADJUVANT TAMOXIFEN IN DCIS

The role of adjuvant medical treatment for DCIS is significantly more controversial. Potential roles for adjuvant treatment include (a) prevention of local recurrence, (b) substitution for another mode of treatment (radiation), or (c) prevention of invasion and metastasis. As DCIS is confined within the basement membrane of the duct, it inherently lacks metastatic potential. Large series of DCIS with axillary dissection reveal few or no examples of positive axillary nodes (16), and therefore, patients with DCIS are generally not offered sentinel lymph node biopsy (SLNB). High-grade extensive lesions, large lesions, and lesions demonstrating micrometastasis constitute a subgroup that may benefit from SLNB (17). However, the overwhelming majority of women are node-negative, and routine examination of the axilla via SLNB or axillary dissection is not indicated (18). Chemotherapy, which is the standard of care for women with invasive carcinoma with nodal involvement or otherwise of sufficient metastatic potential, does not play a role in the treatment of DCIS because its toxicities would outweigh any potential benefit based on the natural history of the disease. The worth of trastuzumab in the management of HER2/neu-overexpressing DCIS is the subject of investigation.

Adjuvant endocrine therapy, which has been well demonstrated to provide benefit in estrogen and progesterone receptor (ER/PR)–positive invasive carcinoma (19), may have a role in the adjuvant treatment of DCIS. This section will examine two major trials, NSABP B-24 and the UK/ANZ trial, that focus on the use of tamoxifen, a selective ER modulator (SERM), with differing conclusions. It will then outline ongoing studies investigating adjuvant and neoadjuvant hormonal therapy in the treatment of DCIS.

NSABP B-24

The NSABP B-24 clinical trial provided the first evidence for a potential role for tamoxifen (20). B-24 was a multicenter trial in the United States conducted between 1990 and 1995 that enrolled 1,804 women with DCIS. The enrollment criteria included a life expectancy greater than 10 years; no involved axillary lymph nodes or, more commonly, unknown axillary nodal status; and no prior diagnosis of cancer. Women with multifocal disease, microscopic positive margins from excision, and scattered calcifications of indeterminate nature deemed "suspicious" and warranting mammographic surveillance were included. The women in both arms of the study received breast-conserving surgery (lumpectomy) plus RT to 50 Gy. They were then randomized to 5 years of tamoxifen 10 mg PO bid (n = 902) or placebo (n = 902). The primary endpoint was the occurrence of invasive or noninvasive tumors in the ipsilateral or contralateral breast.

The results were interpreted as an intention-to-treat analysis, and there was some dropout preferentially in the tamoxifen arm secondary to side effects. Women in the tamoxifen group had fewer breast cancer events at 5 years than did those on placebo (8.2% versus 13.4%, P = 0.0009). The cumulative incidence of all invasive breast cancer events in the tamoxifen group was 4.1% at 5 years: 2.1% in the ipsilateral breast, 1.8% in the contralateral breast, and 0.2% at regional or distant sites. Invasive carcinomas of the ipsilateral breast were significantly reduced by 44% in the tamoxifen arm (P = 0.03). Noninvasive ipsilateral recurrences were reduced by 18%, but this was not statistically significant (P = 0.43). Contralateral invasive events were reduced, but again not significantly (23 versus 15 events, P = 0.22). In subset analysis, the histological finding of comedonecrosis was associated with a higher rate of recurrence. Younger women (under 49 years) also had a much higher rate of ipsilateral recurrence (33.3 per 1,000 versus 13.03 per 1,000).

The NSABP B-24 trial, while critical in advancing our understanding, had several crucial limitations. First was the issue of surgical margins. As noted, positive surgical margins were permitted in the trial, and margins were positive or uncertain in approximately one quarter of subjects. The trial did not require one modern institutional standard of care—excision to negative inked margins, most commonly to more than 2 mm (with adjuvant radiation planned). Thus the role of tamoxifen in the context of excision to negative margins is less clear. In subset analysis, tamoxifen provided a 22% lower recurrence rate among women resected to negative margins and a 44% lower recurrence rate among women resected to positive or unknown margins. The group that drove the significant difference in ipsilateral invasive recurrence was likely influenced by those resected to positive and unknown margins. Therefore, the results of NSABP B-24 provide a rationale for the use of tamoxifen in women with DCIS who are treated with lumpectomy but they do not provide justification for its routine use in all women with DCIS.

A second critical limitation of the NSABP trial, as well as other trials looking at DCIS, is that ER/PR status was not used to select patients who might benefit from endocrine therapy. The estimates of prevalence of ER positivity in DCIS vary widely. Barnes and colleagues analyzed 119 tumors retrospectively and found that 73.0% were ER+ and 61.1% were PR+. Notably, higher tumor grade correlated with a decrease in ER and PR positivity (both $P = 0.002$), and the finding of comedonecrosis was associated with both ER and PR negativity ($P = 0.026$ and 0.033, respectively) (21). In another small retrospective study, Hird and colleagues conducted ER staining of patients with DCIS after excisional biopsy at a single patient care site. Of 55 lesions stained, 76% were ER+, including all grade 1 and 2 lesions, compared with only 54% of high-grade lesions ($P < 0.001$) (22).

A subset analysis of 628 patients enrolled in the NSABP B-24 trial presented at the San Antonio Breast Cancer Symposium in 2002 suggested that the benefit of adjuvant tamoxifen in that study was confined to ER+ patients (23). Among the 628 patients, 77% of the tumors were ER+, a similar prevalence to the Barnes and Hird groups. Among the ER+ patients, tamoxifen was associated with relative risk of recurrence of 0.41 [95% confidence interval (CI) 0.25 to 0.65], while in ER– patients, the relative risk was a nonsignificant 0.8 (95% CI 0.41 to 1.56). If higher-grade lesions are less uniformly ER+ and they are also the most likely to recur (a risk factor second only to adequacy of surgical margins), then tamoxifen may not provide benefit to the most at-risk subset of patients. It is important to note that this analysis was retrospective and not prospectively planned. There are currently no American Society of Clinical Oncology consensus guidelines for ER/PR testing in DCIS.

In summary, the NSABP B-24 trial randomized patients to tamoxifen or placebo after breast conservation surgery and adjuvant radiation for DCIS. The study demonstrated a benefit to adjuvant tamoxifen in preventing invasive carcinoma of the ipsilateral breast—a benefit that appears to be confined to ER+ patients. However, patients with positive and indeterminate surgical margins were included. Therefore, the multidisciplinary need to ensure adequate locoregional treatment can influence the value of systemic treatment in preventing an invasive recurrence.

The UK/ANZ Trial

A second major trial investigating the benefit of adjuvant tamoxifen in DCIS was the UK/ANZ trial (24). The trial was a large, multicenter investigation that enrolled 1,701 patients with DCIS in the United Kingdom, Australia, and New Zealand between 1990 and 1998. Patients with a shortened life expectancy and those with lobular carcinoma in situ were excluded. Patients with positive or unknown surgical margins also were excluded, in contrast to the NSABP B-24 trial. Patients who were excised to positive margins but who subsequently underwent re-excision to negative margins were included, although the method of ascertaining negative margins was not specified. In addition, the trial included patients with tumors with demonstrated microinvasion, defined in the study as less then 1 mm of invasive component, provided tumors were completely excised.

The UK/ANZ trial was conducted with a 2 × 2 factorial design to evaluate both adjuvant tamoxifen and, independently, adjuvant RT. Patients were randomized to four arms: 50 Gy of RT or no RT and tamoxifen 20 mg PO daily × 5 years or no tamoxifen. By this design, one arm received no adjuvant treatment, two arms received one or the other therapy, and one arm received both adjuvant radiotherapy and tamoxifen. The trial's endpoints were recurrence of ipsilateral and contralateral DCIS, as well as invasive recurrence.

The results of the UK/ANZ trial are in sharp contrast to those of the NSABP B-24 trial. While it is one of the key trials supporting the use of adjuvant radiation, it did not demonstrate significant benefit from use of adjuvant tamoxifen alone. The treatment arm that received RT alone, as well as the arm that received RT plus tamoxifen, exhibited a lower ipsilateral recurrence rate, which translated into an absolute risk reduction of 8.9% for all ipsilateral events. Invasive events were reduced by 55%, and in situ ipsilateral events were reduced by 64%. Not surprisingly, RT did not reduce the risk of contralateral events. Tamoxifen, in contrast, did not reach significance in reducing the overall recurrence event rate (which included invasive carcinoma and DCIS). Tamoxifen did reduce the recurrence rate of DCIS alone [hazard ratio (HR) 0.58, 95% CI 0.49 to 0.96, $P = 0.03$]—mainly by reducing ipsilateral recurrence of DCIS in the patients who were not randomized to receive adjuvant RT. It did show a modest, nonsignificant reduction in contralateral overall events (DCIS and invasive carcinoma), but the total number of events, 1% in the treatment arm versus 2% in the control arm, was not high enough to draw definitive conclusions.

There were several limitations to the UK/ANZ trial as well. As in the NSABP B-24 trial, upfront ER/PR testing was not performed. The benefits of tamoxifen may have been diluted by the lack of benefit in ER/PR– patients, as suggested by the subset analysis of NSABP B-24. The 2 × 2 trial design, in which a subset of patients was randomized to adjuvant tamoxifen without RT, demonstrated that tamoxifen can reduce recurrence in nonirradiated patients, but omission of radiation is not considered a standard of care for all patients. In this group, there was a benefit to adjuvant tamoxifen, which may represent a "cleanup" effect in the absence of RT for local control. One major advantage of the UK/ANZ trial was the specification of negative surgical margins—a current standard of care. The lack of demonstrated benefit of adjuvant tamoxifen in the tamoxifen-plus-radiation arm is likely the result of better precision of clear surgical margins compared with NSABP B-24. In addition, the NSABP B-24 study population included more patients under 50 years old (34% of patients versus 10% of patients in the UK/ANZ trial), which constitutes a higher-risk population for whom tamoxifen may be associated with a greater hazard reduction, in accordance with the greater risk of recurrence in younger patients.

NSABP B-35

Building on the conclusion of the NSABP B-24 trial, the NSABP B-35 trial was begun and has completed enrollment. B-35 is a randomized phase III trial that compares the aromatase inhibitor (AI) anastrozole with tamoxifen for the prevention of subsequent breast cancer events: local recurrences, contralateral breast cancers, and distant invasive recurrences. This study was activated in January 2003, closed in 2006, and enrolled 3,104 patients. B-35 will prove an important trial to determine whether an AI is superior to tamoxifen in the prevention of recurrence—and to add credibility to the benefit of antiestrogen therapy to prevent recurrence as a follow-up to NSABP B-24. In addition to comparing the effectiveness of these two agents for cancer recurrence, the trial will evaluate several secondary endpoints: prevention or occurrence of second primary cancers (nonbreast), pathological fractures, disease-free survival, and overall survival.

■ CONCLUSIONS

The role for adjuvant medical treatment in DCIS remains controversial. As discussed above, several major trials have investigated the use of adjuvant tamoxifen in DCIS, with differing results. Since the publication of NSABP B-24 in 1999, tamoxifen has had a presence in the clinic, but it is not uniformly prescribed or accepted by patients. Yen and colleagues reviewed the use of tamoxifen in DCIS at the MD Anderson Cancer Center after the publication (from 1999 to 2002) and found that 60% of patients with surgically proven DCIS were offered tamoxifen, of whom 54% chose to take the drug. Those not offered tamoxifen had a documented reason a significant proportion of the time. Of the 94 patients who received tamoxifen, 20 patients (21%) discontinued use because of side effects or complications—similar to the number of patients in the tamoxifen arm who dropped out of the NSABP trial (25). Major side effects of tamoxifen include phlebitis and venous thromboembolism, irregular menses, menopausal symptoms (hot flashes, vaginal discharge, edema), and irritability. Tamoxifen confers increased risk of endometrial cancer,

and in the NSABP B-24 trial, 1.53 patients per 1,000 per year (versus 0.45 per 1,000 patients per year in the placebo arm) did develop this complication, though with no reported deaths. In an addendum to the 1999 NSABP B-24 study, Fisher and colleagues reported six stroke events, one in the placebo arm and five in the tamoxifen arm, none fatal (26). Tamoxifen, other SERMs, and AIs offer promise but also present a side-effect profile that is not trivial. Without a proven survival advantage, there is reluctance to prescribe these agents.

The multidisciplinary treatment of DCIS consists of surgery (generally breast-conserving surgery) plus RT. The benefits and risks of systemic endocrine therapy must be carefully discussed with patients owing to the conflicting results of two large randomized clinical trials. The results of ongoing clinical trials of aromatase inhibition in patients with DCIS are eagerly awaited. At this time, systemic endocrine therapy with tamoxifen for 5 years in patients with DCIS should be used in selected patients where the benefits outweigh the risks of treatment.

■ SUMMARY

- The natural history of DCIS demonstrates that the majority of patients do not develop a local recurrence, about one half of all recurrences are invasive breast cancer, and nearly all patients with a noninvasive recurrence and more than 90% of those with an invasive recurrence survive their disease after subsequent treatment.
- The multidisciplinary treatment of DCIS consists of surgery (generally breast-conserving surgery) plus RT.
- Available clinical trial data are conflicting as to the benefit of tamoxifen in DCIS.
- At this time, systemic endocrine therapy with tamoxifen in patients with DCIS should be used in selected patients in whom the benefits outweigh the risks of treatment.

■ REFERENCES

1. Welch HG, Woloshin S, Schwartz LM. The sea of uncertainty surrounding ductal carcinoma in situ—the price of screening mammography. *J Natl Cancer Inst.* 2008;100(4):228–229.
2. Jemal A, Siegel R, Ward E, Murray T, Xu J, Thun MJ. Cancer statistics, 2007. *CA Cancer J Clin.* 2007; 57(1):43–66.
3. Calvocoressi L, Sun A, Kasl SV, Claus EB, Jones BA. Mammography screening of women in their 40s: impact of changes in screening guidelines. *Cancer.* 2008;112(3):473–480.
4. Kerlikowske K, Barclay J, Grady D, Sickles EA, Ernster V. Comparison of risk factors for ductal carcinoma in situ and invasive breast cancer. *J Natl Cancer Inst.* 1997;89(1):76–82.
5. Claus EB, Stowe M, Carter D. Breast carcinoma in situ: risk factors and screening patterns. *J Natl Cancer Inst.* 2001;93(23):1811–1817.

6. Lagios MD, Margolin FR, Westdahl PR, Rose MR. Mammographically detected duct carcinoma in situ. Frequency of local recurrence following tylectomy and prognostic effect of nuclear grade on local recurrence. *Cancer.* 1989;15;63:618–624.

7. Silverstein MJ, Poller DN, Waisman JR, et al. Prognostic classification of breast ductal carcinoma-in-situ. *Lancet.* 1995;345: 1154.

8. Morrow M, O'Sullivan MJ. The dilemma of DCIS. *Breast.* 2007;16(Suppl 2):S59–S62.

9. Sanders ME, Schuyler PA, Dupont WD, Page DL. The natural history of low-grade ductal carcinoma in situ of the breast in women treated by biopsy only revealed over 30 years of long-term follow-up. *Cancer.* 2005;103(12):2481–2484.

10. Ernster VL, Barclay J, Kerlikowske K, Grady D, Henderson C. Incidence of and treatment for ductal carcinoma in situ of the breast. *JAMA.* 1996;275(12):913–918.

11. Moore MM. Treatment of ductal carcinoma in situ of the breast. *Semin Surg Oncol.* 1991;7(5):267–270.

12. Silverstein MJ, Cohlan BF, Gierson ED, et al. Duct carcinoma in situ: 227 cases without microinvasion. *Eur J Cancer.* 1992; 28:630–634.

13. Ernster VL, Barclay J, Kerlikowske K, Wilkie H, Ballard-Barbash R. Mortality among women with ductal carcinoma in situ of the breast in the population-based surveillance, epidemiology and end results program. *Arch Intern Med.* 2000;160(7):953–958.

14. Boland GP, Chan KC, Knox WF, Roberts SA, Bundred NJ. Value of the Van Nuys Prognostic Index in prediction of recurrence of ductal carcinoma in situ after breast-conserving surgery. *Br J Surg.* 2003;90(4):426–432.

15. Lagios MD, Margolin FR, Westdahl PR, Rose MR. Mammographically detected duct carcinoma in situ. Frequency of local recurrence following tylectomy and prognostic effect of nuclear grade on local recurrence. *Cancer.* 1989;63(4):618–624.

16. Silverstein MJ, Gierson ED, Colburn WJ, Rosser RJ, Waisman JR, Gamagami P. Axillary lymphadenectomy for intraductal carcinoma of the breast. *Surg Gynecol Obstet.* 1991;172(3): 211–214.

17. Lyman GH, Giuliano AE, Somerfield MR, et al. American Society of Clinical Oncology guideline recommendations for sentinel lymph node biopsy in early-stage breast cancer. *J Clin Oncol.* 2005;23(30):7703–7720.

18. Julian TB, Land SR, Fourchotte V, et al. Is sentinel node biopsy necessary in conservatively treated DCIS? *Ann Surg Oncol.* 2007;14(8):2202–2208.

19. Fisher B, Costantino J, Redmond C, et al. A randomized clinical trial evaluating tamoxifen in the treatment of patients with node-negative breast cancer who have estrogen-receptor-positive tumors. *N Engl J Med.* 1989;320(8):479–484.

20. Fisher B, Dignam J, Wolmark N, et al. Tamoxifen in treatment of intraductal breast cancer: National Surgical Adjuvant Breast and Bowel Project B-24 randomised controlled trial. *Lancet.* 1999;353(9169):1993–2000.

21. Barnes NL, Boland GP, Davenport A, Knox WF, Bundred NJ. Relationship between hormone receptor status and tumour size, grade and comedo necrosis in ductal carcinoma in situ. *Br J Surg.* 2005;92(4):429–434.

22. Hird RB, Chang A, Cimmino V, et al. Impact of estrogen receptor expression and other clinicopathologic features on tamoxifen use in ductal carcinoma in situ. *Cancer.* 2006;106(10):2113–2118.

23. Allred DC, Bryant J, Land S, et al. Estrogen receptor expression as a predictive marker of the effectiveness of tamoxifen in the treatment of DCIS: findings from NSABP protocol B-24. *Breast Cancer Res Treat.* 2002;76(Suppl 1):36.

24. Houghton J, George WD, Cuzick J, et al. Ductal carcinoma in situ working party; DCIS trialists in the UK, Australia, and New Zealand. Radiotherapy and tamoxifen in women with completely excised ductal carcinoma in situ of the breast in the UK, Australia, and New Zealand: randomised controlled trial. *Lancet.* 2003;362(9378):95–102.

25. Yen TW, Hunt KK, Mirza NQ, et al. Physician recommendations regarding tamoxifen and patient utilization of tamoxifen after surgery for ductal carcinoma in situ. *Cancer.* 2004;100(5):942–949.

26. Dignam JJ, Fisher B. Occurrence of stroke with tamoxifen in NSABP B-24. *Lancet.* 2000;355(9206):848–849.

7 Multidisciplinary Approach in the Treatment of Early Breast Cancer

Surgical Management

BARBARA L. SMITH

Until the mid-twentieth century, surgical resection was the only effective treatment option for women with breast cancer. Surgical resection, most often as a radical mastectomy, provided effective local tumor control for most patients and resulted in long-term disease-free survival for many. However, over time it became clear that surgery alone was inadequate treatment for a significant fraction of patients, and it was recognized that incorporation of radiation and systemic therapy into treatment algorithms could improve both local and systemic tumor control. The effectiveness of this multidisciplinary treatment approach allowed the development of less extensive surgical options for breast cancer patients, including modified radical mastectomy and lumpectomy, resulting in decreased surgical morbidity, less disfigurement for patients, and in many cases, improved local control.

There has been continued evolution of surgical approaches for early-stage invasive breast cancer. Widespread adoption of mammographic screening has allowed identification of tumors at smaller and smaller sizes and has required the development of techniques for biopsy and excision of nonpalpable breast cancers. Improvements in diagnostic breast imaging now allow more detailed preoperative assessment of eligibility for breast conservation and enable the surgical procedure to be more accurately tailored to tumor geometry.

As advances in breast cancer detection and treatment have improved overall survival, increasing emphasis has been placed on reducing the impact of treatment on a patient's quality of life. In breast surgery, this has translated into increased awareness of the aesthetic consequences of surgical procedures for breast cancer. Improvements in mastectomy techniques, including use of skin-sparing and nipple-sparing approaches, advances in breast reconstruction options, and the introduction of oncoplastic techniques for lumpectomy have contributed to improved cosmetic outcomes for breast cancer patients.

Surgical staging of the axilla remains critical to determine prognosis and inform systemic and radiation therapy decision making. The development of sentinel node biopsy techniques allows accurate and minimally invasive axillary staging and avoids the morbidity of standard axillary dissection.

This chapter will review current issues in surgical management of patients with early-stage invasive breast cancer.

■ LUMPECTOMY VERSUS MASTECTOMY

Long-term follow-up of prospective randomized clinical trials has confirmed the equivalence of lumpectomy and mastectomy in patients with early-stage breast cancer. No survival advantage was seen with mastectomy over lumpectomy in any of the prospective, randomized trials that compared breast-conserving surgery with mastectomy (1–6). A variety of factors, including tumor size and histology, breast size, potential contraindications to radiation therapy, risk of future breast cancer, and patient preference, are currently evaluated in selecting the best surgical approach.

■ ELIGIBILITY FOR BREAST CONSERVATION

Tumor Size

Tumors up to 5 cm in size were included in randomized trials of lumpectomy versus mastectomy. At the present time, eligibility for lumpectomy is based on the ability to excise the tumor to clear margins while leaving an acceptable cosmetic result rather than on a specific maximum tumor size. Patients with multiple primary tumor nodules close enough together to be included in a single lumpectomy specimen may also be considered for breast conservation.

Margins

Microscopically clear margins of at least 2 to 3 mm must be obtained circumferentially on the lumpectomy specimen because local recurrence rates increase with narrower margins. No additional reduction in local recurrence rates is seen with margin widths greater than 2 mm in patients who receive radiation therapy.

Margins must be clear for both invasive cancer and for ductal carcinoma in situ (DCIS). Atypical hyperplasia and lobular carcinoma in situ at resection margins do not increase local recurrence rates. Although the growth patterns of invasive lobular cancers and cancers with an extensive intraductal component may make achieving clear margins more difficult, tumors with these histological patterns are eligible for lumpectomy if clear margins are achieved.

Nodal Status

Prospective trials of breast conservation included patients with positive axillary nodes. The presence of palpable axillary nodes is not a contraindication to lumpectomy and radiation.

Risk Factors

Tumors in patients with a positive family history of breast cancer, including those with *BRCA* gene mutations, may be considered for breast-conserving surgery. The risk of recurrence in the initial tumor bed is no higher for a patient with multiple risk factors than for the average patient. However, the patient with a risk gene mutation or multiple risk factors may be at significantly higher risk of new primary tumors in the contralateral breast or at other sites distant from the initial tumor location in the ipsilateral breast. The risk of future breast cancers must be weighed into the choice of breast conservation or bilateral mastectomy.

Preoperative Imaging

A complete imaging evaluation is required prior to planning surgery for early-stage breast cancer to assess the extent of disease and inform the decision regarding breast-conserving surgery or mastectomy. At a minimum, this will include a high-quality digital mammogram, often with ultrasound to further define lesion size and guide biopsies. Breast magnetic resonance imaging (MRI) has an increasing role in assessing extent of disease and may identify unsuspected ipsilateral or contralateral lesions in as many as 3% to 5% of newly diagnosed breast cancer patients overall (7,8) and in as many as 12% of women aged 40 or younger at diagnosis (9). Breast MRI may be particularly useful in assessing extent of disease for patients with invasive lobular carcinoma, for patients whose cancers were not visualized by mammography, for *BRCA* and other risk gene mutation carriers, and for young patients with dense breast tissue. Concern has been raised that false-positive MRI findings may incorrectly raise concerns about multifocal disease and lead to an increase in mastectomy rates. Consultation with breast imaging colleagues may be useful in determining which imaging approaches will be best for a given patient.

Core needle biopsy of other remote suspicious lesions identified may be performed prior to a lumpectomy attempt to confirm or rule out eligibility for breast conservation. Multiple localizing wires may be used to bracket larger or more irregularly shaped tumors, and this technique has been shown to reduce the rate of positive margins requiring re-excision (10,11).

For most patients, radiation therapy should follow lumpectomy, and contraindications to breast irradiation must be considered as part of the decision between lumpectomy and mastectomy. In-breast recurrence rates after 20 years' follow-up are as high at 40% without radiation (1), with modern series reporting 5-year local failure rates under 2% after lumpectomy plus radiation (12). Meta-analysis data now demonstrate a survival decrement as a result of locoregional breast cancer recurrence (13), underscoring the importance of radiation after lumpectomy.

An exception to the standard recommendation for radiation after lumpectomy may be made for elderly or medically frail patients for whom tumor biology and comorbid conditions reduce the relative importance of a potential increase in risk of late local recurrence. Prospective, randomized trials have demonstrated excellent local control and survival after lumpectomy plus tamoxifen without radiation for estrogen receptor–positive (ER+) tumors in older women. Hughes and colleagues (14) reported results of Cancer and Leukemia Group B (CALGB) trial 9343, in which women aged 70 and older with ER+ tumors 2 cm or smaller underwent lumpectomy, received tamoxifen, and were randomized to radiation or no radiation. Locoregional recurrence at 5 years was 4% without radiation, compared with 1% with radiation, and survival was no different, suggesting that lumpectomy and hormonal therapy without radiation was reasonable in this setting. These data were updated at 8 years' follow-up with a locoregional recurrence rate of 7% and 1% for the no-radiation and radiation arms, respectively (15).

Fyles and colleagues (16) assessed the impact of radiation added to lumpectomy and tamoxifen in a younger cohort that included women as young as age 50. Although local recurrence rates at 5 years without radiation were low in women over age 60 with ER+ tumors under 2 cm (1.2% without radiation compared with 0% with radiation), in the larger cohort of women aged 50 and older, local recurrence at 5 years was significantly worse without radiation (5.9%) than with radiation (0.4%).

Otherwise fit patients who cannot receive radiation, such as those with a history of prior chest wall or breast radiation or those with active collagen-vascular disease, should be treated with mastectomy. Radiation cannot be delivered during pregnancy, and mastectomy may be required if waiting until after delivery would create an unsafe delay between lumpectomy and initiation of radiation. Mastectomy is also considered for patients for whom personal factors would prevent timely completion of the full course of radiation. Such factors might include multiple medical comorbidities likely to interrupt treatment or excessive travel distance to a radiation facility. Some of these logistic issues may be addressed through use of shorter radiation regimens, such as accelerated partial breast irradiation completed in 1 week (see Chapter 6) or whole breast radiation with Canadian fractionation completed in 3 weeks (17). Eligibility for radiation should be determined prior to surgery in consultation with a radiation oncologist, keeping in mind that some patients will require radiation even after mastectomy, depending on their tumor histology and nodal status.

For male breast cancer patients, lumpectomy with radiation remains an option for tumors far enough away from the areola to permit excision of the lesion with clear margins and preservation of the nipple-areola complex (18).

Patient Preference Issues

Long-term follow-up of prospective randomized clinical trials has confirmed that survival after lumpectomy and radiation is equivalent to that seen after mastectomy (1,2). For most patients, breast conservation will be preferable, with an easier postoperative recovery than mastectomy and without the need for reconstruction or use of a prosthesis, as is required after mastectomy.

However, there are an increasing number of women who elect not just unilateral but bilateral mastectomy, with or without immediate reconstruction, for management of early-stage breast cancer (19). Bilateral mastectomy is often the preferred management option for high-risk gene mutation carriers or other high-risk patients. For women of low or average risk of future contralateral breast cancer, discussion of the basis for the patient's request for a bilateral mastectomy should take place. It is important to ensure that the request is not based on an incorrect overestimation of the risk of future contralateral breast cancer or of the risk of ipsilateral tumor recurrence. It is equally important to be sure that the decision is not based on underestimation of the possible psychological and physical difficulties after bilateral mastectomy and reconstruction or on unrealistic expectations of cosmetic outcome after reconstruction. Frank discussions about risks and benefits of bilateral mastectomy and early plastic surgery consultation can help patients to make an informed decision about

surgical approach and help to decrease postoperative dissatisfaction with decisions and outcomes (20).

■ LUMPECTOMY CONSIDERATIONS

Despite careful preoperative imaging and meticulous surgical technique, microscopic tumor deposits remain at the margins of many lumpectomy specimens, necessitating re-excision or even mastectomy. Although rates of positive margins are highest for invasive lobular cancers and lesions with DCIS, where extent of disease may not be easily assessed by imaging, inspection, or palpation, positive margins can occur for any tumor. As a result, incision placement and specimen orientation become important technical considerations. A review of 2,770 patients who underwent breast-conserving surgery found no association between number of re-excisions and risk of local failure among patients who ultimately achieved clear margins (21).

Incision Placement

Incision placement for every lumpectomy must acknowledge the possibility that clear margins may not be achieved and that mastectomy may ultimately be required. Whenever possible, incisions should be placed so as not to preclude skin-sparing mastectomy, keeping in mind that the lumpectomy incision should be excised as part of the mastectomy. Incisions close to the areola and radial incisions for very medial or lateral lesions are ideal for a lumpectomy that may need to be converted to a skin-sparing mastectomy. Vertical incisions in the medial or lateral positions or incisions high on the breast can require excision of larger amounts of skin or leave devascularized skin bridges when the incision is excised during mastectomy.

Specimen Orientation

The possibility of positive margins makes it essential that the surgeon orient all lumpectomy or biopsy specimens. Specimen orientation permits the pathologist to specify which margins are close or positive, which in turn allows the surgeon to perform a selective re-excision of involved margins rather than a global re-excision of the entire cavity. Selective re-excisions generally result in smaller excision volumes and enhance final cosmetic outcome.

Specimen orientation may be achieved by orientation of the lumpectomy itself with two or more marking sutures followed by six-color inking of the specimen to uniquely identify superior, inferior, medial, lateral, anterior, and deep aspects of the specimen. Alternatively, the surgeon may excise multiple separate, thin or "shaved" final margins from the walls of the lumpectomy cavity after the main lumpectomy specimen has been removed. The use of separate final margins may be particularly useful if there has been tearing or fragmentation of the lumpectomy specimen during excision, making six-color inking of the surface less accurate in reflecting the true specimen edges. It is also useful for needle-localized lumpectomies where specimen compression during imaging may also result in tearing or disruption of the original lumpectomy edges.

Oncoplastic Approaches

A central goal of breast conservation is achievement of good to excellent cosmetic results. As discussed above, this is greatly facilitated by preoperative imaging to guide lumpectomy specimen geometry and by specimen orientation to minimize re-excision volumes. Cosmetic outcome is also greatly influenced by incision closure techniques, which can achieve an excellent cosmetic result even following a large-volume lumpectomy.

For most lumpectomies, local advancement flaps can be created by mobilization of the edges of the lumpectomy cavity off the pectoralis fascia for 2 to 3 cm on all sides, with the option of additional mobilization of skin from breast parenchyma at the superficial cavity edges. Tissue can be advanced and sutured to close at least part of the lumpectomy defect without creating skin dimpling. Such reduction of the size of the lumpectomy cavity can prevent development of an expanding seroma and reduce the risk of a visible tissue defect at the lumpectomy site.

For lumpectomies in patients with large breasts, more advanced oncoplastic approaches that incorporate large-volume excisions with mastopexy and reduction mammoplasty are possible for practitioners with experience in these techniques or in consultation with plastic surgery colleagues.

Other Lumpectomy Considerations

Placement of MRI-compatible metallic clips to mark the edges of the lumpectomy cavity is essential for accurate identification of the cavity margins in patients being considered for external beam partial breast irradiation and may also facilitate delivery of the boost to the tumor bed for patients receiving standard whole breast irradiation. These clips should be large enough to be easily visualized during computed tomography simulation and planning.

■ MASTECTOMY CONSIDERATIONS

Technical Considerations in Mastectomy

While the ideal goal of a mastectomy is to remove all breast tissue, complete removal of breast tissue is not possible. No distinct boundary separates breast tissue from adjacent adipose tissue, and it has been demonstrated that breast structures may extend into pectoralis muscle and along Cooper's ligaments into subcutaneous fat (22,23).

Nevertheless, several anatomical features of the breast can help guide a more thorough removal of breast tissue. A thin but fairly consistent and nearly avascular fibrous plane exists between breast parenchyma and subcutaneous fat. This plane serves as the superficial boundary of a mastectomy dissection and allows separation of the breast from subcutaneous fat while leaving the blood supply to the skin intact. Skin flaps are raised in this plane, dividing Cooper's ligaments superiorly to the clavicle, medially to the sternum, inferiorly to the inframammary fold, and laterally to the border of the latissimus dorsi muscle. Vessels in the skin flap are carefully preserved to maintain flap perfusion. The breast is then removed from the underlying pectoralis muscle, taking pectoral muscle fascia with the breast specimen and creating a well-defined deep margin. All axillary breast tissue superficial to the fascia of the axillary fat pad should be included in the mastectomy specimen. After the breast has been removed, the skin flaps are inspected and any remaining visible breast tissue excised.

The extent of breast tissue removed during a mastectomy should be the same whether or not immediate reconstruction is performed and regardless of the incision used. The extent of skin removed and the extent of axillary node removal may vary in different clinical situations. A simple or total mastectomy includes complete removal of the breast, nipple, and areola, without axillary dissection. A sentinel node biopsy, via the mastectomy incision or through a separate axillary incision, is added for staging in clinically node-negative patients. A modified radical mastectomy includes removal of the breast, nipple, and areola with a level 1 and 2 axillary dissection.

If immediate reconstruction is not performed, sufficient skin should be included in the specimen to allow a smooth closure of the chest wall skin, without redundant skin folds, to facilitate fitting and wearing of a breast prosthesis. For heavier patients, this may require planning the skin incision with the patient in a sitting position to better assess skin tension and accommodate natural skin folds. Use of a diagonal incision that places the medial aspect of the mastectomy incision near the inframammary fold at the sternal border is much more favorable for delayed reconstruction than a horizontal incision higher on the chest wall.

Mastectomy With Immediate Reconstruction

Reconstruction at the time of mastectomy has been shown to be safe for patients with early-stage breast cancer. Compared with delayed reconstruction, immediate reconstruction eliminates the need for a second surgical procedure, provides a better cosmetic outcome, and spares the patient the hardships associated with a prolonged period between mastectomy and reconstruction.

The cosmetic outcome of immediate breast reconstruction is further improved by skin-sparing techniques that excise only nipple and areola skin and preserve the remainder of the breast skin envelope. Several mature studies confirm that local recurrence rates after skin-sparing mastectomy are equivalent to those seen after simple mastectomy without reconstruction (24–29). For patients whose tumor diagnosis has been made with core needle biopsy, only nipple and areola skin is removed, with a lateral skin slit added if required to provide adequate exposure for a thorough resection of breast tissue. For patients undergoing mastectomy after a lumpectomy attempt or after a diagnostic surgical biopsy, the lumpectomy or diagnostic biopsy incision is generally excised, either in continuity with the nipple and areola skin or as a separate specimen.

The efficacy of skin-sparing mastectomy in achieving local control has led to consideration of nipple-sparing mastectomy for selected patients with early-stage breast cancer (30). In nipple-sparing mastectomy all skin, including the nipple and areola, is left in place, with the mastectomy performed through an incision that is closed primarily. Current nipple-sparing techniques differ from prior subcutaneous mastectomy approaches that left a thick flap of tissue under the nipple and areola. Nipple-sparing mastectomy techniques now create standard thin skin flaps and remove all visible breast tissue under the nipple and areola, often including excision of duct tissue from within the nipple papilla (31–33). Early follow-up of nipple-sparing mastectomy in selected patients has shown low rates of nipple recurrence and acceptable rates of nipple necrosis (34–37).

At present, nipple-sparing mastectomy is considered for selected patients at low risk for nipple involvement. This generally includes patients undergoing prophylactic mastectomy and those cancer patients whose tumors are small, are more than 2 cm from the nipple, and do not contain extensive DCIS. Rusby and colleagues have created a calculator to predict risk of nipple involvement for breast cancer patients being considered for nipple-sparing mastectomy (38). Preoperative imaging studies are performed to rule out nipple involvement by tumor or suspicious calcifications. The subareolar margin should be assessed for tumor involvement and the nipple and areola removed if tumor is present at the margin. Petit and colleagues (36) have used a single 16 Gy dose of intraoperative radiation therapy [electron intraoperative therapy (ELIOT)] to the nipple in patients undergoing nipple-sparing mastectomy, with early results showing low rates of recurrence in the retained nipple but rates of nipple necrosis (4.7% total, 10.7% partial) that are higher than are seen without radiation. Breast reconstruction is discussed further in Chapter 9.

■ SURGICAL MANAGEMENT OF THE AXILLA

The pathological status of the axillary lymph nodes remains one of the most important prognostic factors in patients with breast cancer. Identification of metastatic tumor deposits in the axillary nodes indicates a poorer prognosis and often prompts a recommendation for more aggressive systemic and local therapies. Surgical removal of axillary tumor deposits also serves a therapeutic purpose, reducing risks of axillary tumor recurrence.

Unfortunately, axillary dissection is often the main source of morbidity in patients with early-stage breast cancer. Immediate problems include acute pain, the need for hospital stay, reduced range of motion, and the need for a drain in the surgical bed for a week or more. Long-term problems resulting from axillary dissection include permanent lymphedema in 10% to 25%, numbness, chronic pain, and reduced range of motion (39–44). Assessment of patients' subjective symptoms of arm problems shows even higher rates of persistent arm symptoms, with 25% to 50% of patients reporting arm swelling, pain, numbness, or decreased mobility (45–47).

Sentinel Node Biopsy

Although axillary dissection is necessary for patients with clinically involved axillary nodes, sentinel node biopsy provides a less invasive option for axillary staging in clinically node-negative breast cancer patients (48,49). It has been recognized that breast lymphatics converge as they leave the breast, delivering fluid, traveling cells, and dye particles to a small number of "sentinel" nodes first. The sentinel node is identified by injection of technetium-radiolabeled sulfur colloid particles or blue dye, or both, into the breast in a subareolar or peritumoral location, followed by selective excision of the blue or radioactive node(s). If pathological analysis of the sentinel node shows no evidence of metastasis, the likelihood of other nodes being involved is sufficiently low that therapeutic axillary dissection is not required.

Use of the sentinel node biopsy approach dramatically reduces morbidity compared with axillary dissection. Sentinel node biopsy is an outpatient procedure that does not require a drain, allows rapid return to full mobility, and allows rapid return to work and full activity, usually within a week. Rates of long-term lymphedema, numbness, and chronic pain are also greatly reduced.

Sentinel node biopsy has been shown to provide reliable pathological staging of the axilla (50–53). Axillary recurrence rates have been shown to be extremely low after a negative sentinel node biopsy without axillary dissection (54). A negative sentinel node biopsy is now widely accepted as sufficient to establish a patient as node-negative, with no further axillary treatment required.

Although patients with negative sentinel nodes may avoid axillary dissection, completion level 1 and 2 axillary dissection remains the standard of care for patients whose sentinel node is positive for metastases. The need for completion axillary dissection is debated for patients whose sentinel nodes contain only micrometastases or isolated tumor cells, as many such patients are unlikely to have additional positive nodes. Models that predict the risk of additional positive nodes, such as the nomogram designed by Van Zee and colleagues (55) that predicts the risk of additional positive nodes on the basis of features of the primary tumor and sentinel nodes, may be useful in deciding whether axillary dissection is indicated.

Clinical trials addressing use of axillary radiation rather than completion dissection (56,57) or systemic therapy and standard tangent radiation without completion axillary dissection (58) have been conducted, and results are pending.

Eligibility for Sentinel Node Biopsy

There are few contraindications to the use of sentinel node biopsy in patients with early-stage breast cancer. Although concerns were initially raised about sentinel node biopsy in some clinical situations, sentinel node mapping appears reliable in the majority of clinical situations, including in patients with prior open breast biopsies, biopsy site seromas, larger primary tumors, and multifocal tumors. Repeat node mapping is possible after prior axillary sentinel node biopsy or dissection, with lower rates of mapping success but reliable results if a new sentinel node is identified (59,60).

If suspicious axillary nodes are identified by palpation or on imaging studies, confirmation of tumor involvement may be obtained by fine-needle or core biopsy. If the needle biopsy does not confirm node involvement, sentinel node biopsy with frozen section may be considered. Patients with confirmed axillary node involvement should proceed directly to axillary dissection or neoadjuvant therapy.

Axillary Dissection

A level 1 and 2 axillary dissection removes node-bearing axillary fat beneath the hair-bearing skin of the axilla. Its superficial border is formed by subcutaneous fat and the pectoralis major and pectoralis minor muscles, its medial border by the serratus anterior muscle to the medial border of the pectoralis minor muscle, its lateral and deep borders by the latissimus dorsi muscle, its superior border by the axillary vein, and its inferior border by the fascia separating the axillary fat pad from the tail of the breast. The long thoracic, thoracodorsal, and medial pectoral motor nerves are preserved, and every effort is made to preserve the intercostobrachial sensory nerve branches. A level 3 dissection, which adds axillary tissue medial to the pectoralis minor muscle, significantly increases risk of lymphedema and is performed only when palpable nodes are present in level 3.

Patients with extensive axillary node disease will usually receive radiation to the supraclavicular nodes and often to the axilla as well. The placement of MRI-compatible metal clips at the highest point of the surgical dissection may be helpful to delineate dissected from nondissected areas in subsequent radiation planning.

Management of the Axilla in the Elderly

For some clinically node-negative patients, information from axillary staging will not alter treatment decisions, and axillary surgery may be omitted. For example, an elderly or otherwise frail patient with a clinically node-negative, ER+ tumor who is not a candidate for chemotherapy does not require axillary staging if endocrine therapy would be used regardless of nodal status. Axillary recurrence rates are expected to be low for many such patients, even without radiation or axillary surgery. The rate of axillary recurrence was approximately 1% at 5 years among women treated with lumpectomy and tamoxifen without radiation in CALGB 9343, many of whom did not have surgical staging of the axilla (14). For patients who will receive radiation after lumpectomy, use of high tangent radiation without axillary surgery provides excellent local control.

■ PERIOPERATIVE CONSIDERATIONS

Patients undergoing surgery for breast cancer should receive deep venous thrombosis prophylaxis with compression stockings and sequential compression boots. Early ambulation after surgery further reduces risk of thromboembolic disease and also reduces risk of atelectasis.

Prophylactic antibiotics providing coverage for skin flora should be used for patients undergoing breast cancer surgery. A single preoperative antibiotic dose is sufficient for most patients undergoing lumpectomy or mastectomy without reconstruction, although antibiotic coverage may be continued while drains are in place for patients having immediate reconstruction or for patients, such as those with diabetes, who are at higher risk for infection.

For patients undergoing axillary surgery, early shoulder mobilization with range-of-motion exercises can reduce the risk of a frozen shoulder or other long-term shoulder complications.

■ MULTIDISCIPLINARY CONSIDERATIONS

- Planning surgery requires collaboration between the surgeon and the breast imaging team to determine eligibility for breast conservation and to assess extent of disease for lumpectomy planning.
- Incision placement for lumpectomy should not preclude a skin-sparing mastectomy approach should mastectomy and reconstruction be required for positive margins.

- Lumpectomy and biopsy specimens should be oriented by the surgeon to allow the pathologist to identify specific positive margins and allow focal rather than global re-excision. This allows smaller re-excision volumes and optimizes cosmetic result.
- Discussion of potential contraindications to radiation should take place prior to finalizing the decision for lumpectomy versus mastectomy.
- Placement of clips to mark significant surgical landmarks can facilitate subsequent radiation planning. For example, clips at the edges of the lumpectomy cavity are essential for patients being considered for external beam partial breast irradiation and facilitate delivery of the boost to the tumor bed in standard whole breast irradiation. Clips at the site of chest wall tumor involvement or at the apex of an extensive axillary dissection help guide subsequent radiation.

■ REFERENCES

1. Fisher B, Anderson S, Bryant J, et al. Twenty-year follow-up of a randomized trial comparing total mastectomy, lumpectomy, and lumpectomy plus irradiation for the treatment of invasive breast cancer. *New Engl J Med.* 2002;347:1233.
2. Veronesi U, Cascinelli N, Mariani L, et al. Twenty-year follow-up of a randomized study comparing breast-conserving surgery with radical mastectomy for early breast cancer. *New Engl J Med.* 2002;347:1227.
3. Arriagada R, Le M, Rochard F, et al. Conservative treatment versus mastectomy in early breast cancer: patterns of failure with 15 years of follow-up data. *J Clin Oncol.* 1996;14:1558.
4. Jacobson J, Danforth D, Cowan K, et al. Ten-year results of a comparison of conservation with mastectomy in the treatment of stage I and II breast cancer. *New Engl J Med.* 1995;332:907.
5. van Dongen J, Voogd A, Fentiman I, et al. Long-term results of a randomized trial comparing breast-conserving therapy with mastectomy: European Organization for Research and Treatment of Cancer 10801 trial. *J Natl Cancer Inst.* 2000;92: 1143–1150.
6. Blichert-Toft M, Rose C, Andersen J, et al. Danish randomized trial comparing breast conservation therapy with mastectomy: six years of life-table analysis. Danish Breast Cancer Cooperative Group. *J Natl Cancer Inst Monogr.* 1992;11:19.
7. Lehman CD, Gatsonis C, Kuhl CK, et al. MRI evaluation of the contralateral breast in women with recently diagnosed breast cancer. *New Engl J Med.* 2007;356:1295–1303.
8. Liberman L, Morris EA, Kim CM, et al. MR imaging findings in the contralateral breast of women with recently diagnosed breast cancer. *AJR Am J Roentgenol.* 2003;180:333–341.
9. Samphao S, Wheeler AJ, Rafferty E, et al. Diagnosis of breast cancer in women age 40 and younger: delays in diagnosis result from underutilization of genetic testing and breast imaging. *Am J Surg.* In press.
10. Kirstein L, Rafferty E, Moore R, Specht MC, Hughes KS, Smith BL. Outcome of multiple wire localization for larger breast cancers: when can mastectomy be avoided? *J Am Coll Surg.* 2008;207:342–346.
11. Javid S, Kirstein LJ, Rafferty E, et al. Outcome of multiple wire localization for larger breast cancers: do multiple wires translate into additional imaging, biopsies, and recurrences? *Am J Surg.* 2009;198:368–372.
12. Nguyen PL, Taghian AG, Katz MS, et al. Breast cancer subtype approximated by ER, PR, and HER2 receptors is associated with local-regional and distant recurrence after breast-conserving therapy. *J Clin Oncol.* 2008;26:2373–2378.
13. Early Breast Cancer Trialists' Collaborative Group. Effects of radiotherapy and of differences in the extent of surgery for early breast cancer on local recurrence and 15-year survival: an overview of the randomised trials. *Lancet.* 2005;366:2087–2106.
14. Hughes KS, Schnaper L, Berry D, et al. Comparison of lumpectomy plus tamoxifen with and without radiotherapy (rt) in women 70 years of age or older who have clinical stage I, estrogen receptor positive breast carcinoma. *New Engl J Med.* 2004;351:971–977.
15. Hughes KS, Schnaper LA, Berry D, et al. Lumpectomy plus tamoxifen with or without irradiation in women 70 years of age or older with early breast cancer. *Breast Cancer Res Treat.* 2006;100S [Abstract 11].
16. Fyles AW, McCready DR, Manchul LA, et al. Tamoxifen with or without breast irradiation in women 50 years of age or older with early breast cancer. *New Engl J Med.* 2004;351:963–970.
17. Whelan T, Pignol J, Julian J, et al. Long-term results of a randomized trial of accelerated hypofractionated whole breast irradiation following breast conserving surgery in women with node-negative breast cancer. *Int J Radiat Oncol Biol Phys.* 2008;72:S28–S28.
18. Golshan M, Rusby J, Dominguez F, Smith BL. Breast conservation for male breast carcinoma. *Breast.* 2007;16:653–656.
19. Tuttle TM, Habermann EB, Grund EH, Morris TJ, Virnig BA. Increasing use of contralateral prophylactic mastectomy for breast cancer patients: a trend toward more aggressive surgical treatment. *J Clin Oncol.* 2007;25:5203–5209.
20. Frost MH, Slezak JM, Tran NV, et al. Satisfaction after contralateral prophylactic mastectomy: the significance of mastectomy type, reconstructive complications, and body appearance. *J Clin Oncol.* 2005;23:7849–7856.
21. O'Sullivan MJ, Li T, Freedman G, Morrow M. The effect of multiple reexcisions on the risk of local recurrence after breast conserving surgery. *Ann Surg Oncol.* 2007;14:3133–3140.
22. Beer GM, Varga Z, Budi S, Seifert B, Meyer VE. Incidence of the superficial fascia and its relevance in skin-sparing mastectomy. *Cancer.* 2002;94(6):1619–1625.
23. Ho CM, Mak CK, Lau Y, Cheung WY, Chan MC, Hung WK. Skin involvement in invasive breast carcinoma: safety of skin-sparing mastectomy. *Ann Surg Oncol.* 2003;10(2):102–107.
24. Carlson GW, Styblo TM, Lyles RH, et al. The use of skin sparing mastectomy in the treatment of breast cancer: the Emory experience. *Surg Oncol.* 2003;12(4):265–269.
25. Gerber B, Krause A, Reimer T, et al. Skin-sparing mastectomy with conservation of the nipple-areola complex and autologous reconstruction is an oncologically safe procedure. *Ann Surg.* 2003; 238(1):120–127.
26. Greenway RM, Schlossberg L, Dooley WC. Fifteen-year series of skin-sparing mastectomy for stage 0 to 2 breast cancer. *Am J Surg.* 2005;190(6):918–922.
27. Kroll SS, Khoo A, Singletary SE, et al. Local recurrence risk after skin-sparing and conventional mastectomy: a 6-year follow-up. *Plast Reconstr Surg.* 1999;104(2):421–425.
28. Spiegel AJ, Butler CE. Recurrence following treatment of ductal carcinoma in situ with skin-sparing mastectomy and immediate breast reconstruction. *Plast Reconstr Surg.* 2003; 111(2): 706–711.
29. Drucker-Zertuche M, Robles-Vidal C. A 7 year experience with immediate breast reconstruction after skin sparing mastectomy for cancer. *Eur J Surg Oncol.* 2007; 33(2):140–146.
30. Chung A, Sacchini V. Nipple-sparing mastectomy: where are we now? *Surg Oncol.* 2008;7:261–266.
31. Rusby JE, Kirstein. LJ, Brachtel EF, et al. Nipple sparing mastectomy: lessons from ex-vivo procedures. *Breast J.* 2008;14: 464–470.

32. Crowe JP, Kim JA, Yetman R, Banbury J, Patrick RJ, Baynes D. Nipple-sparing mastectomy: technique and results of 54 procedures. *Arch Surg.* 2004;139:148–150.

33. Crowe JP, Patrick RJ, Yetman RJ, Djohan R. Nipple-sparing mastectomy update: one hundred forty-nine procedures and clinical outcomes. *Arch Surg.* 2008;143:1106–1110.

34. Stolier AJ, Sullivan SK, Dellacroce FJ. Technical considerations in nipple-sparing mastectomy: 82 consecutive cases without necrosis. *Ann Surg Oncol.* 2008;15:1341–1347.

35. Caruso F, Ferrara M, Castiglione G, et al. Nipple sparing subcutaneous mastectomy: sixty-six months follow-up. *Eur J Surg Oncol.* 2006; 32(9):937–940.

36. Petit JY, Veronesi U, Orecchia R, et al. Nipple-sparing mastectomy in association with intra operative radiotherapy (ELIOT): a new type of mastectomy for breast cancer treatment. *Breast Cancer Res Treat.* 2006;96:47–51.

37. Sacchini V, Pinotti JA, Barros AC, et al. Nipple-sparing mastectomy for breast cancer and risk reduction: oncologic or technical problem? *J Am Coll Surg.* 2006; 203(5):704–714.

38. Rusby JE, Brachtel EF, Michaelson JS, Koerner FC, Smith BL. Predictors of occult nipple involvement to aid selection of patients for nipple-sparing mastectomy. *Br J Surg.* 2008;95:1356–1361.

39. Erickson VS, Pearson ML, Ganz PA, Adams J, Kahn KL. Arm edema in breast cancer patients. *J Nat Cancer Inst.* 2001; 93:96–111.

40. Blanchard DK, Donohue JH, Reynolds C, Grant CS. Relapse and morbidity in patients undergoing sentinel lymph node biopsy alone or with axillary dissection for breast cancer. *Arch Surg.* 2003;138:482–487.

41. Kwan W, Jackson J, Weir LM, Dingee C, McGregor G, Olivotto IA. Chronic arm morbidity after curative breast cancer treatment: prevalence and impact on quality of life. *J Clin Oncol.* 2002;20:4242–4248.

42. Beaulac SM, McNair LA, Scott TE, LaMorte WW, Kavanah MT. Lymphedema and quality of life in survivors of early-stage breast cancer. *Arch Surg.* 2002;137:1253–1257.

43. Engel J, Kerr J, Schlesinger-Raab A, Sauer H, Holzel D. Axilla surgery severely affects quality of life: results of a 5-year prospective study in breast cancer patients. *Breast Cancer Res Treat.* 2003;79:47–57.

44. Duff M, Hill ADK, McGreal G, Walsh S, McDermott E, O'Higgins NJ. Prospective evaluation of the morbidity of axillary clearance for breast cancer. *Br J Surg.* 2001;88:114–117.

45. Armer JM, Radina ME, Porock D, Culbertson SD. Predicting breast cancer-related lymphedema using self-reported symptoms. *Nurs Res.* 2003;52(6):370–379.

46. Ivens D, Hoe AL, Podd CR, et al. Assessment of morbidity from complete axillary dissection. *Br J Cancer.* 1992;66:136–138.

47. Voogd AC, Ververs JM, Vingerhoets AJ, Roumen RM, Coebergh JW, Crommelin MA. Lymphoedema and reduced shoulder function as indicators of quality of life after axillary lymph node dissection for invasive breast cancer. *Br J Surg.* 2003;90(1):76–81.

48. Giuliano AE, Haigh PI, Brennan MB, et al. Prospective observational study of sentinel lymphadenectomy without further axillary dissection in patients with sentinel node-negative breast cancer. *J Clin Oncol.* 2000;18:2553–2559.

49. Krag D, Weaver D, Ashikaga A, et al. The sentinel node in breast cancer—a multicenter validation study. *New Engl J Med.* 1998; 339:941–946.

50. Lyman GH, Giulians AE, Somerfield MR, et al. American Society of Clinical Oncology guideline recommendations for sentinel node biopsy in early-stage breast cancer. *J Clin Oncol.* 2005;23: 7703–7720.

51. Krag DN, Anderson SJ, Julian TB, et al. Technical outcomes of sentinel lymph node resection and conventional axillary lymph node dissection in patients with clinically node-negative breast cancer: Result from the NSABP B-32 randomised phase III trial. *Lancet Oncol.* 2007;8:881–888.

52. Veronisi U, Paganelli G, Vaile G, et al. A randomized comparison of sentinel node biopsy with routine axillary dissection in breast cancer. *New Engl J Med.* 2003;349:546–553.

53. Mansel RE, Fallowfield L, Kissen M, et al. Randomized multicenter trial of sentinel node biopsy versus standard axillary treatment in operable breast cancer: the ALMANAC Trial. *J Natl Cancer Inst.* 2006;98:599–609.

54. Naik AM, Fey J, Gemignani M, et al. The risk of axillary relapse after sentinel lymph node biopsy for breast cancer is comparable with that of axillary lymph node dissection: a follow-up study of 4008 procedures. *Ann Surg.* 2004;240:462–468.

55. Van Zee KJ, Manasseh DE, Bevilacqua JB, et al. A nomogram for predicting the likelihood of additional nodal metastases in breast cancer patients with a positive sentinel node biopsy. *Ann Surg Oncol.* 2003;10:1140–1151.

56. Gadd M, Harris J, Taghian A, et al. Prospective study of axillary radiation without axillary dissection for breast cancer patients with a positive sentinel node. Oral presentation, San Antonio Breast Cancer Symposium, 2005.

57. Rutgers E, Meijnen P, Bonnefoi H. Clinical trials update of the European Organization for Research and Treatment of Cancer Breast Cancer Group. *Breast Cancer Res.* 2004;6:165–169.

58. Lucy A, Mackie-McCall L, Beitsch PD, et al. Surgical complications associated with sentinel lymph node dissection (SLND) plus axillary lymph node dissection compared with SLND alone in the American college of surgeons oncology group trial Z0011. *J Clin Oncol.* 2007;25:3657–3663.

59. Newman EA, Cimmino VM, Sabel MS, et al. Lymphatic mapping and sentinel lymph node biopsy for patients with local recurrence after breast-conservation therapy. *Ann Surg Oncol.* 2006;13:52–57.

60. Port ER, Garcia-Etienne CA, Park J, Fey J, Borgen PI, Cody HS III. Reoperative sentinel lymph node biopsy: a new frontier in the management of ipsilateral breast tumor recurrence. *Ann Surg Oncol.* 2007;14:2209–2214.

Radiation Treatment of Early-Stage Breast Cancer

JENNIFER R. BELLON

Since the establishment of breast conservation as an alternative to mastectomy (1), the management of early-stage breast cancer has become a prototype for the local treatment of all solid malignancies. When it is combined with systemic therapy, in-breast recurrence rates are now commonly less than 1% per year (2). Not only have in-breast recurrence rates decreased with systemic therapy, but improved control of micrometastatic disease with effective systemic therapy has also increased the importance of local control. As a result, improvements in recurrence rates in the breast have translated, with longer follow-up, into reductions in distant metastases and improved overall survival rates (3). More recent advances have focused on minimizing radiation while maintaining similar local control. These efforts have included omitting radiation in select patients, substituting hormonal therapy for radiation, and accelerated fractionation schedules. The data regarding partial breast irradiation will be discussed elsewhere in this text.

Six randomized trials have compared breast-conserving surgery with mastectomy (1,4–8). These studies have varied in patient selection, margin width, tumor size, and use of systemic therapy but have been markedly consistent in demonstrating similar survival between the surgical approaches (Table 7.1). The largest of these studies, the National Surgical Adjuvant Breast and Bowel Project (NSABP) B-06 trial (1), randomized 1,851 women to total mastectomy, lumpectomy, or lumpectomy with 50 Gy adjuvant radiation. Women with node-positive disease

also received melphalan and fluorouracil. All patients had stage 1 or 2 disease and tumors smaller than 4.0 cm. At the most recent update, in 2002, distant disease-free survival and overall survival were similar among the three groups. Subsequent to this initial work, other institutions have attempted to define appropriate candidates for breast conservation. As this selection process has evolved, the proportion of patients with newly diagnosed breast cancers able to undergo breast conservation has increased, and the risk of local recurrence has continued to fall.

■ PROGNOSTIC FACTORS FOR LOCAL FAILURE

Factors prognostic for local recurrence following breast conservation have been extensively studied. The most significant of these include the width of the surgical margin, patient age, and the use of systemic therapy. While the precise width of the surgical margin necessary to minimize the risk of local recurrence is controversial, positive margins have been consistently associated with a higher risk of in-breast recurrence (8–10). Close margins have been variably defined and have been associated with varying risks of recurrence. Generally, margins greater than 2 mm are associated with a low risk of recurrence (11,12). In patients with an extensive intraductal component (EIC, i.e., ductal carcinoma in situ present as a 25% or larger component of the main tumor and also in the surrounding tissue), clearly negative margins are warranted to minimize the risk of recurrence (13). Young age has also been associated with a higher risk of recurrence in the breast (14–16), although it is unclear whether this finding persists

Table 7.1 Randomized trials of breast-conserving surgery and mastectomy

Study	Median Follow-up (years)	Number of Patients	Overall Survival (%) Conservative Surgery and Radiation	Mastectomy
Danish (Ref. 7)	3.3 (6-yr data)	905	79	82
EORTC (Ref. 8)	13.4 (10-yr data)	868	65	66
NCI (Ref. 6)	10.1 (10-yr data)	247	77	75
NSABP B-06 (Ref. 1)	20	1,851	46	47
Milan (Ref. 5)	20	701	42	41
Institute Gustave-Roussy (Ref. 4)	14.5 (15-yr data)	179	65	73

independently of other high-risk pathological factors that tend to occur in this age group (17). The use of systemic therapy, both hormonal and chemotherapy, has also been consistently associated with a decreased risk of recurrence in the breast (18–22). More recently, attempts have been made to determine the impact of tumor phenotype on risk of local recurrence. Nguyen and colleagues studied the risk of local recurrence in 793 patients treated with breast-conserving surgery and adjuvant radiation therapy (23). At 5 years, local recurrence was 1.8% overall but 7.1% for patients with estrogen receptor–negative, progesterone receptor–negative, and HER-2-negative disease. These results have not been uniformly seen (24,25), although further study of tumor biological characteristics and the risk of local recurrence is clearly warranted.

■ CONTRAINDICATIONS TO BREAST-CONSERVING THERAPY

Contraindications to breast-conserving surgery have also been elucidated. Tumor factors, including persistently positive surgical margins, and multicentric disease (26,27) have been associated with a higher risk of recurrence in the breast. Patient factors such as collagen-vascular disease, particularly scleroderma and active systemic lupus erythematous, are considered to be contraindications to breast conservation, although the literature is incomplete and somewhat contradictory (28,29). Rheumatoid arthritis does not seem to be associated with a higher risk of radiation-induced complications (30). Pregnancy, owing to concerns for scattered dose to the fetus and resulting fetal malformations, is also considered an absolute contraindication to breast conservation. BRCA1 or BRCA2 mutations were thought potentially to increase the risk of radiation-induced malignancies in patients receiving radiation. A multi-institutional review by Pierce and colleagues examined 160 patients with germline BRCA1 or BRCA2 mutations matched to 445 controls. There was no difference in ipsilateral breast cancer recurrence or in radiation toxicity. There was, as expected, a higher risk of new primary cancers in both breasts (31).

The sequencing of radiation and systemic therapy has also been studied. One randomized trial (32) examined chemotherapy followed by radiation and the converse and at 11 years of follow-up found no difference in local recurrence or overall survival. The French ARCOSEIN trial randomized patients to concurrent versus sequential cyclophosphamide, fluorouracil, and mitoxantrone (33). There was no difference in local regional recurrence or overall survival with a median follow-up of 60 months. Select patients, however, may benefit from a concurrent approach. Bellon and colleagues (34) found local recurrence rates of 6% and 4% at 5 years in patients with close and positive margins, respectively, treated with low-dose

radiation (39.6 Gy) and concurrent cyclophosphamide, methotrexate, and fluorouracil. Assersohn and colleagues also reported a 3% recurrence rate in 70 patients with positive margins after lumpectomy who received concurrent mitozantrone, methotrexate, and mitomycin-C (35). Similarly, three nonrandomized trials have shown no difference in outcome when tamoxifen is given concurrently or sequentially with radiation therapy (36–38). Owing to the widespread use of anthracyclines, concurrent radiation and chemotherapy is not commonly used. Further study may still be warranted, however, in high-risk patients or with novel chemotherapeutic agents.

■ BREAST RADIATION DECREASES MORTALITY

Systemic therapy also affects the relationship between breast cancer recurrence and overall survival. Previously, in-breast recurrence was thought to be exclusively a local-only event, potentially a marker of more aggressive histology, but with no potential to impact overall survival. However, two recent meta-analyses changed our view of the relationship between local recurrence and overall survival. Vinh-Hung and colleagues (39) pooled 9,422 patients from 15 trials that randomized patients to radiation therapy following breast-conserving surgery. As expected, radiation decreased the risk of recurrence in the breast, with a relative risk of tumor recurrence of 3.0 [95% confidence interval (CI) 2.65 to 3.40], but also resulted in an 8.6% improvement in overall survival (95% CI 0.3% to 17.5%). The 2005 meta-analysis from the Early Breast Cancer Trialists' Collaborative Group (EBCTCG) has brought considerable attention to this issue mainly owing to its large size and focus on individual patient data (3). A total of 42,000 women were studied from 78 randomized trials from the early 1960s to 1995. Of these, 7,300 women were treated with breast-conserving surgery. Five-year local recurrence was 7% with radiation to the breast and 26% without. This 19% absolute reduction translated into a 5.4% improvement in breast cancer mortality at 15 years (30.5% versus 35.9%, $P = 0.0002$), as well as a 5.3% improvement in 15-year all-cause mortality ($P = 0.005$; Figure 7.1). This has been referred to as the 4:1 ratio (40). For every four local recurrences prevented at 5 years, one additional death owing to breast cancer is avoided. Likely this was not observed in the individual randomized trials of breast radiation owing to insufficient power. In addition, control of microscopic metastatic disease with chemotherapy or hormonal therapy, or both, such as not to overwhelm any effect of local control is likely key. As chemotherapy continues to improve to the extent that it may ultimately be sufficient on its own to control local disease, it is conceivable that radiation therapy will become unnecessary.

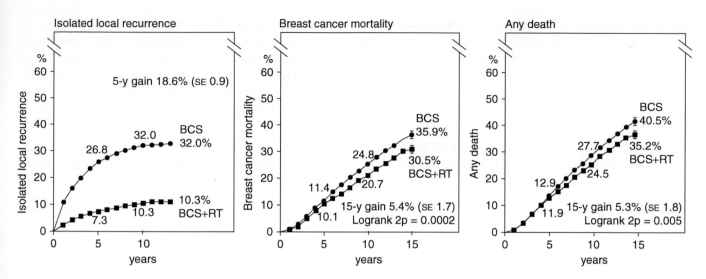

FIGURE 7.1 Isolated local recurrence, breast cancer mortality, and overall survival. (From Ref. 3.)

■ CAN BREAST RADIATION BE OMITTED?

Conventional radiation to the breast typically consists of 45 to 50 Gy to the whole breast over approximately 5 weeks, frequently followed by a lumpectomy site boost of 10 to 16 Gy. Breast radiation usually starts 4 to 6 weeks after the last surgery if no adjuvant chemotherapy is used. While this fractionation does have a long track record of safety and efficacy, it is time-consuming, and living in underserved (41,42) or rural areas (43) may limit access to breast conservation. Nonetheless, radiation has consistently been shown to decrease the risk of recurrence within the breast. The largest trial to study this, NSABP B-06 (1), showed that patients who had lumpectomy with radiation therapy had a lower risk of an in-breast recurrence than those receiving lumpectomy alone (14.3% versus 39.2%, P <0.001). Two single-institution experiences have attempted to select very favorable patients who might be able to avoid radiation. The Joint Center for Radiation Therapy (44) enrolled 87 patients into a single-arm study of women with T1N0 disease. Tumors were required to be lymph-vascular space invasion–negative as well as EIC-negative. Median size was 0.9 cm, and 1.0 cm margins (or a negative re-excision) were required. Mean patient age was 66 years. At 86 months' follow-up, 34% of patients experienced a local recurrence, and the study was closed prematurely when stopping rules were met. Similar results were seen in a randomized trial of select patients from Finland (45). In this study, patients with T1N0 low- or intermediate-grade EIC-negative tumors with margins above 1.0 cm were randomized to 50 Gy whole breast radiation following breast-conserving surgery. Despite these favorable tumor characteristics, 18.1% of patients in the no-radiation arm recurred in the breast, with a mean follow-up of 7.7 years (compared with 7.5% in the radiation arm, P = 0.03).

In the absence of omitting radiation entirely, it may be possible to substitute hormonal therapy. The NSABP, however, in B-21 showed that radiation combined with hormonal therapy was more effective than either alone (2). Moreover, tamoxifen alone still had a substantial recurrence rate. This was a three-armed study comparing radiation with or without tamoxifen to tamoxifen alone in 1,009 women with tumors smaller than 1.0 cm. Even in these smaller T1a and T1b tumors, radiation decreased the risk of recurrence in the breast. Cumulative incidence of local recurrence at 8 years was 16.6% with tamoxifen, 9.3% with radiation, and 2.8% with tamoxifen and radiation. Several other large trials have also looked at substituting tamoxifen for radiation in women with favorable early-stage disease. Fyles and colleagues (46) randomized 769 women older than age 50 to tamoxifen with radiation or tamoxifen alone. All patients had T1 clinically node-negative disease, although only 83% had a pathological evaluation of the axilla. At 5 years, the risk of recurrence in the breast was 0.6% with radiation and tamoxifen and 7.7% with tamoxifen alone (P <0.001). Even in a subgroup (n = 611) with T1 receptor–positive disease, there was still a benefit to radiation (5.9% versus 0.4%, P <.001). On first look, the Cancer and Leukemia Group B (CALGB) experience (47) found results contradictory to these studies. The study design is very similar to the Canadian experience, with a straightforward randomization of 636 women older than age 70 with clinical stage 1 disease to tamoxifen alone for 5 years or tamoxifen with radiation. In this study, however, there was very minimal benefit to radiation. Five-year local recurrence rates were 4% with radiation, compared with 1% without. There was no difference in the two arms between mastectomy-free survival or overall survival. It is prudent, though, to study the patient population in more detail. Overall, 107 patients (17%) in both arms died from other, non–breast cancer causes, likely owing to the high rate of comorbid medical conditions in this elderly population. If a patient has an anticipated prolonged life expectancy, then it is reasonable to consider treatment.

■ SHORTENING OVERALL TREATMENT TIME WITH HYPOFRACTIONATION

Several efforts have been made to shorten the course of whole breast radiation. Whelan and colleagues (48) performed a two-arm randomized trial to compare conventionally fractionated whole breast radiation (50 Gy in 2 Gy fractions) to a hypofractionated accelerated course of 42.5 Gy in 16 fractions. They randomized 1,234 women, and the trial was most recently updated in 2008, with 144 months' median follow-up. At 10 years, local recurrence was 6.2% in the fractionated arm compared with 6.7% in the hypofractionated arm. Long-term cosmetic outcome was also similar, with 70% and 71%, respectively, with a good or excellent outcome. This study did not use a boost dose of radiation in either group, which raises questions about its generalizability to younger patient populations, where the absolute benefit of additional lumpectomy-site radiation is more pronounced. Freedman and colleagues (49) from the Fox Chase Cancer Center used an intensity-modulated radiation therapy technique that employed a concomitant boost to the lumpectomy site. In this way, dose inhomogeneity, which may be amplified by larger doses per fraction, can be minimized. In an initial single-arm study of 75 patients receiving 45 Gy to the whole breast with an additional 11 Gy to the lumpectomy site in 20 fractions, acceptable acute toxicity was seen. In addition, since only 11% of the patients in the Canadian experience received systemic chemotherapy, it is unclear whether the long-term safety is equivalent in patients receiving aggressive chemotherapy regimens, particularly with trastuzumab. There may be increased toxicity, particularly cardiac, that will take a long time to appreciate. Longer follow-up is necessary to determine whether this technique should be used routinely in patients with left-sided disease where the heart cannot be entirely excluded from the radiation fields and in patients who have received chemotherapy.

Others have also attempted a shortened course of radiation. The UK Standardisation of Breast Radiotherapy (START) trials (50,51) consisted of two separate randomizations: 50 Gy in 25 fractions with 41.6 Gy in 13 fractions and 39 Gy in 13 fractions over 5 weeks (START A) and 50 Gy in 25 fractions with 40 Gy in 15 fractions over 3 weeks (START B). Follow-up in both substudies was short, however, at 5.1 years in the three-way randomization and 6.0 years in the second randomization. With this caveat, local control was low in both randomizations (less than 5%), with no significant differences between fractionation arms. While the Canadian experience did not permit treatment to the regional nodes, a single-arm study from Yorkshire (52) included hypofractionation to the supraclavicular/axillary nodes. Both nodes and the breast were treated to 40 Gy in 15 fractions. With 7 years of follow-up, the local-regional recurrence rate is 6.6%.

■ THE VALUE OF THE LUMPECTOMY-SITE BOOST

While the initial NSABP experience delivered radiation to the whole breast without additional dose to the lumpectomy site, examination of patterns of failure has shown that local recurrences are most likely to occur at or near the original tumor (53,54). An additional dose of radiation was therefore given to the lumpectomy site in an attempt to lower further the risk of local recurrence. This is typically accomplished with a superficial en face electron field that can deliver radiation superficially to the lumpectomy site while minimizing radiation dose to underlying normal tissue. Two trials have examined the potential benefit of this extra dose of radiation. Researchers from Lyon (55) randomized 1,024 patients with early-stage disease to 50 Gy to the whole breast with or without an additional 10 Gy to the lumpectomy site. The results were reported with a median follow-up of 3.3 years and have not been updated. Five-year local recurrence was 3.6 % with the additional radiation, compared with 4.5% without ($P = 0.044$). More patients receiving the additional radiation developed telangiectasias, but there was no difference in a patient-assessed cosmetic score. More robust findings were reported by the European Organisation for Research and Treatment of Cancer (EORTC) (16). Following a microscopically complete excision, 5,318 patients were randomized to 50 Gy to the whole breast with or without an additional 16 Gy to the lumpectomy site. Local recurrence at 10 years (median follow-up 10.8 years) was 6.2% and 10.2%, respectively ($P <0.0001$, with a hazard ratio of 0.59 for local recurrence). Severe fibrosis was modestly, but significantly, increased with the boost dose of radiation, from 1.6% to 4.4% ($P <0.0001$). While there was no interaction with age, the risk of local recurrence was higher in younger patients, as was the absolute benefit of the additional radiation. This effect was most pronounced in women under age 40, in whom the risk of local recurrence was decreased from 23.9% to 13.5% ($P = 0.0014$) with additional radiation to the lumpectomy site. Figure 7.2 further demonstrates the impact of the boost dose of radiation by age group. There was no difference in overall survival between groups, but it is possible that follow-up is still too short to see an impact of local recurrence on survival. Omission of the boost may be a reasonable option in elderly patients in whom the absolute benefit is minimal; in all others, however, it remains standard treatment.

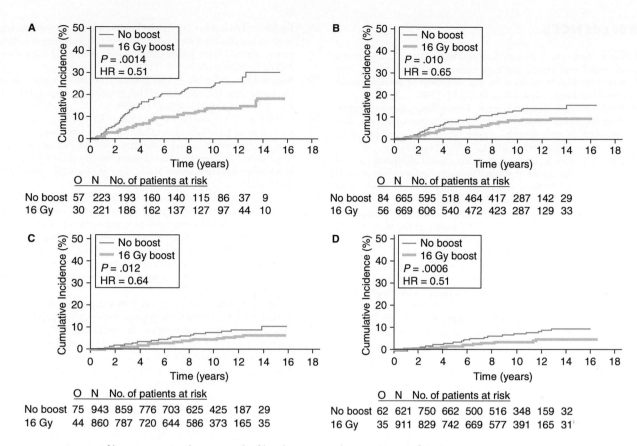

FIGURE 7.2   Impact of lumpectomy-site boost on risk of local recurrence by age. (From Ref. 16.)

In conclusion, breast-conserving surgery with radiation remains a viable alternative to mastectomy, with equivalent survival. Omission of radiation likely compromises overall survival and should be reserved for women with a foreshortened life expectancy. Accelerated whole breast radiation remains a promising alternative, although longer follow-up, particularly regarding long-term toxicity in patients with left-side tumors and those receiving chemotherapy is warranted. For radiation techniques, doses and side effects, see Chapter 6. For a discussion of accelerated partial-breast irradiation, see Chapter 16.

radiation fields and must understand the toxicity of various systemic therapy regimens in order to best integrate radiation with systemic therapy. Multidisciplinary discussion of new patients allows all the disciplines to discuss the optimal integration of the different modalities and in doing so to maximize quality of care for each patient while also increasing learning for each member of the team.

■ THE IMPORTANCE OF THE MULTIDISCIPLINARY APPROACH IN CONSERVATIVE TREATMENT OF BREAST CANCER

Radiation therapists are one part of the team of health care professionals taking care of the patient with early-stage breast. It is essential that all members of the team not only understand the strengths and limitations of their own modality but also have an in-depth understanding of the role of all the other providers. For example, the radiation oncologist must have an idea of the issues relevant to the breast surgeon in order to determine appropriate

■ SUMMARY

- Radiation therapy following breast-conserving surgery remains the standard of care. It not only decreases the chance of recurrence within the breast but also improves overall survival.
- Substitution of hormonal therapy for radiation therapy may be a reasonable option in elderly women with a limited life expectancy.
- Standard fractionation involves extending the radiation over 6 to 6.5 weeks. Shorter courses are currently being investigated, although the optimal candidate for hypofractionated regimens is still being investigated.
- A boost dose of radiation to the lumpectomy site further decreases recurrences within the breast. The absolute benefit of the additional radiation is greater in younger women.

■ REFERENCES

1. Fisher B, Anderson S, Bryant J, et al. Twenty- year follow-up of a randomized trial comparing total mastectomy, lumpectomy, and lumpectomy plus irradiation for the treatment of invasive breast cancer. *New Engl J Med.* 2002;347:1233–1241.

2. Fisher B, Bryant J, Dignam JJ, et al. Tamoxifen, radiation therapy, or both for prevention of ipsilateral breast tumor recurrence after lumpectomy in women with invasive breast cancers of one centimeter or less. *J Clin Oncol.* 2002;20(20):4141–4149.

3. Clarke M, Collins R, Darby S, et al. Effects of radiotherapy and of differences in the extent of surgery for early breast cancer on local recurrence and 15-year survival: an overview of the randomised trials. *Lancet.* 2005;366(9503):2087–2106.

4. Arriagada R, Le MG, Rochard F, et al. Conservative treatment versus mastectomy in early breast cancer: patterns of failure with 15 years of follow-up data. Institute Gustave-Roussy Breast Cancer Group. *J Clin Oncol.* 1996;14(5):1558–1564.

5. Veronsi U, Cascinelli N, Mariani L, et al. Twenty-year follow-up of a randomized study comparing breast-conserving surgery with radical mastectomy for early breast cancer. *New Engl J Med.* 2002;347(16):1227–1232.

6. Jacobson DA, Danforth DN, Cowan KH, et al. Ten-year results of a comparison of conservation with mastectomy in the treatment of stage I and II breast cancer. *New Engl J Med.* 1995;332(14):907–911.

7. Blichert-Toft M, Rose C, Anderson JA, et al. Danish randomized trial comparing breast conservation therapy with mastectomy: six years of life-table analysis. Danish Breast Cancer Cooperative Group. *J Natl Cancer Inst Monogr.* 1992;Aa:19–25.

8. Van Dongen JA, Voogd AC, Fentiman IS, et al Long-term results of a randomized trial comparing breast-conserving therapy with mastectomy: European Organization for Research and Treatment of Cancer 10801 trial. *J Natl Cancer Inst.* 2000;92(14):1143–1150.

9. Freedman G, Fowble B, Hanlon A, et al. Patients with early stage invasive cancer with close of positive margins treated with conservative surgery and radiation have an increased risk of breast recurrence that is delayed by adjuvant systemic therapy. *Int J Radiat Oncol Biol Phys.* 1999;44(5):1005–1015.

10. McIntosh A, Freedman G, Eisenberg D, et al. Recurrence rates and analysis of close or positive margins in patients treated without re-excision before radiation for breast cancer. *Am J Clin Oncol.* 2007;30(2):146–151.

11. Peterson ME, Schultz DJ, Reynolds C, et al. Outcomes in breast cancer patients relative to margin status after treatment with breast-conserving surgery and radiation therapy: the University of Pennsylvania experience. *Int J Radiat Oncol Biol Phys.* 1999;45(5):1029–1035.

12. Borger J, Kemperman H, Hart A, et al. Risk factors in breast-conservation therapy. *J Clin Oncol.* 1994;12(4):653–660.

13. Gage I, Schnitt SJ, Nixon AJ, et al. Pathologic margin involvement and the risk of recurrence in patients treated with breast-conserving therapy. *Cancer.* 1996;78(9):1921–1928.

14. Nixon AJ, Neuberg D, Hayes DF, et al. Relationship of patient age to pathologic features of the tumor and prognosis for patients with stage I and II breast cancer. *J Clin Oncol.* 1994;12(5):888–894.

15. van der Leest M, Evers L, van der Sangen MJ, et al. The safety of breast-conserving therapy in patients with breast cancer aged < or = 40 years. *Cancer.* 2007;109(10):1957–1964.

16. Bartelink H, Horiot JC, Poortsmans PM, et al. Impact of a higher radiation dose on local control and survival in breast-conserving therapy of early stage breast cancer: 10-year results of the randomized boost vs no boost EORTC 22881-10882 trial. *J Clin Oncol.* 2007;25(22):3259–3265.

17. Kurtz JM, Jacquemier J, Amalric, et al. Why are local recurrences after breast-conserving therapy more frequent in younger patients? *J Clin Oncol.* 1990;8(4):591–598.

18. Buchholz TA, Tucker SL, Erwin J, et al. Impact of systemic treatment on local control for patients with lymph node-negative breast cancer treated with breast-conservation therapy. *J Clin Oncol.* 2001;19(8):2240–2246.

19. Romond EH, Perez EA, Bryant J, et al. Trastuzumab plus adjuvant chemotherapy for operable HER2-positive breast cancer. *New Engl J Med.* 2005;353(16):1673–1684.

20. Dahlberg K, Johansson H, Johansson U, et al. A randomized trial of long-term adjuvant tamoxifen plus postoperative radiation therapy versus radiation therapy alone for patients with early stage breast cancinoma treated with breast-conserving surgery. Stockholm Breast Cancer Study Group. *Cancer.* 1998;82(11):2204–2211.

21. Fisher B, Dignam J, Mamounas EP, et al. Sequential methotrexate and fluorouracil for the treatment of node-negative breast cancer patients with estrogen receptor-negative tumors: eight-year results from National Surgical Adjuvant Breast and Bowel Project (NSABP) B-13 and first report of findings from NSABP B-19 comparing methotrexate and fluorouracil with conventional cyclophosphamide, methotrexate, and fluorouracil. *J Clin Oncol.* 1996;14(7):1982–1992.

22. Fisher B, Dignan J, Bryant J, et al. Five versus more than five years of tamoxifen for lymph node negative breast cancer: updated findings form the National Surgical Breast and Bowel Project B-14 randomized trial. *J Natl Cancer Inst.* 2001;93(9):684–90.

23. Nguyen PL, Taghian AG, Katz MS, et al. Breast cancer subtype approximated by estrogen receptor, progesterone receptor and HER-2 is associated with local and distant recurrence after breast-conserving therapy. *J Clin Oncol.* 2008;26(14):2373–2378.

24. Haffty BG, Yang Q, Reiss M, et al. Locoregional relapse and distant metastasis in conservatively managed triple negative early-stage breast cancer. *J Clin Oncol.* 2006;24(36):5652–5657.

25. Dent R, Trudeau M, Pritchard K, et al. Triple-negative breast cancer: clinical features and patterns of recurrence. *Clin Cancer Res.* 2007;13:4429–4434.

26. Kurtz JM, Jacquemier J, Amalric R, et al. Breast-conserving therapy for macroscopically multiple cancers. *Ann Surg.* 1990;212(1):38–44.

27. Hartsell WF, Recine DC, Griem KL, et al. Should multicentric disease be an absolute contraindication to the use of breast-conserving therapy. *Int J Radiat Oncol Biol Phys.* 1994;30(1):49–53.

28. Chen AM, Obedian E, Haffty BG. Breast-conserving therapy in the setting of collagen vascular disease. *Cancer.* 2001;7(6):480–491.

29. Ross JG, Hussey DH, Mayr N, et al. Acute and late reactions to radiation therapy in patients with collagen vascular diseases. *Cancer.* 2006;71(11): 3744–3752.

30. Morris MM, Powell SN. Irradiation in the setting of collagen vascular disease: acute and late complications. *J Clin Oncol.* 1997;15(7):2728–2735.

31. Pierce LJ, Levin AM, Rebbeck TR, et al. Ten-year multi-institutional results of breast-conserving surgery and radiotherapy in BRCA1/2-associated stage I/II breast cancer. *J Clin Oncol.* 2006;24(16):2437–2443.

32. Bellon JR, Come SE, Gelman RS, et al. Sequencing of chemotherapy and radiation therapy in early-stage breast cancer: updated results of a prospective randomized trial. *J Clin Oncol.* 2005;23(9):1934–1940.

33. Toledano A, Azria D, Garaud P, et al. Phase III trial of concurrent or sequential adjuvant chemoradiotherapy after conservative surgery for early-stage breast cancer: final results of the ARCOSEIN trial. *J Clin Oncol.* 2007;25(4):405–410.

34. Bellon JR, Shulman LN, Come SE, et al. A prospective study of concurrent cyclophosphamide/methotrexate/5-fluorouracil and reduced-dose radiotherapy in patients with early-stage breast carcinoma. *Cancer.* 2004;100(7):1358–1364.

35. Assersohn L, Powels TJ, Ashley S, et al. Local relapse in primary breast cancer patients with unexcised positive surgical margins after lumpectomy, radiotherapy and chemoendocrine therapy. *Ann Oncol.* 1999;10(12):1451–1455.

36. Ahn P, Vu HT, Lannin D, et al. Sequence of radiotherapy with tamoxifen in conservatively managed breast cancer does not affect local relapse rates. *J Clin Oncol.* 2005;23:17–23.

37. Harris EER, Christensen VJ, Hwant W-T, et al. Impact of concurrent versus sequential tamoxifen with radiation therapy in early-stage breast cancer. *J Clin Oncol.* 2005;23:11–16.

38. Pierce LJ, Hutchins LF, Green SR, et al. Sequencing of tamoxifen and radiotherapy after breast-conserving surgery in early-stage breast cancer. *J Clin Oncol.* 2005;23:24–29.

39. Vinh-Hung V, Verschraegen C. Breast-conserving surgery with or without radiotherapy: pooled-analysis for risk of ipsilateral breast tumor recurrence and mortality. *J Natl Cancer Inst.* 2004;96(2):115–121.

40. Punglia RS, Morrow M, Winer EP, et al. Local therapy and survival in breast cancer. *New Engl J Med* 2007;356(23):2399–405.

41. Hiotis K, Ye W, Sposto R, et al. Predictors of breast conservation therapy: size is not all that matters. *Cancer.* 2005;103(5):892–899.

42. Dolan JT, Granchi TS, Miller CC, 3rd et al. Low use of breast conservation surgery in medically indigent populations. *Am J Surg.* 1999;178(6):470–474.

43. Answini GA, Woodard WL, Horton HJ, et al. Breast conservation: trends in a major southern metropolitan area compared with surrounding rural counties. *Am Surg.* 2001;67(10):994–998.

44. Lim M, Bellon JR, Gelman R, et al. A prospective study of conservative surgery without radiation therapy in select patients with stage I breast cancer. *Int J Radiat Oncol Biol Phys.* 2006;65(4):1149–1154.

45. Holli K, Saaristo R, Isola J, et al. Lumpectomy with or without postoperative radiotherapy for breast cancer with favourable prognostic features: results of a randomized study. *Br J Cancer.* 2001;84(2):164–169.

46. Fyles AW, McCready DR, Manchul LA, et al. Tamoxifen with or without breast irradiation in women 50 year of age or older with early breast cancer. *New Engl J Med.* 2004;351(10):963–970.

47. Hughes KS, Schnaper LA, Berry D, et al. Lumpectomy plus tamoxifen with or without irradiation in women 70 years of age or older with early breast cancer. *New Engl J Med.* 2004;351(10):971–977.

48. Whelan T, Pignol JP, Julian J, et al. Long-term results of a randomized trial of accelerated hypofractionated whole breast irradiation following breast conserving surgery in women with node negative breast cancer. *Breast Cancer Res Treat.* 2007;106 (suppl 1):S6.

49. Freedman GM, Anderson PR, Goldstein LJ, et al. Four-week course of radiation for breast cancer using hypofractionated intensity modulated radiation therapy with an incorporated boost. *Int J Radiat Oncol Biol Phys.* 2007;68(2):347–353.

50. Start Trialists' Group, Bentzen SM, Agrawal RK, et al. The UK Standarisation of Breast Radiotherapy (START) trial A of radiotherapy hypofractionation for treatment of early breast cancer: a randomized trial. *Lancet Oncol.* 2008;9(4):331–334.

51. Start Trialists' Group, Bentzen SM, Agrawal RK, et al. The UK Standardisation of Breast Radiotherapy (START) trial B of radiotherapy hypofractionation for treatment of early breast cancer: a randomized trial. *Lancet.* 2008;371(9618):1098–1107.

52. Ash DV, Benson EA, Sainsbury JR, et al. Seven-year follow-up on 334 patients treated by breast conserving surgery and short course radical postoperative radiotherapy: a report of the Yorkshire Breast Cancer Group. *Clin Oncol.* 1995;7(2):96.

53. Clark RM, McCulloch PB, Levine MN, et al. Randomized clinical trial to assess the effectiveness of breast irradiation following lumpectomy and axillary dissection for node-negative breast cancer. *J Natl Cancer Inst.* 1992;84(9):683–689.

54. Liljegren G, Holmberg L, Bergh J, et al. 10-year results after sector resection with or without postoperative radiotherapy for stage I breast cancer: a randomized trial. *J Clin Oncol.* 1999;17(8):2326–2333.

55. Romestaing P, Lehingue Y, Carrie C, et al. Role of a 10-Gy boost in the conservative treatment of early breast cancer: results of a randomized clinical trial in Lyon, France. *J Clin Oncol.* 1997;15(3):963–968.

Medical Oncology Treatment of Early-Stage Breast Cancer

JULIE GOLD

HAROLD J. BURSTEIN

The majority of breast cancers (61%) are early stage (1 or 2) at diagnosis (1). The goal of adjuvant therapy is to eradicate possible occult, micrometastatic disease that, if left untreated, is a potential source of disease recurrence. Treatment plans in the adjuvant setting are designed to minimize toxicity while simultaneously reducing the risk of recurrence. Since breast cancer is now considered a heterogeneous group of tumors that all occur in the breast, individual tumor biology should drive the treatment plan. Tumor phenotype [estrogen receptor–positive (ER+)/human epidermal growth factor receptor–negative (HER2–), HER2+, or triple-negative] and TNM staging are weighed together with individual patient characteristics. Over the past decade, gene expression profiling has identified distinct molecular subtypes of breast cancer, each with novel clinical characteristics and treatment needs (2). These tumor subsets have different patterns and rates of recurrence. For instance, while recurrences may be seen well beyond 10 years in women with endocrine-sensitive disease, triple-negative breast cancer tends to recur in the first 3 to 5 years (3). It is also now known that many ER+ cancers are relatively insensitive to chemotherapy. These observations have led clinicians to tailor therapeutic strategies for women with breast cancer.

■ ADJUVANT ENDOCRINE THERAPY

Endocrine therapy plays a critical role in improving disease-free survival (DFS) and overall survival in women with ER+ and progesterone receptor–positive (PR+) tumors. The Early Breast Cancer Trialists' Collaborative Group (EBCTCG) meta-analysis and the National Surgical Adjuvant Breast and Bowel Project (NSABP) B-14 trial suggest that 5 years of tamoxifen therapy offers on average a 40% to 50% relative risk reduction for recurrence in addition to a 34% decrease in the risk of death from breast cancer. There was also a 39% reduction in the risk of contralateral breast cancer observed in tamoxifen-treated women. These benefits were observed across all ages and in both premenopausal and postmenopausal women. Clinical benefits continued after completion of therapy and

extended to at least 15 years of follow-up (4–6). It is also clear than not all patients with hormone receptor–positive tumors benefit equally from adjuvant endocrine therapy. The magnitude of benefit varies substantially but is greatest in women with lower-grade HER2– tumors with high levels of ER and PR expression, tumors that characteristically have lower- or intermediate-range Onco*type* DX recurrence scores. In contrast, such benefits are likely to be more modest in HER2+ cancers or in tumors with high-range Onco*type* DX scores or other features associated with higher grade and proliferative rates, which lowers the threshold for adding chemotherapy in such cases (7,8).

Premenopausal Women

For premenopausal women, the standard of care for initial endocrine treatment is 5 years of tamoxifen, a selective estrogen receptor modulator with mixed agonist/antagonist properties (Table 7.2). Tamoxifen is generally well tolerated and relatively inexpensive. The most common side effects experienced during treatment with tamoxifen are hot flashes, night sweats, and vaginal discharge. Rare but serious toxicities observed in women treated with tamoxifen include thromboembolic events and uterine cancer (9). In the NSABP P-1 trial, these serious events were observed in fewer than 1% of premenopausal women (10).

Ovarian suppression with luteinizing hormone–releasing hormone (LHRH) agonists (or ovarian ablation) may be important in the management of premenopausal women. A variety of direct and indirect evidence suggests that ovarian suppression may be beneficial. The EBCTCG analysis of randomized trials confirmed that ovarian suppression lowers the risk of recurrence compared with no adjuvant therapy (11). Older trials comparing ovarian suppression with cyclophosphamide, methotrexate, and 5-fluorouracil (CMF)–based chemotherapy in ER+, lymph node–negative tumors showed nearly equivalent outcomes for the two approaches (12,13). The benefit of

■ **Table 7.2** Options for endocrine therapy in premenopausal early-stage breast cancer

Tamoxifen × 5 yrs (Ref. 4)
Tamoxifen + OS (goserelin monthly) × 5 yrs (Refs. 15,81)
AI + OS (goserelin monthly)[a] × 5 yrs (Ref. 81)

AI, aromatase inhibitor; OS, ovarian suppression.

[a]This in an option in women with a contraindication to tamoxifen therapy.

chemotherapy in premenopausal women with endocrine-sensitive tumors may be due in large part to its suppression of ovarian function (14). The high rate of chemotherapy-induced amenorrhea has made it difficult to detect the relative benefit from ovarian suppression in women previously treated with chemotherapy. It has therefore been proposed that inhibiting endogenous estradiol production with ovarian suppression can achieve benefits similar to those seen with chemotherapy in a selected population of relatively low-risk women (15). Despite these suggestive findings, the design of these historical trials does not definitively address the question of whether there is benefit from ovarian suppression after chemotherapy or in tamoxifen-treated women. In current practice, ovarian suppression may be offered to high-risk women on tamoxifen who resume their menses after completion of adjuvant chemotherapy, and it may be considered in addition to tamoxifen in women with premenopausal cancers who do not receive chemotherapy. However, outside a clinical trial, the potential benefit and toxicity from ovarian suppression should be considered carefully in each individual given its effects on quality of life and possible long-term effects on skeletal and cardiovascular health. The Suppression of Ovarian Function Trial (SOFT) and Triptorelin with either Exemestane or Tamoxifen (TEXT) trial are currently examining how ovarian suppression can best be used in these populations and, in the case of SOFT, the benefit and toxicity attributable to ovarian suppression (16). Since tamoxifen is potentially teratogenic, women should avoid pregnancy while taking it and discontinue use at least several months prior to planned conception.

Perimenopausal women and women with chemotherapy-induced amenorrhea should be treated as premenopausal women. Such patients may have long durations of residual ovarian function or may recover ovarian function, making the use of aromatase inhibitors (AIs) alone inappropriate. The routine measurement of serum follicle-stimulating hormone (FSH) levels in this population is not reliable enough to dictate treatment decisions and is not recommended (17,18). Women who are perimenopausal at the time of diagnosis can be treated upfront with tamoxifen, with the option of transitioning to an AI as part of sequential or extended endocrine therapy when they are definitively menopausal.

Postmenopausal Women

While tamoxifen is known to be effective in both premenopausal and postmenopausal women, the introduction of AIs for postmenopausal patients offers options in both drug class and treatment schema (Table 7.3). In postmenopausal women, estrogen is produced through aromatization of androgens, testosterone, and androstenedione. Steady-state, low levels of estrogen production occur in tissues including the adrenal glands, adipose tissue, breast, liver, and other sites. AIs block this enzymatic conversion,

■ Table 7.3 Options for endocrine therapy in postmenopausal early-stage breast cancer

Treatment Strategy	Reasons to Consider This Strategy
Tamoxifen × 5 yrs	Lower risk for recurrence Contraindication to AI therapy
AI × 5 yrs	Contraindication to tamoxifen High risk for early recurrence
Tamoxifen × 2–3 yrs → AI × 2–3 yrs	Perimenopausal at diagnosis
Tamoxifen × 5 yrs → AI × 5 yrs	Premenopausal or perimenopausal at diagnosis
AI × 2 yrs → tamoxifen × 3 yrs	Poor tolerance of AI

AI, aromatase inhibitor.

thereby reducing estrogen levels in treated patients to essentially undetectable levels (19). It is through this profound estrogen deprivation that AIs are though to have clinical benefit. Women with persistent ovarian function (i.e., premenopausal women) are not candidates for AI therapy because normal hypothalamic–pituitary–gonadal feedback mechanisms stimulate aromatase production in the ovary when estrogen levels fall.

Evidence for use of AIs in the adjuvant setting has emerged from large-randomized trials comparing 5 years of tamoxifen therapy with treatment plans incorporating AIs—either upfront, as an alternative to tamoxifen; sequentially, after 2 to 3 years of tamoxifen; or as extended adjuvant therapy after 5 years of tamoxifen.

Each of these strategies has shown modest clinical advantages over 5 years of tamoxifen alone, and there are now data to support the use of AIs as part of upfront [Arimidex, Tamoxifen, Alone or in Combination (ATAC), Breast International Group (BIG) 1–98] (19–21), sequenced [Intergroup Exemestane Study (IES), BIG 1–98] (22), or extended endocrine therapy (MA.17) (23) (Table 7.4). In the ATAC trial, 5 years of anastrozole were equal to 5 years of tamoxifen in terms of overall survival, but AI therapy yielded an improvement in DFS, time to distant recurrence, and rate of distant metastases. A recent update from the BIG 1–98 trial presented at the 2008 San Antonio Breast Cancer Symposium found that 5 years of upfront letrozole is superior to 5 years of tamoxifen in terms of event-free survival. Patients who were sequenced with tamoxifen had noninferior outcomes, supporting a switch from an AI to tamoxifen after 2 to 3 years in the small population of women who experience adverse events such as disabling musculoskeletal side effects on AIs. In the IES, women were randomized either to switch to exemestane or to continue on tamoxifen after 2 to 3 years of tamoxifen therapy to complete a 5-year course of endocrine therapy. In the most recent analysis, class switching offered an

■ Table 7.4 Aromatase inhibitor treatment strategies

Trial	Eligibility	Treatment Arms	Number of Patients	DFS Hazard Ratio
Upfront/Primary Therapy				
ATAC (Ref. 19)	Newly diagnosed	Tamoxifen × 5 yrs **Anastrozole × 5 yrs** Tamoxifen + anastrozole × 5 yrs	9,366	0.87
BIG 1–98 (Refs. 21,82)	Newly diagnosed	Tamoxifen × 5 yrs **Letrozole × 5 yrs** (Tamoxifen × 2 yrs → letrozole × 3 yrs) (Letrozole × 2 yrs → tamoxifen × 3 yrs)	8,028	0.82
Sequential/Switching Therapy				
ABCSG 8 (Ref, 83)	Newly diagnosed	Tamoxifen × 5 yrs **Tamoxifen × 2 yrs → anastrozole × 3 yrs**	2,926	0.76
ARNO 95 (Ref. 83)	Disease-free after 2 yrs tamoxifen	Tamoxifen × 3 yrs **Anastrozole × 3 yrs**	979	0.66
IES (Ref. 22)	Disease-free after 2–3 yrs tamoxifen	Tamoxifen × 2–3 yrs **Exemestane × 2–3 yrs**	4,724	0.76
ITA (Ref. 84)	Disease-free after 2–3 yrs tamoxifen	Tamoxifen × 2–3 yrs Anastrozole × 2–3 yrs	448	0.57
Extended Therapy				
MA.17 (Ref. 85)	Disease-free after 5 yrs tamoxifen	Placebo **Letrozole × 5 yrs**	5,187	0.58
NSABP B-33	Disease-free after 5 yrs tamoxifen	Placebo **Exemestane × 5 yrs**	1,598	0.68

DFS, disease-free survival.

Note: Study arms in boldface showed improved DFS.

improvement in DFS that will likely translate into a small improvement in overall survival. Finally, in MA.17, postmenopausal women were treated with letrozole or placebo for 5 years as extended endocrine therapy after 5 years of tamoxifen. Extended endocrine therapy offered an improvement in DFS, but improved overall survival date has been observed only in node-positive patients.

In summary, an upfront AI lowers risk of recurrence by 10% to 20% compared with 5 years of tamoxifen; sequencing tamoxifen and an AI for a total of 5 years lowers risk of recurrence by 24% to 40% compared with 5 years of tamoxifen; extended AI therapy based on MA.17 reduced the risk of recurrence by 30% to 40% compared with no treatment after 5 years of tamoxifen. Because of the generally favorable prognosis for many patients, these significant proportionate risk reductions have translated into only modest absolute differences in event rates. This collective experience has demonstrated superior outcomes for women who receive an AI rather than 5 years of tamoxifen; however, it remains unclear how best to incorporate AI therapy. Therefore, upfront, sequential, and extended AI therapy are all reasonable approaches. The ultimate

decision should take into account patient age, comorbidities, and predicted risk of recurrence.

Tamoxifen and aromatase inhibitors differ with respect to side-effect profiles, a reflection of their different mechanisms of action. The risks of both uterine cancer and venous thromboembolism during treatment with tamoxifen increase with age (9). In the treatment arm of the P-1 trial, the relative risk of invasive endometrial cancer was 5.33 in women aged 50 years or older compared with 1.42 in women under age 50. In addition, rates of deep vein thrombosis (DVT) and pulmonary embolism (PE) were highest in tamoxifen-treated women aged 50 years or older, with a relative risk of 1.49 and 2.16 for DVT and PE, respectively (10).

Concerns also exist for postmenopausal women treated with AIs given the high rate of treatment-associated osteopenia or osteoporosis. Therefore, bone mineral density should be documented prior to AI initiation and followed at regular intervals during treatment. Detrimental effects of AIs on bone mineral density may be mitigated by the use of calcium, vitamin D, weight-bearing exercise, and bisphosphonates, as outlined in the American Society of Clinical Oncology treatment guidelines (24). There are reports of increased cardiovascular events with AIs that warrant further investigation and observation. The AI-associated musculoskeletal syndrome is the most common AI toxicity and manifests as arthralgias, myalgias, or seronegative joint inflammation. AI-associated arthralgias were observed in up to 25% to 30% of AI-treated patients in the large phase III trials, although in practice, many more women seem to be affected by this syndrome. Symptoms of AI-associated arthralgia may be disabling enough to result in treatment interruption or class switching in some women. The exact mechanism underlying this musculoskeletal syndrome is not currently known but is thought to be related to estrogen deprivation.

While tamoxifen and AIs have different side-effect profiles, quality-of-life analyses in the large AI trials showed similar quality of life and tolerability for women receiving tamoxifen and AIs (25). In MA.17, quality of life was similar in the placebo and letrozole arms; however, there was a subgroup of letrozole-treated women who did have appreciable changes in bodily pain and vasomotor domains on quality-of-life analyses that are attributable to estrogen deprivation (26). In postmenopausal women, AI-associated and tamoxifen-associated side effects were both related to local estrogen deprivation; both classes resulted in night sweats and hot flashes, but AI-treated women reported more vaginal dryness and loss of libido.

Unanswered Questions

The optimal duration of adjuvant endocrine therapy remains an area of clinical investigation. Long-term follow-up from the NSABP B-14 rerandomization to 5 versus 10 years of tamoxifen in women with ER+, node-negative tumors failed to show a benefit in the 10-year arm, with a slight advantage in the 5-year arm, establishing 5 years of tamoxifen as the standard (27). Clinicians are currently awaiting the results of the adjuvant Tamoxifen—To offer more? (aTTom) (28) and Adjuvant Tamoxifen—Longer Against Shorter (ATLAS) (29) trials, which looked again at longer durations of tamoxifen beyond 5 years to better define the ideal duration of endocrine therapy. Similar trials comparing duration of AI therapy are under way. With regard to AIs, studies such as MA.17 suggest that extended endocrine treatment with AIs can further lower recurrence risk. At present, there are no data for either the safety or efficacy of AI treatment durations beyond 5 years.

The benefits of AI therapy in postmenopausal women have led to questions as to whether women who are premenopausal at the time of diagnosis should receive upfront AI therapy. The safety and efficacy of AIs in conjunction with ovarian suppression in premenopausal women have been examined by the TEXT and Austrian Breast & Colorectal Cancer Study Group (ABCSG)–12 trials. ABCSG-12 randomized women to AI plus ovarian suppression or tamoxifen plus ovarian suppression and did not detect a difference in outcome between the two arms (30). Therefore, at this time, the standard approach to premenopausal women should remain tamoxifen with consideration of an AI plus ovarian suppression in tamoxifen-intolerant patients or in those with contraindications to tamoxifen.

An emerging area of investigation relates to the metabolism of tamoxifen. It is known that multiple genetic variations in the CYP2D6 allele affect the efficiency of tamoxifen metabolism to its active metabolite, endoxifen. Some patients have a genotype that makes them "poor metabolizers," whereas others will have increased or even ultrahigh rates of drug metabolism. This pharmacogenomic variation likely explains the wide range in endoxifen levels among tamoxifen-treated women. It has been suggested that poor metabolizers do not manifest vasomotor/menopausal symptoms with therapy and that treatment in such patients may be relatively ineffective in the prevention of disease relapse. CYP2D6 testing has been proposed in postmenopausal women because poor metabolizers alternatively could be treated with an AI. The use of CYP2D6 testing in premenopausal women is more controversial because a standard alterative therapy is not available, and ovarian suppression has not been shown to be either equal or superior to tamoxifen in these women (31). Published treatment guidelines do not currently recommend CYP2D6 testing (32), but the effects of drug metabolism are being studied as correlative questions in multiple ongoing clinical trials. In an effort to maximize benefit from tamoxifen, efforts should be made to avoid drugs that inhibit CYP2D6. (33) (Table 7.5).

■ ADJUVANT CHEMOTHERAPY

Cytotoxic chemotherapy plays a significant role in the adjuvant treatment of hormone receptor–negative and HER2+ breast cancer, as well as many cases of hormone

Table 7.5 Drugs to avoid during treatment with tamoxifen: inhibitors of CYP2D6

Strong Inhibitors[a] of CYP2D6	Moderate or Weak Inhibitors of CYP2D6
Fluoxetine	Duloxetine
Paroxetine	Sertraline
Quinidine	Diphenhydramine
Bupropion	Thioridazine
	Trazodone
	Cimetidine
	Amiodarone

[a]A strong inhibitor is one that causes a >5-fold increase in the plasma area under the curve values or more than an 80% decrease in clearance.

Source: From Refs. 86, 87, and 92.

receptor–positive breast cancer when positive lymph nodes or high-risk features are present.

Bonadonna and colleagues were the first to demonstrate a benefit from combination adjuvant chemotherapy (CMF) in breast cancer (34). Long-term follow-up of this and other studies has confirmed the ability of adjuvant chemotherapy to reduce both recurrence of and death from breast cancer (35); its use in a selected patient population is now widely accepted. Follow-up studies by the NSABP and US Intergroup Adjuvant Breast Trial have since broadened the indications for adjuvant chemotherapy to include node-positive, and ER– and higher-risk ER+ node-negative tumors (36,37). Recent trials have worked to identify more effective drug combinations and to shorten treatment courses, particularly through the inclusion of anthracyclines. US and Europeans trials compared CMF with anthracycline-based regimens (CAF and CEF) and showed equivalent but not clearly superior DFS and overall survival in patients treated with either epirubicin or doxorubicin (38,39). NSABP trials (6,40) found that four cycles of doxorubicin and cyclophosphamide (AC) proved equivalent to 6 months of oral CMF. Largely for the sake of convenience, four cycles of AC soon became a standard of care.

The most recent update of the EBCTCG meta-analysis in 2005 provided ongoing support for the use of adjuvant chemotherapy and demonstrated that anthracycline-based chemotherapy reduces the annual rate of death from breast cancer by 38% in women under age 50 and by 20% in women aged 50 to 69. Although not previously detected by individual trials, a statistically significant superiority of anthracycline-based regimens over nonanthracycline regimens, including classical CMF, was also demonstrated in this meta-analysis (41) (Table 7.6).

Newer Regimens: Can Anthracyclines Be Avoided?

Doublet therapy with doxorubicin and cyclophosphamide (AC) or docetaxel and cyclophosphamide (TC) (42) may be appropriate for women who are believed to have chemotherapy-sensitive disease but in whom the risk of recurrence is moderate. For example, women with small triple-negative tumors or T2N0/T1N1 endocrine-sensitive breast cancers may be treated with four cycles of either AC or TC. AC has largely replaced CMF in the adjuvant setting, although CMF remains an acceptable and active regimen, as discussed above. In a single phase III trial, TC demonstrated modest improvements over AC in the adjuvant setting in terms of DFS and overall survival (43). Cardiomyopathy can be avoided by the use of TC, and concerns of secondary bone marrow disorders are minimized by the exclusion of a topoisomerase II inhibitor. The acute toxicities and tolerability of AC and TC are comparable, although different side-effect profiles have

been reported. Febrile neutropenia, myalgias, and arthralgias are more common with TC, whereas nausea, cardiac events, and bone marrow disorders were observed more frequently with AC. Although the phase III trial of AC and TC included women with triple-negative cancers (27% of patients), the study was not powered for definitive subgroup analysis. Therefore, the relative merits of TC in women with triple-negative tumors remain uncertain. Whether an anthracycline is necessary in some women is a question that remains unanswered at this time. This drug class may confer significant benefit in women with HER2+ or triple-negative breast cancer and continues to be used widely by breast oncologists pending further studies. Nonetheless, TC provides an alternative for patients in whom anthracycline-based therapy is not be preferred.

The problem of triple-negative breast cancers deserves brief comment as it is defined at the present time by the lack of hormone receptor expression or overexpression of HER2. In the future, genomic profiling or molecular markers will likely allow subclassification of the triple-negative patients into separate categories that may have specific treatments. Platinum salts have shown promising activity in triple negative breast cancer in both the neoadjuvant and metastatic settings. At present, in the curative setting, triple-negative patients should be treated with the same agents (alkylating, anthracycline, and taxanes) as are used for other types of breast cancer of similar risk of recurrence.

Taxane-containing Regimens

Although the EBCTCG meta-analysis reviewing 2005–2006 data did not look at the effect of taxanes, their benefit in the subset of women at the greatest risk for recurrence has been documented over the past decade through multiple large clinical trials, including CALGB (Cancer and Leukemia Group B) 9344 , NSABP B-28, Breast Cancer International Research Group (BCIRG) 001, and the PACS 01 trial. CALGB 9344, a randomized trial comparing four cycles of AC with escalating doses of A (60, 75, and 90 mg/m^2) to four cycles of AC followed by four cycles of paclitaxel (175 mg/m^2) in node-positive disease, demonstrated an improvement in both DFS and overall survival from the addition of a taxane following AC in women with lymph node–positive breast cancer (44). NSABP B-28 randomized more than 3,000 patients with lymph node–positive breast cancer to AC or to AC followed by four cycles of paclitaxel. The addition of a taxane in this population resulted in an improvement in DFS but not in overall survival (45). These trials and others ultimately led to the approval of paclitaxel and docetaxel for the treatment of lymph node–positive breast cancer. Since that time, multiple taxane-containing regimens have been shown to be effective in the women at greatest risk for local and distant recurrence (46). Taxanes are also likely to benefit women

■ **Table 7.6** Commonly used adjuvant chemotherapy regimens

Regimen (Ref.)	Agents, Dose (mg/m^2), and Schedule	Frequency	Number of Cycles
Oral CMF (classical) (38)	Cyclophosphamide 100, PO days 1–14; methotrexate 40, IV days 1 and 8; fluorouracil 600, IV days 1 and 8	Every 28 d	6
IV CMF (88)	Cyclophosphamide 600, IV day 1; methotrexate 40, IV day 1; fluorouracil 600, IV day 1	Every 21 d	9–12
AC × 4 (89)	Doxorubicin 60, IV day 1; cyclophosphamide 600, IV day 1	Every 21 d	4
TC × 4 (42)	Docetaxel 75, IV day 1; cyclophosphamide 600, IV day 1	Every 21 d	4
CAF × 6 (oral) (38)	Cyclophosphamide 100, PO, days 1–14; doxorubicin 30, IV days 1 and 8; fluorouracil 600, IV days 1 and 8	Every 28 d	6
CAF × 6 (IV) (FAC) (39)	Cyclophosphamide 500, IV day 1; doxorubicin 50, IV day 1; fluorouracil 500, IV day 1 _Or_	Every 28 d	6
	Cyclophosphamide 500, IV days 1 and 8; doxorubicin 50, CI over 72 h; fluorouracil 500, IV day 1	Every 21 d	
CEF (oral, Canadian) (90)	Cyclophosphamide 75, PO days 1–14; epirubicin 60, IV days 1 and 8; fluorouracil 500, IV days 1 and 8	Every 28 d	6
CEF (IV, FEC)	Cyclophosphamide 500, IV day 1; epirubicin 100, IV day 1; fluorouracil 500, IV day 1	Every 21 d	6
AC → P (44)	_Cycles 1–4_ Doxorubicin 60, IV day 1; cyclophosphamide 600, IV day 1 _Cycles 5–8_ Paclitaxel 175, IV day 1	Every 21 d	8
AC → P weekly (49)	_Cycles 1–4_ Doxorubicin 60, IV day 1; cyclophosphamide 600, IV day 1	Every 21 d	
	Weeks 13–24 Paclitaxel 80, IV day 1	Weekly	
Dose dense AC → P^a (52)	_Cycles 1–4_ Doxorubicin 60, IV day 1; cyclophosphamide 600, IV day 1 _Cycles 5–8_ Paclitaxel 175, IV day 1	Every 14 d	8
Dose dense A → P → C^a (52)	_Cycles 1–4_ Doxorubicin 60, IV day 1 _Cycles 5–8_ Paclitaxel 175, IV day 1 _Cycles 9–12_ Cyclophosphamide 600, IV day 1	Every 14 d	12
TAC^a (46)	Cyclophosphamide 500, IV day 1; doxorubicin 50, IV day 1; docetaxel 75, IV day 1	Every 21 d	6

A, doxorubicin; C, cyclophosphamide; E, epirubicin; F, fluorouracil; P, paclitaxel; T, docetaxel. M, methotrexate.

^{a}Requires G-CSF (granulocyte colony-stimulating factor) on days 3 to 10 or pegfilgrastim on day 2 during cycles 1 to 8.

with lymph node–negative disease in whom tumor size, lack of endocrine sensitivity, or other histological features predict a more aggressive biology. A retrospective subset analysis of CALGB 9344 failed to demonstrate a benefit from taxanes in ER+, HER2–, lymph node–positive breast cancer, reinforcing the idea that the greatest benefit of chemotherapy exists in those patients with tumors least sensitive to adjuvant hormonal therapy (47). Not all subset analyses have reached similar conclusions; both a taxane meta-analysis (48) and a prospectively planned subset analysis of BCIRG 001 demonstrated a benefit from the use of taxane in ER+ breast cancer (46).

A 2008 meta-analysis of taxane trials showed a clear benefit in terms of DFS and overall survival with the addition of a taxane to an anthracycline-based regimen, independent of taxane type or schedule of administration (48). Multiple studies have rigorously examined the issues of dose and schedule for optimal administration of adjuvant taxane therapy. When first developed, paclitaxel was added after four cycles of AC chemotherapy and given on an every-3-weeks treatment schedule. The US Intergroup Adjuvant Breast Trial [Eastern Cooperative Oncology Group (ECOG) 1199] was designed to evaluated schedule dependence of two different taxanes (docetaxel and paclitaxel) and used a four-arm design comparing paclitaxel and docetaxel on weekly with every-3-weeks schedules following the completion of AC. The hazard ratio for DFS and overall survival was superior for weekly paclitaxel, but at the expense of increased neuropathy, seen in nearly one third of patients. Patients treated with every-3-weeks docetaxel also demonstrated significantly improved DFS but not overall survival compared with the standard of thrice-weekly paclitaxel. Patients in the docetaxel arms experienced greater toxicity, particularly hematological toxicity, resulting in fewer completed cycles of therapy (49). While patients in the docetaxel arms received similar cumulative doses of taxane, patients in the paclitaxel arm were able to receive significantly more paclitaxel in the weekly arm than in the every-3-weeks arm.

Dose Density

Although initial observations from early adjuvant trials suggested a possible benefit from increased dose intensity, more rigorous evaluations of escalated dose intensity in the CALGB 9344 (anthracycline) and NSABP B-22 and B-25 (cyclophosphamide) trials failed to show improved clinical outcomes, so this approach was abandoned (50).

Dose density was also proposed as a mechanism by which to improve responses to cytotoxic chemotherapy. Dose density is increased when equivalent doses of chemotherapy are administered with a shortened interval between treatments. The Norton-Simon hypothesis states that the rate of regression in tumor volume in response to chemotherapy is proportional to the rate of growth for a given tumor size. It is thought that greater "cell kill" may be achieved by maximizing the rate of drug delivery, not the level of dosing (51). On this reasoning, dose density has been exploited in an effort to optimize adjuvant chemotherapy for breast cancer. CALGB 9741 used a 2´2 factorial design to compare sequential and concurrent AC-T (paclitaxel) on every-3-weeks or every-2-weeks schedules. Fortnightly dosing with filgrastim white blood

cell growth factor support resulted in an improvement in both DFS and overall survival with fewer episodes of febrile neutropenia. There was no perceptible difference between concurrent and sequential therapy (52). A dose-dense schedule for AC-T with pegfilgrastim (GM-CSF) support has since become a standard for women with high-risk, HER2– disease and has being compared with TAC (docetaxel, doxorubicin, and cyclophosphamide) as part of NSABP B-38.

Multiple combination regimens built around taxanes have been developed, including TAC (docetaxel, doxorubicin, and cyclophosphamide), AT (doxorubicin and paclitaxel), and TC (see above). In BCIRG 001, TAC improved DFS and overall survival over FAC for all hormone receptor subtypes in lymph node–positive patients (46). It should be noted that in ECOG 2197, four cycles of doxorubicin anddocetaxel was no more effective than four cycles of AC for lymph node–positive disease; however, the taxane-containing arm had significantly greater toxicity (febrile neutropenia 26% versus 10%), making it an inferior option overall (53). While TC is superior to AC according to one phase III trial (43), head-to-head comparison of third-generation regimens such as dose-dense AC-paclitaxel and docetaxel-AC (TAC) to docetaxel-C (TC) are in progress. Until these data are available, the value of TC in high-risk patients remains uncertain.

In summary, taxanes have proven a useful addition to adjuvant chemotherapy for early-stage breast cancer. Regimens of weekly paclitaxel, every-2-weeks paclitaxel, or every-3-weeks docetaxel are all effective after AC or FEC chemotherapy, and combinations such as TAC or TC also have demonstrated activity.

Patient Selection

The decision to administer chemotherapy in early-stage breast cancer is often difficult due to clinician and patient concerns about acute side effects and long-term toxicities. In women with endocrine-sensitive, HER2– breast cancer, chemotherapy should be considered for lesions larger than 1 cm, lymph node positivity, or both. The threshold for administering chemotherapy to women with HER2-overexpressing or triple-negative tumors is considerably lower because these phenotypes are generally more sensitive to chemotherapy and confer a more aggressive biology (54). In addition, HER2 overexpression likely diminishes the benefit of endocrine therapy among ER+, HER2+ breast cancers, thereby increasing the value of chemotherapy and HER2-directed therapy in such cases. As mentioned, while adjuvant chemotherapy may cut the risk of recurrence by as much as 50% in women with a triple-negative cancer, the benefit of adjuvant chemotherapy may be negligible in women with low-grade, strongly ER+/PR+ cancers.

Historically, many women with breast cancer were treated with chemotherapy; over the past decade it has

■ **Table 7.7** Factors predicting clinical benefit from adjuvant chemotherapy

More Benefit From Chemotherapy	Less Benefit From Chemotherapy
Larger tumor	Smaller tumor
Lymph node positive	Lymph node negative
HER2 overexpressing	HER2 nonoverexpressing
Triple-negative	Stains strongly for estrogen receptor and progesterone receptor
Younger age	Older age
Higher Oncotype DX recurrence score	Lower Oncotype DX recurrence score
High nuclear grade	Low nuclear grade

become increasingly apparent that low-grade, luminal A cancers (55) may be relatively insensitive to chemotherapy. As a result, a recent paradigm shift has focused on endocrine therapy alone for small, low-risk, ER+ breast cancers (Table 7.7).

It is often challenging to identify the women at greatest risk for recurrence and the tumors most likely to be sensitive to chemotherapy. In an effort to ease decisions around chemotherapy administration by identifying high-risk, chemotherapy-sensitive breast cancers, Ravdin and colleagues developed the Adjuvant!Online program (56), a mathematical model to estimate prognosis without treatment and benefit from individual components of therapy. Developed using the Surveillance, Epidemiology and End Results (SEER) database and analysis of the 2000 EBCTCG data, Adjuvant!Online uses a proprietary formula and is widely available online. The model stratifies risk on the basis of clinical and pathological features and has been validated on a large data set (57). A limitation of this model is its failure to incorporate underlying tumor biology in assigning proportionate risk reduction with chemotherapy regimens.

More recently, gene expression assays have increasingly been used to help make chemotherapy decisions in women with ER+, lymph node–negative cancers. As of 2009, Oncotype DX, a reverse-transcriptase/polymerase chain reaction (RT-PCR) assay, is the most commonly used gene expression profile in the United States, despite the lack of completed trials providing level 1 evidence of its predictive capabilities. It can be performed on paraffin-embedded tissue, making it practical for clinical use. The 21-gene assay examines 16 proliferation, ER-related, and HER-2 genes and 5 housekeeping genes and generates a recurrence score (0–100) that predicts the likelihood of benefit from chemotherapy as well as the 10-year risk of recurrence. Oncotype DX has been retrospectively validated within a prospectively conducted clinical trial as prognostic and predictive in a series of patients with ER+,

lymph node–negative, tamoxifen-treated cancers. Women with low recurrence scores (<18) are thought to derive little benefit from chemotherapy. Conversely, women with high recurrence scores (>30) are at increased risk for recurrence and are known to derive significant benefit from adjuvant chemotherapy (58). The ideal management of women with intermediate recurrence scores (defined as 18–30) is not known and is the focus of the ongoing TAILORx trial (59). An important aspect of the trial is its definition of "intermediate risk" to include scores of 11–25. While the cost of Oncotype DX testing currently exceeds US$3,000, it is helpful in some women with ER+, node-negative, intermediate-grade tumors and either low or high recurrence scores; for this reason, it is generally covered by both commercial carriers and Medicare (60). Recent analysis a Southwest Oncology Group (SWOG) trial presented at the 2007 San Antonio Breast Cancer Symposium suggested that Oncotype DX may also have prognostic and predictive value in postmenopausal women with ER+, node-positive breast cancers, with findings that are qualitatively similar to observations among node-negative patients (61).

Once a decision has been made to administer chemotherapy, a standard regimen within the guidelines discussed above should be selected. Large randomized, prospective trials have demonstrated that neoadjuvant chemotherapy is as effective as adjuvant chemotherapy (62). For logistic reasons, chemotherapy is usually administered postoperatively, except in women who require preoperative chemotherapy to facilitate surgery or to make them potential candidates for breast conservation. Many chemotherapeutic agents are known to be active in breast cancer, and randomized, controlled trials have documented the efficacy of multiple regimens (35) (see Table 7.6).

As with the decision to administer chemotherapy, the treatment selection should take into account tumor phenotype, clinicopathological features, and patient comorbidities. Details to consider include duration of therapy, density of therapy, the risk/benefit ratio of using an anthracycline, and whether to include a taxane.

■ TREATMENT OF HER2+ BREAST CANCER

The *HER2* gene encodes for the human epidermal growth factor receptor (HER2), which is known to be overexpressed in 15% to 20% of all breast cancers (63,64). These tumors are associated with many adverse prognostic markers, including high tumor grade and proliferative rate, increased frequency of nodal metastases, and relative resistance to certain classes of chemotherapy (65). In the pretrastuzumab (Herceptin) era, HER2 overexpression was an independent risk factor for shortened DFS and overall survival and a predictor of anthracycline sensitivity (64,66).

The implication of HER2 overexpression as a dominant force in the growth and dissemination of one quarter of breast cancers led to the development of targeted therapy with trastuzumab. A phase III trial of chemotherapy plus trastuzumab for HER2+ metastatic breast cancer showed a striking improvement in both response rate and overall survival, resulting in its approval by the US Food and Drug Administration (67). Trials of trastuzumab in the metastatic setting showed that it is more effective when administered in combination with cytotoxic chemotherapy (68). Since the risk of cardiac toxicity is dramatically increased by the concurrent administration of anthracyclines and trastuzumab, these agents were given sequentially in adjuvant trials.

Trastuzumab was evaluated in the adjuvant setting in women with high-risk, HER2-overexpressing tumors as part of four large randomized, controlled trials that enrolled a total of more than 10,000 women: Hercpetin Adjuvant trial (HERA) (69), North Central Cancer Treatment Group (NCCTG) N-9831 (70), BCIRG 006 (71), and NSABP B-31 (72). Women were randomly assigned to treatment with standard chemotherapy or chemotherapy plus trastuzumab. Most of the patients in these trials also received an anthracycline, since HER2-overexpressing tumors were thought to be particularly sensitive to this drug class (73,74), possibly as a result of the coamplification of the topoisomerase II gene (75). Given the sensitivity of HER2+ tumors to taxanes (47), these trials also included either paclitaxel or docetaxel as the chemotherapy backbone for trastuzumab therapy. In one trial (HERA), trastuzumab was initiated only after all chemotherapy, which was not prospectively defined. The decision to sequence doxorubicin and trastuzumab related to concerns about increased cardiac toxicity from the concurrent use of these agents. Approximately 900 women, as part of the BCIRG study, were treated with docetaxel, carboplatin, and trastuzumab (TCH) and therefore did not receive an anthracycline. The results of these four large phase III trials were nearly uniform, demonstrating an improvement in both DFS and overall survival for women with high-risk, HER2-overexpressing tumors (76). The combination of chemotherapy and trastuzumab, either concurrently or sequentially, was generally well tolerated. The most concerning toxicity observed was symptomatic heart failure and asymptomatic cardiomyopathy. Coadministration of taxanes and trastuzumab has been shown to be safe. The most widely used treatment regimens for women with HER2+ disease are AC → TH and TCH (Table 7.8). Data from BCIRG 006 suggest that TCH is as effective as AC → TH, although the study was underpowered to detect a small difference between the two regimens. While the two regimens are generally well tolerated, the rate of grade 3 to 4 cardiac toxicity in the TCH arm of BCIRG-006 was only 0.4%, compared with approximately 1.8% for AC → TH, making it an attractive option for patients with compromised cardiac function or those perceived to be at increased risk for trastuzumab-associated cardiomyopathy.

The adjuvant trastuzumab trials monitored patients' ejection fractions and evaluated for signs/symptoms of congestive heart failure (CHF) at regular intervals. Treatment with trastuzumab increased the incidence of

Table 7.8 Trastuzumab-containing adjuvant chemotherapy regimens	
Regimen (Ref.)	**Agents, Dose, and Schedule**
AC → TH (72)	Doxorubicin 60 mg/m^2, IV + cyclophosphamide 600 mg/m^2, IV, q3wks × 4 cycles ↓ Paclitaxel 80 mg/m^2, IV + trastuzumab 2 mg/kg weekly × 12 wks[b] ↓ Trastuzumab 6 mg/kg q3wks to complete 52 wks of biological therapy
Dose dense AC → TH[a] (91)	Doxorubicin 60 mg/m^2, IV + cyclophosphamide 600 mg/m^2, q2wks × 4 cycles[a] ↓ Paclitaxel 175 mg/m^2, IV q2wks × 4 cycles[a] + trastuzumab 2 mg/kg, IV weekly × 8 wks[b] ↓ Trastuzumab 6 mg/kg q3wks to complete 52 wks of biological therapy
TCH (71)	Docetaxel, 75 mg/m^2, IV q3wks Carboplatin, AUC 6, IV q3wks Trastuzumab 6 mg/kg IV q3wks[c] ↓ Trastuzumab 6 mg/kg q3wks to complete 52 wks of biological therapy

AC, adriamycin and Cytoxan; TCH, taxotere, carboplatin, and herceptin; TH, taxol and herceptin.

[a]Requires G-CSF (granulocyte colony-stimulating factor) on days 3 to 10 or pegfilgrastim on day 2 during cycles 1 to 4.
[b]4 mg/kg loading dose with first trastuzumab dose.
[c]8 mg/kg loading dose with first cycle.

cardiomyopathy. Identifiable risk factors for cardiomyopathy vary among studies but likely include concurrent/previous anthracycline therapy, age greater than 60 years, underlying cardiac disease, and baseline left ventricular ejection fraction (LVEF) less than 55% (67,72). The rate of New York Heart Association class III or IV CHF was less than 1% in the control arms but ranged from 1.6% to 4.1% in the trastuzumab-treated patients (72). Heart failure rates of 1% to 2% have been reported in the BCIRG 006 TCH treatment. The safety of retreatment with trastuzumab after recovery of left ventricular function remains an unanswered question. Data from the MD Anderson Cancer Center experience suggest that this approach may be considered in a selected population in whom the risk/benefit ratio favors treatment (77–79). Monitoring of the LVEF prior to treatment initiation and at regularly scheduled intervals is recommended for all patients receiving trastuzumab.

The decision to use trastuzumab in women with small, HER2-overexpressing tumors is an area of controversy. The women enrolled in the four large adjuvant trials were generally "high risk," with positive lymph nodes or tumors larger than 2 cm or both. For women with small, lymph node–negative tumors, standard therapy with AC → TH or TCH may be "too much," given its expected side effects and toxicities. Even when these lesions are endocrine sensitive, there is concern that HER2 positivity is associated with relatively poorer prognosis and resistance to endocrine therapy owing to cross-talk between these pathways. Trastuzumab monotherapy lacks proven efficacy. In an effort to address this clinical question, a multicenter phase II trial led by the Dana Farber Cancer Center is examining the efficacy of 12 weeks of paclitaxel and trastuzumab followed by 40 weeks of trastuzumab in women with lower-risk, lymph node–negative, HER2+ breast cancers.

■ EMERGING STRATEGIES

Bisphosphonates

While bisphosphonates have long played a role in the management of bone metastases, there is growing evidence to support their ability to prevent bone demineralization and potentially recurrence in the adjuvant setting. This drug class was initially looked at in the adjuvant setting as part of an effort to counteract bone loss in women receiving ovarian suppression. The Austrian ABCSG-12 trial randomized premenopausal women receiving ovarian suppression plus tamoxifen or an AI to receive zoledronic acid every 6 months for 3 years or to receive no bisphosphonate therapy. In addition to the prevention of bone loss, women treated with zoledronic acid had a significantly improved DFS; interestingly, there was a decreased rate of both bone

and visceral metastases in these women as well as of contralateral breast cancers (30). There is a call for more data to support this practice, and the results of the Adjuvant Zoledronic Acid to Reduce Recurrence (AZURE) trial will be important given the ABCSG-12 findings. The benefit of adjuvant bisphosphonates in premenopausal women treated with chemotherapy or tamoxifen or both or in postmenopausal women remains unknown, and further data are awaited before endorsing bisphosphonate therapy as adjuvant treatment. Bisphosphonates are contraindicated in women who may wish to become pregnant following treatment for breast cancer given the markedly delayed excretion from the body and risk to the fetus.

Inhibitors of Angiogenesis

Bevacizumab, a monoclonal antibody directed against vascular endothelial growth factor (VEGF), in combination with chemotherapy, has been shown to improve progression-free survival in women with metastatic breast cancer (80). Its role in the adjuvant setting is not known but is the subject of ongoing clinical trials such as ECOG 5103, which will treat high-risk women with a third-generation chemotherapy regimen with or without bevacizumab, either for the duration of chemotherapy or for 1 year in total. Given bevacizumab's interference with wound healing and associated risks such as hypertension, thrombosis, and bleeding, it should not be used in the adjuvant setting outside of a clinical trial.

■ SUMMARY

- Breast cancers are a heterogeneous group of tumors. Molecular subtyping has helped to classify breast cancers in an effort to uncover pathophysiology and individualize therapy.
- Endocrine therapy dramatically reduces the risk of recurrence in women with ER+ and PR+ cancers. Premenopausal women should receive tamoxifen, with a consideration of ovarian suppression. Options for postmenopausal women include both tamoxifen and AIs.
- Adjuvant chemotherapy reduces the risk of recurrence in some women with breast cancer. Women with triple-negative, HER2+, or less indolent ER+ cancers are most likely to benefit from chemotherapy.
- Efforts to individualize care for women with breast cancer include gene expression analysis (e.g., Oncotype DX) and targeted therapies (e.g., trastuzumab). This evolving strategy works to minimize unnecessary toxicity and improve clinical benefit.
- Emerging strategies in the treatment of breast cancer are examining the role of ovarian suppression, bisphosphonates, and angiogenesis inhibitors.

■ REFERENCES

1. Jemal A, Siegel R, Ward E, et al. Cancer statistics, 2008. *CA Cancer J Clin.* 2008;58(2):71–96.

2. Sorlie T, Wang Y, Xiao C, et al. Distinct molecular mechanisms underlying clinically relevant subtypes of breast cancer: gene expression analyses across three different platforms. *BMC Genomics.* 2006;7:127.

3. Dent R, Trudeau M, Pritchard KI, et al. Triple-negative breast cancer: clinical features and patterns of recurrence. *Clin Cancer Res.* 2007;13(15):4429–4434.

4. Early Breast Cancer Trialists' Collaborative Group (EBCTCG). Effects of chemotherapy and hormonal therapy for early breast cancer on recurrence and 15-year survival: an overview of the randomised trials. *Lancet.* 2005;365(9472):1687–1717.

5. Fisher B, Costantino J, Redmond C, et al. A randomized clinical trial evaluating tamoxifen in the treatment of patients with node-negative breast cancer who have estrogen-receptor-positive tumors. *New Engl J Med.* 1989;320(8):479–484.

6. Fisher B, Jeong JH, Dignam J, et al. Findings from recent National Surgical Adjuvant Breast and Bowel Project adjuvant studies in stage I breast cancer. *J Natl Cancer Inst Monogr.* 2001(30):62–66.

7. Burstein HJ, Winer EP. HER2 or not HER2: that is the question. *J Clin Oncol.* 2005;23(16):3656–3659.

8. Schiff R, Massarweh S, Shou J, Osborne CK. Breast cancer endocrine resistance: how growth factor signaling and estrogen receptor coregulators modulate response. *Clin Cancer Res.* 2003;9(1):447S–54S.

9. Braithwaite RS, Chlebowski RT, Lau J, George S, Hess R, Col NF. Meta-analysis of vascular and neoplastic events associated with tamoxifen. *J Gen Intern Med.* 2003;18(11):937–947.

10. Fisher B, Costantino JP, Wickerham DL, et al. Tamoxifen for the prevention of breast cancer: current status of the National Surgical Adjuvant Breast and Bowel Project P-1 study. *J Natl Cancer Inst.* 2005;97(22):1652–1662.

11. Ovarian ablation in early breast cancer: overview of the randomised trials. Early Breast Cancer Trialists' Collaborative Group. *Lancet.* 1996;348(9036):1189–1196.

12. Parton M, Smith IE. Controversies in the management of patients with breast cancer: adjuvant endocrine therapy in premenopausal women. *J Clin Oncol.* 2008;26(5):745–752.

13. Castiglione-Gertsch M, O'Neill A, Price KN, et al. Adjuvant chemotherapy followed by goserelin versus either modality alone for premenopausal lymph node-negative breast cancer: a randomized trial. *J Natl Cancer Inst.* 2003;95(24):1833–1846.

14. Walshe JM, Denduluri N, Swain SM. Amenorrhea in premenopausal women after adjuvant chemotherapy for breast cancer. *J Clin Oncol.* 2006;24(36):5769–5779.

15. Cuzick J, Ambroisine L, Davidson N, et al. Use of luteinising-hormone-releasing hormone agonists as adjuvant treatment in premenopausal patients with hormone-receptor-positive breast cancer: a meta-analysis of individual patient data from randomised adjuvant trials. *Lancet* 2007;369(9574):1711–1723.

16. Sharma R, Hamilton A, Beith J. LHRH agonists for adjuvant therapy of early breast cancer in premenopausal women. *Cochrane Database Syst Rev.* 2008(4):CD004562.

17. Burstein HJ, Mayer E, Patridge AH, et al. Inadvertent use of aromatase inhibitors in patients with breast cancer with residual ovarian function: cases and lessons. *Clin Breast Cancer.* 2006;7(2):158–161.

18. Hargis JB, Nakajima ST. Resumption of menses with initiation of letrozole after five years of amenorrhea on tamoxifen: caution needed when using tamoxifen followed by aromatase inhibitors. *Cancer Invest.* 2006;24(2):174–177.

19. Thurlimann B, Keshaviah A, Coates AS, et al. A comparison of letrozole and tamoxifen in postmenopausal women with early breast cancer. *New Engl J Med.* 2005;353(26):2747–2757.

20. Forbes JF, Cuzick J, Buzdar A, Howell A, Tobias JS, Baum M. Effect of anastrozole and tamoxifen as adjuvant treatment for early-stage breast cancer: 100-month analysis of the ATAC trial. *Lancet Oncol.* 2008;9(1):45–53.

21. Mouridsen HT G-HA, Mauriac L, Paridaens R, et al. A randomized double-blind phase III study evaluating letrozole and tamoxifen given in sequence as adjuvant endocrine therapy for postmenopausal women with receptor-positive breast cancer. *Breast Cancer Res Treat.* 2008:A13.

22. Coombes RC, Kilburn LS, Snowdon CF, et al. Survival and safety of exemestane versus tamoxifen after 2–3 years' tamoxifen treatment (Intergroup Exemestane Study): a randomised controlled trial. *Lancet.* 2007;369(9561):559–570.

23. Goss PE, Ingle JN, Martino S, et al. A randomized trial of letrozole in postmenopausal women after five years of tamoxifen therapy for early-stage breast cancer. *New Engl J Med.* 2003;349(19):1793–1802.

24. Hillner BE, Ingle JN, Chlebowski RT, et al. American Society of Clinical Oncology 2003 update on the role of bisphosphonates and bone health issues in women with breast cancer. *J Clin Oncol.* 2003;21(21):4042–4057.

25. Fallowfield L, Cella D, Cuzick J, Francis S, Locker G, Howell A. Quality of life of postmenopausal women in the Arimidex, Tamoxifen, Alone or in Combination (ATAC) Adjuvant Breast Cancer Trial. *J Clin Oncol.* 2004;22(21):4261–4271.

26. Whelan TJ, Goss PE, Ingle JN, et al. Assessment of quality of life in MA.17: a randomized, placebo-controlled trial of letrozole after 5 years of tamoxifen in postmenopausal women. *J Clin Oncol.* 2005;23(28):6931–6940.

27. Fisher B, Dignam J, Bryant J, Wolmark N. Five versus more than five years of tamoxifen for lymph node-negative breast cancer: updated findings from the National Surgical Adjuvant Breast and Bowel Project B-14 randomized trial. *J Natl Cancer Inst.* 2001;93(9):684–690.

28. Gray RG, Rea DW, Handley K, et al. Randomized trial of 10 versus 5 years of adjuvant tamoxifen among 6,934 women with estrogen receptor-positive (ER+) or ER untested breast cancer—preliminary results. *J Clin Oncol.* 2008;26(Suppl):A513.

29. Peto R DC, on Behalf of the ATLAS Collaboration. ATLAS (Adjuvant Tamoxifen, Longer Against Shorter): international randomized trial of 10 versus 5 years of adjuvant tamoxifen among 11,500 women preliminary results. *Breast Cancer Res Treat.* 2007:A48.

30. Gnant M MB, Schippinger W, Luschin-Ebengreuth G, et al. Adjuvant ovarian suppression combined with tamoxifen or anastrozole, alone or in combination with zoledronic acid, in premenopausal women with hormone-responsive, stage I and II breast cancer: first efficacy results from ABCSG-12. *J Clin Oncol.* 2008;26:(Suppl):ALBA4.

31. Goetz MP, Rae JM, Suman VJ, et al. Pharmacogenetics of tamoxifen biotransformation is associated with clinical outcomes of efficacy and hot flashes. *J Clin Oncol.* 2005;23(36):9312–9318.

32. Hayes DF, Stearns V, Rae J, Flockhart D. A model citizen? Is tamoxifen more effective than aromatase inhibitors if we pick the right patients? *J Natl Cancer Inst.* 2008;100(9):610–613.

33. Stearns V, Rae JM. Pharmacogenetics and breast cancer endocrine therapy: CYP2D6 as a predictive factor for tamoxifen metabolism and drug response? *Expert Rev Mol Med.* 2008;10:e34.

34. Bonadonna G, Brusamolino E, Valagussa P, et al. Combination chemotherapy as an adjuvant treatment in operable breast cancer. *New Engl J Med.* 1976;294(8):405–410.

35. Bonadonna G, Valagussa P, Moliterni A, Zambetti M, Brambilla C. Adjuvant cyclophosphamide, methotrexate, and fluorouracil in node-positive breast cancer: the results of 20 years of follow-up. *New Engl J Med.* 1995;332(14):901–916.

36. Fisher B, Dignam J, Mamounas EP, et al. Sequential methotrexate and fluorouracil for the treatment of node-negative breast cancer patients with estrogen receptor-negative tumors: eight-year

results from National Surgical Adjuvant Breast and Bowel Project (NSABP) B-13 and first report of findings from NSABP B-19 comparing methotrexate and fluorouracil with conventional cyclophosphamide, methotrexate, and fluorouracil. *J Clin Oncol.* 1996;14(7):1982–1992.

37. Mansour EG, Gray R, Shatila AH, et al. Survival advantage of adjuvant chemotherapy in high-risk node-negative breast cancer: ten-year analysis—an intergroup study. *J Clin Oncol.* 1998; 16(11):3486–3492.

38. Hutchins LF, Green SJ, Ravdin PM, et al. Randomized, controlled trial of cyclophosphamide, methotrexate, and fluorouracil versus cyclophosphamide, doxorubicin, and fluorouracil with and without tamoxifen for high-risk, node-negative breast cancer: treatment results of Intergroup Protocol INT-0102. *J Clin Oncol.* 2005;23(33):8313–8321.

39. Martin M, Villar A, Sole-Calvo A, et al. Doxorubicin in combination with fluorouracil and cyclophosphamide (i.v. FAC regimen, day 1, 21) versus methotrexate in combination with fluorouracil and cyclophosphamide (i.v. CMF regimen, day 1, 21) as adjuvant chemotherapy for operable breast cancer: a study by the GEICAM group. *Ann Oncol.* 2003;14(6):833–842.

40. Fisher B, Brown AM, Dimitrov NV, et al. Two months of doxorubicin-cyclophosphamide with and without interval reinduction therapy compared with 6 months of cyclophosphamide, methotrexate, and fluorouracil in positive-node breast cancer patients with tamoxifen-nonresponsive tumors: results from the National Surgical Adjuvant Breast and Bowel Project B-15. *J Clin Oncol.* 1990;8(9):1483–1496.

41. EBCTCG. Effects of chemotherapy and hormonal therapy for early breast cancer on recurrence and 15-year survival: an overview of the randomised trials. *Lancet.* 2005;365(9472):1687–1717.

42. Jones SE, Savin MA, Holmes FA, et al. Phase III trial comparing doxorubicin plus cyclophosphamide with docetaxel plus cyclophosphamide as adjuvant therapy for operable breast cancer. *J Clin Oncol.* 2006;24(34):5381–5387.

43. Jones S, Holmes F, O'Shaughnessy J, et al. Docetaxel with cyclophosphamide is associated with an overall survival benefit compared with doxorubicin and cyclophosphamide: 7-Year Follow-Up of US Oncology Research Trial 9735. *J Clin Oncol.* 2009;27(8):1177–183.

44. Henderson IC, Berry DA, Demetri GD, et al. Improved outcomes from adding sequential Paclitaxel but not from escalating Doxorubicin dose in an adjuvant chemotherapy regimen for patients with node-positive primary breast cancer. *J Clin Oncol.* 2003;21(6):976–983.

45. Mamounas EP, Bryant J, Lembersky B, et al. Paclitaxel after doxorubicin plus cyclophosphamide as adjuvant chemotherapy for node-positive breast cancer: results from NSABP B-28. *J Clin Oncol.* 2005;23(16):3686–3696.

46. Martin M, Pienkowski T, Mackey J, et al. Adjuvant docetaxel for node-positive breast cancer. *New Engl J Med.* 2005; 352(22):2302–2313.

47. Hayes DF, Thor AD, Dressler LG, et al. HER2 and response to paclitaxel in node-positive breast cancer. *New Engl J Med.* 2007;357(15):1496–1506.

48. De Laurentiis M, Cancello G, D'Agostino D, et al. Taxane-based combinations as adjuvant chemotherapy of early breast cancer: a meta-analysis of randomized trials. *J Clin Oncol.* 2008;26(1):44–53.

49. Sparano JA, Wang M, Martino S, et al. Weekly paclitaxel in the adjuvant treatment of breast cancer. *New Engl J Med.* 2008;358(16):1663–1671.

50. Fisher B, Anderson S, DeCillis A, et al. Further evaluation of intensified and increased total dose of cyclophosphamide for the treatment of primary breast cancer: findings from National Surgical Adjuvant Breast and Bowel Project B-25. *J Clin Oncol.* 1999;17(11):3374–3388.

51. Norton L, Simon R. The Norton-Simon hypothesis revisited. *Cancer Treat Rep.* 1986;70(1):163–169.

52. Citron ML, Berry DA, Cirrincione C, et al. Randomized trial of dose-dense versus conventionally scheduled and sequential versus concurrent combination chemotherapy as postoperative adjuvant treatment of node-positive primary breast cancer: first report of Intergroup Trial C9741/Cancer and Leukemia Group B Trial 9741. *J Clin Oncol.* 2003;21(8):1431–1439.

53. Goldstein LJ, O'Neill A, Sparano JA, et al. Concurrent doxorubicin plus docetaxel is not more effective than concurrent doxorubicin plus cyclophosphamide in operable breast cancer with 0 to 3 positive axillary nodes: North American Breast Cancer Intergroup Trial E 2197. *J Clin Oncol.* 2008;26(25):4092–4099.

54. Clarke M, Coates AS, Darby SC, et al. Adjuvant chemotherapy in oestrogen-receptor-poor breast cancer: patient-level meta-analysis of randomised trials. *Lancet.* 2008;371(9606):29–40.

55. Sorlie T, Perou CM, Tibshirani R, et al. Gene expression patterns of breast carcinomas distinguish tumor subclasses with clinical implications. *Proc Natl Acad Sci USA.* 2001;98(19):10869–10874.

56. Ravdin, PM, Siminoff, LA, Davis, GJ, et al. Computer program to assist in making decisions about adjuvant therapy for women with early breast cancer. *J Clin Oncol.* 2001;19:980.

57. Olivotto IA, Bajdik CD, Ravdin PM, et al. Population-based validation of the prognostic model ADJUVANT! for early breast cancer. *J Clin Oncol.* 2005;23(12):2716–2725.

58. Paik S, Shak S, Tang G, et al. A multigene assay to predict recurrence of tamoxifen-treated, node-negative breast cancer. *New Engl J Med.* 2004;351(27):2817–2826.

59. Sparano JA. TAILORx: trial assigning individualized options for treatment (Rx). *Clin Breast Cancer.* 2006;7(4):347–350.

60. Harris L, Fritsche H, Mennel R, et al. American Society of Clinical Oncology 2007 update of recommendations for the use of tumor markers in breast cancer. *J Clin Oncol.* 2007;25(33):5287–5312.

61. Albain K BW, Shak S, Hortobagyi G, et al. Prognostic and predictive value of the 21-gene recurrence score assay in postmenopausal, node-positive, ER-positive breast cancer (S8814,INT0100). *Breast Cancer Res Treat.* 2007:Abstract 10.

62. Mauri D, Pavlidis N, Ioannidis JP. Neoadjuvant versus adjuvant systemic treatment in breast cancer: a meta-analysis. *J Natl Cancer Inst.* 2005;97(3):188–194.

63. Revillion F, Bonneterre J, Peyrat JP. ERBB2 oncogene in human breast cancer and its clinical significance. *Eur J Cancer.* 1998;34(6):791–808.

64. Slamon DJ, Clark GM, Wong SG, Levin WJ, Ullrich A, McGuire WL. Human breast cancer: correlation of relapse and survival with amplification of the HER-2/neu oncogene. *Science.* 1987; 235(4785):177–182.

65. Paik S, Hazan R, Fisher ER, et al. Pathologic findings from the National Surgical Adjuvant Breast and Bowel Project: prognostic significance of erbB-2 protein overexpression in primary breast cancer. *J Clin Oncol.* 1990;8(1):103–112.

66. Press MF, Pike MC, Chazin VR, et al. Her-2/neu expression in node-negative breast cancer: direct tissue quantitation by computerized image analysis and association of overexpression with increased risk of recurrent disease. *Cancer Res.* 1993;53(20): 4960–4970.

67. Slamon DJ, Leyland-Jones B, Shak S, et al. Use of chemotherapy plus a monoclonal antibody against HER2 for metastatic breast cancer that overexpresses HER2. *New Engl J Med.* 2001; 344(11):783–792.

68. Vogel CL, Cobleigh MA, Tripathy D, et al. Efficacy and safety of trastuzumab as a single agent in first-line treatment of HER2-overexpressing metastatic breast cancer. *J Clin Oncol.* 2002;20(3):719–726.

69. Piccart-Gebhart MJ, Procter M, Leyland-Jones B, et al. Trastuzumab after Adjuvant Chemotherapy in HER2-Positive Breast Cancer. *New Engl J Med.* 2005;353(16):1659–1672.

70. Perez E. Further analysis of NCCTG-N9831. Data presented at the 41st Annual Meeting of the American Society of Clinical Oncology. Orlando, FL, May 16th, 2005.

71. Slamon D EW, Robert N, Pienkowski T, et al. BCIRG 006: 2nd interim analysis phase III randomized trial comparing doxorubicin and cyclophosphamide followed by docetaxel (ACT) with doxorubicin and cyclophosphamide followed by docetaxel and trastuzumab (ACTH) with docetaxel, carboplatin and trastuzumab (TCH) in Her2neu positive early breast cancer patients. *Breast Cancer Res Treat.* 2006:A52.

72. Romond EH, Perez EA, Bryant J, et al. Trastuzumab plus adjuvant chemotherapy for operable HER2-positive breast cancer. *New Engl J Med.* 2005;353(16):1673–1684.

73. Pritchard KI, Shepherd LE, O'Malley FP, et al. HER2 and responsiveness of breast cancer to adjuvant chemotherapy. *New Engl J Med.* 2006;354(20):2103–2111.

74. Paik S, Bryant J, Tan-Chiu E, et al. HER2 and choice of adjuvant chemotherapy for invasive breast cancer: National Surgical Adjuvant Breast and Bowel Project Protocol B-15. *J Natl Cancer Inst.* 2000;92(24):1991–1998.

75. Pritchard KI, Messersmith H, Elavathil L, Trudeau M, O'Malley F, Dhesy-Thind B. HER-2 and topoisomerase II as predictors of response to chemotherapy. *J Clin Oncol.* 2008;26(5):736–744.

76. Perez EA, Suman VJ, Jeong J, et al. NCCTG/NSABP. Updated results of the combined analysis of NCCTG N9831 and NSABP B-31 adjuvant chemotherapy with/without trastuzumab in patients with HER2-positive breast cancer. *J Clin Oncol.* 2007 ASCO Annual Meeting Proceedings Part I Vol 25, No 18S (June 20 Supplement), 2007 2007:A512.

77. Ewer MS, Vooletich MT, Durand JB, et al. Reversibility of trastuzumab-related cardiotoxicity: new insights based on clinical course and response to medical treatment. *J Clin Oncol.* 2005; 23(31):7820–7826.

78. Chien KR. Herceptin and the heart—a molecular modifier of cardiac failure. *New Engl J Med.* 2006;354(8):789–790.

79. Tan-Chiu E, Yothers G, Romond E, et al. Assessment of cardiac dysfunction in a randomized trial comparing doxorubicin and cyclophosphamide followed by paclitaxel, with or without trastuzumab as adjuvant therapy in node-positive, human epidermal growth factor receptor 2-overexpressing breast cancer: NSABP B-31. *J Clin Oncol.* 2005;23(31):7811–7819.

80. Miller K, Wang M, Gralow J, et al. Paclitaxel plus bevacizumab versus paclitaxel alone for metastatic breast cancer. *New Engl J Med.* 2007;357(26):2666–2676.

81. Gnant M, Mlineritsch B, Schippinger W, et al. Endocrine therapy plus zoledronic acid in premenopausal breast cancer. *New Engl J Med.* 2009;360(7):679–691.

82. Coates AS, Keshaviah A, Thurlimann B, et al. Five years of letrozole compared with tamoxifen as initial adjuvant therapy for postmenopausal women with endocrine-responsive early breast cancer: update of study BIG 1–98. *J Clin Oncol.* 2007;25(5):486–492.

83. Jakesz R, Jonat W, Gnant M, et al. Switching of postmenopausal women with endocrine-responsive early breast cancer to anastrozole after 2 years' adjuvant tamoxifen: combined results of ABCSG trial 8 and ARNO 95 trial. *Lancet.* 2005;366(9484):455–462.

84. Boccardo F, Rubagotti A, Puntoni M, et al. Switching to anastrozole versus continued tamoxifen treatment of early breast cancer: preliminary results of the Italian Tamoxifen Anastrozole Trial. *J Clin Oncol.* 2005;23(22):5138–5147.

85. Goss PE, Ingle JN, Martino S, et al. Randomized trial of letrozole following tamoxifen as extended adjuvant therapy in receptor-positive breast cancer: updated findings from NCIC CTG MA.17. *J Natl Cancer Inst.* 2005;97(17):1262–1271.

86. Drug Interactions: Cytochrome P450 Drug Interaction Table. 2007 http://www.atforum.com/SiteRoot/pages/addiction_resources/P450%20Drug%20Interactions.PDF; accessed December 30, 2008.

87. Borges S, Desta Z, Li L, et al. Quantitative effect of CYP2D6 genotype and inhibitors on tamoxifen metabolism: implication for optimization of breast cancer treatment. *Clin Pharmacol Ther.* 2006;80(1):61–74.

88. Weiss RB, Valagussa P, Moliterni A, Zambetti M, Buzzoni R, Bonadonna G. Adjuvant chemotherapy after conservative surgery plus irradiation versus modified radical mastectomy. Analysis of drug dosing and toxicity. *Am J Med.* 1987;83(3):455–463.

89. Fisher B, Jeong JH, Anderson S, Wolmark N. Treatment of axillary lymph node-negative, estrogen receptor-negative breast cancer: updated findings from National Surgical Adjuvant Breast and Bowel Project clinical trials. *J Natl Cancer Inst.* 2004; 96(24):1823–1831.

90. Levine MN, Pritchard KI, Bramwell VH, Shepherd LE, Tu D, Paul N. Randomized trial comparing cyclophosphamide, epirubicin, and fluorouracil with cyclophosphamide, methotrexate, and fluorouracil in premenopausal women with node-positive breast cancer: update of National Cancer Institute of Canada Clinical Trials Group Trial MA5. *J Clin Oncol.* 2005;23(22):5166–5170.

91. Dang C, Fornier M, Sugarman S, et al. The safety of dose-dense doxorubicin and cyclophosphamide followed by paclitaxel with trastuzumab in HER-2/neu overexpressed/amplified breast cancer. *J Clin Oncol.* 2008;26(8):1216–1222.

92. Consortium on Breast Cancer Pharmacogenomics. *Drug Interactions with Tamoxifen. A Guide for Breast Cancer Patients and Physicians.* Indiana University School of Medicine; January 2008. Available at www.medicine.iupui.edu/clinpharm/COBRA/Tamoxifen%20and%202D6v7.pdf.

Multidisciplinary Approach in the Treatment of Locally Advanced Breast Cancer

Surgical Treatment of Locally Advanced Breast Cancer

BARBARA L. SMITH

Locally advanced breast cancer includes large primary tumors, bulky axillary node disease, inflammatory carcinoma, and tumors with direct skin involvement. Patients with supraclavicular and internal mammary node involvement are now considered to have local regional disease and are now classified as having locally advanced rather than metastatic disease.

In contrast to patients with metastatic disease, patients with locally advanced breast cancer are potentially curable. Surgery, radiation, and systemic therapies are all essential components of successful treatment of locally advanced breast cancer, and appropriate integration and sequencing of therapeutic modalities is essential.

■ INITIAL EVALUATION

The initial diagnosis for a locally advanced breast cancer should be obtained with core needle biopsy for histological diagnosis and determination of hormone receptor and HER2 status to guide systemic therapy choices. Incisional biopsy should be avoided whenever possible. Small skin biopsies may be obtained as needed if documentation of dermal lymphatic invasion is required.

Patients presenting with locally advanced breast cancer are at significant risk of harboring metastatic disease. A full staging workup to rule out the presence of metastatic disease is critical prior to initiation of treatment. Patients found to have metastatic disease should be referred for participation in metastatic disease protocols.

As part of the initial evaluation of a patient with locally advanced breast cancer, it is determined whether the patient is operable or inoperable. Those with inoperable disease include patients with inflammatory carcinoma, extensive skin involvement by tumor, fixed or very bulky axillary nodes, supraclavicular or internal mammary node disease, or ipsilateral arm edema. Patients with operable disease are those where all identifiable tumor may be removed in a standard lumpectomy or mastectomy and axillary dissection.

■ LOCALLY ADVANCED INOPERABLE TUMORS

For patients whose tumors are inoperable at presentation, systemic therapy is the first treatment modality administered. The decision to use systemic chemotherapy or endocrine therapy is based on features of the primary tumor as well as the patient's general medical condition and comorbidities.

When chemotherapy is used first, a complete standard course of chemotherapy is generally administered prior to consideration of surgery. Most initially inoperable patients will be converted to an operable category by therapy, and the subsequent decision for lumpectomy or mastectomy is made on the basis of the initial tumor presentation and extent of response. Breast conservation may be reasonable in patients who were initially considered inoperable on the basis of bulky lymph node disease or large primary tumors. However, some patients with extensive involvement of the breast by tumor may be better served by with mastectomy. A 2007 National Cancer Institute Conference concluded that "Patients with inflammatory breast cancer should not be considered for breast conservation therapy if they are being treated with curative intent" (1).

Occasionally, the initial systemic therapy administered will not convert the tumor to an operable state. Additional systemic therapy may be administered to try to obtain a more robust tumor response. In rare cases, radiation may be administered prior to consideration of surgery to try to produce sufficient tumor response to permit surgical resection. Such patients have increased risks of surgical complications, including prolonged seroma formation.

The radiological assessment recommended prior to consideration of breast conservation is discussed below.

■ LOCALLY ADVANCED OPERABLE BREAST CANCER

For patients whose tumors are operable at presentation, either surgery or systemic therapy may be considered as the initial treatment. Systemic therapy is often given first for patients whose tumors would currently require mastectomy but might become eligible for breast conservation with preoperative therapy. Use of systemic therapy first may also be considered for patients eligible for participation in neoadjuvant treatment protocols. Surgery may be considered first for patients unlikely to be converted to breast conservation or for whom complete pathological staging would be helpful for making systemic therapy decisions. A variety of patients and tumor factors are considered in making these decisions.

■ SELECTION OF INITIAL THERAPY IN OPERABLE PATIENTS: SYSTEMIC THERAPY OR SURGERY

As part of the initial evaluation of a patient with locally advanced breast cancer, thorough breast imaging is required to document the extent of disease and assess eligibility for breast conservation. Digital mammography, supplemented by ultrasound as necessary, is performed. Breast magnetic resonance imaging (MRI) has an increasing role in assessing extent of disease and may identify unsuspected ipsilateral or contralateral lesions in as many as 3% to 5% of newly diagnosed breast cancer patients overall (2,3) and in as many as 12% of women aged 40 or younger at diagnosis (4). MRI is also helpful in defining extent of disease in women with dense breast tissue and those with invasive lobular carcinoma (5,6).

It should be recognized that MRI, mammography and ultrasound, all have substantial rates of false positive findings, making accurate documentation of malignant and benign findings important before proceeding with mastectomy. Additional core needle biopsies are performed to document histological findings at any suspicious areas identified on imaging. Radioopaque marking clips should be placed at all biopsy sites to document tumor location and to guide surgical excision in case of a complete clinical and radiological response following preoperative therapy.

For patients whose tumors are likely to require mastectomy despite preoperative therapy, it may be preferable to proceed directly to mastectomy to obtain complete histological tumor staging, with systemic therapy then delivered in an adjuvant fashion. Patients with extensive calcifications suggesting extensive ductal carcinoma in situ (DCIS) are unlikely to be converted to breast conservation by preoperative chemotherapy as DCIS does not generally regress with chemotherapy. Patients with extensive invasive lobular carcinoma masses are also unlikely to have sufficient tumor shrinkage with preoperative therapy to allow lumpectomy. Patients found to have multiple separate tumor masses spanning more than one quadrant will not likely become eligible for breast conservation with preoperative therapy. Tumors with direct involvement of the nipple and areola skin at presentation will likely require nipple and areola resection, limiting the feasibility of breast conservation.

For patients where breast conservation remains a possibility, preoperative therapy to obtain tumor shrinkage may be preferable. Preoperative therapy should be considered for patients with a single large breast mass where moderate tumor shrinkage would allow breast conservation. Patients with superficial central tumors close to the nipple and areola, but not directly involving nipple or areola skin, may also benefit from tumor shrinkage with preoperative therapy to allow a more cosmetic lumpectomy.

■ ASSESSMENT OF TUMOR RESPONSE AFTER PREOPERATIVE THERAPY

At completion of systemic therapy, breast imaging studies should be repeated to document the extent of residual disease and assess the feasibility of breast conservation. Multiple localizing wires may prove helpful in guiding lumpectomy for large or eccentrically shaped lesions, and have been shown to reduce re-excision rates (7).

■ RESULTS OF BREAST CONSERVATION AFTER NEOADJUVANT THERAPY

Several studies have examined rates of breast conservation and rates of local recurrence in patients receiving preoperative systemic therapy. The National Surgical Adjuvant Breast and Bowel Project (NSABP) B-18 trial randomized 1,523 women with operable T1–3,N0–1 breast cancers to surgery followed by Adriamycin/Cytoxan chemotherapy versus Adriamycin/Cytoxan chemotherapy followed by surgery (8). A total of four cycles of chemotherapy were given to each group.

Although no survival advantage was seen with preoperative over postoperative systemic therapy, some advantages were seen with preoperative therapy. The majority of women receiving preoperative chemotherapy did show tumor shrinkage. Breast tumor size was reduced in 80% of patients after preoperative therapy, with 36% showing a clinical complete response with no residual palpable primary tumor mass. Clinical nodal response occurred in 89% of node-positive patients, with 73% showing a clinical complete response in their lymph nodes. There was a 37% increase in the incidence of pathologically negative nodes in the group receiving preoperative therapy. Overall, 12% more lumpectomies were performed in the preoperative chemotherapy group. In women with tumors larger than 5 cm, there was a 175% increase in successful lumpectomy in the preoperative chemotherapy group.

There was no significant difference in local recurrence rates after lumpectomy with preoperative or postoperative chemotherapy in the NSABP B-18 trial at a median follow-up of 9.5 years (10.7% in the preoperative chemotherapy group, 7.6% in the group receiving chemotherapy postoperatively, P = not significant) (9). When analyzed by initial tumor size, the difference in local recurrence rates after breast conservation became greater, with those patients who would have required mastectomy prior to chemotherapy showing a 15.7% local recurrence rate, compared with a 9.9% local recurrence rate in those whose tumors were eligible for breast conservation at presentation (P = 0.04). These findings may be the result of less thorough tumor excision following preoperative chemotherapy or, alternatively, more aggressive biological behavior of initially larger tumors (1).

Similar results were seen in the European Organisation for Research and Treatment of Cancer (EORTC) 10902 trial, which randomized 698 women with T1c–T4,N0–1 breast cancers to four cycles of fluorouracil, epirubicin, and cyclophosphamide (CEF) chemotherapy followed by surgery or to surgery followed by CEF chemotherapy (10). At 56 months' follow-up, there was no significant difference in overall survival, progression-free survival, or time to local-regional recurrence. There was a higher rate of breast conservation in patients who received preoperative chemotherapy.

A meta-analysis of 3,946 patients with breast cancer in nine randomized trials comparing neoadjuvant and adjuvant chemotherapy found no statistical or clinically significant difference between neoadjuvant therapy and adjuvant therapy with respect to overall survival, progression-free survival, or distant disease recurrence (11). However, neoadjuvant therapy was statistically significantly associated with an increased risk of locoregional disease recurrences [relative risk (RR) 1.22, 95% confidence interval (CI) 1.04 to 1.43] compared with adjuvant therapy, especially in trials where more patients in the neoadjuvant than the adjuvant arm received radiation therapy without surgery (RR 1.53, 95% CI 1.11 to 2.10). These results confirm the importance of surgical resection

of the primary tumor site prior to radiation, even in those patients who have a clinical complete response after preoperative therapy.

Chen and colleagues reported the MD Anderson Cancer Center experience with breast conservation after neoadjuvant chemotherapy in 340 patients (12). Surgery included gross excision of the residual primary tumor with a margin of normal tissue, with no attempt to excise the full preoperative tumor volume. Clear margins were obtained in all but 4% of cases, and whole breast radiation was administered.

At 60 months' follow-up, higher rates of ipsilateral breast and local-regional recurrence were seen in patients with clinical N2 or N3 nodal disease at diagnosis, residual tumor masses larger than 2 cm after neoadjuvant therapy, multifocal residual disease, or lymphovascular space invasion.

Patients with multifocal residual tumor, defined as noncontiguous tumor on histological examination or nests of tumor interspersed among fibrosis, necrosis, granulomas, and giant cells, had an increased risk of local recurrence after breast conservation compared with those with a single tumor mass. However, initial primary tumor size (T1–2 versus T3–4) did not impact ipsilateral breast recurrence rates (local control rate 96% versus 92%, respectively, P = 0.19).

Additional analysis led to the design of a prognostic index to better predict risk of ipsilateral breast tumor recurrence after neoadjuvant chemotherapy and breast conservation (13). These authors concluded that breast conservation therapy after neoadjuvant chemotherapy results in acceptably low rates of local recurrence in appropriately selected patients, even those initially presenting with T3 or T4 disease. Lumpectomy may be performed with excision to clear margins rather than excision of the initial tumor volume.

■ SENTINEL NODE BIOPSY IN LOCALLY ADVANCED BREAST CANCER

The best use and optimal timing of sentinel lymph node biopsy (SLNB) in the setting of neoadjuvant chemotherapy remains controversial. In clinically node-negative patients, an SLNB prior to neoadjuvant chemotherapy allows accurate and early nodal staging and provides information useful in selecting systemic therapy and radiation fields. Rates of sentinel node identification may be higher before preoperative chemotherapy, and false negative rates may be lower.

SLNB after preoperative therapy allows axillary staging to be performed at the time of definitive surgery, without the need for a separate surgical procedure. In addition, a significant number of clinically node-positive patients may become node-negative following chemotherapy (14,15), and SLNB following chemotherapy may allow such patients to avoid complete axillary dissection. For those who consider the axillary node status following preoperative chemotherapy to be a key indicator of prognosis, SLNB after preoperative therapy is favored.

A number of authors have addressed these issues. Jones and colleagues (16) compared SLNB before and after neoadjuvant chemotherapy. The sentinel node mapping rate prior to chemotherapy was 100% among 52 clinically node-negative patients with a mean tumor size of 4 cm, and only 81% in 36 patients who underwent mapping after neoadjuvant therapy. Failure to map following chemotherapy correlated with clinically positive nodes at presentation and residual disease at axillary lymph node dissection. Among patients who mapped successfully, the false negative rate was 11%.

Breslin and colleagues (17) reported results of SLNB following preoperative therapy in 51 stage 2 to 3 breast cancer patients. Overall, 84% of patients had successful mapping, with mapping success increasing with time and surgeon experience over the duration of the study. The false negative rate was 14%.

The NSABP B-27 study provided the largest cohort of patients undergoing SLNB following preoperative chemotherapy (18). SLNB was attempted before the required axillary dissection in 428 patients who had received preoperative chemotherapy. The success rate for identification and removal of a sentinel lymph node was 84.8%. Among 218 patients with negative sentinel lymph nodes, the false-negative rate was 10.7%. The false-negative rate did not appear to be influenced by patient or tumor characteristics, method of lymphatic mapping, or breast tumor response to chemotherapy. These results were felt to be comparable to those obtained from multicenter studies evaluating SLNB before systemic therapy. The authors concluded that the sentinel lymph node approach is applicable following neoadjuvant chemotherapy.

Newman and colleagues (15) reported a 98% rate of sentinel lumph node identification in 54 patients with biopsy-confirmed positive nodes prior to neoadjuvant chemotherapy, with a false-negative rate of 8.6%. Of 54 patients, 17 (32%) were converted to node-negative following chemotherapy and were correctly identified as such by SLNB.

Classe and colleagues (19) reported results of SLNB after preoperative chemotherapy in 195 patients with advanced, large operable breast cancers. The SLNB detection rate was 90%, and the false-negative rate was 11.5%. Patients without palpable axillary nodes (N0) before neoadjuvant chemotherapy had a better detection rate than patients with suspicious N1 axillary nodes (N0 94.6% versus N1 81.5%, $P = 0.008$). The false-negative rate was not correlated with clinical nodal status before preoperative chemotherapy (9.4% versus 15%, $P = 0.66$).

A recent National Cancer Institute Conference reviewing locoregional treatments after preoperative chemotherapy for breast cancer concluded that SLNB can be performed either before or after preoperative chemotherapy for patients with clinically negative axillary nodes (1). It may be advantageous to perform SLNB prior to neoadjuvant chemotherapy for clinically node-negative patients with earlier-stage disease, where systemic therapy and radiation decisions may be influenced by initial nodal status. SLNB after neoadjuvant therapy may be preferable for patients whose systemic and radiation therapy decisions have been made, to avoid an additional surgical procedure, and where downstaging of nodal disease by systemic therapy may eliminate the need for complete axillary dissection.

It has been suggested that SLNB is not appropriate for patients with inflammatory breast carcinoma owing to low mapping success rates and the overall high risk of axillary node involvement (20).

■ AXILLARY DISSECTION

A standard level 1 and 2 axillary dissection is performed in patients with locally advanced breast cancers who present with palpable nodes or positive sentinel nodes at the time of definitive surgery. A level 3 dissection is performed only when palpable nodes are present in level 3. Patients with extensive axillary node disease will usually receive radiation to the supraclavicular nodes and often to the axilla as well. Placement of MRI-compatible radio-opaque clips at the highest point of the surgical dissection may be helpful to delineate dissected versus nondissected areas for subsequent radiation planning.

■ INTERNAL MAMMARY NODE ISSUES

Clinically evident recurrence in the internal mammary nodes is rare (21–25) but has been associated with a poor prognosis (26). In the past, internal mammary node involvement was considered stage 4 metastatic disease. Early studies assessing the value of extended radical mastectomy with removal of the internal mammary nodes found that routine excision of internal mammary nodes did not improve survival or reduce locoregional relapse. Veronesi and Valagussa reported results of 716 evaluable patients randomized to radical mastectomy or radical mastectomy with internal mammary node dissection (27). None received systemic therapy or radiation. Internal mammary node involvement was seen in 20.5% of patients who had internal mammary node dissection (24.6% in cases with tumor in medial or central quadrants and 17.7% in cases with tumor in lateral quadrants). However, at 10 years' follow-up, only 3.7% of patients with standard radical mastectomy developed parasternal tumor recurrences, suggesting that the majority of internal mammary node metastases did not produce clinically significant recurrences even in the absence of adjuvant systemic therapy or radiation. At 30 years' follow-up of this series, overall and disease-specific survival was not improved by internal mammary node dissection (28).

The role of internal mammary node evaluation and treatment has been revisited with new anatomical data derived from sentinel node mapping and other anatomical studies (29). Sentinel node mapping techniques have demonstrated that the internal mammary or other regional nodes outside the axilla may be the primary drainage site for a number of breast cancers. Krag and colleagues used technetium-99m sulfur colloid for sentinel node mapping and found sentinel nodes outside the axilla in 8% of patients, with a positive sentinel node outside the axilla in 3% (30). More than half the extra-axillary sentinel nodes were in the internal mammary chain.

American Joint Committee on Cancer staging now recognizes internal mammary and supraclavicular node involvement as local-regional disease rather than distant metastases (31). Meta-analysis suggesting that local-regional failure is associated with decreased breast cancer survival (32) has prompted a review of internal mammary node issues. Principles for management of axillary node disease are increasingly being applied to internal mammary node disease.

Approximately 20% of internal mammary sentinel nodes show metastases when excised (33), and in 3% to 10% the internal mammary sentinel nodes are positive and the axillary nodes negative (26,30,34). The feasibility of internal mammary SLNB has been reported by a number of authors (26,30,34,35), but concerns remain about potential morbidity, the lack of evidence supporting improved survival with preemptive internal mammary node treatment, and the low observed rate of internal mammary node recurrence with current standard local and systemic therapies.

There are no modern data on resection of grossly involved isolated internal mammary and supraclavicular nodes prior to regional nodal irradiation, although extrapolation from axillary node data might suggest that this would be beneficial if it is possible to perform internal mammary node resection with minimal morbidity.

The impact of internal mammary node irradiation has also been addressed, although results to date do not clarify the importance of local therapy for internal mammary node involvement. Most series find no survival benefit from internal mammary node irradiation (36–39). However, it has been suggested that select groups of patients, such as those with medial or central tumors and positive axillary nodes, might benefit from preemptive treatment of the internal mammary nodes. The Institut Gustave-Roussy series of 1,195 patients treated for breast cancer found that internal mammary node irradiation was associated with a reduction in the risk of distant metastasis for patients with medial or central primary tumors and positive axillary lymph nodes (38,40). Two studies are under way to address this issue in a modern patient cohort. An ongoing EORTC trial randomizes patients with positive axillary nodes and node negative patients with high-risk, medially and centrally located tumors to treatment with or without internal mammary node and supraclavicular irradiation (41), and a Canadian trial randomizes axillary node–positive patients to breast irradiation with or without ipsilateral supraclavicular, axillary, and internal mammary node irradiation (42).

■ MASTECTOMY TECHNIQUES

Modified radical mastectomy or simple mastectomy with SLNB is performed when mastectomy is required in patients with locally advanced breast cancer. Radical and extended radical mastectomy procedures have been abandoned as they increase morbidity without improving survival. However, a portion of the pectoralis muscle may be resected during simple or modified radical mastectomy to obtain clear margins when tumor directly involves muscle. Surgical clips should be placed to mark areas of muscle resection or other close margins to allow identification of these sites during radiation planning. If delayed breast reconstruction is a possibility, use of a diagonal incision that places the medial aspect of the mastectomy incision near the inframammary fold at the sternal border is more favorable than a horizontal incision higher on the chest wall.

■ BREAST RECONSTRUCTION IN PATIENTS WITH LOCALLY ADVANCED BREAST CANCER

The safety of immediate breast reconstruction is well established for patients with early-stage breast cancer (43–45), with no increase in local recurrence and no decrement in survival associated with the treatment delays associated with immediate reconstruction. However, patients undergoing mastectomy for locally advanced breast cancer nearly always require additional postoperative systemic therapy and postmastectomy radiation. Unlike patients with early-stage disease, for whom immediate reconstruction is routine, locally advanced patients have high rates of both local and systemic recurrence. There is concern that recurrence risks for locally advanced patients would be increased by delays in the delivery of radiation and systemic therapy associated with scheduling and recuperating from a reconstruction, or from complications of reconstructive surgery. As a result, delayed reconstruction is usually the preferred approach for women who require mastectomy for locally advanced breast cancers.

Immediate reconstruction may be considered for selected patients with locally advanced breast cancer. A rare patient may require a vascularized tissue flap for closure of the mastectomy defect in cases where extensive skin resection is required or after mastectomy in heavily irradiated tissue. Very thin patients who do not have sufficient donor-site tissue to allow delayed autologous tissue reconstruction may have no viable delayed reconstruction options. Such thin patients may be considered for immediate tissue expander reconstruction to maximize preservation of chest wall skin and allow a delayed implant reconstruction. For other patients with locally advanced breast cancer, the advantages of immediate reconstruction must be weighed against potential treatment delays and negative effects associated with radiation of the reconstruction.

Multidisciplinary input is essential in making decisions about the feasibility and timing of breast reconstruction for patients undergoing treatment for locally advanced breast cancer. The breast surgeon and plastic surgeon should discuss systemic therapy and radiation issues with medical oncology and radiation oncology colleagues prior to any definitive surgical procedures. Challenges for the plastic surgeon and radiation oncologist associated with postmastectomy radiation and reconstruction are discussed in more detail in Chapter 9.

■ MULTIDISCIPLINARY CONSIDERATIONS

- Surgery, radiation, and systemic therapy are all essential components of successful treatment of locally advanced breast cancer, and collaborative integration and sequencing of therapeutic modalities is essential.
- SLNB may be performed before or after neoadjuvant systemic therapy, with timing based on individual patient and treatment factors.
- Lumpectomy after neoadjuvant systemic therapy may be performed with excision to clear margins rather than excision of the initial tumor volume.
- Intraoperative placement of radioopaque marking clips at the apex of the axillary dissection, at sites of muscle resection, at close margins, and at other key locations will facilitate radiation planning for locally advanced breast cancers.
- Delayed breast reconstruction is the preferred approach for locally advanced breast cancers, although immediate reconstruction may be considered in selected patients.

■ REFERENCES

1. Buchholz TA, Lehman CD, Harris JR, et al. Statement of the science concerning locoregional treatments after preoperative chemotherapy for breast cancer: a National Cancer Institute Conference. *J Clin Oncol.* 2008;26:791–797.
2. Lehman CD, Gatsonis C, Kuhl CK, et al. MRI evaluation of the contralateral breast in women with recently diagnosed breast cancer. *New Eng J Med.* 2007;356:1295–1303.
3. Liberman L, Morris EA, Kim CM, et al. MR imaging findings in the contralateral breast of women with recently diagnosed breast cancer. *AJR Am J Roentgenol.* 2003;180:333–341.
4. Samphao S, Wheeler AJ, Rafferty E. Diagnosis of breast cancer in women age 40 and younger: delays in diagnosis result from underutilization of genetic testing and breast imaging. *Am J Surg.* In press.
5. Bedrosian I, Mick R, Orel SG, et al. Changes in the surgical management of patients with breast carcinoma based on preoperative magnetic resonance imaging. *Cancer.* 2003;98:468–473.
6. Quan ML, Sclafani L, Heerdt AS, Fey JV, Morris EA, Borgen PI. Magnetic Resonance imaging detects unsuspected disease in patients with invasive lobular cancer. *Ann Surg Oncol.* 2003;10:1048–1053.
7. Kirstein L, Rafferty E, Moore R, Specht MC, Hughes KS, Smith BL. Outcome of multiple wire localization for larger breast cancers: when can mastectomy be avoided? *J Am Coll Surg.* 2008; 207:342–346.
8. Fisher B, Brown A, Mamounas E, et al. Effect of preoperative chemotherapy on local-regional disease in women with operable breast cancer: findings from National Surgical Adjuvant Breast and Bowell Project B-18. *J Clin Oncol.* 1997;15:2483–2493.
9. Wolmark N, Wang J, Mamounas E, et al. Preoperative chemotherapy in patients with operable breast cancer: nine-year results from National Surgical Adjuvant Breast and Bowel Project B-18. *Cancer.* 2001;30:96–102.
10. van der Hage JA, Cornelis JH, van de Velde CJ, et al. Preoperative chemotherapy in primary operable breast cancer: results from the European Organization for Research and Treatment of Cancer trial 10902. *J Clin Oncol.* 2001;19:4224–4237.
11. Mauri D, Pavlidis N, Ioannidis JP. Neoadjuvant versus adjuvant systemic treatment in breast cancer: a meta-analysis. *J Natl Cancer Inst.* 2005;97:188–194.
12. Chen AM, Meric-Bernstam F, Hunt KK, et al. Breast-conserving therapy after neoadjuvant chemotherapy: the M. D. Anderson Cancer Center experience. *J Clin Oncol.* 2004;22:2303–2312.
13. Huang EH, Strom EA, Perkins GH, et al. Comparison of risk of local-regional recurrence after mastectomy or breast conservation therapy for patients treated with neoadjuvant chemotherapy and radiation stratified according to a prognostic index score. *Int J Radiat Oncol Biol Phys.* 2006;66:352–357.
14. Kuerer HM, Sahin AA, Hunt KK, et al. Incidence and impact of documented eradication of breast cancer axillary lymph node metastases before surgery in patients treated with neoadjuvant chemotherapy. *Ann Surg.* 1999;230:72–78.
15. Newman EA, Sabel MS, Nees AV, et al. Sentinel lymph node biopsy performed after neoadjuvant chemotherapy is accurate in patients with documented node-positive breast cancer at presentation. *Ann Surg Oncol.* 2007;14:2946–2952.
16. Jones JL, Zabicki, K, Christian RL, et al. A comparison of sentinel node biopsy before and after neoadjuvant chemotherapy: timing is important. *Am J Surg.*2005;190:517–520.
17. Breslin TM, Cohen L, Sahin A, et al. Sentinel lymph node biopsy is accurate after neoadjuvant chemotherapy for breast cancer. *J Clin Oncol.* 2000;20:3480–3486.
18. Mamounas EP, Brown A, Anderson S, et al. Sentinel node biopsy after neoadjuvant chemotherapy in breast cancer: results from National Surgical Adjuvant Breast and Bowel Project Protocol B-27. *J Clin Oncol.* 2005; 23:2694–2702.

19. Classe J-M, Bordes V, Campion L, et al. Sentinel lymph node biopsy after neoadjuvant chemotherapy for advanced breast cancer: results of ganglion sentinelle et chimiothérapie neoadjuvante, a French prospective multicentric study. *J Clin Oncol*. 2009; 27:726–732.

20. Sterns V, Ewing CA, Slack R, et al. Sentinel lymph node biopsy after neoadjuvant chemotherapy for breast cancer may reliably represent the axilla except for inflammatory breast cancer. *Ann Surg Oncol*. 2002;9:235–242.

21. Katz A, Strom EA, Buchholz TA, et al. Locoregional recurrence patterns after mastectomy and doxorubicin-based chemotherapy: implications for postoperative irradiation. *J Clin Oncol*. 2000; 18(15):2817–2827.

22. Recht A, Gray R, Davidson NE, et al. Locoregional failure 10 years after mastectomy and adjuvant chemotherapy with or without tamoxifen without irradiation: experience of the Eastern Cooperative Oncology Group. *J Clin Oncol*. 1999; 17(6):1689–1700.

23. Strom EA, Woodward WA, Katz A, et al. Clinical investigation: regional nodal failure patterns in breast cancer patients treated with mastectomy without radiotherapy. *Int J Radiat Oncol Biol Phys*. 2005;63(5):1508–1513.

24. Schwaibold F, Fowble BL, Solin LJ, Schultz DJ, Goodman RL. The results of radiation therapy for isolated local regional recurrence after mastectomy. *Int J Radiat Oncol Biol Phys*. 1991; 21(2):299–310.

25. Halverson KJ, Taylor ME, Perez CA, et al. Regional nodal management and patterns of failure following conservative surgery and radiation therapy for stage I and II breast cancer. *Int J Radiat Oncol Biol Phys*. 1993;26:709–710.

26. Morrow M, Foster RS. Staging of breast cancer. A new rationale for internal mammary node biopsy. *Arch Surg*. 1981;116:748–751.

27. Veronesi U, Valagussa P. Inefficacy of internal mammary nodes dissection in breast cancer surgery. *CA Cancer J Clin*. 1981;47:170–175.

28. Veronesi U, Marubini E, Mariani L, Valagussa P, Zucali R. The dissection of internal mammary nodes does not improve the survival of breast cancer patients. 30-year results of a randomised trial. *Eur J Cancer*. 1999;35:1320–1325.

29. Suami H, Pan W-R, Mann GB, Taylor GI. The lymphatic anatomy of the breast and its implications for sentinel lymph node biopsy: a human cadaver study. *Ann Surg Oncol*. 2008;15:863–871.

30. Krag D, Weaver D, Ashikaga A, et al. The sentinel node in breast cancer—a multicenter validation study. *New Engl J Med*. 1998;339:941–946.

31. Singletary SE, Allred C, Ashley P, et al. Revision of the American Joint Committee on Cancer Staging System for breast cancer. *J Clin Oncol*. 2002;20:3628–3636.

32. Early Breast Cancer Trialists' Collaborative Group. Effects of radiotherapy and of differences in the extent of surgery for early breast cancer on local recurrence and 15-year survival: an overview of the randomised trials. *Lancet*. 2005;366:2087–2106.

33. Chen RC, Lin NU, Golshan M, Harris JR, Bellon JR. Internal mammary nodes in breast cancer: diagnosis and implications for patient management—a systematic review. *J Clin Oncol*. 2008;26:4981–4989.

34. van der Ent FWC, Kengen RAM, van der Pol HAG, et al. Halsted revisited: internal mammary sentinel lymph node biopsy in breast cancer. *Ann Surg*. 2001;234:79–84.

35. Dupont, E, Cox CE, Nguyen K, et al. Utility of internal mammary lymph node removal when noted by intraoperative gamma probe detection. *Ann Surg Oncol*. 2001;8:833–836.

36. Fowble B, Hanlon A, Freedman G, et al. Internal mammary node irradiation neither decreases distant metastases nor improves survival in stage I and II breast cancer. *Int J Radiat Oncol Biol Phys*. 2000;47:883–894.

37. Obedian E, Haffty BG. Internal mammary nodal irradiation in conservatively-managed breast cancer patients: is there a benefit? *Int J Radiat Oncol Biol Phys*. 1999;44:997–1003.

38. Arriagada R, Le MG, Mouriesse H, et al. Long-term effect of internal mammary chain treatment: results of a multivariate analysis of 1195 patients with operable breast cancer and positive axillary nodes. *Radiother Oncol*. 1988;11:213–222.

39. Stemmer SM, Rizel S, Hardan I, et al. The role of irradiation of the internal mammary lymph nodes in high-risk stage II to IIIA breast cancer patients after high-dose chemotherapy: a prospective sequential nonrandomized study. *J Clin Oncol*. 2003; 21:2713–2718.

40. Arriagada R, Rutqvist LE, Mattsson A, Kramar A, Rotstein S. Adequate locoregional treatment for early breast cancer may prevent secondary dissemination. *J Clin Oncol*. 1995;13(12): 2869–2878.

41. Phase III randomized trial investigating the role of internal mammary and medial supraclavicular (IM-MS) lymph node chain irradiation in stage I–III breast cancer (joint study of the EORTC Radiotherapy Cooperative Group and the EORTC Breast Cancer Cooperative Group). EORTC Study No. 10925/22922 Available at http://journalscambridgeorg/downloadphp?file=%2FBCO%2FBCO9_S1%2FS147090310600 9126apdf&code=ff6fdd98cb2f5726417e3dfa463249ff

42. A phase III study of regional radiation therapy in early breast cancer. NCIC CTG trial MA.20. Available at http://journals.cambridge.org/download.php?file=%2FBCO%2FBCO9_S1%2FS1470903106009308a.pdf&code=6dd5cf7a40e57b2a9a01ec5fab104dcd

43. Carlson GW, Bostwick J III, Styblo TM, et al. Skin-sparing mastectomy. Oncologic and reconstructive considerations. *Ann Surg*. 1997;225:570–575.

44. Cunnick GH, Mokbel K. Skin-sparing mastectomy. *Am J Surg*. 2004;188:78–84.

45. Greenway RM, Schlossberg L, Dooley WC. Fifteen-year series of skin-sparing mastectomy for stage 0 to 2 breast cancer. *Am J Surg*. 190: 918–922.

Radiation Treatment of Locally Advanced Breast Cancer

MOHAMED A. ALM EL-DIN

ALPHONSE G. TAGHIAN

Locally advanced breast cancer (LABC) generally is defined by bulky primary breast tumors (larger than 5 cm) or extensive adenopathy (1). It also includes tumors with direct involvement of the underlying chest wall or skin with edema (including peau d'orange), tumors considered inoperable but without distant metastasis (including involvement of the supraclavicular lymph nodes), and skin ulceration or satellitosis confined to the same breast (2), as well as inflammatory breast cancer (IBC). Other discrete skin changes, such as dimpling or nipple retraction, may occur in T1–3 disease; they do not constitute evidence of a locally advanced tumor. In the TNM staging classification, LABC is represented by stage 3A (T0–N2; T1/2–N2; T3–N1/2), 3B (T4, N0–2), and 3C disease (any T, N3) (3) and a subset of stage 2B (T3–N0). IBC represents a T4d primary tumor designation and, therefore, stage 3B disease. Recent studies demonstrate that prolonged survival can be achieved in patients with metastatic disease limited to the supraclavicular nodes after appropriate multimodality breast cancer treatment (4,5). Consequently, isolated supraclavicular metastasis is included in the stage 3/LABC disease category (6).

The management of patients with LABC is complex because most of the treatment guidelines are derived from phase II studies or retrospective reviews of single-institution experience rather than controlled randomized trials, although there are some exceptions (7–11). A multidisciplinary approach employing combinations of systemic and locoregional therapy had been developed as the treatment of choice by the 1980s (8,10,12–14). The sequence of combined modality treatment can be different from one patient to another, depending on disease characteristics. In general, patients with operable disease usually undergo surgery first (mostly mastectomy), whereas those with advanced/inoperable disease should receive preoperative systemic therapy to allow for mastectomy or even breast-conserving surgery in patients with good response to systemic treatment.

It is important to distinguish between two groups of patients: those with noninflammatory LABC and those with IBC. Although treatment guidelines are generally the same for both groups, there are some exceptions. Breast conservation therapy is considered inappropriate for IBC, as is sentinel lymph node biopsy (15).

■ MANAGEMENT OF NONINFLAMMATORY LABC

Operable LABC

By definition, patients with operable LABC are not good candidates for breast-conserving surgery; therefore, mastectomy and sentinel lymph node biopsy with or without axillary dissection would be the treatment of choice for these patients. The exception would be the patient desirous to keep her breast; here, preoperative chemotherapy is indicated in an attempt to downstage the tumor to allow for breast conservation. Breast-conserving surgery following neoadjuvant chemotherapy for LABC is discussed later in this chapter. The results of surgical pathology after mastectomy will identify patients at high risk of disease failure who would benefit from adjuvant therapy. Generally, almost all women with positive axillary lymph nodes and/or tumor size larger than 1 cm will receive adjuvant systemic therapy, with combination chemotherapy, hormone therapy, or both. The details of postmastectomy radiotherapy (PMRT) are discussed in this chapter.

Risk Factors for Locoregional Recurrence

Clinical and pathological factors predicting high risk (i.e., greater than 20%), moderate risk (10% to 20%), and low risk (less than 10%) for locoregional failure are used to categorize the potential locoregional benefit from comprehensive PMRT. The number of positive nodes and the size of the primary tumor have been considered consistent independent risk factors for locoregional recurrence. Several studies have documented higher rates of locoregional failure in patients with greater numbers of involved axillary nodes (16–26). For example, in a report from the MD Anderson Cancer Center, 10-year actuarial rates of isolated locoregional failure and locoregional failure as a component of relapse, for patients who underwent mastectomy, doxorubicin-based chemotherapy, and no radiation, were 10% and 14% for one to three involved nodes, 21% and 25% for four to nine nodes, and 22% and 34% for 10 or more nodes, respectively (17).

Tumor size is one of the most powerful predictors of breast tumor behavior (27), reported by several studies as an independent risk factor for postmastectomy locoregional failure (18,19,28). In the report from the Eastern Cooperative Oncology Group (ECOG), the 10-year risk of locoregional failure in women with T3 versus T1–2 lesions was significantly higher in patients with one to three positive nodes (31% versus 12%) and for those with four to seven positive nodes (45% versus 20%) (18). In addition, the extent of axillary dissection as measured by the number of nodes in the pathological specimen has been shown to affect the cumulative rate of locoregional failure. Among women with one to three positive nodes, the rate of axillary failure was significantly higher when only two to five nodes were examined, compared with six to 10 and 11 or more nodes. In patients with more than four positive nodes, the risk of supraclavicular failure was greater when only four to five nodes were examined, compared with six to 10 and 11 or more nodes. The authors concluded that larger tumor size, higher number of involved nodes, negative estrogen receptors, and fewer nodes examined were predictive for a higher locoregional recurrence rate, with or without simultaneous distant failure.

In a recursive partitioning analysis of 1,031 women treated with mastectomy without radiotherapy, the 8-year locoregional recurrence for women with tumors larger than 3.5 cm and metastatic involvement of more than 20% of the removed nodes was 41%, compared with 10% in those with tumors smaller than 5 cm and less than 20% involved nodes (29). Therefore, combined use of tumor size and number of involved nodes may give a better estimate of the likelihood of locoregional recurrence. Other factors that may predict for locoregional recurrence include young age at diagnosis, the presence of lymphovascular invasion (LVI), positive deep margin status, and microscopic extracapsular extension (16,17,28–31). It should be noted that when the number of involved axillary nodes was taken into account, extracapsular extension was not solely associated with a higher rate of axillary failure (31,32).

Impact of Systemic Therapy on Locoregional Control

The reduction in risk of locoregional failure as an effect of systemic therapy has been controversial. Some studies document a reduction in the risk with chemotherapy and tamoxifen (33–37), whereas others show no effect of systemic treatment on local control (38,39). Some authors have reported that the absolute rates of isolated locoregional failure remained 15% or higher in most node-positive series, depending upon the baseline estimate of risk, regardless of the risk reduction induced by systemic therapy (32,40).

In the most recent meta-analysis from the Early Breast Cancer Trialists' Collaborative Group (EBCTCG), polychemotherapy reduced the local recurrence rate, irrespective of hormone receptor status, by about one third (ratios 0.63 and 0.70 for women aged below 50 and aged 50 to 69, respectively), whereas 5 years of tamoxifen reduced the local recurrence rate by about one half in women with hormone receptor–positive disease (local recurrence ratio 0.47) (36). Nevertheless, a later report from the EBCTCG showed a similar reduction in the incidence

of locoregional failure from chest wall radiotherapy in patients who received adjuvant systemic therapy compared with those who did not (41). Furthermore, several studies suggest that dose-dense regimens and newer systemic agents do not significantly reduce the risk of locoregional failure beyond that achieved with standard chemotherapy (42–45). In the Cancer and Leukemia Group B 9433 trial, locoregional control was significantly better with the addition of paclitaxel to anthracycline and cyclophosphamide following breast conservation, whereas the reduction in locoregional recurrence rate was not statistically significant for mastectomy patients who received additional paclitaxel (44). Radiotherapy was required if breast-conserving surgery was performed but was elective after mastectomy. Retrospective analyses demonstrate locoregional failure rates of approximately 33% to 40% in the absence of radiotherapy despite administration of high-dose chemotherapy with peripheral stem-cell support (17,46). Collectively, these studies suggest that while systemic therapy can reduce rates of locoregional failure, considerable risk for recurrence persists, particularly in high-risk patients, further reinforcing the potential role of PMRT in these patients.

PMRT: Rationale

The goal of PMRT is to eradicate subclinical disease within the chest wall and the peripheral lymphatics for high-risk patients. This could potentially be translated into a decrease in the rate of locoregional recurrence and an increase in long-term disease-free and overall survival. A recent review of seven key early trials conducted in the United Kingdom, the United States, Norway, and Sweden evaluating PMRT in the absence of adjuvant chemotherapy showed a threefold decrease in locoregional recurrence (47).

Prevention of locoregional failure has a potential role in oncology management, as, on average, only approximately 50% of locoregional recurrences can be subsequently controlled (48). In addition, there is substantial evidence that optimal locoregional control results in meaningful survival gains, as women who develop local recurrence have shown a higher rate of distant metastases, and most of these women will die of their cancer (47). Some of the most important data linking better local control to enhanced survival come from the EBCTCG overview analyses (41).

PMRT: Indications

Four or More Positive Axillary Nodes. The results of the Danish and Canadian trials suggest that both premenopausal and postmenopausal women with node-positive operable breast cancer may benefit from radiotherapy following mastectomy in terms of both breast cancer–specific and overall survival (22–24). Therefore, many major groups, including the American Society for Therapeutic Radiology and Oncology (ASTRO), the American Society of Clinical Oncology (ASCO), the National Comprehensive Cancer Network (NCCN), and the Canadian Practice Guidelines, recommend the routine use of PMRT for all premenopausal and postmenopausal women with four or more positive nodes (49–53). The treatment field should include the chest wall and supraclavicular and infraclavicular regions, with or without internal mammary nodes.

The first Danish Breast Cancer Cooperative Group trial included 1,708 women who had undergone mastectomy for pathological stage 2 or 3 breast cancer who were randomly assigned to receive eight cycles of cyclophosphamide, methotrexate, and fluorouracil (CMF) plus irradiation of the chest wall and regional lymph nodes (852 women) or nine cycles of CMF alone (856 women) (22). With a median follow-up of just under 10 years, PMRT was associated with a significant reduction in locoregional failure (32% versus 9%) and significantly improved disease-free survival (48% versus 34%) as well as overall survival (54% versus 45%). The improvement in disease-free survival and overall survival associated with radiotherapy was independent of tumor size, number of positive nodes, or histopathological grade.

The low number of dissected axillary lymph nodes (median of seven) was a major concern in the Danish trial. This issue was underscored with the observations that 44% of the locoregional recurrences in the CMF-alone arm were in axillary lymph nodes (54). This rate of axillary failure is higher than that expected with level 1 or 2 axillary dissection (55), raising the possibility of disease left behind in the axilla in many women following axillary sampling. Thus the improved survival rates might be attributed to treatment of such residual axillary disease by both radiotherapy and chemotherapy as compared with chemotherapy alone.

The benefit of PMRT among postmenopausal women at high risk for locoregional recurrence was examined in a second Danish trial (23). Between 1982 and 1990, postmenopausal women with stage 2 or 3 breast cancer were randomly assigned to adjuvant tamoxifen (30 mg daily for 1 year) alone (689 patients) or with postoperative radiotherapy to the chest wall and regional lymph nodes (686 patients). The use of radiotherapy was associated with a decreased risk of locoregional recurrence (8% versus 35%, $P < 0.001$) and a significant improvement in 10-year disease-free survival (36% versus 24%, $P < 0.001$) and overall survival (45% versus 36%, $P = 0.03$) in high-risk postmenopausal breast cancer patients after mastectomy and limited axillary dissection. The benefit from PMRT was similar in patients with one to three positive axillary nodes (58% of the study population) and those with four or more positive axillary nodes.

A long-term follow-up was performed among the 3,083 patients from the Danish Breast Cancer Cooperative Group 82b and c trials, except in those already recorded with distant metastases or contralateral breast cancer (56). Radiotherapy was associated with significantly lower 18-year probability of any first breast cancer event (59% versus 73%, $P < 0.001$) and locoregional failure (14% versus 49%, $P < 0.001$). In addition, the 18-year probability of distant metastasis subsequent to locoregional recurrence was 35% with no radiotherapy arm compared with 6% in the radiotherapy arm ($P < 0.001$), whereas the probability of any distant metastasis was 64% and 53% ($P < 0.001$) after no radiotherapy and radiotherapy, respectively.

In the British Columbia trial, from 1978 through 1986, 318 premenopausal women with node-positive breast cancer were randomly assigned, after modified radical mastectomy, to receive chemotherapy plus radiotherapy or chemotherapy alone (24). Radiotherapy was given to the chest wall and locoregional lymph nodes, including the internal mammary nodes, between the fourth and fifth cycles of CMF. At median follow-up of 15 years, PMRT was associated with a 33% reduction in the rate of recurrence and a 29% reduction in mortality from breast cancer. As reported in the Danish trial, the beneficial effects of radiotherapy were noted in women with one to three positive lymph nodes, as well as in those with four or more positive nodes. The median number of dissected axillary lymph nodes was higher than in the Danish trial (11 versus 7, respectively). Nevertheless, among the no radiotherapy group, the rates of locoregional recurrence-free survival at 5, 10, and 15 years (79%, 75%, and 67%, respectively) were higher than expected and were also higher than the corresponding rates in the radiotherapy group (90%, 87%, and 87%, respectively). There was a trend toward improved survival associated with radiotherapy in the 15-year follow-up (54% versus 46%). The update at a median follow-up of 20 years demonstrated a significant survival benefit in favor of PMRT (overall survival 47% versus 37%, hazard ratio 0.73, 95% confidence interval 0.55 to 0.98) (57). The significant improvement with radiotherapy plus chemotherapy compared with chemotherapy alone was confirmed in all other end points, including survival free of isolated locoregional recurrences (74% versus 90%, respectively, $P = 0.002$), systemic relapse-free survival (31% versus 48%, $P = 0.004$), breast cancer–free survival (48% versus 30%, $P = 0.001$), event-free survival (35% versus 25%, $P = 0.009$), and breast cancer–specific survival (53% versus 38%, $P = 0.008$). The absolute improvement in overall survival associated with radiotherapy was 14% (31% versus 17%) in patients with four or more positive nodes and 7% (57% versus 50%) in those with one to three positive nodes.

Positive Deep Margins. In one series, the pathological reports from 789 patients treated by mastectomy between

1985 and 1994 were retrospectively reviewed (58). The study population consists of 34 patients with close or positive margins whose primary tumor size was less than 5 cm, who had zero to three positive axillary nodes, and who received no postoperative radiation. Premenopausal women with a close or positive margin were shown to be at high risk of chest wall recurrence (28% at 8 years), regardless of the use of adjuvant systemic therapy, and therefore should be considered for PMRT. In another study of 94 patients with a positive surgical margin after mastectomy, trends for higher cumulative locoregional relapse rates (LRRs) without PMRT were identified in the presence of age under 50 years (LRR 20% without versus 0% with PMRT), T2 tumor size (19.2% versus 6.9%), grade 3 disease (23.1% versus 6.7%), and LVI (16.7% versus 9.1%) (59). The authors suggested that, for selected patients with node-negative breast cancer, improvements in locoregional control with radiotherapy could justify the judicious, but not routine, use of PMRT for positive margins after mastectomy.

PMRT: One to Three Positive Axillary Lymph Nodes

There is far less agreement on the benefit of PMRT in patients with one to three positive nodes. Nevertheless, most of the guidelines were based on data prior to subset analyses from the Danish and British Columbia trials, which specifically looked at the subset with one to three positive nodes. Both the British Columbia trial and a subgroup analysis of the Danish trials demonstrated similar survival benefit after PMRT in patients with one to three and four or more positive lymph nodes, underscoring the benefit of radiotherapy for all node-positive subsets (57,60). Due to concerns regarding the inadequate axillary dissection among the last-mentioned studies, particularly the Danish trials, PMRT for one to three positive node breast cancer patients is not a routine practice in several institutions in the United States. It should be noted that the distinction between one to three and four or more positive nodes as two different groups is no longer used in the setting of adjuvant chemotherapy of breast cancer, and the concept that node-positive breast cancer represents a continuum is now more acceptable. Therefore, the assumption that patients with one to three positive nodes are not at substantial enough risk of locoregional failure to justify the use of PMRT, as would be done for four or more nodes, does not appear to be reasonable. In addition, the Oxford meta-analysis has shown that for patients after mastectomy and axillary lymph node dissection, radiotherapy produced similar proportional reductions in local recurrence rate, irrespective of patient age, tumor size and grade, hormone receptor status, or number of nodes involved (41).

Therefore, recently, many have recommended PMRT for the majority of patients with node-positive breast cancer (61). In addition, the most recent NCCN guidelines suggest that PMRT to the chest wall and supraclavicular area should be strongly considered after chemotherapy in women with one to three positive nodes (53). There was no consensus regarding the irradiation of internal mammary nodes. A recent study has suggested chest wall radiotherapy alone as a middle ground for treatment of patients with one to three positive lymph nodes after mastectomy (62). The authors reported similar benefit of PMRT and chest wall radiotherapy alone in terms of 10-year locoregional recurrence rate (0% for both) and disease-free survival (93% and 96%, respectively).

The identification of patients at higher risk of locoregional failure on the basis of genetic expression profiling is an area of ongoing research that might help in proper selection of patients who would benefit from PMRT (63). Higher nodal ratio (a ratio of the number of positive nodes to the total number of excised nodes of 0.2 or above) might also permit the identification of patients who have the highest risk of locoregional recurrence in the setting of one to three positive nodes and who are consequently expected to get the most benefit from PMRT (64).

PMRT: Large Node-negative Breast Tumor

Another challenge in the context of PMRT is large breast tumors (larger than 5 cm) without lymph node metastases. This clinical scenario is relatively uncommon, with an incidence ranging from 0.5% to 4% (17,65–69). The management of these patients is complex in view of the paucity of data addressing this issue, which complicates evidence-based clinical decisions. Several studies have reported a local recurrence rate of 7% to 60% in T3N0 breast cancer patients with no PMRT (12,17,22,23,65–67,70). The wide variation in the reported results is likely due to the limited number of patients with large breast tumors and negative lymph nodes included in these studies. In the Danish trial for premenopausal women, the local failure among node-negative tumors without irradiation was 17%, while the rate among those treated with radiation was 3% (22). Similarly, among postmenopausal women, local failure without radiation was 26%, compared with 6% in the irradiated group (23). While interpreting the data from the Danish trials, two major concerns should be considered. The first is related to the low number of dissected axillary lymph nodes, and the second is the entry criteria, which were such that node-negative women were eligible only with tumor size greater than 5 cm or invasion of the skin or pectoral fascia. Results in these studies were reported by nodal status and tumor size. Therefore, the statistics reported for node-negative women are based on a mixture of T3N0 tumors and tumors with skin or fascia invasion. Two more recent publications have addressed local recurrence rates for T3N0 breast cancer patients. These studies have included those with tumors of 5 cm, categorized as T2 lesions, among patients with large tumors and negative lymph nodes. This has allowed the assembly of a tri-institutional retrospective review of 71 patients (66) and of the largest data set reported to date pooled from several National Surgical Adjuvant Breast and Bowel Project (NSABP) trials (313 patients) (65). The axillary dissection was considered adequate, with a median number of 16 lymph nodes examined in both studies. In addition, the study using the NSABP data indicated that there was a nonsignificant trend toward a correlation between the number of dissected lymph nodes at surgery and the local recurrence rate (65), further emphasizing the importance of adequate lymph node dissection to ensure node-negative status. The isolated local recurrence rate was around 7% in both the tri-institutional series and the NSABP series, which is clearly lower than the previously reported recurrence rates for T3N0 breast cancer patients. LVI was found to have an impact on the rate of locoregional failure in the tri-institutional study, while the combined NSABP series was unable to address LVI as a risk factor for recurrence due to the fact that this variable was not recorded in the data sets from these trials. The results of these two studies suggest that large breast tumors in the presence of actual negative axillary nodes are not associated with rates of local failure that justify routine PMRT for all patients included in this category. Although this issue was not addressed by the 1999 ASTRO guidelines (49), the treatment guidelines from the NCCN and Canada recommend PMRT (but not of the supraclavicular or infraclavicular regions) in women with tumors larger than 5 cm, regardless of the status of the axillary nodes (52,53).

Ongoing trials, such as the MRC/EORTC/SUPREMO (Medical Research Council/European Organisation for Research and Treatment of Cancer/Selective Use of Postoperative Radiotherapy after Mastectomy) trial, may help determine whether PMRT is advantageous for patients with high-risk node-negative tumors and one to three positive nodes, but it will be years before the outcomes are available (71).

PMRT: Clinical Targets

The choice of radiation fields following mastectomy has been based on studies that have shown patterns of locoregional failures in these patients. The chest wall and the supraclavicular/infraclavicular regions have been identified as the most common sites of failure following mastectomy and adequate axillary dissection (i.e., 10 or more nodes removed) (17,18,72–74). Donegan and colleagues reported that more than 50% of locoregional failures following mastectomy occur at the chest wall, with the scar and the surrounding skin are at greatest risk for recurrence (16).

The second most common site of locoregional failure is the supraclavicular/infraclavicular (axillary apex) region. Following a level 1 or 2 axillary dissection, 20% to 41% of locoregional recurrence occurs in this region

(17–19,72,73). The risk of axillary failure is greatly influenced by the extent of axillary surgery; that is, with level 1 or 2 dissection, the 10-year risk of axillary failure is only 2% to 4% in contemporary series (17,18). This percentage does not warrant full axillary irradiation for such women.

Whether to include the internal mammary chain (IMC) in PMRT remains controversial. The strongest support for the use of IMC irradiation comes from the Institut Gustave-Roussy. On multivariate analysis of 1,195 patients treated over a 20-year period, IMC irradiation was independently associated with a reduction in the risk of distant metastasis ($P = 0.02$) for patients with medial or central primary tumors and positive axillary lymph nodes (47,75). In addition, pathological involvement has been reported in up to 37% of axillary node–positive breast cancers that are located in the inner or central breast (76). Nevertheless, evident recurrence at this site is not a common clinical scenario (17,18,72,73).

Given the possible benefit from IMC irradiation in certain subsets of breast cancer patients, ongoing prospective randomized studies are addressing the role of locoregional irradiation. EORTC 10925/22922 randomized 4,000 patients with positive axillary nodes or high-risk lymph node–negative medially and centrally located tumors to treatment with or without IMC and supraclavicular irradiation (77). The study was closed to accrual in 2004 and is in follow-up for analysis. The National Cancer Institute of Canada Clinical Trials Group (NCIC CTG) MA.20 study randomizes axillary node positive patients to breast irradiation with or without ipsilateral supraclavicular, axillary, and IMC irradiation (78).

PMRT: Toxicity

Immediate side effects during irradiation may include fatigue and skin soreness. Skin toxicity is usually mild and transient, with complete resolution of symptoms within a few weeks of completion of treatment. Radiation pneumonitis (a clinical syndrome of cough, fever, and shortness of breath accompanied by radiographic changes consistent with a noninfectious infiltrate) is uncommon following PMRT; the incidence rises significantly with an increase in irradiated lung volume within tangential fields (79) as well as with the presence of adjuvant or concomitant chemotherapy (80), and specifically taxanes (81).

Late radiation toxicities include possible cardiac toxicity (82–85), lymphedema (86), and, rarely, brachial plexopathy (87), and second malignancies such as radiation-induced sarcoma (88). Although the clinical significance of incidental irradiation of the heart during breast or chest wall radiotherapy has yet to be defined, modern techniques are expected to minimize the cardiac exposure to radiation (89,90). The incidence and grade of lymphedema are related to the extent of axillary surgery as well as the type of breast surgery; both are increased with the addition of axillary radiotherapy (86,91,92).

Inoperable LABC

Historically, surgery has been at the forefront of investigating LABC treatment. In 1943, Haagensen and Stout provided early data regarding the dismal results of radical mastectomy alone as treatment for LABC, reporting five-year local recurrence and survival rates of 46% and 6%, respectively (93). The authors defined grave local signs as poor prognostic factors. These included ulceration, limited skin edema, fixation to the pectoralis muscle, and bulky axillary adenopathy.

Similarly, therapeutic doses of chest wall radiotherapy had been tried in the setting of LABC, with unsatisfactory results. Several studies from the 1970s and 1980s reported excessively high failure rates, with five-year local recurrence rates ranging from 46% to 72% and survival rates of 16% to 30% (48,94,95). Combined treatment of radiation plus surgery was also attempted, with no significant improvement in disease control (96–98).

With the concept of breast cancer as a systemic disease at presentation, chemotherapy was introduced into the treatment of LABC in the 1970s. Given that survival is similar for both preoperative and postoperative systemic treatment (45,99–103), in addition to tumor downstaging and the improved resectability that can be achieved with neoadjuvant chemotherapy, the sequence of neoadjuvant chemotherapy followed by surgery and radiation has become the common approach for LABC, including IBC (101,104).

Breast-conserving Surgery Following Neoadjuvant Chemotherapy for LABC

Resection is essential for documenting chemotherapy response and achieving optimal locoregional control (105). The choice of type of surgery depends on several factors—most importantly the tumor response to neoadjuvant chemotherapy as well as the patient's acceptance of mastectomy as a treatment decision. Breast-conserving surgery has been reported as feasible in patients with LABC whose tumors demonstrate adequate downstaging in response to neoadjuvant chemotherapy to allow for acceptable cosmetic outcome. In this setting, prechemotherapy clip placement is absolutely necessary, especially for those patients who might show complete clinical and radiological response after neoadjuvant chemotherapy. Proper selection of patients plays a key role in the success of this treatment modality, as it will affect the treatment outcome in terms of locoregional control, disease-free survival, and overall survival. The eligibility criteria for breast conservation after induction chemotherapy in LABC are similar to those applied in early-stage breast cancer. Presence of multicentric disease, extensive microcalcification, extensive skin changes, and lymphatic permeation are generally considered contraindications for breast conservation (106). For those patients, mastectomy would be the treatment of choice. As in early breast cancer, postoperative radiotherapy is an integral part of the management of patients with LABC undergoing breast conservation. The technique of irradiation is generally the same; however, existing data are limited regarding whether comprehensive irradiation is absolutely necessary to achieve optimal locoregional control in patients whose tumors achieve a substantial degree of downstaging in response to chemotherapy.

Radiation Therapy Following Neoadjuvant Chemotherapy and Mastectomy

In most uncontrolled series and at least one randomized trial, local control rates appear to be higher when both surgery and radiotherapy are included in the treatment strategy for LABC (14,102,107–114), even for women who have a pathological response to neoadjuvant chemotherapy (115). While the survival impact for chest wall irradiation in this setting is unclear (14,116), the improvement in locoregional control in these women who are at high risk for chest wall failure makes radiotherapy an important part of their management.

Nevertheless, the question is whether comprehensive radiation is needed for every patient undergoing mastectomy after neoadjuvant chemotherapy. The results of surgical pathology have traditionally been used to estimate the odds of locoregional recurrence following surgery in breast cancer patients and hence to identify those who would benefit from nodal irradiation. However, this could not be applied for patients undergoing preoperative chemotherapy with an expected response rate up to 80%. Therefore, it has been suggested that, in the context of preoperative chemotherapy, both the initial clinical stage and the final pathological extent of disease independently predict the risk of a locoregional recurrence (112).

The investigators at the MD Anderson Cancer Center retrospectively analyzed the outcomes of 542 patients treated on six consecutive institutional prospective trials with neoadjuvant chemotherapy, mastectomy, and radiation (110). These data were compared with those for 134 patients who received similar treatment in these same trials but without radiation. Patients who presented with clinically advanced stage 3 or 4 disease but subsequently achieved a complete pathological response to neoadjuvant chemotherapy still had a high rate of locoregional recurrence, which was significantly reduced with radiation (10-year rates 33% versus 3%, $P = 0.006$). Comprehensive radiation improved cause-specific survival in the following subsets: stage 3B or higher disease, clinical T4 tumors, and four or more positive nodes ($P \leq 0.007$ for all comparisons). The 5-year locoregional rate in 12 patients with stage 3 disease who achieved a complete pathological remission remained high when radiation was not used (33.3% ± 15.7%) (115).

Although definitive guidelines have not been established for PMRT in patients undergoing neoadjuvant chemotherapy, interpretation of the data from different studies would be helpful in determining the optimal approach. Patients undergoing mastectomy after neoadjuvant chemotherapy with complete pathological response in both breast tumors and axillary nodes should receive radiotherapy to chest wall and supraclavicular nodes, with or without internal mammary nodes. For those who achieve only a partial response in the primary tumor or who have residual positive lymph nodes, comprehensive radiotherapy should include axillary fields.

■ MANAGEMENT OF IBC

IBC (stage T4d) is an aggressive form of LABC that is defined by the American Joint Committee on Cancer as a clinicopathological entity characterized by diffuse erythema and edema (peau d'orange) of the breast, often without an underlying palpable mass (117). Patients with IBC typically present with pain and a tender, firm, and enlarged breast. The skin over the breast is reddened, warm, and thickened. Historically, treatment with surgery or radiation therapy, or both, resulted in fewer than 5% of IBC patients surviving beyond five years (118). The integration of chemotherapy, surgery, and radiation therapy has evolved to become a standard approach to treating IBC, with primary systemic chemotherapy being the initial component. The success of the multimodality approach to the management of IBC has been confirmed by several reports (75,119–131).

In a study from the MD Anderson Cancer Center, a total of 178 patients were treated with upfront doxorubicin-based chemotherapy then local therapy with irradiation with or without mastectomy followed by adjuvant chemotherapy (132). The results of this study highlighted two important aspects of IBC management. First, with a combined modality approach, 28% of the patients were alive and without evidence of disease beyond 15 years. Median survival was 37 months, with an overall survival of 40% at 5 years and 33% at 10 years. Second, 71% of all IBC patients had an objective response to the doxorubicin-based primary chemotherapy, with 12% achieving a complete pathological response. Disease-free survival at 15 years was 44% in patients who attained a complete pathological response, 31% in those who attained a partial response, and 7% in those who did not respond to primary systemic chemotherapy. These two aspects of the study demonstrate how combined modality therapy has essentially changed the natural history of IBC. Furthermore, this study and also other reports (125,133,134) confirm that, as with LABC, the assessment of response to primary chemotherapy is a powerful predictor of patients who would have better survival.

Several reports suggest higher locoregional failure rates when surgery is not a component of therapy for IBC (124,131,135,136). Flemming and colleagues retrospectively reviewed the effectiveness of mastectomy in patients with IBC treated at the MD Anderson Cancer Center (136). Of the 178 patients treated, those who had a response to primary chemotherapy and underwent a mastectomy had significantly lower rates of local recurrence and exhibited improved disease-specific survival compared with those who responded to primary chemotherapy but did not undergo mastectomy. Five-year disease-free survival rates in patients treated with chemotherapy followed by surgery and radiotherapy ranged from 22% to 49%, and the overall survival from 30% to 70%. In another report, locoregional control was significantly better in women who underwent surgery as part of their multimodality treatment for IBC (76% vs 30%) The combined local approach of surgery and radiotherapy provides optimal locoregional control; the impact on overall survival is questionable (137,138).

Nonsurgical Approach

As mentioned earlier, surgery plays an integral role in the context of multidisciplinary management of IBC. Nevertheless, two European groups have questioned the necessity of mastectomy in this setting (75,139). In the first study, from the Institute Gustave-Roussy (France), 99 patients presenting with nonmetastatic IBC were treated with an alternating protocol of radiotherapy and chemotherapy (75). The alternating schedule consisted of eight courses of combined chemotherapy, including doxorubicin, vincristine, cyclophosphamide, methotrexate, and 5-fluorouracil, and three series of locoregional radiotherapy delivering a total dose of 65 to 75 Gy to the breast tumor, 65 Gy to the axilla, and 50 Gy to the supraclavicular and IMC lymph nodes. Radiotherapy was started after the third course of chemotherapy. Five-year overall survival and disease-free survival rates were 50% and 38%, respectively, and the cumulative rates of local failure and distant metastases were 27% and 53%, respectively. These results appear comparable to those achieved by mastectomy and radiotherapy. The study from the Royal Marsden Hospital showed similar results (139). Fifty-four patients who had responsive or stable disease following primary chemotherapy went on to have either radiotherapy alone (*n* = 35) or surgery plus radiotherapy (*n* = 19). In the group treated with radiotherapy alone, durations of median progression-free survival and overall survival were 16 and 35 months, respectively. Of the 69% who relapsed, half relapsed locally. In the surgically treated patients, the median progression-free survival and overall survival were 20 and 35 months, respectively, and more than half relapsed locally. These results do not suggest a clinical advantage for surgery in addition to chemotherapy and radiotherapy for patients with IBC.

Nevertheless, mastectomy remains an integral component of therapy for most women with IBC, as long as it is feasible after neoadjuvant chemotherapy.

Altered Fractionation Schemes

IBC has been recognized as having a rapid proliferative potential compared with non-IBC, and one mechanism of developing resistance to standard radiation therapy protocols is the repopulation of tumor cells between radiation treatments. Therefore, hyperfractionated accelerated radiotherapy has been evaluated as a means of improving locoregional control (138,140–142).

In one report, 54 patients, previously untreated, with nonmetastatic IBC were entered in an alternating protocol consisting of eight courses of combined chemotherapy and two series of locoregional hyperfractionated accelerated radiotherapy with twice-daily fractions of 1.5 Gy to a total dose of 66 Gy (140). Of the 53 patients evaluated at the end of the treatment, 44 (83%) had a complete clinical response, 7 (13%) had a partial response (above 50%), and 2 (4%) had tumor progression. With a median follow-up of 39 months, the 3- and 5-year overall survival rates were 66% and 45%, respectively, and the corresponding disease-free survival rates were 45% and 36%, respectively. The authors concluded that alternating a combination of chemotherapy and hyperfractionated accelerated radiotherapy is well tolerated and provides acceptable local control.

A second study supported the use of postmastectomy accelerated hyperfractionated radiation to 66 Gy in twice-daily fractions of 1.5 Gy, with target volumes including the chest wall and lymph nodes within the axillary, infraclavicular, supraclavicular, and internal mammary regions (141). Between 1986 and 1993, 39 patients underwent multimodality treatment for IBC that included twice-daily fractions of 1.5 Gy to a dose of 66 Gy. When treatment results were compared with historical controls treated between 1977 and 1985 with 60 Gy conventional fractionation radiotherapy, there was a significant improvement in the rate of locoregional control in favor of the accelerated fractionation group (84% versus 58%) and in overall survival (77% versus 58%).

Although altered fractionation schemes appear to be promising on the basis of the expected biology of IBC, conventional fractionation following mastectomy remains the standard in this setting.

■ CONCLUSIONS

The management of LABC has been revolutionized by the movement from single-modality treatment to the combined use of surgery, chemotherapy, and radiation therapy. The combined modality approach has improved the outcome of patients with LABC in terms of better rates of locoregional control, enhanced disease-free survival and overall survival. The optimal sequence of such treatment modalities should be individualized, as it can differ from one patient to another according to the clinical scenario.

While surgery has been at the forefront in patients with operable LABC, neoadjuvant chemotherapy comes first in those with inoperable LABC and IBC. The exception is the patient who wants to keep her breast, for whom preoperative chemotherapy will be indicated, with the goal of tumor downstaging prior to surgery. Breast conservation and sentinel lymph node biopsy appear to be inadequate for patients with IBC.

■ MULTIDISCIPLINARY APPROACH IN THE TREATMENT OF LABC

Evidence-based data show that combined modality treatment employing surgery, chemotherapy, and radiation therapy is the standard of care for patients with LABC. The optimal sequence of such treatment modalities should be discussed in a multidisciplinary clinic that includes surgical, medical, and radiation oncology, as well as breast radiology and pathology. For example, some patients would be suitable for surgery first, whereas others should receive chemotherapy prior to surgery. Patients undergoing neoadjuvant chemotherapy with the goal of breast conservation should be referred to a radiologist for clip placement around the tumor prior to the start of treatment. Nevertheless, certain tumor characteristics preclude a breast-conserving approach in patients with LABC. Therefore, review of the pathology and the imaging as a group appears to be beneficial. This ensures that all aspects of treatment are adequately addressed at presentation. In addition, multidisciplinary discussion allows better understanding of the role of each specialty in the management and helps in the delivery of quality care for each patient.

■ SUMMARY

- Operable LABC
  - The traditional approach is upfront mastectomy with axillary staging, followed by adjuvant therapy as indicated.
  - Breast-conserving surgery appears to be feasible for appropriately selected patients following neoadjuvant chemotherapy.
  - Almost all women with positive axillary lymph nodes will receive adjuvant systemic therapy.
  - American Society for Therapeutic Radiology and Oncology practice guidelines recommend PMRT for patients with four or more positive axillary lymph nodes; for T3 and T4 tumors; where there is no substantial evidence of routine chest wall radiotherapy for women with one to three positive axillary nodes.

- Inoperable LABC
  - Owing to the high risk of locoregional failure, PMRT is indicated for women undergoing neoadjuvant chemotherapy and mastectomy; however, the impact on survival is unclear.
  - In patients whose tumors and axillary nodes show a complete pathological response to neoadjuvant chemotherapy, PMRT should include chest wall and supraclavicular nodes, with or without internal mammary nodes.
  - For those who show only a partial response in the primary tumor or who have residual positive lymph nodes, comprehensive PMRT should include axillary fields.
- IBC
  - The management of IBC is generally the same as for inoperable LABC, except that conservative surgery and sentinel lymph node biopsy seem to be inadequate.
  - Nonsurgical approaches and altered fractionation schemes have been tried, with good results, yet neoadjuvant chemotherapy followed by mastectomy and radiotherapy using conventional fractionation remains the standard of care for IBC.

■ REFERENCES

1. Lee MC, Newman LA. Management of patients with locally advanced breast cancer. *Surg Clin North Am.* 2007;87(2):379–398, ix.
2. Gueth U, Wight E, Schoetzau A, et al. Non-inflammatory skin involvement in breast cancer, histologically proven but without the clinical and histological T4 category features. *J Surg Oncol.* 2007;95(4):291–297.
3. Greene, FL, Page, DL, Fleming, ID, et al. *AJCC Cancer Staging Manual.* New York: Springer-Verlag;2002:223.
4. Brito RA, Valero V, Buzdar AU, et al. Long-term results of combined-modality therapy for locally advanced breast cancer with ipsilateral supraclavicular metastases: the University of Texas M.D. Anderson Cancer Center experience. *J Clin Oncol.* 2001;19(3):628–633.
5. Olivotto IA, Chua B, Allan SJ, Speers CH, Chia S, Ragaz J. Long-term survival of patients with supraclavicular metastases at diagnosis of breast cancer. *J Clin Oncol.* 2003;21(5):851–854.
6. Singletary SE, Allred C, Ashley P, et al. Revision of the American Joint Committee on Cancer staging system for breast cancer. *J Clin Oncol.* 2002;20(17):3628–3636.
7. Bartelink H, Rubens RD, van der Schueren E, Sylvester R. Hormonal therapy prolongs survival in irradiated locally advanced breast cancer: a European Organization for Research and Treatment of Cancer randomized phase III trial. *J Clin Oncol.* 1997;15(1):207–215.
8. Gazet JC, Ford HT, Coombes RC. Randomised trial of chemotherapy versus endocrine therapy in patients presenting with locally advanced breast cancer (a pilot study). *Br J Cancer.* 1991;63(2):279–282.
9. Heys SD, Sarkar T, Hutcheon AW. Primary docetaxel chemotherapy in patients with breast cancer: impact on response and survival. *Breast Cancer Res Treat.* 2005;90(2):169–185.
10. Rubens RD, Bartelink H, Engelsman E, et al. Locally advanced breast cancer: the contribution of cytotoxic and endocrine treatment to radiotherapy. An EORTC Breast Cancer Co-operative Group Trial (10792). *Eur J Cancer Clin Oncol.* 1989;25(4):667–678.
11. Smith IC, Heys SD, Hutcheon AW, et al. Neoadjuvant chemotherapy in breast cancer: significantly enhanced response with docetaxel. *J Clin Oncol.* 2002;20(6):1456–1466.
12. Klefstrom P, Grohn P, Heinonen E, Holsti L, Holsti P. Adjuvant postoperative radiotherapy, chemotherapy, and immunotherapy in stage III breast cancer. II. 5-year results and influence of levamisole. *Cancer.* 1987;60(5):936–942.
13. Spangenberg JP, Nel CJ, Anderson JD, Doman MJ. A prospective study of the treatment of stage III breast cancer. *S Afr J Surg.* 1986;24(2):57–60.
14. Olson JE, Neuberg D, Pandya KJ, et al. The role of radiotherapy in the management of operable locally advanced breast carcinoma: results of a randomized trial by the Eastern Cooperative Oncology Group. *Cancer.* 1997;79(6):1138–1149.
15. Lyman GH, Giuliano AE, Somerfield MR, et al. American Society of Clinical Oncology guideline recommendations for sentinel lymph node biopsy in early-stage breast cancer. *J Clin Oncol.* 2005;23(30):7703–7720.
16. Donegan WL, Perez-Mesa CM, Watson FR. A biostatistical study of locally recurrent breast carcinoma. *Surg Gynecol Obstet.* 1966;122(3):529–540.
17. Katz A, Strom EA, Buchholz TA, et al. Locoregional recurrence patterns after mastectomy and doxorubicin-based chemotherapy: implications for postoperative irradiation. *J Clin Oncol.* 2000;18(15):2817–2827.
18. Recht A, Gray R, Davidson NE, et al. Locoregional failure 10 years after mastectomy and adjuvant chemotherapy with or without tamoxifen without irradiation: experience of the Eastern Cooperative Oncology Group. *J Clin Oncol.* 1999;17(6):1689–1700.
19. Taghian A, Jeong JH, Mamounas E, et al. Patterns of locoregional failure in patients with operable breast cancer treated by mastectomy and adjuvant chemotherapy with or without tamoxifen and without radiotherapy: results from five National Surgical Adjuvant Breast and Bowel Project randomized clinical trials. *J Clin Oncol.* 2004;22(21):4247–4254.
20. Stefanik D, Goldberg R, Byrne P, et al. Local-regional failure in patients treated with adjuvant chemotherapy for breast cancer. *J Clin Oncol.* 1985;3(5):660–665.
21. Griem KL, Henderson IC, Gelman R, et al. The 5-year results of a randomized trial of adjuvant radiation therapy after chemotherapy in breast cancer patients treated with mastectomy. *J Clin Oncol.* 1987;5(10):1546–1555.
22. Overgaard M, Hansen PS, Overgaard J, et al. Postoperative radiotherapy in high-risk premenopausal women with breast cancer who receive adjuvant chemotherapy. Danish Breast Cancer Cooperative Group 82b Trial. *New Engl J Med.* 1997;337(14):949–955.
23. Overgaard M, Jensen MB, Overgaard J, et al. Postoperative radiotherapy in high-risk postmenopausal breast-cancer patients given adjuvant tamoxifen: Danish Breast Cancer Cooperative Group DBCG 82c randomised trial. *Lancet.* 1999;353(9165):1641–1648.
24. Ragaz J, Jackson SM, Le N, et al. Adjuvant radiotherapy and chemotherapy in node-positive premenopausal women with breast cancer. *New Engl J Med.* 1997;337(14):956–962.
25. Mentzer SJ, Osteen RT, Wilson RE. Local recurrence and the deep resection margin in carcinoma of the breast. *Surg Gynecol Obstet.* 1986;163(6):513–517.
26. Fowble B, Gray R, Gilchrist K, Goodman RL, Taylor S, Tormey DC. Identification of a subgroup of patients with breast cancer and histologically positive axillary nodes receiving adjuvant chemotherapy who may benefit from postoperative radiotherapy. *J Clin Oncol.* 1988;6(7):1107–1117.

27. Leitner SP, Swern AS, Weinberger D, Duncan LJ, Hutter RV. Predictors of recurrence for patients with small (one centimeter or less) localized breast cancer (T1a,b N0 M0). *Cancer.* 1995;76(11):2266–2274.

28. Jagsi R, Raad RA, Goldberg S, et al. Locoregional recurrence rates and prognostic factors for failure in node-negative patients treated with mastectomy: implications for postmastectomy radiation. *Int J Radiat Oncol Biol Phys.* 2005;62(4):1035–1039.

29. Katz A, Buchholz TA, Thames H, et al. Recursive partitioning analysis of locoregional recurrence patterns following mastectomy: implications for adjuvant irradiation. *Int J Radiat Oncol Biol Phys.* 2001;50(2):397–403.

30. Cheng SH, Horng CF, Clarke JL, et al. Prognostic index score and clinical prediction model of local regional recurrence after mastectomy in breast cancer patients. *Int J Radiat Oncol Biol Phys.* 2006;64(5):1401–1409.

31. Mignano JE, Zahurak ML, Chakravarthy A, Piantadosi S, Dooley WC, Gage I. Significance of axillary lymph node extranodal soft tissue extension and indications for postmastectomy irradiation. *Cancer.* 1999;86(7):1258–1262.

32. Gruber G, Bonetti M, Nasi ML, et al. Prognostic value of extracapsular tumor spread for locoregional control in premenopausal patients with node-positive breast cancer treated with classical cyclophosphamide, methotrexate, and fluorouracil: long-term observations from International Breast Cancer Study Group Trial VI. *J Clin Oncol.* 2005;23(28):7089–7097.

33. Fisher B, Fisher ER, Redmond C. Ten-year results from the National Surgical Adjuvant Breast and Bowel Project (NSABP) clinical trial evaluating the use of l-phenylalanine mustard (l-PAM) in the management of primary breast cancer. *J Clin Oncol.* 1986;4(6):929–941.

34. Richards MA, O'Reilly SM, Howell A, et al. Adjuvant cyclophosphamide, methotrexate, and fluorouracil in patients with axillary node-positive breast cancer: an update of the Guy's/Manchester trial. *J Clin Oncol.* 1990;8(12):2032–2039.

35. Castiglione M, Gelber RD, Goldhirsch A. Adjuvant systemic therapy for breast cancer in the elderly: competing causes of mortality. International Breast Cancer Study Group. *J Clin Oncol.* 1990;8(3):519–526.

36. Effects of chemotherapy and hormonal therapy for early breast cancer on recurrence and 15-year survival: an overview of the randomised trials. *Lancet.* 2005;365(9472):1687–1717.

37. Falkson HC, Gray R, Wolberg WH, et al. Adjuvant trial of 12 cycles of CMFPT followed by observation or continuous tamoxifen versus four cycles of CMFPT in postmenopausal women with breast cancer: an Eastern Cooperative Oncology Group phase III study. *J Clin Oncol.* 1990;8(4):599–607.

38. Morrison JM, Howell A, Kelly KA, et al. West Midlands Oncology Association trials of adjuvant chemotherapy in operable breast cancer: results after a median follow-up of 7 years. I. Patients with involved axillary lymph nodes. *Br J Cancer.* 1989;60(6):911–918.

39. Misset JL, di Palma M, Delgado M, et al. Adjuvant treatment of node-positive breast cancer with cyclophosphamide, doxorubicin, fluorouracil, and vincristine versus cyclophosphamide, methotrexate, and fluorouracil: final report after a 16-year median follow-up duration. *J Clin Oncol.* 1996;14(4):1136–1145.

40. Zambetti M, Valagussa P, Bonadonna G. Adjuvant cyclophosphamide, methotrexate and fluorouracil in node-negative and estrogen receptor-negative breast cancer. Updated results. *Ann Oncol.* 1996;7(5):481–485.

41. Clarke M, Collins R, Darby S, et al. Effects of radiotherapy and of differences in the extent of surgery for early breast cancer on local recurrence and 15-year survival: an overview of the randomised trials. *Lancet.* 2005;366(9503):2087–2106.

42. Bellon JR, Harris JR. Chemotherapy and radiation therapy for breast cancer: what is the optimal sequence? *J Clin Oncol.* 2005;23(1):5–7.

43. Citron ML, Berry DA, Cirrincione C, et al. Randomized trial of dose-dense versus conventionally scheduled and sequential versus concurrent combination chemotherapy as postoperative adjuvant treatment of node-positive primary breast cancer: first report of Intergroup Trial C9741/Cancer and Leukemia Group B Trial 9741. *J Clin Oncol.* 2003;21(8):1431–1439.

44. Sartor CI, Peterson BL, Woolf S, et al. Effect of addition of adjuvant paclitaxel on radiotherapy delivery and locoregional control of node-positive breast cancer: cancer and leukemia group B 9344. *J Clin Oncol.* 2005;23(1):30–40.

45. Fisher B, Anderson S, Wickerham DL, et al. Increased intensification and total dose of cyclophosphamide in a doxorubicin-cyclophosphamide regimen for the treatment of primary breast cancer: findings from National Surgical Adjuvant Breast and Bowel Project B-22. *J Clin Oncol.* 1997;15(5):1858–1869.

46. Hoeller U, Heide J, Kroeger N, Krueger W, Jaenicke F, Alberti W. Radiotherapy after high-dose chemotherapy and peripheral blood stem cell support in high-risk breast cancer. *Int J Radiat Oncol Biol Phys.* 2002;53(5):1234–1239.

47. Arriagada R, Rutqvist LE, Mattsson A, Kramar A, Rotstein S. Adequate locoregional treatment for early breast cancer may prevent secondary dissemination. *J Clin Oncol.* 1995;13(12):2869–2878.

48. Rao DV, Bedwinek J, Perez C, Lee J, Fineberg B. Prognostic indicators in stage III and localized stage IV breast cancer. *Cancer.* 1982;50(10):2037–2043.

49. Harris JR, Halpin-Murphy P, McNeese M, Mendenhall NP, Morrow M, Robert NJ. Consensus Statement on postmastectomy radiation therapy. *Int J Radiat Oncol Biol Phys.* 1999; 44(5):989–990.

50. Recht A, Edge SB, Solin LJ, et al. Postmastectomy radiotherapy: clinical practice guidelines of the American Society of Clinical Oncology. *J Clin Oncol.* 2001;19(5):1539–1569.

51. Eifel P, Axelson JA, Costa J, et al. National Institutes of Health Consensus Development Conference Statement: adjuvant therapy for breast cancer, November 1–3, 2000. *J Natl Cancer Inst.* 2001;93(13):979–989.

52. Truong PT, Olivotto IA, Whelan TJ, Levine M. Clinical practice guidelines for the care and treatment of breast cancer: 16. Locoregional post-mastectomy radiotherapy. *CMAJ.* 2004;170(8): 1263–1273.

53. National Comprehensive Cancer Network (NCCN) guidelines. Available at www.nccn.org/professionals/physician_gls/default. asp. Accessed May 12, 2009.

54. Overgaard M, Christensen JJ, Johansen H, et al. Postmastectomy irradiation in high-risk breast cancer patients. Present status of the Danish Breast Cancer Cooperative Group trials. *Acta Oncol.* 1988;27(6A):707–714.

55. Recht A, Houlihan MJ. Axillary lymph nodes and breast cancer: a review. *Cancer* 1995;76(9):1491–1512.

56. Nielsen HM, Overgaard M, Grau C, Jensen AR, Overgaard J. Study of failure pattern among high-risk breast cancer patients with or without postmastectomy radiotherapy in addition to adjuvant systemic therapy: long-term results from the Danish Breast Cancer Cooperative Group DBCG 82 b and c randomized studies. *J Clin Oncol.* 2006;24(15):2268–2275.

57. Ragaz J, Olivotto IA, Spinelli JJ, et al. Locoregional radiation therapy in patients with high-risk breast cancer receiving adjuvant chemotherapy: 20-year results of the British Columbia randomized trial. *J Natl Cancer Inst.* 2005;97(2):116–126.

58. Freedman GM, Fowble BL, Hanlon AL, et al. A close or positive margin after mastectomy is not an indication for chest wall irradiation except in women aged fifty or younger. *Int J Radiat Oncol Biol Phys.* 1998;41(3):599–605.

59. Truong PT, Olivotto IA, Speers CH, Wai ES, Berthelet E, Kader HA. A positive margin is not always an indication for radiotherapy after mastectomy in early breast cancer. *Int J Radiat Oncol Biol Phys.* 2004;58(3):797–804.

60. Overgaard M, Nielsen HM, Overgaard J. Is the benefit of post-mastectomy irradiation limited to patients with four or more positive nodes, as recommended in international consensus reports? A subgroup analysis of the DBCG 82 b&c randomized trials. *Radiother Oncol.* 2007;82(3):247–253.

61. Marks LB, Zeng J, Prosnitz LR. One to three versus four or more positive nodes and postmastectomy radiotherapy: time to end the debate. *J Clin Oncol.* 2008;26(13):2075–2057.

62. Macdonald SM, Abi-Raad RF, Alm El-Din MA, et al. Chest wall radiotherapy: middle ground for treatment of patients with one to three positive lymph nodes after mastectomy. *Int J Radiat Oncol Biol Phys.* In press.

63. Cheng SH, Horng CF, West M, et al. Genomic prediction of locoregional recurrence after mastectomy in breast cancer. *J Clin Oncol.* 2006;24(28):4594–4602.

64. Truong PT, Woodward WA, Thames HD, Ragaz J, Olivotto IA, Buchholz TA. The ratio of positive to excised nodes identifies high-risk subsets and reduces inter-institutional differences in locoregional recurrence risk estimates in breast cancer patients with 1–3 positive nodes: an analysis of prospective data from British Columbia and the M. D. Anderson Cancer Center. *Int J Radiat Oncol Biol Phys.* 2007;68(1):59–65.

65. Taghian AG, Jeong JH, Mamounas EP, et al. Low locoregional recurrence rate among node-negative breast cancer patients with tumors 5 cm or larger treated by mastectomy, with or without adjuvant systemic therapy and without radiotherapy: results from five national surgical adjuvant breast and bowel project randomized clinical trials. *J Clin Oncol.* 2006;24(24):3927–3932.

66. Floyd SR, Buchholz TA, Haffty BG, et al. Low local recurrence rate without postmastectomy radiation in node-negative breast cancer patients with tumors 5 cm and larger. *Int J Radiat Oncol Biol Phys.* 2006;66(2):358–364.

67. Helinto M, Blomqvist C, Heikkila P, Joensuu H. Post-mastectomy radiotherapy in pT3N0M0 breast cancer: is it needed? *Radiother Oncol.* 1999;52(3):213–217.

68. Wallgren A, Bonetti M, Gelber RD, et al. Risk factors for locoregional recurrence among breast cancer patients: results from International Breast Cancer Study Group Trials I through VII. *J Clin Oncol.* 2003;21(7):1205–1213.

69. Trudeau ME, Pritchard KI, Chapman JA, et al. Prognostic factors affecting the natural history of node-negative breast cancer. *Breast Cancer Res Treat.* 2005;89(1):35–45.

70. Mignano JE, Gage I, Piantadosi S, Ye X, Henderson G, Dooley WC. Local recurrence after mastectomy in patients with T3pN0 breast carcinoma treated without postoperative radiation therapy. *Am J Clin Oncol.* 2007;30(5):466–472.

71. Kunkler IH, Canney P, van Tienhoven G, Russell NS. Elucidating the role of chest wall irradiation in 'intermediate-risk' breast cancer: the MRC/EORTC SUPREMO trial. *Clin Oncol (R Coll Radiol).* 2008;20(1):31–34.

72. Strom EA, Woodward WA, Katz A, et al. Clinical investigation: regional nodal failure patterns in breast cancer patients treated with mastectomy without radiotherapy. *Int J Radiat Oncol Biol Phys.* 2005;63(5):1508–1513.

73. Schwaibold F, Fowble BL, Solin LJ, Schultz DJ, Goodman RL. The results of radiation therapy for isolated local regional recurrence after mastectomy. *Int J Radiat Oncol Biol Phys.* 1991;21(2):299–310.

74. Toonkel LM, Fix I, Jacobson LH, Wallach CB. The significance of local recurrence of carcinoma of the breast. *Int J Radiat Oncol Biol Phys.* 1983;9(1):33–39.

75. Arriagada R, Mouriesse H, Spielmann M, et al. Alternating radiotherapy and chemotherapy in non-metastatic inflammatory breast cancer. *Int J Radiat Oncol Biol Phys.* 1990;19(5):1207–1210.

76. Lacour J, Le M, Caceres E, Koszarowski T, Veronesi U, Hill C. Radical mastectomy versus radical mastectomy plus internal mammary dissection. Ten year results of an international cooperative trial in breast cancer. *Cancer.* 1983;51(10):1941–1943.

77. Phase III randomized trial investigating the role of internal mammary and medial supraclavicular (IM-MS) lymph node chain irradiation in stage I–III breast cancer (joint study of the EORTC Radiotherapy Cooperative Group and the EORTC Breast Cancer Cooperative Group). EORTC Study No. 10925/22922 Available at http://journalscambridgeorg/downloadphp?file=%2FBCO%2FBCO9_S1%2FS1470903106009126apdf&code=ff6fdd98cb2f5726417e3dfa463249ff Accessed May 12, 2009.

78. A phase III study of regional radiation therapy in early breast cancer. NCIC CTG trial MA.20. Available at http://journals.cambridge.org/download.php?file=%2FBCO%2FBCO9_S1%2FS1470903106009308a.pdf&code=6dd5cf7a40e57b2a9a01ec5fab104dcd Accessed May 12, 2009.

79. Rothwell RI, Kelly SA, Joslin CA. Radiation pneumonitis in patients treated for breast cancer. *Radiother Oncol.* 1985;4(1):9–14.

80. Lingos TI, Recht A, Vicini F, Abner A, Silver B, Harris JR. Radiation pneumonitis in breast cancer patients treated with conservative surgery and radiation therapy. *Int J Radiat Oncol Biol Phys.* 1991;21(2):355–360.

81. Taghian AG, Assaad SI, Niemierko A, et al. Risk of pneumonitis in breast cancer patients treated with radiation therapy and combination chemotherapy with paclitaxel. *J Natl Cancer Inst.* 2001;93(23):1806–1811.

82. Gyenes G. Radiation-induced ischemic heart disease in breast cancer—a review. *Acta Oncol.* 1998;37(3):241–246.

83. Paszat LF, Mackillop WJ, Groome PA, Boyd C, Schulze K, Holowaty E. Mortality from myocardial infarction after adjuvant radiotherapy for breast cancer in the surveillance, epidemiology, and end-results cancer registries. *J Clin Oncol.* 1998;16(8):2625–2631.

84. Rutqvist LE, Lax I, Fornander T, Johansson H. Cardiovascular mortality in a randomized trial of adjuvant radiation therapy versus surgery alone in primary breast cancer. *Int J Radiat Oncol Biol Phys.* 1992;22(5):887–896.

85. Darby S, McGale P, Peto R, Granath F, Hall P, Ekbom A. Mortality from cardiovascular disease more than 10 years after radiotherapy for breast cancer: nationwide cohort study of 90 000 Swedish women. *BMJ* 2003;326(7383):256–257.

86. Meek AG. Breast radiotherapy and lymphedema. *Cancer.* 1998; 83(12 Suppl American):2788–2797.

87. Powell S, Cooke J, Parsons C. Radiation-induced brachial plexus injury: follow-up of two different fractionation schedules. *Radiother Oncol.* 1990;18(3):213–220.

88. Taghian A, de Vathaire F, Terrier P, et al. Long-term risk of sarcoma following radiation treatment for breast cancer. *Int J Radiat Oncol Biol Phys.* 1991;21(2):361–367.

89. Krueger EA, Schipper MJ, Koelling T, Marsh RB, Butler JB, Pierce LJ. Cardiac chamber and coronary artery doses associated with postmastectomy radiotherapy techniques to the chest wall and regional nodes. *Int J Radiat Oncol Biol Phys.* 2004; 60(4):1195–1203.

90. Pierce LJ, Butler JB, Martel MK, et al. Postmastectomy radiotherapy of the chest wall: dosimetric comparison of common techniques. *Int J Radiat Oncol Biol Phys.* 2002;52(5):1220–1230.

91. Violet JA, Harmer C. Breast cancer: improving outcome following adjuvant radiotherapy. *Br J Radiol.* 2004;77(922):811–820.

92. Larson D, Weinstein M, Goldberg I, et al. Edema of the arm as a function of the extent of axillary surgery in patients with stage I-II carcinoma of the breast treated with primary radiotherapy. *Int J Radiat Oncol Biol Phys.* 1986;12(9):1575–1582.

93. Haagensen CD, Stout AP. Carcinoma of the Breast: II. Criteria of operability. *Ann Surg.* 1943;118(5):859–870.

94. Harris JR, Sawicka J, Gelman R, Hellman S. Management of locally advanced carcinoma of the breast by primary radiation therapy. *Int J Radiat Oncol Biol Phys.* 1983;9(3):345–349.

95. Rubens RD, Armitage P, Winter PJ, Tong D, Hayward JL. Prognosis in inoperable stage III carcinoma of the breast. *Eur J Cancer.* 1977;13(8):805–811.

96. Townsend CM, Jr., Abston S, Fish JC. Surgical adjuvant treatment of locally advanced breast cancer. *Ann Surg.* 1985;201(5): 604–610.

97. Arnold DJ, Lesnick GJ. Survival following mastectomy for stage III breast cancer. *Am J Surg.* 1979;137(3):362–366.

98. Montague ED, Fletcher GH. Local regional effectiveness of surgery and radiation therapy in the treatment of breast cancer. *Cancer.* 1985;55(9):2266–2272.

99. Mauriac L, Durand M, Avril A, Dilhuydy JM. Effects of primary chemotherapy in conservative treatment of breast cancer patients with operable tumors larger than 3 cm. Results of a randomized trial in a single centre. *Ann Oncol.* 1991;2(5):347–354.

100. Mauriac L, MacGrogan G, Avril A, et al. Neoadjuvant chemotherapy for operable breast carcinoma larger than 3 cm: a unicentre randomized trial with a 124-month median follow-up. Institut Bergonie Bordeaux Groupe Sein (IBBGS). *Ann Oncol.* 1999;10(1):47–52.

101. Schwartz GF, Hortobagyi GN. Proceedings of the consensus conference on neoadjuvant chemotherapy in carcinoma of the breast, April 26–28, 2003, Philadelphia, Pennsylvania. *Cancer.* 2004;100(12):2512–2532.

102. Makris A, Powles TJ, Ashley SE, et al. A reduction in the requirements for mastectomy in a randomized trial of neoadjuvant chemoendocrine therapy in primary breast cancer. *Ann Oncol.* 1998;9(11):1179–1184.

103. Wolmark N, Wang J, Mamounas E, Bryant J, Fisher B. Preoperative chemotherapy in patients with operable breast cancer: nine-year results from National Surgical Adjuvant Breast and Bowel Project B-18. *J Natl Cancer Inst Monogr.* 2001(30):96–102.

104. Shenkier T, Weir L, Levine M, Olivotto I, Whelan T, Reyno L. Clinical practice guidelines for the care and treatment of breast cancer: 15. Treatment for women with stage III or locally advanced breast cancer. *CMAJ.* 2004;170(6):983–994.

105. Hortobagyi GN, Ames FC, Buzdar AU, et al. Management of stage III primary breast cancer with primary chemotherapy, surgery, and radiation therapy. *Cancer.* 1988;62(12):2507–2516.

106. Rustogi A, Budrukkar A, Dinshaw K, Jalali R. Management of locally advanced breast cancer: evolution and current practice. *J Cancer Res Ther.* 2005;1(1):21–30.

107. Rivkin SE, Green S, Metch B, et al. Adjuvant CMFVP versus melphalan for operable breast cancer with positive axillary nodes: 10-year results of a Southwest Oncology Group Study. *J Clin Oncol.* 1989;7(9):1229–1238.

108. Armstrong DK, Fetting JH, Davidson NE, Gordon GB, Huelskamp AM, Abeloff MD. Sixteen week dose intense chemotherapy for inoperable, locally advanced breast cancer. *Breast Cancer Res Treat.* 1993;28(3):277–284.

109. Schwartz GF, Cantor RI, Biermann WA. Neoadjuvant chemotherapy before definitive treatment for stage III carcinoma of the breast. *Arch Surg.* 1987;122(12):1430–1434.

110. Huang EH, Tucker SL, Strom EA, et al. Postmastectomy radiation improves local-regional control and survival for selected patients with locally advanced breast cancer treated with neoadjuvant chemotherapy and mastectomy. *J Clin Oncol.* 2004; 22(23):4691–4699.

111. Abdel-Wahab M, Wolfson A, Raub W, et al. The importance of postoperative radiation therapy in multimodality management of locally advanced breast cancer: a phase II trial of neoadjuvant MVAC, surgery, and radiation. *Int J Radiat Oncol Biol Phys.* 1998;40(4):875–880.

112. Buchholz TA, Tucker SL, Masullo L, et al. Predictors of local-regional recurrence after neoadjuvant chemotherapy and mastectomy without radiation. *J Clin Oncol.* 2002;20(1):17–23.

113. Panades M, Olivotto IA, Speers CH, et al. Evolving treatment strategies for inflammatory breast cancer: a population-based survival analysis. *J Clin Oncol.* 2005;23(9):1941–1950.

114. Ring A, Webb A, Ashley S, et al. Is surgery necessary after complete clinical remission following neoadjuvant chemotherapy for early breast cancer? *J Clin Oncol.* 2003;21(24):4540–4545.

115. McGuire SE, Gonzalez-Angulo AM, Huang EH, et al. Postmastectomy radiation improves the outcome of patients with locally advanced breast cancer who achieve a pathologic complete response to neoadjuvant chemotherapy. *Int J Radiat Oncol Biol Phys.* 2007;68(4):1004–1009.

116. McCammon R, Finlayson C, Schwer A, Rabinovitch R. Impact of postmastectomy radiotherapy in T3N0 invasive carcinoma of the breast: a Surveillance, Epidemiology, and End Results database analysis. *Cancer.* 2008;113(4):683–689.

117. Green FL, Page DL, Flemming ID, et al. Breast. In: *AJCC Cancer Staging Manual*, 6th ed. New York, NY: Springer-Verlag; 2002:225–281.

118. Giordano S, Hortobagyi G. Locally advanced breast cancers: role of medical oncology. In: Bland KI, Copeland EM (eds). *The Breast*, 3rd ed. Philadelphia, PA: WB Saunders; 2004:1283–1300.

119. Buzdar AU, Singletary SE, Booser DJ, Frye DK, Wasaff B, Hortobagyi GN. Combined modality treatment of stage III and inflammatory breast cancer. M.D. Anderson Cancer Center experience. *Surg Oncol Clin N Am.* 1995;4(4):715–734.

120. Swain SM, Sorace RA, Bagley CS, et al. Neoadjuvant chemotherapy in the combined modality approach of locally advanced nonmetastatic breast cancer. *Cancer Res.* 1987;47(14):3889–3894.

121. Merajver SD, Weber BL, Cody R, et al. Breast conservation and prolonged chemotherapy for locally advanced breast cancer: the University of Michigan experience. *J Clin Oncol.* 1997; 15(8):2873–2881.

122. Jacquillat C, Baillet F, Weil M, et al. Results of a conservative treatment combining induction (neoadjuvant) and consolidation chemotherapy, hormonotherapy, and external and interstitial irradiation in 98 patients with locally advanced breast cancer (IIIA-IIIB). *Cancer.* 1988;61(10):1977–1982.

123. Cristofanilli M, Buzdar AU, Sneige N, et al. Paclitaxel in the multimodality treatment for inflammatory breast carcinoma. *Cancer.* 2001;92(7):1775–1782.

124. Perez CA, Fields JN, Fracasso PM, et al. Management of locally advanced carcinoma of the breast. II. Inflammatory carcinoma. *Cancer.* 1994;74(1 Suppl):466–476.

125. Thoms WW, Jr., McNeese MD, Fletcher GH, Buzdar AU, Singletary SE, Oswald MJ. Multimodal treatment for inflammatory breast cancer. *Int J Radiat Oncol Biol Phys.* 1989;17(4):739–745.

126. Smoot RL, Koch CA, Degnim AC, et al. A single-center experience with inflammatory breast cancer, 1985–2003. *Arch Surg.* 2006;141(6):567–572; discussion 72–73.

127. Baldini E, Gardin G, Evagelista G, Prochilo T, Collecchi P, Lionetto R. Long-term results of combined-modality therapy for inflammatory breast carcinoma. *Clin Breast Cancer.* 2004;5(5):358–363.

128. Bauer RL, Busch E, Levine E, Edge SB. Therapy for inflammatory breast cancer: impact of doxorubicin-based therapy. *Ann Surg Oncol.* 1995;2(4):288–294.

129. Fein DA, Mendenhall NP, Marsh RD, Bland KI, Copeland EM, 3rd, Million RR. Results of multimodality therapy for inflammatory breast cancer: an analysis of clinical and treatment factors affecting outcome. *Am Surg.* 1994;60(3):220–225.

130. Chevallier B, Bastit P, Graic Y, et al. The Centre H. Becquerel studies in inflammatory non metastatic breast cancer. Combined modality approach in 178 patients. *Br J Cancer.* 1993;67(3):594–601.

131. Brun B, Otmezguine Y, Feuilhade F, et al. Treatment of inflammatory breast cancer with combination chemotherapy and mastectomy versus breast conservation. *Cancer.* 1988;61(6):1096–1103.

132. Ueno NT, Buzdar AU, Singletary SE, et al. Combined-modality treatment of inflammatory breast carcinoma: twenty years of experience at M. D. Anderson Cancer Center. *Cancer Chemother Pharmacol.* 1997;40(4):321–329.

133. Harris EE, Schultz D, Bertsch H, Fox K, Glick J, Solin LJ. Ten-year outcome after combined modality therapy for inflammatory breast cancer. *Int J Radiat Oncol Biol Phys.* 2003;55(5):1200–1208.

134. Palangie T, Mosseri V, Mihura J, et al. Prognostic factors in inflammatory breast cancer and therapeutic implications. *Eur J Cancer.* 1994;30A(7):921–927.

135. Curcio LD, Rupp E, Williams WL, et al. Beyond palliative mastectomy in inflammatory breast cancer—a reassessment of margin status. *Ann Surg Oncol.* 1999;6(3):249–254.

136. Fleming RY, Asmar L, Buzdar AU, et al. Effectiveness of mastectomy by response to induction chemotherapy for control in inflammatory breast carcinoma. *Ann Surg Oncol.* 1997;4(6):452–461.

137. Jaiyesimi IA, Buzdar AU, Hortobagyi G. Inflammatory breast cancer: a review. *J Clin Oncol.* 1992;10(6):1014–1024.

138. Pisansky TM, Schaid DJ, Loprinzi CL, Donohue JH, Schray MF, Schomberg PJ. Inflammatory breast cancer: integration of irradiation, surgery, and chemotherapy. *Am J Clin Oncol.* 1992; 15(5):376–387.

139. De Boer RH, Allum WH, Ebbs SR, et al. Multimodality therapy in inflammatory breast cancer: is there a place for surgery? *Ann Oncol.* 2000;11(9):1147–1153.

140. Hasbini A, Le Pechoux C, Roche B, et al. [Alternating chemotherapy and hyperfractionated accelerated radiotherapy in nonmetastatic inflammatory breast cancer]. *Cancer Radiother.* 2000; 4(4):265–273.

141. Liao Z, Strom EA, Buzdar AU, et al. Locoregional irradiation for inflammatory breast cancer: effectiveness of dose escalation in decreasing recurrence. *Int J Radiat Oncol Biol Phys.* 2000; 47(5):1191–1200.

142. Gurney H, Harnett P, Kefford R, Boyages J. Inflammatory breast cancer: enhanced local control with hyperfractionated radiotherapy and infusional vincristine, ifosfamide and epirubicin. *Aust NZ J Med.* 1998;28(3):400–402.

Medical Oncology Treatment of Locally Advanced Breast Cancer

STEVEN J. ISAKOFF

The medical oncology management of locally advanced breast cancer (LABC) presents unique challenges particularly well suited for a multidisciplinary team approach. Treatment of patients with LABC requires careful pathological review; close coordination among medical, surgical, and radiation oncologists; and collaboration with breast radiologists in order to obtain the necessary information to make the most appropriate treatment decisions. When reconstruction is being considered, coordination is critical to ensure that planned anticancer therapy can be adequately delivered, along with appropriate reconstruction to achieve the best cosmetic result. The expertise of each discipline has a direct and important impact on the potential interventions that may be offered by the other specialties. Success therefore requires effective communication among healthcare team members. The treatment of LABC involving large tumors or inflammatory breast cancer (IBC) often requires neoadjuvant chemotherapy (also called primary systemic therapy) followed by definitive local and regional therapy with surgery and radiation.

■ DIAGNOSIS AND STAGING EVALUATION

The term "locally advanced breast cancer" generally refers to stage 3 breast cancer (any tumor size with 4 or more nodes or supraclavicular nodes, or T3N1, or any T4, including IBC; see Section 4.4 for details on staging). Alternatively, LABC may also refer to any breast cancer for which primary surgery with lumpectomy or mastectomy is unlikely to yield clear margins, such as a large T3N0 tumor. The incidence of LABC has declined in populations with adequate screening programs and with the increased use of mammography. However, in underserved and uninsured populations LABC presents in up to 50% of patients according to some estimates and therefore remains a significant problem in the United States and other countries. For example, one study of patients at a large public city hospital in the United States noted that 16% of Caucasian and 19% of African American patients presented with LABC, compared with national statistics from the Surveillance, Epidemiology and End Results (SEER) data of 4.2% and 6.5%, respectively (1).

LABC often presents on clinical exam or by patient identification of a mass, although routine mammographic screening remains an important tool and may be the initial method of detection. Clinical staging by physical exam may reveal T4 tumors extending to the chest wall or skin, with ulceration, skin nodules, edema, or signs of IBC (see below). In addition, matted ipsilateral axillary nodes or palpable infraclavicular or supraclavicular nodes may be identified. Commonly, however, the presence of stage 3 disease is not evident by clinical exam and is realized only after definitive surgery, when the full extent of the lymph node involvement is known.

The initial diagnosis and workup of LABC should include history, physical exam, blood work to assess liver function and blood counts, and diagnostic mammogram and ultrasound. All suspicious ipsilateral or contralateral lesions should be biopsied before initiating neoadjuvant therapy. At the time of initial diagnosis, patients with LABC should be staged with imaging according to the guidelines of the National Comprehensive Cancer Network (NCCN). Generally, most patients with LABC should undergo chest and abdominal computed tomography (CT) imaging and radionucleotide bone scan. The utility of positron-emission tomography (PET)/CT scans is the subject of ongoing investigation, but they are generally considered unnecessary in the initial evaluation of LABC unless there is a specific clinical question left unanswered by other imaging studies. Because of the relatively higher risk of stage 4 disease in patients who present with LABC and the potential impact on treatment decisions, suspicious sites identified on staging scans should be biopsied if clinically feasible. Each member of the multidisciplinary team should have an opportunity to evaluate the patient before definitive treatment plans are made to ensure that the necessary pathology, clinical information, and other data will be obtained prior to making final treatment plans.

■ TREATMENT OVERVIEW

Combined modality treatment is the mainstay of modern approaches to effective therapy for LABC. This approach was introduced by the Milan group, who demonstrated that induction chemotherapy produced very high rates of clinical objective responses (2). The decision to proceed with primary surgery depends on the initial clinical staging and imaging. LABC can be further divided into a subset considered operable that is likely to achieve pathologically negative margins and initial disease control, and a subset deemed inoperable, where initial surgery is unlikely to achieve disease control. Generally, operable LABC includes clinical stage 3A limited to T3N1 disease, whereas inoperable LABC includes the remainder of stage 3A and stages 3B and 3C. Patients with operable LABC who proceed to initial surgery are treated with adjuvant therapy similarly to patients with stage 2 disease. An underlying theme in the treatment of LABC is that effective systemic therapies are required given the high rates of systemic recurrence. Traditionally, the initial systemic therapy of choice for patients requiring neoadjuvant treatment has been chemotherapy. However, endocrine therapy is being recognized increasingly as a reasonable option for selected patients with hormone receptor (HR)–positive cancer.

■ NEOADJUVANT OR ADJUVANT THERAPY

Neoadjuvant chemotherapy is the preferred approach in many patients with LABC in order to accomplish several goals. A major goal is to allow breast-conserving therapy (BCT) in women who present with large tumors who would otherwise be candidates for mastectomy. In this setting, preoperative chemotherapy may reduce the tumor size and increase the chance of obtaining clear margins. A second goal is to convert an inoperable tumor to one that can be successfully removed with surgery. This may occur in cases where even a mastectomy is unlikely to result in clear margins. This situation commonly arises when the chest wall is involved or with IBC. Additional theoretical advantages of preoperative chemotherapy include: earlier initiation of systemic treatment to prevent micrometastatic growth, inhibition of metastatic tumor growth that has been described to occur after the primary tumor is removed, ability to assess response to therapy in vivo, and the ability to deliver chemotherapy through an intact vasculature. However, potential disadvantages of neoadjuvant therapy include delay of definitive local therapy in patients who are nonresponders and selection for resistance in the setting of a larger tumor burden. Furthermore, full local-regional staging in this setting is limited to clinical findings rather than pathological staging. Other than improvement in rates of breast conservation, additional clinical advantages have not yet been universally demonstrated for the patient. The benefits and challenges of neoadjuvant therapy were the subject of a National Cancer Institute Consensus Panel Conference that concluded that a multidisciplinary approach improves outcomes for patients who are candidates for neoadjuvant therapy (3).

One additional potential benefit from preoperative therapy is to provide prognostic information about a tumor. The concept proposed decades ago that micrometastases are present at the time of diagnosis leads to the prediction that response to neoadjuvant therapy may be a surrogate marker for response of the micrometastatic deposits. This is supported by the dramatic improvement in long-term outcome among patients who achieve a pathological complete response (pCR) after neoadjuvant therapy. Numerous studies have shown that patients who achieve a pCR have an excellent prognosis in all subgroups of breast cancer. For example, one retrospective study demonstrated that in patients unselected for breast cancer subtype, the 5- and 10-year overall survival was 91.1% and 91.1%, respectively, among patients who achieved a pCR, compared with 79.7% and 45%, respectively, among those who did not achieve a pCR (4). When broken down by subgroup, only 8% of HR+ patients achieved a pCR, compared with 24% of HR– patients. Nevertheless, HR+ patients who achieved a pCR had a 96.4% 5-year overall survival, compared with 84.5% for those without a pCR. In the HR– group, a pCR resulted in a 5-year overall survival of 83.9%, compared with 67.4% in those without a pCR (4). Studies of triple-negative breast cancer (TNBC) revealed a statistically non-significant difference in 3-year overall survival of 98% and 94% for non-TNBC and TNBC patients achieving a pCR, respectively (5). However, for TNBC patients who did not achieve a pCR, the 3-year overall survival was significantly worse than for non-TNBC patients who did not achieve a pCR (overall survival 68% versus 88%). With the demonstration of robust activity of trastuzumab in the metastatic setting, numerous phase II studies with trastuzumab in the neoadjuvant setting have consistently shown a pCR rate in the range of 25% with 12 weeks of therapy (6–8) but as high as 67% to 75% (9,10) with prolonged therapy.

The definition of pCR has varied among studies and continues to evolve, but the most rigorous current definition requires that no residual invasive cancer remains at the primary tumor site or in the ipsilateral axillary lymph nodes. Residual ductal carcinoma in situ (DCIS) following neoadjuvant therapy is not considered in the determination of pCR. The presence of positive axillary nodes after neoadjuvant therapy is an important predictor of adverse long-term outcome (11,12). In one study of 152 patients with cytologically proven positive axillary nodal disease by fine-needle aspiration prior to treatment, the presence of residual invasive tumor in axillary nodes following therapy reduced the 5-year distant disease-free survival (DFS) from 73.5% to 48.7% (12).

The multidisciplinary approach to neoadjuvant therapy allows patients to be carefully monitored so that an ineffective treatment program can be modified to a more effective strategy. Patients who progress during neoadjuvant therapy represent a particularly worrisome group, and monitoring by the team may prompt earlier salvage therapy. Patients with operable breast cancer may be able to proceed directly to mastectomy in order to achieve clear margins and can then complete adjuvant chemotherapy. Inoperable patients who progress after neoadjuvant therapy may proceed to palliative radiation to attempt local control and then continue to receive additional adjuvant chemotherapy. Certain chemotherapy agents, such as capecitabine, may be used as a radiosensitizer in such cases, but the overall benefit of such approaches is not well established in these refractory tumors.

During the course of neoadjuvant chemotherapy, the medical oncologist is generally responsible for the overall monitoring of the clinical response to neoadjuvant therapy. The clinical utility of imaging compared with physical exam to monitor response to neoadjuvant therapy is not proven. Outside of a clinical trial, following RECIST (Response Evaluation Criteria in Solid Tumors) guidelines to monitor tumor response is not clinically very useful when making management decisions. Several studies have evaluated mammography, ultrasonography, magnetic resonance imaging (MRI), and PET imaging to predict pathological response (13,14). PET imaging after two cycles of therapy had reasonably high sensitivity (89%), specificity (95%), and negative predictive value (85%) as a surrogate marker to predict pathological response, allowing for relatively early assessment of treatment efficacy (13). However, PET has not been correlated with long-term clinical outcomes. Preoperative MRI after neoadjuvant therapy had a 55% concordance with the degree of pathological response (14). Preoperative imaging after neoadjuvant therapy may assist in surgical planning in certain cases.

Although one theoretical benefit of neoadjuvant treatment mentioned above is earlier initiation of systemic therapy to treat potential micrometastatic disease, data from several large studies comparing neoadjuvant with adjuvant therapy demonstrate no significant difference in long-term outcomes. Recent updates from the National Surgical Adjuvant Breast and Bowel Project (NSABP) B-18 and B-27 trials continue to demonstrate no difference in outcome in patients who received chemotherapy before or after surgery (15). A meta-analysis of nearly 4,000 patients confirmed that neoadjuvant and adjuvant therapies had equivalent DFS and overall survival (16).

Numerous studies have also shown that breast-conserving surgery can be appropriate for a subset of patients treated for LABC. Patients selected for breast conservation after neoadjuvant treatment of LABC should meet certain criteria, including resolution of skin changes, residual tumor size less than 5 cm, no chest wall involvement, no extensive microcalcifications, and predicted likelihood of clear margins. Observation by the breast surgeon throughout the course of treatment, alongside the medical oncologist, is often very useful for optimizing choice of surgery and reconstructive options. Although many studies support the improvement in breast conservation rates

after neoadjuvant therapy, a large phase III randomized study designed to directly compare outcomes after neoadjuvant therapy for LABC treated with breast conservation or mastectomy closed early for poor accrual (17). Local recurrence rates at 5 and 10 years after breast-conserving surgery following neoadjuvant therapy were 16% and 22%, compared with 6% and 12% in those who had mastectomy. Nevertheless, long-term survival among patients with conservative surgery is similar to that following mastectomy. Factors affecting the risk of local recurrence include the presence of lymphatic and vascular invasion, lymph node status, and whether radiation therapy was delivered to the lumpectomy site. Patients experiencing local-regional recurrence remain at high risk for systemic relapse.

■ CHEMOTHERAPY

The benefit of polychemotherapy for long-term outcome in LABC is now well established from the Oxford overview meta-analyses, which showed that all subgroups of breast cancer receive benefit (18). Randomized data from the NSABP demonstrate that long-term outcomes are similar regardless of whether the same regimen is given either before or after surgery. Participation in a clinical trial should be encouraged when available; in the absence of a clinical trial, there are numerous regimens that have been explored in the neoadjuvant setting. A standard approach that we favor and that is supported by the NCCN guidelines is to select the most appropriate regimen that otherwise would be given in the adjuvant setting and simply deliver the regimen preoperatively. The rationale for this approach is that the selection of a regimen supported by large randomized adjuvant trials is reasonable to serve as the backbone of neoadjuvant therapy. There is no evidence to date that tailoring a regimen to response during treatment affords a DFS or overall survival advantage. However, prospectively defined programs do differ in effectiveness in terms of long-term results.

In many centers the standard regimens include anthracycline-based polychemotherapy. Regional differences may guide the choice of doxorubicin or epirubicin, but results are generally similar. Common combinations include doxorubicin and cyclophosphamide with or without fluorouracil (CAF), or epirubicin, cyclophosphamide, and fluorouracil (FEC). The use of taxanes in the neoadjuvant setting also should follow recommendations for adjuvant chemotherapy regimens. Taxanes are often added to anthracycline-based regimens in either sequential or concurrent fashion. For example, the adjuvant use of sequential paclitaxel for four cycles following doxorubicin and cyclophosphamide (AC) was established in the Cancer and Leukemia Group B (CALGB) 9344 trial (19), and the benefit of administering the regimen in a dose-dense fashion was further supported in CALGB 9741 (20). The concurrent use of docetaxel, doxorubicin, and cyclophosphamide (TAC) is also a well-established regimen that may be delivered in the neoadjuvant setting (21).

The use of taxanes in the neoadjuvant setting has had conflicting results. The TAX-301 study randomized patients to four cycles of doxorubicin, cyclophosphamide, vincristine, and prednisolone (CAVP) followed by randomization to either an additional four cycles of CAVP or to four cycles of docetaxel. The results of the docetaxel arm were superior, with a pCR rate of 34%, compared with 16%, an increased clinical response rate, and improved 5-year overall survival of 97%, compared with 78% (22). On the other hand, the NSABP B-27 trial showed no long-term benefit from the addition of docetaxel to AC therapy. Patients in this study were randomized into three arms. All arms received preoperative AC with either no further chemotherapy, sequential docetaxel and then surgery, or surgery with adjuvant docetaxel. Addition of docetaxel did increase the response rate twofold, but there was no overall survival benefit with the addition of docetaxel in either arm compared with AC alone (23). A number of factors may explain these results, which are not consistent with many other studies showing a benefit of adjuvant taxanes. Thus, for patients with LABC who are at high risk for recurrence, the addition of taxanes remains an integral component of therapy.

How long to treat with neoadjuvant chemotherapy remains unknown. On the one hand, treatment with a standard adjuvant regimen in the neoadjuvant setting may be sufficient to achieve a desired clinical response. However, several studies suggest that prolonged neoadjuvant treatment may result in increased pCR rates, raising the question of whether they would result in improvements in overall survival. The GeparTrio study is important to help define the effect of different treatment lengths and strategies (24,25). In this trial, all patients received two cycles of TAC chemotherapy. Patients were then stratified into responders and nonresponders. The responders were then randomized to receive either four or six additional cycles of TAC. The nonresponders were randomized to receive four more cycles of TAC or to switch to vinorelbine plus capecitabine. In the responder group, the extended TAC regimen achieved a similar pCR rate to the shorter regimen, suggesting more cycles of chemotherapy may not result in higher pCR. Interestingly, however, in the nonresponder group, 20% of the patients randomized to the TAC arm achieved a clinical complete response, though the pCR rate was similar in the TAC and vinorelbine/capecitabine arms (5.3% and 6%, respectively). Despite the relatively low pCR, continued chemotherapy resulted in similar rates of breast conservation. The benefit of extended neoadjuvant therapy remains less studied with targeted therapy. The ongoing CALGB 40601

study compares preoperative paclitaxel with trastuzumab alone, lapatinib alone, or the combination. The weekly regimen has been extended in this trial to 16 weeks from the standard 12 on the hypothesis that prolonged neoadjuvant therapy with targeted biologics will improve the response rate.

In most situations, regimens in the neoadjuvant setting that have not been validated in randomized long-term studies are best left for use only in the context of clinical trials. When no trial exists, selection of an established adjuvant regimen in the neoadjuvant setting is usually the most appropriate choice of therapy. However, with the recognition that different subtypes of breast cancer have different responses to neoadjuvant chemotherapy, and with improvements in understanding which tumors benefit most from different adjuvant regimens, treatment for LABC is now most appropriately individualized to the specific breast cancer subtype (see below).

Endocrine Receptor–Positive/HER2-Negative Breast Cancer

The relative value of chemotherapy in HR+, HER2– tumors has been the subject of much controversy. In the adjuvant setting, for example, a meta-analysis of eight studies suggested that few if any HR+, HER2– tumors derive benefit from anthracycline-based regimens (26), and a meta-analysis of three CALGB studies suggested HR+ patients derive significantly less relative benefit than HR– patients (27). In the neoadjuvant setting, a retrospective analysis of more than 1,700 patients found that only 8% of HR+ tumors achieved a pCR compared with 24% in HR– tumors (4). Similarly, the European Cooperative Trial found that among patients who received doxorubicin and paclitaxel followed by CMF, the HR+ group achieved a pCR rate of 12% compared with 42% in the HR– group. Subgroup analysis from several studies have called into question the value of adding taxanes to anthracyclines in HR+ tumors, suggesting that the estrogen receptor (ER)–positive tumors derived relatively little benefit from the addition of paclitaxel following AC (28). However, other studies suggest the addition of taxanes does improve outcome in the adjuvant setting and pCR in the HR+ tumors in the neoadjuvant setting. The NSABP B-27 trial looked at pCR rates by ER status in each arm (29). In the HR+ patients who received preoperative AC, the pCR was 5.7%, compared with 14.1% when docetaxel was added preoperatively. The HR– subgroup had higher overall pCR but also had a similar improvement with the addition of docetaxel (13.6% versus 22.8%). Interestingly, the improved pCR rate with the addition of docetaxel in either HR+ or HR– settings did not translate into improvements in overall survival, in disagreement with other studies in which pCR correlates with overall survival (23). A pooled analysis of seven studies including 1,079 patients found that HR+ patients had pCR rates of 8.8% and 2% with and without taxanes, though HR– patients had pCR rates of 29% and 15% with and without taxanes. Therefore, although pCR rates are generally lower in the HR+ subgroup, clinically meaningful responses are seen, and taxanes appear to improve response rates, supporting the use of polychemotherapy regimens in HR+ LABC. The exception may be invasive lobular LABC, which demonstrated only 3% pCR in a retrospective study in which more than 90% of the tumors were HR+ (30).

Triple-Negative Breast Cancer

TNBC accounts for approximately 15% of all new breast cancer diagnoses. The recognition that this subtype of breast cancer has a relatively worse prognosis than HR+ or HER2+ breast cancer has spurred efforts to identify the optimal regimen for triple-negative LABC. No specific therapies yet exist that are validated for TNBC, though identification of potential targets is an active area of research. TNBC paradoxically demonstrates a higher response rate to neoadjuvant chemotherapy yet has a higher risk of recurrence. In a study of 107 patients who received neoadjuvant AC, 32% of tumors were basal-like and 58% were luminal (which are approximate surrogates for TNBC and HR+ tumors, respectively). The pCR rate for the basal tumors was 27%, compared with only 7% of the ER+ tumors. However, the basal tumors had worse overall survival and DFS, while the subgroup of patients who achieved a pCR had a significantly improved outcome. These data support the notion that TNBC represent a heterogeneous group of cancers with variable sensitivity to established chemotherapy regimens.

Recently, platinum agents have been reemerging as chemotherapeutics for breast cancer that may have particular activity in the TNBC subtype. This trend arises in part from the observation that most *BRCA1* carriers develop TNBC and that in vitro *BRCA1* tumors are platinum sensitive. This observation has led to the hypothesis that sporadic TNBC and *BRCA1*-deficient breast cancer may behave functionally as phenocopies. A neoadjuvant study in 28 patients with TNBC examined the pCR rate after treatment with four cycles of single-agent cisplatin and found that 6 (24%) achieved a pCR, including 2 of 2 *BRCA1* mutation carriers (31). A subsequent study of 51 patients with TNBC who received neoadjuvant cisplatin and bevacizumab resulted in a pCR rate of 16%, and 37% had a pCR or near-complete response (32). A provocative study from Poland treated 25 patients with *BRCA1*-associated breast cancer with four cycles of neoadjuvant cisplatin and reported a 72% pCR rate (33). While these single-agent responses are encouraging, outside of a clinical trial there is insufficient evidence to recommend routine use of platinum agents for TNBC in the adjuvant or neoadjuvant setting.

HER2-Positive Breast Cancer

The integration of trastuzumab into the adjuvant and neoadjuvant settings has dramatically improved outcomes for HER2+ tumors. The treatment of HER2+ LABC should include trastuzumab-based chemotherapy regimens. There have been many studies evaluating the benefit of preoperative trastuzumab using a variety of combinations and schedules. The common theme among all of the HER2+ neoadjuvant trials is that the addition of trastuzumab has resulted in increased clinical and pathological responses. For example, the MD Anderson group demonstrated an increase in pCR from 25% to 67% with the addition of trastuzumab to four cycles of paclitaxel followed by four cycles of fluorouracil, epirubicin, and cyclophosphamide in a phase III trial (9). Most studies, however, demonstrate more modest pCR rates, which may be due to overall shorter courses of neoadjuvant therapy, with the remainder given as adjuvant therapy. Additional examples of regimens that have been explored in the phase II setting include: weekly vinorelbine plus trastuzumab, FEC/trastuzumab, docetaxel/carboplatin/trastuzumab (TCH), and paclitaxel weekly plus trastuzumab. Ongoing clinical trials are evaluating the use of the newer anti-HER2 agent lapatinib with or without trastuzumab as neoadjuvant chemotherapy.

■ INFLAMMATORY BREAST CANCER

IBC represents approximately 1.3% to 2.5% of new breast cancer diagnoses, and the incidence has been increasing slowly in the United States (34). Some populations, such as that of Tunisia, may have an IBC incidence of up to 50%. Whether IBC represents a clinical subset of LABC or is a distinct molecular and pathological entity remains controversial and is the subject of much research. Nevertheless, it is more common in African Americans and younger patients and has a relatively poor prognosis compared with other forms of LABC. Median survival after a diagnosis of IBC is approximately 2.9 years in some studies. The diagnosis of IBC is based solely on clinical evidence, although a uniform definition is lacking. IBC is characterized by invasive breast cancer with erythema and edema of the breast, with a classic peau d'orange appearance involving more than one third of the skin that develops relatively rapidly over a few weeks. Many patients may have no discrete mass on clinical exam. Histopathological analysis of the skin may reveal dermal lymphatic invasion, but this is not required for the clinical diagnosis. IBC may be of ductal or lobular histology, as well as the rare small cell, large cell, or medullary carcinomas. Overexpression of HER2 occurs more frequently in IBC, as does lack of HR expression and high-grade histology. The clinical findings are the result of tumor emboli in dermal lymphatics and a propensity for cells to disseminate systemically, accounting for the high rates of distant metastases. A tissue diagnosis of invasive breast cancer must be made to confirm the diagnosis.

Combined multimodality treatment with neoadjuvant chemotherapy, surgery, and radiation has emerged as the backbone of treatment for IBC. The optimal chemotherapy regimen for IBC is not established, although anthracycline-containing regimens have emerged as a standard. Patients who achieve a pCR to neoadjuvant therapy for IBC have significantly improved five-year survival of nearly 90%. The sequential use of anthracyclines and taxanes is an effective strategy, with an overall response rate of 82% achieved in a neoadjuvant study of four cycles of fluorouracil, doxorubicin, and cyclophosphamide followed by four cycles of paclitaxel. Although not specifically evaluated in IBC, the adjuvant regimen of dose-dense AC followed by paclitaxel either every 2 weeks or weekly is a reasonable option to treat IBC. For IBC overexpressing HER2, the addition of trastuzumab to chemotherapy has improved pCR rates. Trastuzumab delivered with three cycles of FEC followed by three cycles of paclitaxel results in an impressive 55% pCR rate. A phase II study evaluating lapatinib and paclitaxel for 12 weeks resulted in a clinical response rate of 95%, leading to further studies to validate this approach. Following neoadjuvant therapy the multidisciplinary team should work together to ensure adequate local therapy is achieved with mastectomy followed by radiation and continuation of appropriate adjuvant therapy.

■ ADJUVANT THERAPY AFTER NEOADJUVANT THERAPY

Residual disease after neoadjuvant therapy predicts high likelihood for distant recurrence. Therefore, an important unanswered question is whether additional chemotherapy would improve outcomes for these patients with apparent chemotherapy-resistant disease despite having received an appropriate standard regimen. In patients who did not receive a full course of a standard adjuvant therapy preoperatively, it is reasonable to complete the course of treatment in the adjuvant setting. For patients who do complete an acceptable standard regimen preoperatively but have significant residual disease, there are no clear data to guide clinical management, and the standard approach is to offer no further therapy. A pilot study demonstrated that an antiangiogenic approach using additional chemotherapy with metronomic oral cyclophosphamide and methotrexate with bevacizumab postoperatively was well tolerated (35). Additional trials are needed to answer the important question of whether additional chemotherapy will improve recurrence-free survival in patients with poor response to neoadjuvant therapy. In patients who progress

during neoadjuvant therapy and who do not complete their intended course of preoperative chemotherapy, additional adjuvant chemotherapy is considered standard to allow patients the opportunity to complete an established adjuvant regimen, although data providing proof of efficacy of this approach are lacking.

■ ENDOCRINE THERAPY

Patients with endocrine-responsive tumors (ER+ or progesterone receptor–positive) should receive adjuvant endocrine therapy with either tamoxifen or an aromatase inhibitor. The use of adjuvant endocrine therapy is discussed in Section 7.3. In HR+ LABC, neoadjuvant endocrine therapy is emerging as a viable treatment option that may have outcomes comparable to those of chemotherapy. The ideal setting to use neoadjuvant endocrine therapy is not established, but for carefully selected patients it may be a treatment of choice. For example, chemotherapy may be contraindicated in certain patients with LABC due to comorbid conditions, patient age, or preference. Several studies have evaluated the utility of neoadjuvant endocrine therapy in the management of LABC. Together, the studies suggest that while response rates may be acceptable, endocrine therapy is unlikely to yield pCR. In addition, because of the often prolonged time to elicit a response to neoadjuvant endocrine therapy compared with chemotherapy, most patients receiving neoadjuvant endocrine therapy will often wait at least four to six months before definitive surgery can be achieved. The timing of surgery after neoadjuvant endocrine therapy is based on physical exam findings. Therefore, close coordination between medical and surgical oncology is required, and patients should follow closely with both so that a collaborative decision can be made regarding timing of surgery.

Several studies demonstrate the potential benefits of neoadjuvant endocrine therapy. In one study, 239 postmenopausal women with large HR+ LABC were randomized to doxorubicin and paclitaxel for four cycles or an aromatase inhibitor for three months. Clinical response by palpation was 64% in each group, and pCR rate was similar between chemotherapy and endocrine therapy (6% and 3%, respectively). Local recurrence at three years was 3% in each group. However, the rate of breast-conserving surgery was actually greater in the endocrine therapy group (33% versus 24%). This study suggests that hormone therapy may be at least as good as chemotherapy in this population. The superiority of aromatase inhibitors over tamoxifen seen in the adjuvant and metastatic setting is replicated in the neoadjuvant setting. A meta-analysis of more than 1,100 patients revealed an improvement in clinical response and breast-conserving surgery in favor of aromatase inhibitors over tamoxifen (36). Furthermore, the IMPACT (immediate preoperative anastrozole, tamoxifen, or combined with tamoxifen) study compared neoadjuvant anastrozole with tamoxifen or the combination in 330 women with operable or LABC (37). There was no significant difference in the objective response. However, twice as many women were deemed candidates for breast conservation in the anastrozole arm as in the tamoxifen arm (44% versus 22%). Interestingly, in the HER2+ subgroup, the objective response was higher in the anastrozole arm, although the difference was not statistically significant (58% versus 22%, $P = 0.18$). Aromatase inhibitor therapy is effective in lobular LABC. In 59 LABC lobular cancers, a 68% reduction in ultrasound-measured volume was seen. The ongoing ACOSOG Z1031 study is randomizing 375 patients to one of three aromatase inhibitors to receive 16 to 18 weeks of neoadjuvant therapy. This study will be followed by a phase III study designed to compare neoadjuvant endocrine therapy with neoadjuvant chemotherapy. Until the planned phase III trial comparing neoadjuvant endocrine therapy and chemotherapy is completed, neoadjuvant endocrine therapy should be considered an effective approach for the treatment of HR+ LABC and may be preferred in select patients with contraindications to chemotherapy.

FOLLOW-UP AND RECURRENT DISEASE

Although patients with LABC who are able successfully to undergo surgery to clear margins are still at high risk for systemic recurrence, current guidelines do not recommend routine screening for recurrence with imaging or tumor markers. Patients should be followed closely by the multidisciplinary team according to consensus group guidelines, and new areas of concern should be evaluated with biopsy and imaging as necessary. The management of metastatic breast cancer is discussed in Chapter 10. However, for local-regional recurrence, a variety of treatment options exist, depending on the course of prior therapy. At diagnosis of a local or regional recurrence, full staging studies are recommended to assess for systemic disease. The absence of overt metastatic disease does not diminish the high risk of systemic recurrence that exists in these patients. Nevertheless, in the absence of evidence of metastatic disease, aggressive local treatment should be pursued.

CONCLUSIONS

LABC remains a significant problem, particularly in medically underserved populations. A multidisciplinary team approach is important to provide combined modality treatment involving chemotherapy, surgery, and radiation. Inoperable disease upfront can often be rendered

operable with neoadjuvant chemotherapy. Potential advantages of neoadjuvant therapy include: increased likelihood of successful surgery, increased rates of breast conservation, assessment of treatment effect to provide prognostic information, and earlier treatment of micrometastatic disease. Treatment should be individualized for patients on the basis of the subtype of breast cancer (HR and HER2 status), extent of disease, and individual patient features. Polychemotherapy with anthracycline-based and taxane-based regimens remains the standard of care for most patients with LABC and has shown benefit in all subgroups regardless of receptor status. In general, standard adjuvant treatment regimens are reasonable options to deliver as neoadjuvant therapy. HER2+ patients should receive trastuzumab-based neoadjuvant therapy, which has shown dramatic improvements in outcome. The use of platinum agents for TNBC is not established and is still considered investigational. Patients who experience a pCR to neoadjuvant chemotherapy have significantly improved DFS and overall survival. Patients who do not respond to neoadjuvant chemotherapy are at high risk for local and systemic recurrence and should proceed to salvage therapy with alternative neoadjuvant systemic therapy or radiation therapy followed by surgery if possible. Patients with IBC should proceed to mastectomy and radiation following neoadjuvant therapy and are not appropriate candidates for breast conservation. Neoadjuvant endocrine therapy may be appropriate for patients with reduced organ function, older age, or other characteristics that present excess risk from initial chemotherapy or surgery. Although pCR rates are low with endocrine therapy, clinical responses and long-term outcomes may be similar to those for chemotherapy in select populations. Following the upfront combined modality therapy, patients should receive appropriate adjuvant therapy, with endocrine therapy for HR+ tumors and trastuzumab for HER2+ tumors. The benefit of additional adjuvant chemotherapy in patients with significant residual disease after neoadjuvant therapy is unknown, but currently additional chemotherapy is generally not delivered. Despite its challenges, the treatment of LABC with neoadjuvant therapy presents robust opportunities to conduct translational research studies to help improve therapeutic strategies and enhance our basic understanding of breast cancer biology (discussed in the next section).

SUMMARY

- LABC should be assessed by surgeons, medical oncologists, and radiation oncologists prospectively prior to initiation of therapy. Medical oncologists will play a leading role in determining initial systemic treatment.
- Radiological staging studies per NCCN guidelines are advised for LABC patients, as for stage 3 patients.

- Chemotherapy should be initiated as an attempt to attain a major clinical response. Treatment should be individualized on the basis of breast cancer subtype to achieve the highest chance of pCR.
- pCR in general predicts improved DFS and overall survival, although many patients with HR+ disease who do not achieve a pCR will have prolonged DFS with adjuvant endocrine therapy.
- Trials with translational science incorporated should be considered wherever possible when patients are to be treated with neoadjuvant chemotherapy.

■ REFERENCES

1. Naik AM, Joseph K, Harris M, Davis C, Shapiro R, Hiotis KL. Indigent breast cancer patients among all racial and ethnic groups present with more advanced disease compared with nationally reported data. *Am J Surg.* 2003;186(4):400–403.

2. De Lena M, Zucali R, Viganotti G, Valagussa P, Bonadonna G. Combined chemotherapy-radiotherapy approach in locally advanced (T3b-T4) breast cancer. *Cancer Chemother Pharmacol.* 1978;1(1):53–59.

3. Buchholz TA, Lehman CD, Harris JR, et al. Statement of the science concerning locoregional treatments after preoperative chemotherapy for breast cancer: a National Cancer Institute conference. *J Clin Oncol.* 2008;26(5):791–797.

4. Guarneri V, Broglio K, Kau SW, et al. Prognostic value of pathologic complete response after primary chemotherapy in relation to hormone receptor status and other factors. *J Clin Oncol.* 2006;24(7):1037–1044.

5. Liedtke C, Mazouni C, Hess KR, et al. Response to neoadjuvant therapy and long-term survival in patients with triple-negative breast cancer. *J Clin Oncol.* 2008;26(8):1275–1281.

6. Burstein HJ, Harris LN, Gelman R, et al. Preoperative therapy with trastuzumab and paclitaxel followed by sequential adjuvant doxorubicin/cyclophosphamide for HER2 overexpressing stage II or III breast cancer: a pilot study. *J Clin Oncol.* 2003;21(1):46–53.

7. Harris LN, You F, Schnitt SJ, et al. Predictors of resistance to preoperative trastuzumab and vinorelbine for HER2-positive early breast cancer. *Clin Cancer Res.* 2007;13(4):1198–1207.

8. Kelly H, Kimmick G, Dees EC, et al. Response and cardiac toxicity of trastuzumab given in conjunction with weekly paclitaxel after doxorubicin/cyclophosphamide. *Clin Breast Cancer.* 2006;7(3):237–243.

9. Buzdar AU, Ibrahim NK, Francis D, et al. Significantly higher pathologic complete remission rate after neoadjuvant therapy with trastuzumab, paclitaxel, and epirubicin chemotherapy: results of a randomized trial in human epidermal growth factor receptor 2-positive operable breast cancer. *J Clin Oncol.* 2005; 23(16):3676–3685.

10. Paluch-Shimon S, Wolf I, Goldberg H, et al. High efficacy of pre-operative trastuzumab combined with paclitaxel following doxorubicin & cyclophosphamide in operable breast cancer. *Acta Oncol (Stockholm).* 2008;47(8):1564–1569.

11. McCready DR, Hortobagyi GN, Kau SW, Smith TL, Buzdar AU, Balch CM. The prognostic significance of lymph node metastases after preoperative chemotherapy for locally advanced breast cancer. *Arch Surg.* 1989;124(1):21–25.

12. Rouzier R, Extra JM, Klijanienko J, et al. Incidence and prognostic significance of complete axillary downstaging after primary chemotherapy in breast cancer patients with T1 to T3 tumors and cytologically proven axillary metastatic lymph nodes. *J Clin Oncol.* 2002;20(5):1304–1310.

13. Rousseau C, Devillers A, Sagan C, et al. Monitoring of early response to neoadjuvant chemotherapy in stage II and III breast cancer by [^{18}F]fluorodeoxyglucose positron emission tomography. *J Clin Oncol.* 2006;24(34):5366–5372.

14. Yeh E, Slanetz P, Kopans DB, et al. Prospective comparison of mammography, sonography, and MRI in patients undergoing neoadjuvant chemotherapy for palpable breast cancer. *AJR.* 2005;184(3):868–877.

15. Rastogi P, Anderson SJ, Bear HD, et al. Preoperative chemotherapy: updates of National Surgical Adjuvant Breast and Bowel Project Protocols B-18 and B-27. *J Clin Oncol.* 2008;26(5):778–785.

16. Mauri D, Pavlidis N, Ioannidis JP. Neoadjuvant versus adjuvant systemic treatment in breast cancer: a meta-analysis. *J Natl Cancer Inst.* 2005;97(3):188–194.

17. Sinacki M, Jassem J, van Tienhoven G. Conservative local treatment versus mastectomy after induction chemotherapy in locally advanced breast cancer: a randomised phase III study (EORTC 10974/22002, LAMANOMA)—why did this study fail? *Eur J Cancer.* 2005;41(18):2787–2788.

18. Effects of chemotherapy and hormonal therapy for early breast cancer on recurrence and 15-year survival: an overview of the randomised trials. *Lancet.* 2005;365(9472):1687–1717.

19. Henderson IC, Berry DA, Demetri GD, et al. Improved outcomes from adding sequential Paclitaxel but not from escalating Doxorubicin dose in an adjuvant chemotherapy regimen for patients with node-positive primary breast cancer. *J Clin Oncol.* 2003;21(6):976–983.

20. Citron ML, Berry DA, Cirrincione C, et al. Randomized trial of dose-dense versus conventionally scheduled and sequential versus concurrent combination chemotherapy as postoperative adjuvant treatment of node-positive primary breast cancer: first report of Intergroup Trial C9741/Cancer and Leukemia Group B Trial 9741. *J Clin Oncol.* 2003;21(8):1431–1439.

21. Martin M, Pienkowski T, Mackey J, et al. Adjuvant docetaxel for node-positive breast cancer. *New Engl J Med.* 2005; 352(22):2302–2313.

22. Heys SD, Sarkar T, Hutcheon AW. Primary docetaxel chemotherapy in patients with breast cancer: impact on response and survival. *Breast Cancer Res Treat.* 2005;90(2):169–185.

23. Bear HD, Anderson S, Smith RE, et al. Sequential preoperative or postoperative docetaxel added to preoperative doxorubicin plus cyclophosphamide for operable breast cancer: National Surgical Adjuvant Breast and Bowel Project Protocol B-27. *J Clin Oncol.* 2006;24(13):2019–2027.

24. von Minckwitz G, Kummel S, Vogel P, et al. Intensified neoadjuvant chemotherapy in early-responding breast cancer: phase III randomized GeparTrio study. *J Natl Cancer Inst.* 2008;100(8):552–562.

25. von Minckwitz G, Kummel S, Vogel P, et al. Neoadjuvant vinorelbine-capecitabine versus docetaxel-doxorubicin-cyclophosphamide in early nonresponsive breast cancer: phase III randomized GeparTrio trial. *J Natl Cancer Inst.* 2008;100(8):542–551.

26. Gennari A, Sormani MP, Pronzato P, et al. HER2 status and efficacy of adjuvant anthracyclines in early breast cancer: a pooled analysis of randomized trials. *J Natl Cancer Inst.* 2008; 100(1):14–20.

27. Berry DA, Cirrincione C, Henderson IC, et al. Estrogen-receptor status and outcomes of modern chemotherapy for patients with node-positive breast cancer. *JAMA.* 2006;295(14):1658–1667.

28. Hayes DF, Thor AD, Dressler LG, et al. HER2 and response to paclitaxel in node-positive breast cancer. *New Engl J Med.* 2007;357(15):1496–1506.

29. Bear HD, Anderson S, Brown A, et al. The effect on tumor response of adding sequential preoperative docetaxel to preoperative doxorubicin and cyclophosphamide: preliminary results from

National Surgical Adjuvant Breast and Bowel Project Protocol B-27. *J Clin Oncol.* 2003;21(22):4165–4174.

30. Cristofanilli M, Gonzalez-Angulo A, Sneige N, et al. Invasive lobular carcinoma classic type: response to primary chemotherapy and survival outcomes. *J Clin Oncol.* 2005;23(1):41–48.

31. Garber JE, Richardson A, Harris LN, et al. Neo-adjuvant cisplatin (CDDP) in triple-negative breast cancer (BC). San Antonio Breast Cancer Symposium, 2006;Abstract 3074.

32. Ryan PD, Tung NM, Isakoff SJ, et al. Neoadjuvant cisplatin and bevacizumab in triple negative breast cancer (TNBC): safety and efficacy. *J Clin Oncol.* 2009;27(Suppl.):15s.Abstract 551.

33. Gronwald J, Byrski T, Huzarski T, et al. Neoadjuvant therapy with cisplatin in BRCA1-positive breast cancer patients. *J Clin Oncol,* 2009; 27:15s.

34. Hance KW, Anderson WF, Devesa SS, Young HA, Levine PH. Trends in inflammatory breast carcinoma incidence and survival: the surveillance, epidemiology, and end results program at the National Cancer Institute. *J Natl Cancer Inst.* 2005;97(13):966–975.

35. Mayer EL, Miller KD, Rugo HS, et al. A pilot study of adjuvant bevacizumab and chemotherapy after neoadjuvant chemotherapy for high-risk breast cancer. *J Clin Oncol.* 2008;26(Suppl.): Abstract 519.

36. Seo JH, Kim YH, Kim JS. Meta-analysis of pre-operative aromatase inhibitor versus tamoxifen in postmenopausal woman with hormone receptor-positive breast cancer. *Cancer Chemother Pharmacol.* 2009;63(2):261–266.

37. Smith IE, Dowsett M, Ebbs SR, et al. Neoadjuvant treatment of postmenopausal breast cancer with anastrozole, tamoxifen, or both in combination: the immediate preoperative anastrozole, tamoxifen, or combined with tamoxifen (IMPACT) multicenter double-blind randomized trial. *J Clin Oncol.* 2005;23(22):5108–5116.

Incorporating Translational Research in the Treatment of Locally Advanced Breast Cancer

STEVEN J. ISAKOFF

LEIF W. ELLISEN

The neoadjuvant setting provides a rich opportunity to carry out translational studies that can directly lead to advances in both understanding the basic biology of breast cancer and improving patient outcomes. The successful conduct of neoadjuvant translational studies requires close collaboration between members of the multidisciplinary team in order to ensure that the most fruitful research data can be obtained without compromising the best clinical care for patients. This is particularly important in the neoadjuvant setting because patients can potentially be cured of their disease. Therefore, the selection of patients appropriate for preoperative trials requires a careful balance between asking an important experimental question and providing optimal clinical care. Most importantly, translational research studies must be careful to minimize the potential risk of interfering with the delivery of therapy with curative intent. Although neoadjuvant therapy is most often used clinically to treat locally advanced breast cancer (LABC), because of the rich research opportunities neoadjuvant clinical trials will often include patients with stage 1 or 2 disease who might not otherwise require preoperative therapy.

Because the neoadjuvant treatment strategy developed in response to the need to shrink tumors in patients with inoperable LABC, clinical and pathological response rates have traditionally been the primary endpoint in these studies. Increasingly, however, modern studies are being designed with translational primary endpoints. In addition, even traditional neoadjuvant studies increasingly incorporate a number of correlative studies as secondary and exploratory endpoints. The facile acquisition of tumor tissue for research purposes is of fundamental importance in designing such studies, and many of these translational studies require pretreatment and posttreatment tissue to be collected during the course of neoadjuvant therapy. These studies therefore require the establishment of an infrastructure to obtain breast tumor tissue in a timely fashion and with uniform handling, which involves cooperation among medical oncologists, breast radiologists, breast surgeons, and pathologists. Standard procedures should be developed to ensure that specimens are collected and processed according to the demands of the protocol in as uniform a process as possible. Because tissue collection

is often a key part of the trial, the selection of patients with appropriate tumor size is important; if tumors are too small, they may not be amenable to repeat biopsies for research purposes. In addition, because many of these studies are designed for a specific histological subtype of breast cancer and have stricter eligibility criteria, they often require multi-institutional participation, which makes it even more important to develop standard tissue handling and banking procedures. A variety of translational opportunities exist in neoadjuvant studies, and examples of some of these will be described below.

Molecular and histological analysis of tumor tissue usually constitutes a major translational component in neoadjuvant studies. One of the most appealing aspects of such studies is the opportunity to evaluate response to therapies on treatment-naïve tumors and to collect tissue samples both before and after treatment. This approach allows investigation into several distinct clinical and translational questions. First, putative biomarkers can be identified in the primary tumor that correlate with pathological response rates following definitive surgery. Second, research biopsies performed during the course of treatment allow assessment of whether the therapy has had its intended biological effect. This question is most relevant in trials involving novel pathway–targeted agents, in which it may be critical to determine whether the agent has "hit" its intended target within the tumor cell. Such interval research biopsies also provide the opportunity to uncover early biomarkers that may correlate with the ultimate pathological response. Third, comparison of the primary tumor to the posttreatment residual tumor in cases in which pathological complete response (pCR) is not achieved has the potential to yield insight into biological mechanisms of treatment resistance. For example, the potential to observe changes in expression of HER2 or phosphorylation of its downstream signaling components following targeted therapy makes such translational studies in the neoadjuvant setting extremely valuable.

The variety of techniques available for molecular analysis of tumors is expanding rapidly while at the same time becoming more amenable to applications using small amounts of frozen or, in some cases, fixed tumor tissue. For example, primary tumor biopsies can now be subject to DNA analysis to identify specific mutations, gene copy number alterations, or epigenetic changes that may predict tumor response or long-term outcome. Several of the currently available platforms for these assays allow assessment on a genome-wide scale using even the small amounts of tissue available from research biopsies. Similarly, tumor RNA can be used for analyses, including whole genome gene expression arrays, real-time polymerase chain reaction analysis, or microRNA analysis in order to uncover predictors of response. Proteomic analysis from tumor tissue or blood samples before and after treatment may also lead to identification of early predictors of response. Immunohistochemistry to assess changes in markers of proliferation, phosphoproteins, or protein expression can also be informative in preoperative tissue samples. New techniques for highly quantitative immunohistochemistry are likely to increase its usefulness as a research tool (1).

An important underlying question in translational research involving preoperative studies is whether the results of these studies might predict the long-term outcome data obtained from adjuvant studies but at far less cost, over a much shorter time period, and with a dramatically smaller sample size. This possibility was suggested by the results of a neoadjuvant study comparing letrozole and tamoxifen (2). The Letrozole 024 study was a double-blind randomized trial in 324 patients and demonstrated that neoadjuvant letrozole was more effective than tamoxifen, with a higher response rate and higher incidence of breast-conserving surgery. Translational correlative studies using samples collected from that study revealed that reductions in mean Ki67 staining (a marker of proliferation) were greater in the letrozole arm (87% versus 75%). These results correlate well with the findings from the ATAC (Arimidex, Tamoxifen Alone or in Combination) study in 9,366 patients randomized to receive 5 years of adjuvant anastrozole, tamoxifen, or both, which demonstrated that anastrozole had superior disease-free survival (hazard ratio 0.87), time to recurrence, and distant metastatic recurrence. Identifying the optimal biomarker(s) to predict long-term response and determining whether the same markers are useful in patients treated with chemotherapy or biologics remain important challenges. Nevertheless, the principle of using translational work in the neoadjuvant setting to complement long-term data obtained from traditional adjuvant studies has great potential.

In addition to the molecular studies described above, neoadjuvant studies offer the opportunity to assess the ability of functional imaging modalities to correlate early changes in tumor physiology with pathological response. For example, positron emission tomography (PET) scans can assess tumor metabolism and have been shown to predict response with good sensitivity and specificity (3). However, limited useful physiological and biological information is acquired during those studies. Newer functional imaging, such as near-infrared optical imaging and functional magnetic resonance imaging (MRI), is being studied as a way to identify changes in the physiology of tumors. A preliminary report demonstrated that changes in deoxyhemoglobin detected by optical imaging within one week after treatment predicted pathological response to neoadjuvant therapy (4).

The ongoing I-SPY trial sponsored by the National Cancer Institute (NCI) and several cooperative groups is a tour de force multidisciplinary collaboration whose overall goal is to identify biomarkers that predict response of LABC to preoperative chemotherapy with doxorubicin, cyclophosphamide, and paclitaxel (5). This trial serves as a comprehensive example of the type of study that can be carried out in the neoadjuvant setting in patients with LABC. The trial collects data from serial breast MRI studies, research core biopsies, and blood samples, and then correlates them with pathological response by traditional histology and the residual cancer burden (RCB) approach. Tumor tissue is analyzed using a variety of methods. Primary tumor specimens are first categorized by genomic expression array into groups corresponding to the intrinsic subtypes of luminal A and B, basal, HER2, and normal; patients are then evaluated for pCR rate, RCB score, and MRI response. The pCR rate in each subtype group was 2%, 15%, 34%, 52%, and 43%, respectively, in agreement with previous studies showing the predictive value of intrinsic subtype profiles. Subsequent analysis of the 21-gene recurrence score signature (Oncotype DX) revealed that the low- and intermediate-risk scores were associated with a mere 3% and 10% response rate, respectively, compared with the high-risk group (36%). These analyses were then compared with standard immunohistochemistry, demonstrating that estrogen receptor (ER)–negative subgroups had the highest pCR rates, as the ER+/HER2– (10%) and ER+/HER2+ (28%) subgroups experienced significantly lower rates than the ER–/HER2– (36%) and ER–/HER2+ (48%) subgroups. Importantly, among the groups with very low pCR rates, there is a subset with excellent disease-free survival, calling into question the value of pCR in all subgroups. Additional correlative studies will involve comparative genomic hybridization, p53 gene chip studies, immunohistochemistry, and reverse-phase protein microarray (RPMA) to assess a variety of phosphoproteins, as well as serum proteomics. Ultimately, it is hoped that such trials will help to determine the relative value of newer molecular diagnostics compared with standard clinical and pathological analysis. At the very least, this trial demonstrates the vast array of studies that can be accomplished in the preoperative setting.

One of the most promising translational opportunities is in the evaluation of novel targeted therapies. Because these agents are designed to affect specific cellular pathways, translational studies focusing on the relevant pathways have the ability to obtain important pharmacodynamic data and to provide key insights into the biological activity of these agents in vivo. Thus, such studies can address specifically whether an agent has the intended effect (e.g., a change in phosphorylation of a target protein). In addition, translational work on targeted agents allows the testing of specific hypotheses regarding particular mechanisms of resistance. As an example, many growth factor receptor pathways cross-talk with HER2 signaling, and it has therefore been postulated that activation of such pathways might be associated with treatment resistance in HER2-positive tumors. Indeed, one study found that HER2-positive tumors that expressed higher levels of insulin-like growth factor 1 receptor (IGF1R) were more likely to be resistant to neoadjuvant trastuzumab and vinorelbine (6). The availability of an increasing number of novel targeted therapies, together with our increasing understanding of the fundamental biology of breast cancer, suggests that more focused, hypothesis-driven, and productive translational studies of these agents will be pursued in years to come. Translational work in the preoperative setting will be essential for maximizing the efficiency with which these new agents can be tested in clinical trials and ultimately utilized in clinical practice.

Many challenges remain in realizing the translational opportunities that neoadjuvant therapy affords. Practical challenges involve the development of the infrastructure to carry out the studies, while conceptual challenges lie in understanding how to interpret the data collected from neoadjuvant trials. Neoadjuvant trials are, by their very nature, fairly demanding in what they require both of patients and of caregivers. Systems need to be in place to adequately collect and process tissue, an effort which requires careful input from pathologists and radiologists. Patient recruitment can be difficult without close collaboration between surgeons and medical oncologists, particularly as patients with operable tumors are increasingly eligible for neoadjuvant studies. For this reason the multidisciplinary new patient clinic is the ideal environment to identify these patients in most centers. For many studies, the consent process may be time consuming, given that the potential benefit to individual patients is limited and that explaining the scientific merit of providing additional research biopsies is complex. Cost is also a significant issue in conducting neoadjuvant studies, as research biopsies, tissue processing, and specimen analysis each involve distinct teams of specialists. As centers become more accustomed to conducting translational studies, many of these issues can be managed and will be mitigated.

As neoadjuvant trials and associated translational studies are being designed for the future, there remain many additional unanswered questions regarding data collection and interpretation. For example: Which method of assessing pathological response is a more useful correlate of active therapy? Does response to neoadjuvant therapy correlate with future risk of relapse in all subgroups of patients? Will early biomarker predictors of response after treatment initiation (such as functional imaging or changes evident in tumor biopsies) translate into valid surrogate markers of long-term outcome? Will predictors of response developed on the basis of chemotherapy apply to novel agents? Which patients are most appropriate to enter neoadjuvant studies—those with LABC only or those with smaller operable tumors as well? What role will preoperative "window of opportunity" trials (in which short-term treatment is given before surgery for translational studies but without therapeutic intent) play in informing or validating therapeutic neoadjuvant trials? These and many other questions are being actively pursued, and there is no doubt that translational studies in the preoperative setting will contribute importantly to addressing them.

■ REFERENCES

1. Chung GG, Zerkowski MP, Ghosh S, Camp RL, Rimm DL. Quantitative analysis of estrogen receptor heterogeneity in breast cancer. *Lab Invest.* 2007;87(7):662–669.
2. Ellis MJ, Coop A, Singh B, et al. Letrozole inhibits tumor proliferation more effectively than tamoxifen independent of HER1/2 expression status. *Cancer Res.* 2003;63(19):6523–6531.
3. Rousseau C, Devillers A, Sagan C, et al. Monitoring of early response to neoadjuvant chemotherapy in stage II and III breast cancer by [18F]fluorodeoxyglucose positron emission tomography. *J Clin Oncol.* 2006;24(34):5366–5372.
4. Cerussi A, Hsiang D, Shah N, et al. Predicting response to breast cancer neoadjuvant chemotherapy using diffuse optical spectroscopy. *Proc Natl Acad Sci USA.* 2007;104(10):4014–4019.
5. Esserman LJ, Perou C, Cheang M, et al. Breast cancer molecular profiles and tumor response of neoadjuvant doxorubicin and paclitaxel: The I-SPY TRIAL (CALGB 150007/150012, ACRIN 6657). *J Clin Oncol.* 2009;27:18s(Suppl; Abstract LBA515).
6. Harris LN, You F, Schnitt SJ, et al. Predictors of resistance to preoperative trastuzumab and vinorelbine for HER2-positive early breast cancer. *Clin Cancer Res.* 2007;13(4):1198–1207.

9 Multidisciplinary Approach in Breast Reconstruction

Surgical Considerations in Breast Reconstruction

LIZA S. KIM

ANUJA KANDANATT ANTONY

ERIC C. LIAO

WILLIAM G. AUSTEN, JR.

The ideal breast reconstruction creates a natural appearing and feeling construct to replace the breast tissue removed by mastectomy (1). Many studies have demonstrated the beneficial effects of breast reconstruction after mastectomy, with improvement in a patient's psychological health as well as body image (2–4). Some studies have suggested that preexisting psychological health may influence postreconstruction patient satisfaction; thus, psychological assessment should be included as part of a complete preoperative history and physical prior to proceeding with breast reconstruction (5–7).

Breast reconstruction can be carried out immediately, at the same time as the breast removal, or in a delayed fashion, months to years after the mastectomy. Although there is an increasing trend toward immediate reconstruction, the decision to carry out an immediate or delayed reconstruction depends on many different factors (discussed below). Regardless of timing, reconstructive methods can be categorized into three groups: (a) prosthetic, utilizing a saline or silicone implant, (b) autologous, created by manipulation of a patient's own tissue, or (c) combination. Alternatively, a patient may choose to forgo the reconstructive process altogether, opting for an external breast prosthesis.

The decision to proceed with any one of these options must take into consideration the particular risks and benefits of an individual type of reconstruction, the patient's expectations, the urgency of implementing adjuvant therapy, the long-term anticipated reconstructive outcome, and the individual characteristics of the patient [e.g., body mass index (BMI), comorbidities, and breast cancer risk profile]. Each of these factors is weighed by the plastic surgeon and the patient and is coordinated with the cancer team's treatment plan. Thus an optimal reconstruction requires a multidisciplinary effort appropriately to accommodate the patient's cancer treatment requirements and reconstruction expectations (Figure 9.1).

■ GENERAL CONSIDERATIONS IN BREAST RECONSTRUCTION

As methods of breast reconstruction have developed over the years, and as our knowledge of risks and outcomes has improved, reconstructive algorithms guiding treatment have become more complex. Patient factors and risk profiles impact the decision to proceed with any particular type of reconstruction. Integrating the patient's reconstructive goals with her lifestyle and comorbidities is critical to a successful reconstruction. Studies have demonstrated the devastating effects of poor lifestyle and health, such as tobacco use and obesity, in certain types of breast reconstruction, with higher rates of necrosis and infection, flap loss, abdominal donor-site morbidity, and mastectomy skin flap necrosis (8–14).

Tobacco use is well known to be detrimental to microvascular circulation (15,16). A mastectomy skin flap depends on the tenuous subdermal blood supply that remains after removal of the underlying breast tissue. Tobacco use increases the risk of mastectomy skin flap necrosis and infection, which is especially problematic in a prosthesis-based reconstruction (9,12–14,17). Autologous reconstruction also carries increased risks in smokers, with higher rates of fat necrosis, flap loss, wound dehiscence, and donor-site complications (abdominal flap and umbilical necrosis, hernia/bulge formation) (8,9,12). Patients should discontinue all tobacco use for a minimum of 4 weeks prior to surgery and refrain from smoking after surgery (9,18).

Another important consideration in breast reconstruction is the patient's BMI. Obesity is defined as a BMI greater than 30. Multiple studies have corroborated that complications such as fat necrosis, flap loss, mastectomy skin flap

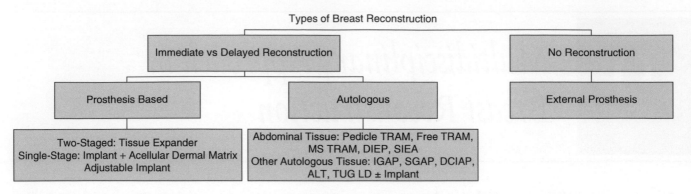

FIGURE 9.1 Overview of breast reconstruction. *Abbreviations:* ALT, anterior lateral thigh flap; DCIAP, deep circumflex iliac artery perforator flap; DIEP, deep inferior epigastric perforator flap; IGAP, inferior gluteal artery perforator flap; LD, latissimus dorsi flap; MS TRAM, muscle-sparing TRAM flap; SGAP, superior gluteal artery perforator flap; SIEA, superficial inferior epigastric artery flap; TRAM, transverse rectus abdominis myocutaneous flap; TUG, transverse upper gracilis flap.

necrosis, seroma, wound infection, and donor-site wound problems are significantly increased in obese patients (8,10,11,19). In particular, autologous flap complications are usually more common than donor-site complications in obese patients, and there is an increased potential for deep vein thrombosis and pulmonary embolism, although rates of clinically symptomatic thromboembolic events are less than 1% (10,11,18,19). Reconstruction complications are amplified when a reconstructive candidate is obese and smokes.

In addition, aspects of the mastectomy operation itself can significantly influence the reconstructive outcome. The viability of the mastectomy skin flaps must be determined prior to flap transfer or placement of a prosthetic device. Use of fluorescein or indocyanine green dye to assess intraoperative skin viability has been described, but neither is used routinely owing to their inconsistent results (20–25). Depending on the status of the mastectomy flap, the reconstructive plan may change from immediate to delayed or from a single-stage implant reconstruction to a two-stage tissue expander reconstruction. In cases of autologous reconstruction where the viability of the skin flaps at the time of the mastectomy is unclear, a skin-banking approach can be used by preserving the transferred flap's skin for use in the event that mastectomy skin flap necrosis and loss ensues (26,27). In addition, the integrity of the inframammary fold (IMF) and the lateral and medial borders of the breast should be assessed. If the IMF or the breast borders have been violated during the course of the mastectomy dissection, recreation of these anatomical landmarks is carried out to prevent migration and distortion of the reconstructed breast. Suture technique and the use of acellular dermal matrix have been described for correction of postreconstruction asymmetry and symmastia, where there is a communication between the two breasts over the sternum owing to overdissection medially, giving the appearance of one continuous breast (28–31).

Finally, most, if not all, types of breast reconstructions frequently require more than one surgical procedure to achieve the desired aesthetic result. The initial reconstruction provides the basis for the breast mound. The subsequent surgeries, such as revisions, nipple reconstruction, and symmetry procedures, are less involved and can be performed as an outpatient (see below). These secondary procedures are timed to avoid interference with adjuvant therapy and can provide lasting, aesthetically pleasing results (32).

Prosthesis-based Reconstruction

Prosthesis-based methods of breast reconstruction remain the mainstay for most breast reconstructive surgeons. Compared with autologous tissue methods, prosthesis-based reconstruction offers the advantages of a shorter postoperative recovery period, the greatest flexibility in determining breast size (not dependent on donor tissues), and no additional morbidity at the surgical or donor site (17,33,34). Prosthesis-based reconstruction is favored for patients with comorbid conditions that preclude a lengthy procedure and in patients who lack sufficient autologous tissue to reconstruct a breast (18,33–34). Most patients who undergo prosthesis-based reconstruction require approximately 1 to 2 postoperative days in the hospital (mean length of stay 1.76 days) and approximately 2 to 4 weeks for a full recovery (mean 15.09 days) (36,37). In addition, cost analysis of prosthetic and autologous reconstruction has identified significant differences: Implant reconstructions are generally less expensive earlier, though longer-term comparisons demonstrate variable results in institutional resource cost differences over time (Figure 9.2) (37,38).

There are two main types of permanent prosthetic devices: saline and silicone breast implants (Figure 9.3). All implants have a silicone elastomer outer shell. In November 2006, the Food and Drug Administration approved the use of cohesive silicone gel–filled implants after two major implant manufacturing companies, Allergan/Inamed and Mentor, conducted rigorous clinical and preclinical trials demonstrating safety (39–42). Despite previous concerns, no association was found between silicone implants and risk of developing autoimmune disease, such as rheumatoid

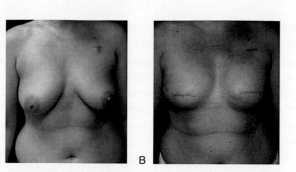

FIGURE 9.2 Bilateral breast reconstruction with tissue expanders followed by implant exchange. (A) Preoperative; (B) postoperative.

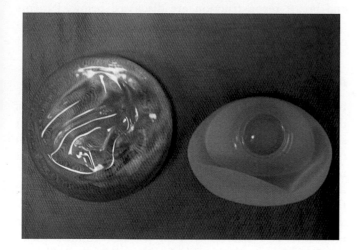

FIGURE 9.3 (*Left*) Silicone gel–filled implant. (*Right*) Mentor tissue expander.

arthritis, systemic lupus erythematosus, or chronic fatigue syndrome (18,17,34,39,43). Silicone implants also have been shown to be durable. Recently published studies have shown that 98% of implants remain intact 5 years after placement, and 83% to 85% remain intact at 10 years, although these data may differ depending on the generation of the implant as well as the manufacturer (40,43,44). When compared with saline implants, silicone implants produce a more natural feel and appearance and are less likely to show rippling caused by implant wrinkling visible through the thin soft tissue coverage over the implant. Use of silicone implants has been associated with higher patient satisfaction rates in recent reports (18). However, compared with saline implants, silicone implants are more costly and do not allow intraoperative size adjustment, and implant ruptures are more difficult to detect (18,45,46).

The most common method of carrying out a prosthesis-based reconstruction involves a two-stage approach, with initial placement of a tissue expander (see Figure 9.3), followed by a period of expansion, and ending with an exchange of the expander for a permanent implant. Staging of a prosthetic reconstruction is recommended if there is concern regarding mastectomy skin viability or if the patient wishes to increase her breast size.

Tissue expanders are typically placed into a musculofascial pocket consisting of the pectoralis major muscle superiorly and medially, the serratus anterior muscle laterally, and the rectus fascia inferiorly (33,47). The expander can be left empty or filled to tissue tolerance intraoperatively with sterile saline (48). Approximately 2 to 3 weeks postoperatively, weekly (or as tolerated by the patient) injections of the tissue expander are initiated in the office until the desired volume is attained. Since recreation of the natural ptotic appearance of the breast is a challenging aspect of an implant-based method of reconstruction, the lower pole of the breast can be preferentially expanded by appropriate tissue expander selection and placement (17). In addition, tissue expanders can be overexpanded by up to 20% to 30% to create a larger skin envelope, thereby aiding in the illusion of breast ptosis (17). After 1 to 3 months, the tissue expander is exchanged for a permanent implant as an outpatient surgical procedure. At the time of the implant exchange, capsulotomy, capsulectomy, and/or capsulorrhaphy are performed to tailor the breast position and symmetry and to optimize the aesthetic results (18,35,49).

Disadvantages of the two-stage implant reconstruction approach include attenuation and thinning of the muscle layer during expansion, the additional time required for the expansion process and final reconstruction, and risk of infection from repeated needle placement during the filling process (17,50). However, this method does give the patient an increased freedom to determine final breast size.

Recently, with the increasing popularity of skin-sparing mastectomy and nipple-sparing techniques, single-stage reconstruction has become a viable alternative to the more traditional two-stage approach (18). Nipple-sparing techniques have become more common, largely due to studies demonstrating oncologic resection with nipple preservation to be as effective as more traditional procedures for certain breast cancers, particularly for smaller peripheral cancers without nodal involvement or lymphatic vascular invasion (51–54).

The preferred patient for a single-stage implant reconstruction is one with moderate breast size, adequate excess skin to drape over the implant, and a preference for a similar or smaller breast size. The single-stage implant reconstruction often requires the use of acellular dermal matrix, a biologically processed product created from cadaveric skin/dermis, which retains the native basement membrane and cellular matrix but removes the cellular components involved in rejection and infection (55–58). The acellular dermal sheet is fashioned as a lower lateral sling, or hammock, for complete implant coverage (28,50,59,60–62), supplementing the inferior and lateral aspects of a retropectoral pocket by suturing it to the IMF inferiorly, the serratus laterally, and the elevated pectoral muscle edge. The resulting pocket allows immediate implant placement with sufficient ptosis, eliminating the need for multiple operations for breast mound creation (28,50,59,62). Alternatively, a serratus anterior muscle flap can be raised to cover the lateral aspect of the implant (28,33,50).

Although there is a longer learning curve for the single-stage implant reconstruction approach, a well-executed single-stage reconstruction can produce results resembling the native breast in a more cost-effective and time-efficient manner than a two-stage approach (28,59,62). This technique obviates the need for multiple office visits for expansion, reduces the overall number of operations, and decreases the pain and morbidity associated with these procedures (62,63). In addition, immediate single-stage reconstruction after nipple-sparing mastectomy, despite unique challenges with described nipple-sparing mastectomy incisions (periareolar, inframammary, lateral) and intraoperative nipple positioning, can produce high-quality, aesthetically pleasing results (64–67) (Figure 9.4).

Adjustable implant breast reconstruction is an approach similar to single-stage reconstruction in that a permanent implant, such as the Becker implant, is placed at the time of the initial surgery (17,68–71). The implant comes with a removable port that can be accessed postoperatively for volume adjustment. A separate procedure is required for port removal, which can be performed in the office. Proposed advantages of the Becker implant include patient control over final size, with decreased incidence of patient disappointment, correction of greater degrees of breast ptosis, treatment of early capsular contracture, correction of congenital breast disorders, and correction of symmastia (68,72–75). Complications of the Becker implant are similar to those of implant-based reconstruction, with the addition of possible fill-port failure (76).

There are several limitations of prosthesis-based reconstruction. In unilateral breast reconstruction, breast symmetry can be more difficult to achieve than with autologous reconstruction, especially for those patients with ptotic, pendulous breasts. Symmetry and cosmesis is more easily obtained when bilateral implant reconstructions are performed, as the contour and degree of ptosis of both breasts are controlled simultaneously. Other disadvantages of implant-based reconstruction include capsular contracture, implant rupture, rippling, migration/malposition, extrusion/exposure, symmastia, lack of projection, thinning of the overlying skin over time, and "bottoming out" of the implant over time, with movement of the implant inferiorly to a location below the inframammary crease, which requires surgical correction (1,12,18,35,50,77). In addition, patients who require adjuvant chemotherapy or radiation after reconstruction may have a higher risk for significant short-term and long-term complications (12,35,77–79). Issues related to coordination of radiation and breast reconstruction are discussed below. Patients should be made aware of these potential risks prior to proceeding with any type of implant-based reconstruction.

Abdominal Tissue–based Reconstruction

Breast reconstruction using abdominal tissue provides the most natural appearance and produces a texture most similar to that of the native breast (1,80,81). The abdomen typically affords the most abundant supply of tissue for reconstruction. Described and popularized by Hartrampf, the transverse rectus abdominis myocutaneous (TRAM) flap and its derivatives remain the most common autologous tissue options for breast reconstruction (82). The procedure is often referred to as the "tummy tuck" breast reconstruction since redundant abdominal tissue is removed and used for the reconstruction. However, the incision often lies superior to what would be expected for a true cosmetic abdominoplasty (Figure 9.5).

The infraumbilical soft tissue is based on two main blood supplies: the deep superior and the deep inferior epigastric vessels. The deep superior epigastric vessel connects to the inferior epigastric vessel via a system of anastomotic vessels termed the choke vessels (18,83,84,85). The deep inferior epigastric vessel provides the dominant blood supply, accounting for a greater percentage of the

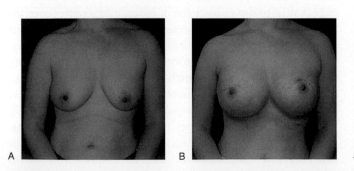

FIGURE 9.4 Bilateral nipple-sparing mastectomy with immediate tissue expander placement and staged silicone implant reconstruction. (A) Preoperative; (B) postoperative.

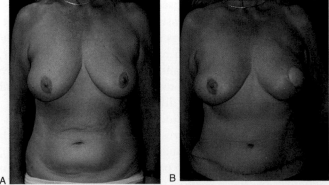

FIGURE 9.5 Left breast reconstruction with pedicled TRAM flap. Note the transverse abdominal scar but improved abdominal contour. (A) Preoperative; (B) postoperative.

infraumbilical soft tissue perfusion (1,18,19,85–87). Thus a myocutaneous flap based on the deep inferior epigastric vessel has a higher survival rate with less fat necrosis or partial flap loss and the potential to harvest more tissue volume than the same flap supplied by the deep superior epigastric vessel (1,18,19,86,87).

In a unilateral breast reconstruction using a TRAM flap, the loss of one rectus abdominis muscle has minimal adverse long-term effects due to the compensatory increase in strength of other muscle groups. However, the loss of both rectus abdominis muscles, required for bilateral TRAM flap reconstruction, can significantly weaken and decrease abdominal flexion (18,88,89). For those patients requiring bilateral reconstruction, methods that minimize morbidity to the muscle, such as the deep inferior epigastric perforator (DIEP) flap, muscle-sparing TRAM (MS TRAM) flap, or superficial inferior epigastric artery (SIEA) flap, may be preferred, although the functional benefits of these muscle-sparing approaches remain controversial (80,90–92). These flaps will be discussed in detail in the following sections.

Pedicled TRAM Flap

The blood supply to the pedicled TRAM flap is the deep superior epigastric vessels. Infraumbilical abdominal skin and fat, and one rectus muscle, are transposed on the superior pedicle to reconstruct the breast. There are many ways to close the resulting abdominal fascial defect, including primary closure, prosthetic mesh interposition, and onlay (93–97). Most patients stay in the hospital for 3 to 5 days; the mean length of stay after this procedure has been reported as 4.67 days, with a return to normal activities after 4 to 6 weeks (mean of 33.27 days) (19,36,98).

Prior to the surgery, the patient should be examined for any surgical scars, rectus diastasis, and abdominal wall hernias. Paramedian incisions, subcostal Kocher incisions, and multiple abdominal scars are potential contraindications to a pedicled TRAM reconstruction, as transection of the superior blood supply may have occurred. However, flap design strategies have been described, including flap splitting (hemi-TRAM), flap skewing to avoid abdominal scars (to avoid poor perfusion across scars), minimal abdominoplasty flap undermining, and selective use of DIEP, SIEA, free, and pedicled TRAM flaps to obtain satisfactory results (18,99). Prior abdominoplasty is considered a relative contraindication to this procedure (100). Rectus perforators, which are undermined during an abdominoplasty, have been shown by color-duplex scanning and power ultrasound to undergo perforator vessel reperfusion to as much as 40% of the caliber of their original diameter within 6 months of surgery. These vessels may or may not be sufficient to supply the flap adequately (101). Liposuction, which does not necessarily disrupt the perforators, is not an absolute contraindication to TRAM flap reconstruction. Unilateral breast reconstruction using TRAM flap after abdominal liposuction has been described, though discriminating use is recommended (102). Caution should also be taken with patients who smoke or are obese as they are at risk for higher rates of fat necrosis and partial flap failures (9,10,11).

In those patients with risk factors, such as tobacco use or obesity, associated with poor tissue perfusion, flap survival can be improved by a delay procedure (47,103–105). Here, the dominant deep inferior epigastric system is divided, allowing augmentation of the superior blood supply through the recruitment of choke vessels and angiogenesis. The procedure can be performed as an open procedure or laparoscopically (103,105). The patient is brought back to the operating room for the definitive operation ideally 2 to 4 weeks later. "Supercharging" of the flap is sometimes undertaken to augment the blood supply to a flap; here, a secondary blood supply is added through anastomosis of the deep inferior epigastric vessels or the superficial inferior epigastric vessels of the flap to recipient vessels in proximity to the breast, such as the thoracodorsal artery and vein (18,106,107).

After transfer of the pedicled TRAM flap, a bulge may be created in the inferomedial aspect of the breast from the rotation of the rectus abdominis muscle, especially when the contralateral rectus muscle is used. Breast reconstruction using an ipsilateral TRAM flap can provide superior results by preserving the medial IMF and eliminating the perixiphoid bulge (108). However, bulge irregularities resulting from contralateral transposition often attenuate and become less visible over time as the muscle atrophies from the denervation that routinely occurs during flap harvest. Other perceived advantages of the ipsilateral TRAM flap include simplicity and versatility of flap shaping and a lower rate of partial flap necrosis than with the contralateral TRAM flap (109). Complications with either of the described pedicled TRAM flaps include abdominal wall hernia or laxity, fat necrosis, partial flap loss, abdominal wall weakness, mesh infection, pulmonary embolism, and seroma (10,18,36,82). Complete flap loss is rare.

Free TRAM Flap

The blood supply to the free TRAM flap is the deep inferior epigastric vessels. This flap takes advantage of the dominant blood supply to the abdominal tissue, allowing transfer of a larger volume of tissue (84,85). The deep inferior epigastric vessels are completely transected from their origin and a microvascular anastomosis is performed to the thoracodorsal or internal mammary vessels. Currently, anastomosis with the internal mammary vessels is more common, which requires resection of either the second or the third costal cartilage for vessel exposure (110). Alternatively, perforator branches from the internal mammary vessels in these interspaces can be used for anastomosis, provided that vessel caliber is suitable. This obviates the need for rib resection and resulting contour deformity and avoids sacrifice of the internal mammary vessels, leaving them available for later use in myocardial revascularization (111–115). An additional benefit of the free TRAM flap is the ability to perform this flap in certain patients with prior superior abdominal surgical scars or poor tissue perfusion. A free TRAM requires a longer operative time and may not be appropriate for patients with significant comorbidities. The procedure also requires appropriate training in microsurgical techniques. Complications of a free TRAM flap are similar to those of a pedicled TRAM flap but also include the possibility of complete flap loss, with loss rates of 0.3% to 0.9% or higher in less experienced hands (8,18,116,117).

Postoperatively, close monitoring, especially in the first 24 hours, is essential. The nursing care required for frequent assessment of flap viability may necessitate a short stay in the intensive care unit or on a specialty floor. If there is any question of flap compromise, the patient should be taken back to the operating room immediately for exploration of the microanastomosis. Most patients spend approximately 4 to 7 days in the hospital and require 4 to 6 weeks for full recovery (118,119).

DIEP Flap and MS TRAM Flap

The DIEP flap and MS TRAM flaps are derivatives of the free TRAM flap that have evolved largely to address concerns of abdominal morbidity and functional deficits after harvest of the rectus muscle(s). The DIEP flap is supplied by one or more perforators from the deep inferior epigastric system. Ideally, the rectus abdominis muscles remain intact, innervated, and functional, and only abdominal skin and fat based on a dominant perforator vessel or vessels is harvested. The concept behind the MS TRAM flap is similar to that of the DIEP flap, where only a portion of the rectus abdominis muscle is harvested and the residual rectus abdominis muscle continues to function. By sparing most, if not all, of the rectus abdominis musculature, the morbidity to the abdominal wall is minimized and the chance of a bulge or a hernia is significantly decreased (92,117,119,120). Both DIEP and MS TRAM flaps are performed as free flaps with complete transection of the inferior blood supply and subsequent anastomosis to the internal mammary or thoracodorsal vessels. Primary closure of the abdominal fascia is usually possible, avoiding the need for mesh.

Potential disadvantages of DIEP flaps are technical difficulty, longer operative time, and higher rates of fat necrosis (117,119). Accordingly, some have advocated use of preoperative imaging such as computed tomography–angiogram, Doppler ultrasound, or magnetic resonance imaging/magnetic resonance angiogram to better delineate the location of these perforators (121–125) and guide surgical dissection, ensuring better perfusion and decreased dissection times (126). Although theoretical advantages of the DIEP flap over the TRAM flap, including decreased abdominal wall morbidity and reduced risks of herniation, pain, and bulge, have been described (18,92,119,120), the advantages of the DIEP flap over the MS TRAM flap have not been clearly demonstrated (127). However, some studies have shown shorter hospital stay with the DIEP flap than with TRAM flaps in bilateral breast reconstruction, possibly owing to less pain and abdominal wall morbidity (80).

SIEA Flap

The free SIEA flap is supplied by the superficial inferior epigastric vessel, which is a branch of the femoral vessels. The SIEA crosses superiorly over the inguinal ligament to perfuse the tissue to the abdomen. The SIEA flap has distinct advantages for bilateral breast reconstruction as it does not violate the abdominal fascia or take muscle, so there is no associated abdominal wall morbidity (128,116).

The use of this flap may be limited by the variability in presence and caliber of the SIEA vessels. Approximately 30% to 35% of the population has an absent or inadequate SIEA for use in microvascular anastomosis (117,129,130). The exact territory that the SIEA perfuses is also unclear, potentially limiting the amount of tissue that can be harvested (129–132). The available tissue for SIEA flap breast reconstruction is usually less than that of the DIEP/TRAM flaps, as the SIEA usually cannot supply tissue past the midline (131,132). Despite the presence of larger-caliber SIEA vessels in the obese abdomen (92,128), the chance of fat necrosis and flap loss is higher in the obese patient because of poor fat microcirculation. Use of this flap in patients who are obese generally should be avoided, although it has shown some promise in patients who have undergone massive weight loss (133). The dissection for the SIEA flap is also challenging, potentially increasing operative time. The vessels, however, always should be considered for anastomosis for augmenting or "supercharging" the blood supply in other abdominal tissue–based reconstructions to improve perfusion when needed (18,106,134,135).

Other Free-Flap Reconstruction Options

Other options for free-flap breast reconstruction include the inferior or superior gluteal artery perforator (IGAP and SGAP) flaps (117,136), the deep circumflex iliac artery perforator (DCIAP) flap (137,138), the anterior lateral thigh (ALT) flap (139,140), and the transverse upper gracilis (TUG)/transverse myocutaneous gracilis (TMG) flap (141,142–145), to name a few. These free flaps are usually used as alternative flaps when the abdominal tissue is not available for the breast reconstruction (110). The aforementioned flaps can be technically more challenging to harvest and may be associated with donor-site asymmetry (in unilateral reconstruction), limited amounts of tissue for reconstruction, shorter pedicle lengths with inconsistent vessel anatomy, and longer operative times, and may require repositioning of the patient for harvesting and inset (110). However, the potential benefits of each individual flap must be weighed for a patient with a paucity of abdominal fat or preferential distribution of fat in the region of an alternate flap. The major benefits of these alternative flaps are a different donor site with potentially less morbidity and functional loss, donor-site scars in less conspicuous locations, and the opportunity for capitalization of a relative abundance of skin and fat in an alternate location.

Latissimus Dorsi Musculocutaneous Flap

In patients where microsurgical reconstruction is not favored or where abdominal tissue is not available, or for reasons relating to surgeon preference, the latissimus dorsi musculocutaneous (LDM) flap is a dependable source of nonirradiated neighboring tissue that can be used for pedicled flap breast reconstruction. The LDM flap is based on the thoracodorsal vessels. A skin paddle is designed that allows the donor site to be closed primarily, with the residual scar hidden under the lines of the patient's bra straps. Typically, the latissimus dorsi muscle harvest proceeds with full muscle elevation and transposition to the breast region. An implant can be used to achieve the requisite breast volume. The latissimus dorsi muscle is draped over the implant, providing complete muscle coverage for the prosthetic device. For a smaller-breasted patient, the extended LDM flap has been described to supplement the amount of tissue available for reconstruction, obviating the need for an implant (146).

The latissimus dorsi muscle assists in adduction, extension, and medial rotation of the humerus and plays a part in stabilization of the pelvis. While there is some loss of upper-extremity strength and range of motion in the immediate postoperative period, most patients do not notice any functional loss once fully recovered from surgery, although this recovery may take up to a year (1,18,147–149). Some patients may require physical therapy to achieve full recovery. Patients who are elite athletes and those who require significant upper extremity strength (avid rowers, cross-country skiers, paraplegics) are less optimal candidates for an LDM flap reconstruction (1,18,147–149). Patients usually stay 1 to 4 days in the hospital (mean 2.67 days) and return to normal activities in 2 weeks (mean reported 16.5 days) (36,150).

The LDM flap should be used with caution in patients with prior thoracotomy and axillary incisions since damage to the latissimus dorsi muscle or the thoracodorsal vascular pedicle may have occurred. The integrity of the muscle can be assessed by having the patient adduct her arms against resistance (18,151). If the thoracodorsal vessels are ligated during the axillary dissection, it may still be possible to harvest the flap and support it by reverse flow off of the serratus branch (151).

The LDM flap has a robust blood supply, adequate even for patients with contraindications to other flaps or medical concerns (tobacco use, radiation treatment, obesity) (150,152). Thus many surgeons prefer to use the LDM flap for salvage situations (152).

One of the most significant complications after LDM transposition is seroma fluid accumulation in the back donor site, which may require repeated aspirations. Preventive strategies include closed suction drainage for as long as 6 weeks postoperatively (150) and quilting sutures to decrease the dead space (153). The donor-site scar also may widen owing to constant tension placed on the wound with movement. Another disadvantage of this flap is the requirement for multiple intraoperative patient repositioning steps (supine to prone to decubitus), which add to operative time and difficulty.

■ RECONSTRUCTION IN THE CONTEXT OF OVERALL ONCOLOGIC TREATMENT

Timing of Reconstruction

Breast reconstruction can be performed in two ways, immediately or in a delayed fashion months or years after a mastectomy procedure. Immediate reconstruction is thought to have a positive psychological benefit by reducing the stigma and disfigurement resulting from a loss of a breast following a cancer diagnosis (3,17,154). An immediate reconstruction can be aesthetically superior to a delayed reconstruction owing to a more pliable skin envelope, an intact IMF, and more abundant availability of native breast skin, especially after skin-sparing mastectomy (3,154). The overall surgical morbidity is also decreased because the reconstructive surgery is performed at the same time as the mastectomy, and thus the recovery is shortened with fewer total surgical procedures (154).

The disadvantages of an immediate reconstruction include higher patient expectations, as the patient does not experience a period with complete absence of the breast, and higher surgical complication rates, especially relating to mastectomy skin flap necrosis. Rates of mastectomy skin flap necrosis have been reported to be as high as 10% and may be even higher in skin-sparing mastectomies (155,156). Tissue loss from the mastectomy skin flap can lead to exposure and infection, especially when an implant-based reconstruction is performed. This, in turn, may require removal of the implant or expander followed by a period of healing prior to attempting reconstruction again. Such wound healing issues can delay adjuvant therapy and may require additional mastectomy skin flap revisions (154). Depending on the viability of the mastectomy skin flaps intraoperatively, a reconstruction may need to be converted from an immediate to a delayed procedure. Pathological analysis of surgical margins and axillary nodes is also not finalized at the time of an immediate reconstruction, thus complicating the reconstruction process. If the final pathology results indicate the need for postmastectomy radiation or adjuvant chemotherapy, this may further delay the reconstructive process, resulting in delays in exchanging a tissue expander for a permanent implant or nipple reconstruction, which is deferred until after completion of adjuvant treatments.

Delayed reconstruction is sometimes recommended for patients with locally advanced tumors who may require more urgent administration of adjuvant chemotherapy or postmastectomy radiation, or both (3). Lower complication rates have been reported with delayed reconstruction with regard to mastectomy skin flaps, as skin flap viability is more certain and there is a decreased risk of seroma formation (154).

In general, aesthetic results tend to be inferior when the breast is reconstructed in a delayed fashion. Poorer results are due to a loss of the skin envelope from contraction of the breast skin, obliteration of the IMF, and loss of suppleness and elasticity of the breast skin and subcutaneous tissue over time. It is significantly more difficult to create a natural breast contour with appropriate ptosis in this setting. Also, in the case of a free flap reconstruction, the dissection of the recipient vessels may be technically more challenging due to scarring. Importantly, patients have expressed greater anxiety and depression and decreased sense of sexual attractiveness when breast reconstruction is delayed (154).

Chemotherapy

Chemotherapy in breast cancer patients may be administered prior to definitive surgery, as neoadjuvant therapy, or following definitive surgery, as adjuvant therapy (3). Some studies have suggested an increase in tissue expander and implant failure in those undergoing immediate reconstruction following neoadjuvant therapy. In particular, higher infection rates, higher rates of implant extrusion and tissue necrosis, and an increased tendency for wound healing problems have been reported (8,77).

For patients who have undergone reconstruction with tissue expanders, adjuvant chemotherapy can be initiated during the expansion process (157). Some surgeons recommend timing the expansion to the day prior to the patient's chemotherapy so that fluid injections take place when blood counts are at optimum levels to reduce risks of infection and bleeding. The exchange of the tissue expander for a permanent implant is performed after the completion of the chemotherapy, following the return of normal lab values (33). Despite the increased risks, chemotherapy is not an absolute contraindication for immediate reconstruction. However, if the patient has extensive disease and urgent adjuvant therapy is warranted, delaying reconstruction is often recommended.

Radiation

Adjuvant radiation therapy provides improved local control and survival among patients with locally advanced or node-positive breast cancer (78,158). It has also been shown to prevent local recurrence in patients with close or positive mastectomy margins and to provide long-term regional control in those with chest wall recurrence (78,158). Thus postmastectomy radiation therapy has become an increasingly common practice in the treatment of breast cancer.

The effects of radiation on surrounding tissues vary, and thus may add complexity to breast reconstruction. The effects of radiation are thought to be permanent and progressive. Tissues that have been radiated can be contracted and less elastic and can show color mismatch relative to surrounding tissue (152,159–164). In addition, radiation impairs wound healing and predisposes individuals to infection (159–164). Radiation also increases the risk of complications in any type of reconstruction, with potential for less pleasing aesthetic results (12,17,35,78,79,154,165,166). For these reasons, delayed autologous tissue reconstruction has often been recommended in patients requiring postmastectomy radiation in order to bring in healthy vascularized, nonirradiated tissue to replace the tissues damaged by the radiation process (152,165,167).

More recently, studies have shown that prosthesis-based reconstruction can be attempted with satisfactory results even if postmastectomy radiation is planned (3,12,35,48,78,168). In addition, studies have shown that implants do not interfere with the radiation dosage delivered to the desired location (169,170). At our institution, a two-stage approach is often recommended. Here, tissue expanders are placed at the time of the mastectomy. The tissue expanders are filled to completion prior to initiation of the radiotherapy (78). The tissue expander is exchanged for a permanent implant after the completion of the radiotherapy.

Tangential radiation fields are often used in breast cancer therapy. Thus, surrounding structures may be included as part of the radiated field, which may cause injury to vital structures such as the heart and the lung (171–174). To decrease this complication, in a bilateral breast reconstruction, the radiation oncologist may request the contralateral tissue expander to be deflated.

Prosthesis-based reconstruction can be considered in patients with prior radiation when postradiation changes are minimal and tissues are still supple and soft (166,168). Rates of complications such as infection, seroma, implant exposure/extrusion, capsular contracture (Baker grades 3 and 4), and failed reconstruction can range from 20% to 60%, often requiring additional autologous tissue for salvage or aesthetic reasons (158,165,166,168). When a tissue expander is used for breast reconstruction in previously irradiated tissue, radiation damage to tissue may limit the expansion process and restrict the final breast size (159,160,165,166,175).

If postoperative radiation therapy is anticipated, some surgeons recommend delayed reconstruction with autologous tissue. Autologous tissue breast reconstructions that are subsequently radiated have unpredictable outcomes, with higher complication rates and potentially unfavorable aesthetic outcomes (158,167). Although most studies have not demonstrated an increase in early surgical complications (vessel thrombosis, partial flap loss, total flap loss, or mastectomy skin flap necrosis), late complications (fat necrosis, volume loss, and flap contracture) have been reported and may require additional prosthetic or autologous reconstructive procedures (161,165,167).

■ ADJUNCT PROCEDURES

Revision Procedures to Improve Symmetry

Approximately 3 months after the primary reconstruction, wound healing is complete, swelling has subsided, and the tissues become more malleable. At this time, minor revisional surgeries as well as symmetry procedures to the contralateral breast can be performed more easily. In addition, the reconstructed breast or the contralateral breast may be augmented, reduced, or lifted (mastopexy). Fat grafts or injections can be used to fill in smaller contour defects. Nipple reconstruction may be performed at the same time as symmetry procedures.

Nipple Reconstruction

There are multiple ways to reconstruct the nipple, including using local flaps. In patients with large contralateral nipples, a portion of that nipple can be borrowed for use in the nipple-sharing reconstruction. Composite grafts from the earlobe and toes have been used for nipple reconstruction, although this has fallen out of favor owing to donor-site morbidity (18). With time, virtually all the techniques used for nipple reconstruction lose volume, necessitating that the nipple be reconstructed to be larger than the expected final size required (176). Once the flap is completely healed, soft-tissue fillers and cartilage can be used to maintain projection if desired by the patient. The pigmented nipple-areola complex can be constructed by using full-thickness skin grafts from the inner thigh or labia majora or more simply by a tattoo (177,178).

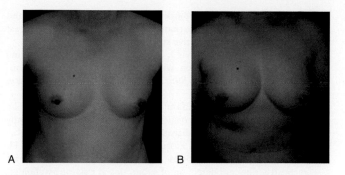

FIGURE 9.6 Immediate left breast reconstruction with pedicled TRAM flap, followed by nipple reconstruction and tattoo. (A) Preoperative; (B) postoperative.

The patient may also choose to forgo nipple reconstruction, choosing to wear a prosthetic nipple or nothing at all. Typically, nipple and areola reconstructions are preformed under local anesthesia. After nipple reconstruction and tattoo, satisfactory breast reconstruction result can be achieved (Figure 9.6).

■ MULTIDISCIPLINARY CONSIDERATIONS

- Despite the overall benefits of breast reconstruction, continuous advances in breast reconstruction techniques, and improved understanding of reconstruction benefits, the surgeon and the patient must not be distracted from the primary goal—namely, treatment of the breast cancer.
- Achieving the desired cosmetic result in a breast reconstruction should be secondary to achieving optimal breast cancer treatment.
- Careful coordination and planning that involves the patient, the reconstructive surgeon, and the entire cancer care team, including the radiation oncologist, medical oncologist, and surgical oncologist, is required to determine the best type of breast reconstruction as well as the best time for reconstruction. This becomes especially important when adjuvant radiation therapy or chemotherapy is required.

■ REFERENCES

1. Association of Breast Surgery at BASO; Association of Breast Surgery at BAPRAS; Training Interface Group in Breast Surgery, Baildam A, Bishop H, Boland G, et al. Oncoplastic breast surgery-a guide to good practice. *Eur J Surg Oncol.* 2007;33:S1–S23.
2. Wilkins EG, Cederna PS, Lowery JC, et al. Prospective analysis of psychosocial outcomes in breast reconstruction: One-year postoperative results from the Michigan breast reconstruction outcome study. *Plast Reconstr Surg.* 2000;106(5):1014–1025.
3. Gouy S, Rouzier R, Missana MC, Atallah D, Youssef O, Barreau-Pouhaer L. Immediate reconstruction after neoadjuvant chemotherapy: effect on adjuvant treatment starting and survival. *Ann Surg Oncol.* 2005;12:161–166.

4. Elder EE, Brandberg Y, Bjorklund T, et al. Quality of life and patient satisfaction in breast cancer patients after immediate breast reconstruction: a prospective study. *Breast*. 2005;14:201–208.

5. Roth RS, Lowery JC, Davis J, Wilkins EG. Psychological factors predict patient satisfaction with postmastectomy breast reconstruction. *Plast Reconstr Surg*. 2007;119:2008–2015; discussion 2016–2017.

6. Holmberg L, Zaren E, Adami HO, Bergstrom R, Burns T. The patient's appraisal of the cosmetic result of segmental mastectomy in benign and malignant disease. *Ann Surg*. 1988;207:189–194.

7. Gilboa D, Borenstein A, Floro S, Shafir R, Falach H, Tsur H. Emotional and psychosocial adjustment of women to breast reconstruction and detection of subgroups at risk for psychological morbidity. *Ann Plast Surg*. 1990;25:397–401.

8. Mehrara BJ, Santoro TD, Arcilla E, Watson JP, Shaw WW, Da Lio AL. Complications after microvascular breast reconstruction: experience with 1,195 flaps. *Plast Reconstr Surg*. 2006; 118:1100–1109.

9. Chang DW, Reece GP, Wang B, et al. Effect of smoking on complications in patients undergoing free TRAM flap breast reconstruction. *Plast Reconstr Surg*. 2000;105:2374–2380.

10. Spear SL, Ducic I, Cuoco F, Taylor N. Effect of obesity on flap and donor-site complications in pedicled TRAM flap breast reconstruction. *Plast Reconstr Surg*. 2007;119:788–795.

11. Chang DW, Wang B, Robb GL, et al. Effect of obesity on flap and donor-site complications in free transverse rectus abdominis myocutaneous flap breast reconstruction. *Plast Reconstr Surg*. 2000;105:1640–1648.

12. McCarthy CM, Mehara BJ, Riedel E, et al. Predicting complications following expander/implant breast reconstruction: an outcome analysis based on preoperative clinical risk. *Plast Reconstr Surg*. 2008;121:1886–1892.

13. Goodwin SJ, McCarthy CM, Pusic AL, et al. Complications in smokers after postmastectomy tissue expander/implant breast reconstruction. *Ann Plast Surg*. 2005;55:16–19.

14. Padubidri AN, Yetman R, Browne E, et al. Complications of postmastectomy breast reconstructions in smoker, ex-smokers, and nonsmokers. *Plast Reconstr Surg*. 2001;107:342–349.

15. Netscher DT, Wigoda P, Thornby J, Yip B, Rappaport NH. The hemodynamic and hematologic effects of cigarette smoking versus a nicotine patch. *Plast Reconstr Surg*. 1995;96:681–688.

16. Reus WF, Colen LB, Straker DJ. Tobacco smoking and complication in elective microsurgery. *Plast Reconstr Surg*. 1992;89: 490–494.

17. Mesbahi AN, McCarthy, CM, Disa JJ. Breast reconstruction with prosthetic implants. *Cancer J*. 2008;14:230–235.

18. Sigurdson L, Lalonde DH. MOC-PS CME article: breast reconstruction. *Plast Reconstr Surg*. 2008;121:1–12.

19. Moran SL, Serletti JM. Outcome comparison between free and pedicled TRAM flap breast reconstruction in the obese patient. *Plast Reconstr Surg*. 2001;108:1954–1960.

20. Losken A, Styblo TM, Schaefer TG, Carlson GW. The use of fluorescein dye as a predictor of mastectomy skin flap viability following autologous tissue reconstruction. *Ann Plast Surg*. 2008;61:24–29.

21. Yamaguchi S, De Lorenzi F, Petit JY, et al. The "Perfusion Map" of the unipedicled TRAM flap to reduce postoperative partial necrosis. *Ann Plast Surg*. 2004; 53:205–209.

22. Giunta RE, Holzbach T, Taskov C, et al. Prediction of flap necrosis with laser induced indocyanine green fluorescence in a rat model. *Br J Plast Surg*. 2005; 58:695–701.

23. Singer R, Lewis CM, Franklin JD, Lynch JB. Fluorescein test for prediction of flap viability during breast reconstruction. *Plast Reconstr Surg*. 1978;61:371–375.

24. Thorvaldsson SE, Grabb WC. The intravenous flourescein test as a measure of skin flap viability. *Plast Reconstr Surg*. 1974; 53:576–578.

25. Graham BH, Walton RL, Elings VB, Lewis FR. Surface quantification of injected fluorescent as a predictor of flap viability. *Plast Reconstr Surg*. 1983;71:826–831.

26. Liao EC, Labow BI, May JW. Skin banking closure technique in immediate autologous breast reconstruction. *Plast Reconstr Surg*. 2007;120:1133–1136.

27. Kovach SJ, Georgiade GS. The "Banked" TRAM: a method to ensure mastectomy skin flap survival. *Ann Plast Surg*. 2006;57:366–369.

28. Breuing KH, Colwell AS. Inferolateral alloderm hammock for implant coverage in breast reconstruction. *Ann Plast Surg*. 2007;59:250–255.

29. Baxter RA. Intracapsular allogenic dermal grafts for breast implant-related problems. *Plast Reconstr Surg*. 2003;112:1692–1696.

30. Ryan JJ. The lower thoracic advancement technique in breast reconstruction. *Clin Plast Surg*. 1984;11:277–286.

31. Ryan JJ. A lower thoracic advancement flap in breast reconstruction after mastectomy. *Plast Reconstr Surg*. 1982;70:153–160.

32. Burk RW, Grotting JC. Conceptual considerations in breast reconstruction. *Clin Plast Surg*. 1995;22:141–152.

33. Spear SL, Spittler, CJ. Breast reconstruction with implants and expanders. *Plast Reconstr Surg*. 2001;107:177–187.

34. Handel N, Cordray T, Gutierrez J, Jensen JA. A long-term study of outcomes, Complications, and patient satisfaction with breast implants. *Plast Reconstr Surg*. 2006;117:757–767.

35. Cordeiro PG, McCarthy CM. A single surgeon's 12-year experience with tissue expander/implant breast reconstruction: part ii. an analysis of long-term complications, aesthetic outcomes, and patient satisfaction. *Plast Reconstr Surg*. 2006;118:832–839.

36. Spear SL, Newman MK, Bedford MS, Schwartz KA, Cohen M, Schwartz JS. A retrospective analysis of outcomes using three common methods for immediate breast reconstruction. *Plast Reconstr Surg*. 2008;122:340–347.

37. Spear SL, Mardini S, Ganz JC. Resource cost comparison of implant-based breast reconstruction versus TRAM flap breast reconstruction. *Plast Reconstr Surg*. 2003;112:101–115.

38. Kroll SS, Evans GR, Reece GP, et al. Comparison of resource costs between implant-based and TRAM reconstruction. *Plast Reconstr Surg*. 1996;97:364–372.

39. Cunningham B. The mentor core study on silicone memorygel breast implants. *Plast Reconstr Surg*. 2007;120:19S–29S.

40. Spear SL, Murphy DK, Slicton A, Walker PS. Inamed silicone breast implant U.S. Study Group. Inamed silicone breast implant core study results at 6 years. *Plast Reconstr Surg*. 2007;120:8S–16S.

41. Spear SL, Parikh PM, Goldstein JA. History of breast implants and the food and drug administration. *Clin Plast Surg*. 2009; 36:15–21.

42. Silicone gel-filled breast implants approved. *FDA Consumer Magazine*. 2007;41:8–9.

43. McLaughlin JK, Lipworth L, Murphy DK, Walker PS. The safety of silicone gel-filled breast implants: a review of the epidemiologic evidence. *Ann Plast Surg*. 2007;59:569–580.

44. Holmich LR, Friis S, Fryzek JP, et al. Incidence of silicone breast implant rupture. *Arch Surg*. 2003;138:801–806.

45. Rohrich RJ, Reece EM. Breast augmentation today: saline versus silicone-what are the facts? *Plast Reconstr Surg*. 2008;121: 669–672.

46. Kelleher JC. Saline versus silicone for breast augmentation today. *Plast Reconstr Surg*. 2008;122:990–991.

47. Weiss PR. Breast reconstruction after mastectomy. *Am J Manag Care*. 1997;3:932–937.

48. Cordeiro PG, McCarthy CM. A single surgeon's 12-year experience with tissue expander/implant breast reconstruction: Part I. A prospective analysis of early complications. *Plast Reconstr Surg*. 2006;118:825–831.

49. Loustau HD, Mayer HF, Sarrabayrouse M. Pocket work for optimising outcomes in prosthetic breast reconstruction. *J Plast Reconstr Aesthet Surg*. 2008.

50. Zienowicz RJ, Karacaoglu E. Implant-based breast reconstruction with allograft. *Plast Reconstr Surg.* 2007;120:373–381.

51. Gulben, K, Yildirim E, Berberoglu U. Prediction of occult nipple-areola complex involvement in breast cancer patients. *Neoplasma.* 2009;56:72–75.

52. Laronga C, Kemp B, Johnston D, Robb GL, Singletary SE. The incidence of occult nipple-areola complex involvement in breast cancer patients receiving a skin-sparing mastectomy. *Ann Surg Oncol.* 1999;6:609–613.

53. Vlajcic Z, Zic R, Stanec S, Lambasa S, Petrovecki M, Stanec Z. Nipple-areola complex preservation: predictive factors of neoplastic nipple-areola complex invasion. *Ann Plast Surg.* 2005;55:240–244.

54. Cense HA, Rutgers EJ, Lopes Cardozo M, Van Lanschott JJ. Nipple-sparing mastectomy in breast cancer: a viable option? *Eur J Surg Oncol.* 2001;27:521–526.

55. Livesey SA, Herndon DN, Hollyoak MA, Atkinson YH, Nag A. Transplanted acellular allograft dermal matrix. potential as template for the reconstruction of viable dermis. *Transplantation.* 1995;60:1–9.

56. Milburn ML, Holton LH, Chung TL, et al. Acellular dermal matrix compared with synthetic implant material for repair of ventral hernia in the setting of peri-operative staphylococcus aureus implant contamination: a rabbit model. *Surg Infect.* 2008;9:433–442.

57. Luczyszyn SM, Grisi MF, Novaes AB, Palioto DB, Souza SL, Taba M. Histologic analysis of the acellular dermal matrix graft incorporation process: a pilot study in dogs. *Int J Periodont Restor Dent.* 2007;27:341–347.

58. Buinewicz B, Rosen B. Acellular cadaveric dermis (alloderm): a new alternative for abdominal hernia repair. *Ann Plast Surg.* 2004;52:188–194.

59. Breuing KH, Warren SM. Immediate bilateral breast reconstruction with implants and inferolateral alloderm slings. *Ann Plast Surg.* 2005;55:232–239.

60. Ashikari RH, Ashikari AY, Kelemen PR, Salzberg CA. Subcutaneous mastectomy and immediate reconstruction for prevention of breast cancer for high-risk patients. *Breast Cancer.* 2008;15:185–191.

61. Zienowicz RJ, Karacaoglu E. Implant-based breast reconstruction with allograft. *Plast Reconstr Surg.* 2007;120:373–381.

62. Salzberg CA. Nonexpansive immediate breast reconstruction using human acellular tissue matrix graft (AlloDerm). *Ann Plast Surg.* 2006;57:1–5.

63. Maguina P, Grubb K, Kalimuthu R. Single-stage immediate reconstruction after skin-sparing mastectomy. *Plast Reconstr Surg.* 2008;122:223e–224e.

64. Kiluk JV, Santillan AA, Kaur P, et al. Feasibility of sentinel lymph node biopsy through an inframammary incision for a nipple-sparing mastectomy. *Ann Surg Oncol.* 2008;15:3402–346.

65. Regolo L, Ballardini B, Gallarotti E, Scoccia E, Zanini V. Nipple sparing mastectomy: an innovative skin incision for an alternative approach. *Breast.* 2007;17:8–11.

66. Simmons RM, Hollenbeck ST, Latrenta GS. Areola-sparing mastectomy with immediate breast reconstruction. *Ann Plast Surg.* 2003;51:547–551.

67. Topol BM, Dalton EF, Ponn T, Campbell CJ. Immediate single-stage breast reconstruction using implants and human acellular dermal tissue matrix with adjustment of the lower pole of the breast to reduce unwanted lift. *Ann Plast Surg.* 2008;61:494–499.

68. Becker H. The permanent tissue expander. *Clin Plast Surg.* 1987;14:519–527.

69. Becker H. Breast reconstruction using an inflatable breast implant with detachable reservoir. *Plast Reconstr Surg.* 1984;73:678–683.

70. Becker H, Maraist F. Immediate breast reconstruction after mastectomy using a permanent tissue expander. *South Med J.* 1987;80:154–160.

71. Becker H. The expandable mammary implant. *Plast Reconstr Surg.* 1987;79:631–637.

72. Persoff MM. Expansion-augmentation of the breast. *Plast Reconstr Surg.* 1993;91:393–403.

73. Becker H, Van Leeuwen JB. The correction of breast ptosis with the expander mammary prosthesis. *Ann Plast Surg.* 1990;24:489–497.

74. Becker H, Shaw KE, Kara M. Correction of symmastia using an adjustable implant. *Plast Reconstr Surg.* 2005;115:2124–2126.

75. Kneafsey B, Crawford DS, Khoo CT, Saad MN. Correction of developmental breast abnormalities with a permanent expander/implant. *Br J Plast Surg.* 1996;49:302–306.

76. Camilleri IG, Malata CM, Stavrianos S, McLean NR. A review of 120 Becker permanent tissue expanders in reconstruction of the breast. *Br J Plast Surg.* 1996;49:346–351.

77. Mitchem J, Herrmann D, Margenthaler JA, Aft RL. Impact of neoadjuvant chemotherapy on rate of tissue expander/implant loss and progression to successful breast reconstruction following mastectomy. *Am J Surg.* 2008;196(4):519–522.

78. Cordeiro PG, Pusic AL, Disa JJ, McCormick B, VanZee K. Irradiation after immediate tissue expander/implant breast reconstruction: outcomes, complications, aesthetic results, and satisfaction among 156 Patients. *Plast Reconstr Surg.* 2004;113:877–881.

79. McCarthy CM, Pusic AL, Disa JJ, McCormick BL, Montgomery LL, Cordeiro PG. Unilateral postoperative chest wall radiotherapy in bilateral tissue expander/implant reconstruction patients: a prospective outcome analysis. *Plast Reconstr Surg.* 2005;116:1642–1647.

80. Vega, SJ, Bossert RP, Serletti JM. Improving outcomes in bilateral breast reconstruction using autogenous tissue. *Ann Plast Surg.* 2006;56:487–491.

81. Cordeiro, PG. Breast reconstruction after surgery for breast cancer. *New Eng J Med.* 2008;359:1590–1601.

82. Hartrampf CR, Scheflan M, Black PW. Breast reconstruction with a transverse abdominal island flap. *Plast Reconstr Surg.* 1982;69:216–224.

83. Cederna PS, Chang P, Pittet-Cuenod BM, Razaboni RM, Cram AE. The effect of the delay phenomenon on the vascularity of rabbit rectus abdominis muscles. *Plast Reconstr Surg.* 1997;99:194–205.

84. Moon HK, Taylor GI. The vascular anatomy of rectus abdominis musculocutaneous flap based on the deep superior epigastric system. *Plast Reconstr Surg.* 1988;82:815–832.

85. Boyd JB, Taylor GI, Corlett R. The vascular territories of the superior epigastric and the deep inferior epigastric systems. *Plast Reconstr Surg.* 1984;73:1–16.

86. Tuominen HP, Asko-Seljavaara S, Svartling NE. Cutaneous blood flow in the free TRAM flap. *Br J Plast Surg.* 1993;46:665–669.

87. Tuominen HP, Asko-Seljavaara S, Svartling NE, Harma MA. Cutaneous blood flow in the tram flap. *Br J Plast Surg.* 1992;45:261–269.

88. Dulin WA, Avila RA, Verheyden CN, Grossman L. Evaluation of abdominal wall strength after TRAM Flap Surgery. *Plast Reconstr Surg.* 2004;113:1662–1665.

89. Simon AM, Bouwense CL, McMillan S, Lamb S, Hammond DC. Comparison of unipedicled and bipedicled TRAM flap breast reconstructions: assessment of physical function and patient satisfaction. *Plast Reconstr Surg.* 2004;113:136–140.

90. Bonde CT, Lund H, Fridberg M, Danneskiold-Samsoe B, Elberg JJ. Abdominal strength after breast reconstruction using a free abdominal flap. *J Plast Reconstr Aesthet Surg.* 2007;60:519–523.

91. Futter CM, Webster MH, Hagen S, Mitchell SL. A retrospective comparison of abdominal muscle strength following breast reconstruction with free TRAM or DIEP flap. *Br J Plast Surg.* 2000;53:578–583.

92. Vyas RM, Dickinson BP, Fastekjian JH, Watson JP, Dalio AL, Crisera CA. Risk factors for abdominal donor-site morbidity in

free flap breast reconstruction. *Plast Reconstr Surg.* 2008;121: 1519–1526.

93. Zienowicz RJ, May JW. Hernia prevention and aesthetic contouring of the abdomen following TRAM flap breast reconstruction by the use of polypropylene mesh. *Plast Reconstr Surg.* 1995;96:1346–1350.

94. Kroll SS, Marchi M. Comparison of strategies for preventing abdominal-wall weakness after TRAM flap breast reconstruction. *Plast Reconstr Surg.* 1992;89:1045–1051.

95. Paterson P, Sterne GD, Fatah F. Mesh assisted direct closure of bilateral TRAM flap donor sites. *J Plast Reconstr Aesthet Surg.* 2006;59:347–351.

96. Moscona RA, Ramon Y, Toledano H, Barzilay G. Use of synthetic mesh for the entire abdominal wall after TRAM flap transfer. *Plast Reconstr Surg.* 1998;101:706–710.

97. Bucky LP, May JW. Synthetic mesh. Its use in abdominal wall reconstruction after the TRAM. *Clin Plast Surg.* 1994;21:273–277.

98. Dell DD, Weaver C, Kozempel J, Barsevick A. Recovery after transverse rectus abdominis myocutaneous flap breast reconstruction surgery. *Oncol Nurs Forum.* 2008;35:189–196.

99. Hsieh F, Kumiponjera D, Malata CM. An algorithmic approach to abdominal flap breast reconstruction in patients with pre-existing scars-results from a single surgeon's experience. *J Plast Reconstr Aesthet Surg.* 2008.

100. Sozer SO, Cronin ED, Biggs TM, Gallegos ML. The use of transverse rectus abdominis musculocutaneous flap after abdominoplasty. *Ann Plast Surg.* 1995;35:409–411.

101. Ribuffo D, Marcellino M, Barnett GR, Houseman ND, Scuderi N. Breast reconstruction with abdominal flaps after abdominoplasties. *Plast Reconstr Surg.* 2001;108:1604–1608.

102. Hess CL, Gartside RL, Ganz JC. TRAM flap breast reconstruction after abdominal liposuction. *Ann Plast Surg.* 2004;53: 166–169.

103. O'Shaughnessy KD, Mustoe TA. The surgical TRAM flap delay: reliability of zone III using a simplified technique under local anesthesia. *Plast Reconstr Surg.* 2008;122:1627–1630.

104. Ribuffo D, Muratori L, Antoniadou K, et al. A hemodynamic approach to clinical results in the TRAM flap after selective delay. *Plast Reconstr Surg.* 1997;99:1706–1714.

105. Taylor GI, Corlett RJ, Caddy CM, Zelt RG. An anatomic review of the delay phenomenon: II. Clinical applications. *Plast Reconstr Surg.* 1992;89:408–416.

106. Marck KW, Van Der Biezen JJ, Dol JA. Internal mammary artery and vein supercharge in TRAM flap breast reconstruction. *Microsurgery.* 1996;17:371–374.

107. Wu LC, Iteld L, Song DH. Supercharging the transverse rectus abdominis musculocutaneous flap: breast reconstruction for the overweight and obese population. *Ann Plast Surg.* 2008; 60:609–613.

108. Olding M, Emory RE, Barrett WL. Preferential use of the ipsilateral pedicle in TRAM flap breast reconstruction. *Ann Plast Surg.* 1998;40:349–353.

109. Clugston PA, Gingrass MK, Azurin D, Fisher J, Maxwell GP. Ipsilateral pedicled TRAM flaps: the safer alternative? *Plast Reconstr Surg.* 2000;105:77–82.

110. Beckenstein MS, Grotting JC. Breast reconstruction with free-tissue transfer. *Plast Reconstr Surg.* 2001;108:1345–1353.

111. Rad AN, Flores JI, Rosson GD. Free DIEP and SIEA breast reconstruction to internal mammary intercostal perforating vessels with arterial microanastomosis using a mechanical coupling device. *Microsurgery.* 2008;28:407–411.

112. Saint-Cyr M, Chang DW, Robb GL, Chevray PM. Internal mammary perforator recipient vessels for breast reconstruction using free TRAM, DIEP, and SIEA flaps. *Plast Reconstr Surg.* 2007;120:1769–1773.

113. Haywood RM, Raurell A, Perks AG, Sassoon EM, Logan AM, Phillips J. Autologous free tissue breast reconstruction using the

internal mammary perforators as recipient vessels. *Br J Plast Surg.* 2003;56:689–691.

114. Hamdi M, Blondeel P, Van Landuyt K, Monstrey S. Algorithm in choosing recipient vessels for perforator free flap in breast reconstruction: the role of the internal mammary perforators. *Br J Plast Surg.* 2004;57:258–265.

115. Munhoz AM, Ishida LH, Montag E, et al. Perforator flap breast reconstruction using internal mammary perforator branch as a recipient site: an anatomical and clinical analysis. *Plast Reconstr Surg.* 2004;114:62–68.

116. Selber JC, Samra F, Bristol M, et al. A head-to-head comparison between the muscle-sparing free TRAM and the SIEA Flaps: is the rate of flap loss worth the gain in abdominal wall function? *Plast Reconstr Surg.* 2008;122:348–355.

117. Granzow JW, Levine JL, Chiu ES, Allen RJ. Breast reconstruction using perforator flaps. *J Surg Oncol.* 2006;94:441–454.

118. Serletti JM, Moran SL. Free versus the pedicled TRAM flap: a cost comparison and outcome analysis. *Plast Reconstr Surg.* 1997;100:1418–1428.

119. Garvey PB, Buchel EW, Pockaj BA, Casey WJ, Hernandez JL, Samson TD. DIEP and pedicled TRAM flaps: a comparison of outcomes. *Plast Reconstr Surg.* 2006;117:1711–1719.

120. Futter CM, Webster MH, Hagen S, Mitchell SL. A retrospective comparison of abdominal muscle strength following breast reconstruction with a free TRAM or DIEP flap. *Br J Plast Surg.* 2000;53:578–583.

121. Alonso-Burgos A, Garcia-Tutor E, Bastarrika G, Benito A, Dominguez PD, Zubieta JL. Preoperative planning of DIEP and SGAP flaps: preliminary experience with magnetic resonance angiography using 3-tesla equipment and blood-pool contrast medium. *J Plast Reconstr Aesthet Surg.* 2009.

122. Rozen WM, Ashton MW. Improving outcomes in autologous breast reconstruction. *Aesthetic Plast Surg.* 2008.

123. Rozen WM, Garcia-Tutor E, Alonso-Burgos A, et al. Planning and optimising DIEP flaps with virtual surgery: the Navarra experience. *J Plast Reconstr Aesthet Surg.* 2008.

124. Smit JM, Dimopoulou A, Liss AG, et al. Preoperative CT angiography reduces surgery time in perforator flap reconstruction. *J Plast Reconstr Aesthet Surg.* 2008.

125. Phillips TJ, Stella DL. Rozen WM, Ashton M, Taylor GI. Abdominal wall CT angiography: a detailed account of a newly established preoperative imaging technique. *Radiology.* 2008; 249:32–44.

126. Phillips TJ, Stella DL, Rozen WM, Ashton M, Taylor GI. Abdominal wall ct angiography: a detailed account of a newly established preoperative imaging technique. *Radiology.* 2008;249:32–44.

127. Nahabedian MY, Tsangaris T, Momen B. Breast reconstruction with the DIEP flap or the muscle-sparing (MS-2) free TRAM flap: is there a difference? *Plast Reconstr Surg.* 2005;115:436–444.

128. Wu LC, Bajaj A, Chang DW, Chevray PM. Comparison of donor-site morbidity of SIEA, DIEP, and muscle-sparing TRAM flaps for breast reconstruction. *Plast Reconstr Surg.* 2008;122:702–709.

129. Fathi M, Hatamipour E, Fathi HR, Abbasi A. The anatomy of superficial inferior epigastric artery flap. *Acta Cir Bras.* 2008; 23:429–434.

130. Taylor GI, Daniel RK. The anatomy of several free flap donor sites. *Plast Reconstr Surg.* 1975;56:243–253.

131. Holm, C, Mayr M, Hofter E, Ninkovic M. The versatility of the SIEA Flap: a clinical assessment of the vascular territory of the superficial epigastric inferior artery. *J Plast Reconstr Aesthet Surg.* 2007;60:946–951.

132. Holm C, Mayr M, Hofter E, Raab N, Ninkovic M. Interindividual variability of the SIEA angiosome: effects on operative strategies in breast reconstruction. *Plast Reconstr Surg.* 2008;122:1612–1620.

133. Gusenoff JA, Coon D, De La Cruz C, Rubin JP. Superficial inferior epigastric vessels in the massive weight loss population:

implications for breast reconstruction. *Plast Reconstr Surg.* 2008;122:1621–1626.

134. Groth AK, Campos AC, Goncalves CG, et al. Effects of venous supercharging in deep inferior epigastric artery perforator flap. *Acta Cir Bras.* 2007;22:474–478.

135. Semple JL. Retrograde microvascular augmentation (turbo-charging) of a single-pedicle TRAM flap through a deep inferior epigastric arterial and venous loop. *Plast Reconstr Surg.* 1994;93:109–117.

136. Granzow JW, Levine JL, Chiu ES, Allen RJ. Breast reconstruction with gluteal artery perforator flaps. *J Plast Reconstr Aesthet Surg.* 2006;59:614–621.

137. Offman SL, Geddes CR, Tang M, Morris SF. The vascular basis of perforator flaps based on the source arteries of the lateral lumbar region. *Plast Reconstr Surg.* 2005;115:1651–1659.

138. Kimata Y. Deep circumflex iliac perforator flap. *Clin Plas Surg.* 2003;30:433–438.

139. Nojima K, Brown SA, Acikel C, et al. Defining vascular supply and territory of thinned perforator flaps: part 1. Anterolateral thigh perforator flap. *Plast Reconstr Surg.* 2005;116:182–193.

140. Rosenberg JJ, Chandawarkar R, Ross MI, Chevray PM. Bilateral anterolateral thigh flaps for large-volume breast reconstruction. *Microsurgery.* 2004;24:281–284.

141. Fattah A, Figus A, Mathur B, Ramakrishnan VV. The transverse myocutaneous gracilis flap: technical refinements. *J Plast Reconstr Aesthet Surg.* 2009.

142. Schoeller T, Huemer GM, Wechselberger G. The transverse musculocutaneous gracilis flap for breast reconstruction: guidelines for flap and patient selection. *Plast Reconstr Surg.* 2008;122: 29–38.

143. Hasen KV, Gallegos ML, Dumanian GA. Extended approach to the vascular pedicle of the gracilis muscle flap: anatomical and clinical study. *Plast Reconstr Surg.* 2003;111:2203–2208.

144. Fansa H, Schirmer S, Warnecke IC, Cervelli A, Frerichs Onno. The transverse myocutaneous gracilis muscle flap: a fast and reliable method for breast reconstruction. *Plast Reconstr Surg.* 2008;122:1326–1333.

145. Yousif NJ, Matloub HS, Kolachalam R, Grunert BK, Sanger JR. The transverse gracilis musculocutaneous flap. *Ann Plast Surg.* 1992;29:482–490.

146. Heitmann C, Pelzer M, Kuentscher M, Menke H, Germann G. The extended latissimus dorsi flap revisited. *Plast Reconstr Surg.* 2003;111:1697–1701.

147. Glassey N, Perks GB, McCulley SJ. A prospective assessment of shoulder morbidity and recovery time scales following latissimus dorsi breast reconstruction. *Plast Reconstr Surg.* 2008; 122:1334–1340.

148. Clough KB, Louis-Sylvestre C, Fitoussi A, Couturaud B, Nos C. Donor site sequelae after autologous breast reconstruction with an extended latissimus dorsi flap. *Plast Reconstr Surg.* 2002; 109:1904–1911.

149. Russell RC, Pribaz J, Zook EG, Leighton WD, Eriksson E, Smith CJ. Functional evaluation of latissimus dorsi donor site. *Plast Reconstr Surg.* 1986;78:336–344.

150. Hammond DC. Postmastectomy reconstruction of the breast using the latissimus dorsi musculocutaneous flap. *Cancer J.* 2008;14:248–252.

151. Fisher J, Bostwick, J, Powell RW. Latissimus dorsi blood supply after thoracodorsal vessel division: the serratus collateral. *Plast Reconstr Surg.* 1983;72:502–509.

152. Disa JJ, McCarthy CM, Mehara BJ, Pusic AL, Cordeiro PG. Immediate latissimus dorsi/prosthetic breast reconstruction following salvage mastectomy after failed lumpectomy/irradiation. *Plast Reconstr Surg.* 2008;121:159e–165e.

153. Titley OG, Spyrou GE, Fatah MF. Preventing seroma in the latissimus dorsi flap donor site. *Br J Plast Surg.* 1997;50:106–108.

154. Chevray PM. Timing of breast reconstruction: immediate versus delayed. *Cancer J.* 2008;14:223–229.

155. Carlson GW, Bostwick J, Styblo TM, et al. Skin sparing mastectomy oncologic and reconstructive considerations. *Ann Surg.* 1997;225:570–578.

156. Rainsbury RM. Skin-sparing mastectomy. *Br J Surg.* 2006; 93:276–281.

157. Disa JJ, Ad-El D, Cohen SM, Cordeiro PG, Hidalgo DA. The premature removal of tissue expanders in breast reconstruction. *Plast Reconstr Surg.* 1999;104:1662–1665.

158. Jhaveri JD, Rush SC, Kostroff K, et al. Clinical outcomes of post-mastectomy radiation therapy after immediate breast reconstruction. *Int J Radiat Oncol Biol Phys.* 2008;72:859–865.

159. Kao JT, Dagum AB, Mahoney JL, Gardiner GW, Beaton D. The histopathological changes in irradiated vs. nonradiated tissue-expanded skin in the porcine model. *Ann Plast Surg.* 1997;39:287–291.

160. Dvali LT, Dagum AB, Pang CY, et al. Effects of radiation on skin expansion and skin flap viability in pigs. *Plast Reconstr Surg.* 2000;106:624–629.

161. Forman DL, Chiu J, Restifo RJ, Ward BA, Haffty B, Ariyan S. Breast reconstruction in previously irradiated patients using tissue expanders and implants: a potentially unfavorable result. *Ann Plast Surg.* 1998;40:360–363.

162. Mansfield C. Effects of radiation therapy on wound healing after mastectomy. *Clin Plast Surg.* 1979;6:19–26.

163. Bristol SG, Lennox PA, Clugston PA. A comparison of ipsilateral pedicled TRAM with and without previous irradiation. *Ann Plast Surg.* 2006;56:589–592.

164. Ruvalcaba-Limon E, Robles-Vidal C, Poitevin-Chacon A, Chavez-Macgregor M, Gamboa-Vignolle C, Vilar-Compte D. Complications after breast cancer surgery in patients treated with concomitant preoperative chemoradiation: a case-control analysis. *Breast Cancer Res Treat.* 2006;95:147–152.

165. Chang DW, Barnea Y, Robb GL. Effects of an autologous flap combined with an implant for breast reconstructions: an evaluation of 1000 consecutive reconstructions of previously irradiated breasts. *Plast Reconstr Surg.* 2008;122:356–362.

166. Spear SL, Onyewu C. Staged breast reconstruction with saline-filled implants in the irradiated breast: recent trends and therapeutic implications. *Plast Reconstr Surg.* 2000;105:930–942.

167. Tran NV, Chang DW, Gupta A, Kroll SS, Robb GL. Comparison of immediate and delayed free TRAM flap breast reconstruction in patients receiving postmastectomy radiation therapy. *Plast Reconstr Surg.* 2001;108:78–82.

168. Spear SL, Boehmler JH, Bogue DP, Mafi AA. Options in reconstructing the irradiated breast. *Plast Reconstr Surg.* 2008;122: 379–388.

169. McGinley PH, Powell WR, Bostwick J. Dosimetry of a silicone breast prosthesis. *Radiology.* 1980;135:223–224.

170. Moni J, Graves-Ditman M, Cederna P, Griffith K, Kruegar EA, Fraass BA, Pierce LJ. Dosimetry around metallic ports in tissue expanders in patients receiving postmastectomy radiation therapy: an ex vivo evaluation. *Medical Dosimetry.* 2004;1:49–54.

171. Hardman PD, Tweeddale PM, Kerr GR, Anderson ED, Rodger A. The effects of pulmonary function of local and loco-regional irradiation for breast cancer. *Radiother Oncol.* 1994;30:33–42.

172. Kimsey FC, Mendenhall NP, Ewald LM, Coons TS, Layon AJ. Is radiation treatment volume a predictor for acute or late effect on pulmonary function? A prospective study of patients treated with breast-conserving surgery and postoperative irradiation. *Cancer.* 1994;73:2549–2555.

173. Raj KA, Marks LB, Prosnitz RG. Late effects of breast radiotherapy in young women. *Breast Dis.* 2005-2006;23:53–65.

174. Miles EA, Venables K, Hoskin PJ, Aird EG, on behalf of the START Trial Management Group. Dosimetry and field matching

for radiotherapy to the breast and supraclavicular fossa. *Radiother Oncol.* 2009;91:42–48.

175. Percec I, Bucky LP. Successful prosthetic breast reconstruction after radiation therapy. *Ann Plast Surg.* 2008; 60:527–531.

176. Shestak KC, Gabriel A, Landecker A, Peters S, Shestak A, Kim J. Assessment of long-term nipple projection: a comparison of three techniques. *Plast Reconstr Surg.* 2002;110:780–786.

177. Hammond DC, Khuthaila D, Kim J. The skate flap purse-string technique for nipple-areola complex reconstruction. *Plast Reconstr Surg.* 2007;120:399–406.

178. Vendemia N, Mesbahi AN, McCarthy CM, Disa JJ. Nipple areola reconstruction. *Cancer J.* 2008;14:253–257.

179. Vega S, Smartt JM, Jiang S, et al. 500 consecutive patients with free TRAM flap breast reconstruction: a single surgeon's experience. *Plast Reconstr Surg.* 2008;122:329–339.

Radiation Therapy Considerations in Breast Reconstruction

ABRAM RECHT

Postmastectomy radiotherapy (PMRT) is very effective at preventing local-regional failure and thereby increases relapse-free breast cancer–specific and overall survival rates (1,2). However, several questions must be addressed in order to optimize the integration of radiation therapy and reconstructive surgery. First, how does PMRT or prior radiation therapy given for breast-conserving therapy affect the outcome of different types of reconstructive surgery? Second, how does the timing between radiation therapy and reconstruction affect these interactions? Finally, does reconstruction affect the effectiveness or risk of complications of PMRT?

This chapter will focus on these issues for patients undergoing mastectomy as primary treatment. Since results for patients treated with mastectomy for local failure following breast-conserving therapy who undergo breast reconstruction appear similar to those of patients having reconstruction following PMRT, data from studies of such patients will also be included when useful. Further discussion of these topics may be found elsewhere (3,4).

■ PROSTHETIC RECONSTRUCTIVE TECHNIQUES

Most studies have shown that PMRT substantially increased rates of capsular fibrosis and other complications for patients undergoing prosthetic reconstructions performed either directly or with the intermediate step of tissue expansion (5–15). For example, Spear and colleagues at Georgetown University in Washington examined results in 40 patients treated from 1990 to 1998 who underwent staged breast reconstruction with an expander and implant and received radiation before, during, or after the expansion (7). Of these, 47.5% required an additional flap procedure to improve, correct, or salvage the implant. Their overall complication rate was 52.5%, compared with 10% for a control group of 40 patients who did not undergo irradiation who were randomly sampled from 200 such patients treated during the same period. In a study from Memorial Sloan-Kettering Cancer Center in New York, with a mean follow-up of 34 months, 11% of the 81 irradiated patients required removal of their

implants (of which 1 of 9 was replaced), compared with 6% of 542 nonirradiated patients (with 26 of 33 implants being replaced) (12). The rate of capsular contracture in 68 patients undergoing PMRT who had a minimum follow-up of 1 year was 68%, compared with 40% for a control group of 75 unirradiated patients. "Acceptable" cosmetic results in the two groups were 80% and 88%, respectively, with 72% and 85% of respective patients saying they would choose the same form of reconstruction again. A study from Columbia University in New York found that 18% of irradiated patients (5 of 27) required removal or replacement of their implant, compared with 4% of nonirradiated patients (4 of 96) (13).

Not all studies show such severe effects from PMRT. The risk of major complications at 3 years was only 5% in 50 patients undergoing PMRT at Fox Chase Cancer Center in Philadelphia after placement of a tissue expander and implant, with two patients requiring removal of the prosthesis (16). Overall cosmetic results were good or excellent in 82% of patients. The reasons for the differences between this study and those described above are not clear.

Complication rates in the studies from Georgetown University and Columbia University were the same whether patients had PMRT before or after reconstruction (7,13). However, an update of the Memorial Sloan-Kettering Cancer Center experience found that the rate of grade 3 or 4 capsular contracture was 20% among patients undergoing prior radiotherapy, compared with 51% among patients irradiated following exchange of the tissue expander for the permanent prosthesis and 10% for nonirradiated patients (15).

Tissue expanders or implants are also poorly tolerated by patients initially undergoing breast-conserving therapy (11,17,18). For example, a group in Marseille, France, found complications in five of eight patients undergoing reconstruction as a part of salvage surgery for a local recurrence (11). One patient developed a concave deformity of the chest wall following tissue expansion (19). Again, some studies have reported lower rates of complications, at least in carefully selected individuals (20–22).

■ AUTOLOGOUS FLAP RECONSTRUCTIVE TECHNIQUES

Complication rates in patients who undergo reconstruction with a pure myocutaneous flap *following* PMRT are only slightly higher than those for nonirradiated patients (23–28). For example, Williams and colleagues described results in patients treated with pedicled transverse rectus abdominus muscle (TRAM) flaps from 1981 to 1993 at Emory University in Atlanta (29). The risk of complications was little different between the 572 unirradiated patients (17%) and the 108 patients irradiated prior to reconstruction (25%).

The type of flap used may influence the risk of complications in patients irradiated prior to reconstruction. Complication rates in one series of patients undergoing reconstruction after local recurrence following breast-conserving therapy were higher when latissimus flaps were used (47%) than when TRAM flaps were employed (25%) (23), but many of these complications were minor. No patient in this series suffered complete flap loss.

For patients who undergo reconstruction *before* PMRT, the risk of complications depends heavily on the type of reconstruction performed. Several studies show that pedicled TRAM flaps tolerate PMRT well, although there may be small differences in cosmetic outcome from nonirradiated patients (10,16,25–28,30,31). For example, a recent study from Emory University found the risk of any complication to be 34% among 149 patients who underwent immediate reconstruction without subsequent PMRT, compared with 44% among 25 patients receiving PMRT (28). There was no difference in the need for remedial surgery (19% versus 12%, respectively). However, the incidence of fat necrosis was higher in the irradiated group (32%, compared with 15% on the unirradiated patients), and overall cosmetic results were slightly worse as judged from photographs.

The risk of complications may be substantially increased for patients undergoing PMRT after reconstruction with "free" flaps (i.e., those in which the flap's vessels are severed and anastamosed to vessels at the recipient site). For example, Tran and colleagues at the MD Anderson Cancer Center in Houston compared results among 32 patients undergoing immediate free TRAM flap reconstructions followed by PMRT and 70 patients having reconstruction after PMRT (30). They found significantly higher rates of fat necrosis (44% versus 9%), volume loss (88% versus nil), and flap contracture (75% versus nil) when PMRT was given after reconstruction. The effects were substantial enough to require repair with a second flap in 28% of the patients irradiated after reconstruction, compared with none of the patients having PMRT first.

Poor results have also been reported for patients who undergo irradiation after a deep inferior epigastric perforator (DIEP) flap compared with nonirradiated patients. For example, a case-control study from Memorial Medical Center in New Orleans comparing 30 patients receiving PMRT following reconstruction with 30 patients have DIEP flap reconstruction alone found substantially higher rates of fat necrosis (23% versus nil), fibrosis or shrinkage (57% versus nil), and contracture (17% versus nil) at

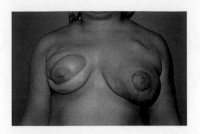

FIGURE 9.7 Fibrosis and shrinkage owing to volume loss in a patient undergoing a right-sided superior gluteal artery perforator flap followed by postmastectomy radiotherapy. (Courtesy of Dr. Bernard Lee, Beth Israel Deaconess Medical Center, Boston, Massachusetts.)

any time during follow-up in the irradiated patients, with respective mean follow-up periods of 20 and 17 months (32). There were no significant differences in the rates of flap revision (67% versus 87%) or flap dehiscence (37% versus 27%). Other perforator free flaps are probably equally vulnerable to the effects of PMRT (Figure 9.7). However, patients irradiated *before* DIEP flap reconstruction do not appear to have increased rates of complications compared with nonirradiated patients (31).

■ MIXED PROSTHESIS/FLAP RECONSTRUCTIVE TECHNIQUES

One option for patients wishing to avoid the potential donor-site morbidity of a TRAM flap is to use a latissimus dorsi flap with a prosthesis in order to achieve greater bulk than the flap alone can provide while having a more natural consistency than a prosthesis alone. However, the use of a prosthesis does not seem to prevent complications when PMRT is given following reconstruction. In a study from the MD Anderson Cancer Center, the risk of significant complications was 40% for 25 for patients undergoing reconstruction with a latissimus dorsi flap plus prosthesis who were then irradiated, compared with 8% for nonirradiated patients (5).

The interval between irradiation and reconstruction may have an impact on the risk of complications in patients undergoing a latissimus dorsi flap and expander/implant approach. In a study from Georgetown University, two of four patients undergoing reconstruction immediately *following* PMRT required implant exchanges owing to infection or deflation (33). However, results were much more acceptable when such reconstruction was done in patients who had received radiation 1 year or more earlier.

■ RADIOTHERAPY TECHNIQUE AND THE RISK OF COMPLICATIONS

There are few data on how details of radiotherapy technique affect the risk of complications after reconstruction.

Relevant variables include the daily dose (fraction size), the total dose given to the chest wall as a whole, whether a boost dose is given to the mastectomy scar or a portion of the chest wall, the use of tissue-equivalent material placed on the skin (bolus) to increase the skin dose, the homogeneity of the dose deposited within the treated area (which, in turn, depends on the patient's body size, the photon or electron beam energy used, and the dose-prescription convention), and the possible adverse affects of overlaps between treatment fields. In addition, chemotherapy (especially if given concurrently with radiotherapy) and tamoxifen might potentially increase the risk of complications.

The most careful study of how these parameters impact results was performed by investigators in the Michigan Breast Reconstruction Outcome study (9). The risks of complications and reconstruction failure after expander/implant reconstruction were not substantially affected by whether regional nodes were irradiated, by total dose (less than or greater than 60 Gy), by the use of a boost or bolus, or by the timing of radiotherapy and reconstruction. They did find that the use of tamoxifen increased the risk of complications (75% versus 57%) and reconstruction failure (58% versus 0%). However, there were only 19 irradiated patients in this study (of whom 12 received tamoxifen). In contrast, a study from Massachusetts General Hospital and Boston Medical Center of 48 patients treated with either tissue/expander implant or TRAM flap and radiotherapy found that tamoxifen did not affect the risk of complications (34).

■ THE EFFECT OF RECONSTRUCTION ON RADIATION TECHNIQUE

One concern often raised in the past to discourage the use of immediate breast reconstruction was that it might reduce the effectiveness of PMRT. However, this has not been seen to date (1). For example, a recent study of patients treated in Kaohsiung, Taiwan, from 1997 to 2001 found that the crude rate of chest wall recurrence was 4% for 82 patients undergoing PMRT following TRAM flap reconstruction, compared with 2% for 109 patients who did not have reconstruction (35).

Immediate reconstruction can reduce the technical options available to the radiation oncologist (36). This could result in increasing the exposed volumes of the heart and lung and hence the risk of complications. There are no published data showing whether such effects are seen clinically. However, the exact degree to which this is a problem depends on the patient's anatomy, the chosen target volume (especially whether the internal mammary nodes are included), and the choice of treatment techniques available. Alternatives such as intensity-modulated radiation

therapy (37) and deep-inspiration breath holding (38,39) can reduce or eliminate such exposure.

■ STRATEGIES TO HELP MINIMIZE DELETERIOUS INTERACTIONS BETWEEN RADIOTHERAPY AND RECONSTRUCTIVE SURGERY

A major obstacle to optimally integrating PMRT and reconstructive surgery is that, for many patients, the decision as to whether PMRT is indicated cannot be made until after mastectomy. One strategy to avoid this problem is to place a tissue expander at the time of mastectomy to preserve the skin envelope and then wait for the pathology to decide whether PMRT is indicated. If it is not, then definitive reconstruction can be completed during the same hospitalization (the so-called delayed-immediate approach) (3,4). If PMRT will be needed, reconstruction can be completed 4 to 6 months after PMRT. However, this approach has the disadvantage of requiring two operations in quick succession.

Since pathological nodal status is the single most important factor in making this decision, another strategy is to perform sentinel node biopsy before mastectomy. If the nodes are involved, then the chance that PMRT will be indicated is much greater than if the nodes are negative, and hence a more informed decision can be made between different reconstructive procedures and about when reconstruction should be performed. For example, a group in Norwich, England, found that 30% of 67 patients having immediate reconstruction unexpectedly required PMRT (40). They then implemented a policy of premastectomy sentinel node biopsy, which resulted in 15% of 72 patients being offered a temporary subpectoral expander, to be followed by definitive reconstruction later.

Finally, the most critical factor in avoiding deleterious interactions between reconstructive surgery and radiation therapy is early communication and interaction between all those involved in the patient's care. This is most easily accomplished by seeing patients in multidisciplinary clinics or discussing them in tumor boards where oncologic surgeons, plastic surgeons, radiation oncologists, and medical oncologists can jointly discuss the issues outlined above before irreversible decisions are made. However, the absence of such formalized multispecialty conferences or clinics does not relieve physicians of their duty to talk with each other to create a joint treatment plan that will optimize the patient's oncologic, cosmetic, and psychological outcomes.

■ CONCLUSIONS

PMRT substantially increases the risks of capsular fibrosis and complications following reconstruction with a prosthesis in most studies, whether given before or after surgery. However, such reconstructions are less difficult to perform than pure myocutaneous procedures and hence are more widely available; they are often easier for patients to endure; and some patients may not be candidates for alternative procedures. Since complications do not occur in all patients undergoing prosthetic reconstruction who receive PMRT, it is reasonable to use such techniques for patients who have been or will be irradiated, reserving myocutaneous procedures for later use if needed. Pedicled TRAM flaps appear to tolerate PMRT well and hence can be used for immediate reconstruction in patients known to require PMRT before mastectomy. Giving PMRT after reconstruction substantially increases the risk of complications and poor cosmetic results following procedures requiring microvascular anastamoses. Performing immediate reconstruction does not interfere with the effectiveness of PMRT and is unlikely to affect the risk of long-term cardiac or pulmonary complications. Strategies such as "delayed-immediate" reconstruction and premastectomy sentinel node biopsy may help patients and their physicians make better choices regarding the optimal reconstructive procedure. Optimizing patients' outcomes requires close cooperation between all specialists from the beginning of diagnosis and treatment.

■ SUMMARY

- PMRT substantially increases the risks of capsular fibrosis and complications following reconstruction with a prosthesis in most studies, whether given before or after surgery.
- Pedicled TRAM flaps appear to tolerate PMRT well and hence can be used for immediate reconstruction in patients known to require PMRT before mastectomy.
- Giving PMRT after reconstruction substantially increases the risk of complications and poor cosmetic results following procedures requiring microvascular anastomoses.
- Performing immediate reconstruction does not interfere with the effectiveness of PMRT and is unlikely to affect the risk of long-term cardiac or pulmonary complications.
- Strategies such as "delayed-immediate" reconstruction and premastectomy sentinel node biopsy may help patients and their physicians choose the optimal reconstructive procedure.
- Optimizing patients' outcomes requires close cooperation between all specialists from the beginning of diagnosis and treatment.

■ REFERENCES

1. Recht A, Edge SB, Solin LJ, et al. Postmastectomy radiotherapy: guidelines of the American Society of Clinical Oncology (Special Article). *J Clin Oncol.* 2001;19:1539–1569.
2. Early Breast Cancer Trialists' Collaborative Group. Effects of radiotherapy and of differences in the extent of surgery for early breast cancer on local recurrence and 15-year survival: an overview of the randomised trials. *Lancet.* 2005;366:2087–2106.
3. Kronowitz SJ, Robb GL. Breast reconstruction with postmastectomy radiation therapy: current issues. *Plast Reconstr Surg.* 2004;114:950–960.
4. Pomahac B, Recht A, May JW, Hergrueter CA, Slavin SA. New trends in breast cancer management: is the era of immediate breast reconstruction changing? *Ann Surg.* 2006;244:282–288.
5. Evans GRD, Schusterman MA, Kroll SS, et al. Reconstruction and the irradiated breast: is there a role for implants? *Plast Reconstr Surg.* 1995;96:1111–1115.
6. Spear SL, Majidian A. Immediate breast reconstruction in two stages using textured, integrated-valve tissue expanders and breast implants: a retrospective review of 171 consecutive breast reconstructions from 1989 to 1996. *Plast Reconstr Surg.* 1998;101:53–63.
7. Spear SL, Onyewu C. Staged breast reconstruction with saline-filled implants in the irradiated breast: recent trends and therapeutic implications. *Plast Reconstr Surg.* 2000;105:930–942.
8. Contant CME, van Geel AN, van der Holt B, Griep C, Tjong Joe Wai R, Wiggers T. Morbidity of immediate breast reconstruction (IBR) after mastectomy by a subpectorally placed silicone prosthesis: the adverse effect of radiotherapy. *Eur J Surg Oncol.* 2000;26:344–350.
9. Krueger EA, Wilkins EG, Strawderman M, et al. Complications and patient satisfaction following expander/implant breast reconstruction with and without radiotherapy. *Int J Radiat Oncol Biol Phys.* 2001;49:713–721.
10. Wong JS, Kaelin CM, Ho A, et al. Incidence of subsequent major corrective surgery after postmastectomy breast reconstruction and radiation therapy (Abstract). *Int J Radiat Oncol Biol Phys.* 2002;54 (2 Suppl):4–5.
11. Tallet AV, Salem N, Moutardier V, et al. Radiotherapy and immediate two-stage breast reconstruction with a tissue expander and implant: complications and esthetic results. *Int J Radiat Oncol Biol Phys.* 2003;57:136–142.
12. Cordeiro PG, Pusic AL, Disa JJ, McCormick B, VanZee K. Irradiation after immediate tissue expander/implant breast reconstruction: outcomes, complications, aesthetic results, and satisfaction among 156 patients. *Plast Reconstr Surg.* 2004;113:877–881.
13. Ascherman JA, Hanasono MM, Newman MI, Hughes DB. Implant reconstruction in breast cancer patients treated with radiation therapy. *Plast Reconstr Surg.* 2006;117(2):359–365.
14. Cordeiro PG, McCarthy CM. A single surgeon's 12-year experience with tissue expander/implant breast reconstruction: I. A prospective analysis of early complications. *Plast Reconstr Surg.* 2006;118:825–831.
15. Cordeiro PG, McCarthy CM. A single surgeon's 12-year experience with tissue expander/implant breast reconstruction: II. An analysis of long-term complications, aesthetic outcomes, and patient satisfaction. *Plast Reconstr Surg.* 2006;118:832–839.
16. Anderson PR, Hanlon AL, Fowble BL, McNeeley SW, Freedman GM. Low complication rates are achievable after postmastectomy breast reconstruction and radiation therapy. *Int J Radiat Oncol Biol Phys.* 2004;59:1080–1087.
17. Dickson MG, Sharpe DT. The complications of tissue expansion in breast reconstruction: a review of 75 cases. *Br J Plast Surg.* 1987;40:629–635.
18. Olenius M, Jurell G. Breast reconstruction using tissue expansion. *Scand J Plast Reconstr Hand Surg.* 1992;26:83–90.

19. Fodor PB, Swistel AJ. Chest wall deformity following expansion of irradiated soft tissue for breast reconstruction. *NY State J Med.* 1989;89:419–420.

20. Fowble B, Solin L, Schultz D, Rubenstein J, Goodman RL. Breast recurrence following conservative surgery and radiation: patterns of failure, prognosis, and pathologic findings from mastectomy specimens with implications for treatment. *Int J Radiat Oncol Biol Phys.* 1990;19:833–842.

21. LaRossa D. Reconstructive surgery. In: Fowble B, Goodman RL, Glick JH, Rosato EF, eds. *Breast Cancer Treatment: A Comprehensive Guide to Management.* St Louis: Mosby–Year Book; 1991:311–324.

22. Barreau-Pouhaer L, Lê MG, Rietjens M, et al. Risk factors for failure of immediate breast reconstruction with prosthesis after total mastectomy for breast cancer. *Cancer.* 1992;70: 1145–1151.

23. Kroll SS, Schusterman MA, Reece GP, Miller MJ, Smith B. Breast reconstruction with myocutaneous flaps in previously irradiated patients. *Plast Reconstr Surg.* 1994;93:460–469.

24. Jacobsen WM, Meland NB, Woods JE. Autologous breast reconstruction with use of transverse rectus abdominis musculocutaneous flap: Mayo clinic experience with 147 cases. *Mayo Clinic Proc.* 1994;69(7):635–640.

25. Williams JK, Carlson GW, Bostwick J, Bried JT, Mackay G. The effects of radiation treatment after TRAM flap breast reconstruction. *Plast Reconstr Surg.* 1997;100:1153–1160.

26. Mehta VK, Goffinet D. Postmastectomy radiation therapy after TRAM flap breast reconstruction. *Breast J.* 2004;10:118–122.

27. Spear SL, Ducic I, Low M, Cuoco F. The effect of radiation on pedicled TRAM flap breast reconstruction: outcomes and implications. *Plast Reconstr Surg.* 2005;115:84–95.

28. Carlson GW, Page AL, Peters K, Ashinoff R, Schaefer T, Losken A. Effects of radiation therapy on pedicled transverse rectus abdominis myocutaneous flap breast reconstruction. *Ann Plast Surg.* 2008;60:568–572.

29. Williams JK, Bostwick J, Bried JT, Mackay G, Landry J, Benton J. TRAM flap breast reconstruction after radiation treatment. *Ann Surg.* 1995;221:756–766.

30. Tran NV, Chang DW, Gupta A, Kroll SS, Robb GL. Comparison of immediate and delayed free TRAM flap breast reconstruction in patients receiving postmastectomy radiation therapy. *Plast Reconstr Surg.* 2001;108:78–82.

31. Gill PS, Hunt JP, Guerra AB, et al. A 10-year retrospective review of 758 DIEP flaps for breast reconstruction. *Plast Reconstr Surg.* 2004;113:1153–1160.

32. Rogers NE, Allen RJ. Radiation effects on breast reconstruction with the deep inferior epigastric perforator flap. *Plast Reconstr Surg.* 2002;109:1919–1926.

33. Spear SL, Boehmler JH, Taylor NS, Prada C. The role of the latissimus dorsi flap in reconstruction of the irradiated breast. *Plast Reconstr Surg.* 2007;119:1–9.

34. Chawla AK, Kachnic LA, Taghian AG, Niemierko A, Zapton DT, Powell SN. Radiotherapy and breast reconstruction: complications and cosmesis with TRAM versus tissue expander/implant. *Int J Radiat Oncol Biol Phys.* 2002;54:520–526.

35. Huang CJ, Hou MF, Lin SD, et al. Comparison of local recurrence and distant metastases between breast cancer patients after postmastectomy radiotherapy with and without immediate TRAM flap reconstruction. *Plast Reconstr Surg.* 2006;118:1079–1086.

36. Motwani SB, Strom EA, Schechter NR, et al. The impact of immediate breast reconstruction on the technical delivery of postmastectomy radiotherapy. *Int J Radiat Oncol Biol Phys.* 2006; 66:76–82.

37. Krueger EA, Fraass BA, McShan DL, Marsh R, Pierce LJ. Potential gains for irradiation of chest wall and regional nodes with intensity modulated radiotherapy. *Int J Radiat Oncol Biol Phys.* 2003;56:1023–1037.

38. Pedersen AN, Korreman S, Nyström H, Specht L. Breathing adapted radiotherapy of breast cancer: reduction of cardiac and pulmonary doses using voluntary inspiration breath-hold. *Radiother Oncol.* 2004;72:53–60.

39. Frazier RC, Vicini FA, Sharpe MB, et al. Impact of breathing motion on whole breast radiotherapy: a dosimetric analysis using active breathing control. *Int J Radiat Oncol Biol Phys.* 2004;58:1041–1047.

40. Navi A, Mirza AN, Anwar E, Fuchs G, Pain S, Hussien M. Impact of sentinel lymph node biopsy before mastectomy and immediate reconstruction in predicting post mastectomy adjuvant radiotherapy. Does it improve the choice of the reconstruction? (abstract 2090). *EJC.* 2007;5(4):210.

10 Multidisciplinary Approach in the Treatment of Metastatic Disease

Surgical Management of Metastatic Disease

COLLEEN D. MURPHY

MEHRA GOLSHAN

In the United States, nearly 200,000 women are diagnosed annually with invasive breast cancer, of whom up to 6% will present with stage 4 disease (1). Traditional oncologic teaching dictates that in metastatic breast cancer, as in the majority of solid tumors, there is limited role for surgical excision of the primary tumor, as survival will remain unchanged in this incurable stage. Recently, this concept has been challenged, as there is an increasing body of evidence that suggests that removal of the primary breast cancer may improve overall survival in those with stage 4 disease. This chapter will review the studies central to this controversy. Data from each study are summarized in Table 10.1.

Systemic therapies, including chemotherapy, endocrine therapy, and targeted biological therapy, have long been considered to be the cornerstone of treatment for stage 4 disease (2). The main goals of systemic treatment are to maintain or improve quality of life, with some patients achieving improved disease-free or overall survival. Radiation also has an important role in the palliation of metastatic breast cancer, particularly for brain and bone metastases. Surgery at the primary tumor site is generally reserved for palliation of patients with symptomatic or uncontrolled local disease. Figure 10.1 shows a patient with metastatic breast cancer who requires surgical palliation for symptomatic control.

Resection of an intact primary tumor could potentially improve overall survival through several mechanisms. It has been hypothesized that shedding of tumor cells from an intact primary tumor leads to ongoing seeding of metastatic sites, and resection thereby eliminates the primary source. In addition, it is thought that adjuvant therapies may be more effective if there is a smaller overall tumor burden. Finally, it has been suggested that removal of the primary tumor also eliminates the source of a yet undiscovered molecule that may promote tumor growth at metastatic sites.

The notion that overall survival in patients with stage 4 breast cancer could be improved by primary tumor resection was first introduced by a large retrospective study published in 2002 by Khan and colleagues (3). Using the American College of Surgeon's National Cancer Data Base, treatment patterns and survival data of 16,023 women diagnosed with metastatic breast cancer from 1990 to 1993 were identified and analyzed. Specifically, surgical excision of the primary tumor, margin status, metastatic burden, type of metastases, and use of systemic therapies were analyzed. Of this cohort, 42.8% of patients did not undergo surgical resection of the primary tumor, whereas 57.2% underwent either mastectomy or partial mastectomy. Axillary surgery was inconsistently performed in those undergoing surgery. Of the total cohort, 7,779 patients received systemic therapy. For the entire study population, 3-year survival was 24.9%. When stratified by surgery status, the mean survival was 19.3 months for patients who did not undergo surgery, 26.9 months for those undergoing partial mastectomy, and 31.9 months for those undergoing total mastectomy. On multivariate analysis, systemic therapy, location of metastatic disease, metastatic burden, and surgical resection were independent predictors of survival. For those patients having surgery, further analysis showed patients with negative margins had better survival than those with involved margins.

In a population-based study from the Geneva, Switzerland tumor registry, 317 patients were identified who presented with stage 4 breast cancer from 1977 to 1996, of whom 42% underwent surgical resection of the primary tumor (4). Similar to the Khan study, data on primary tumor size, margin status, metastatic site, metastatic burden, and use of systemic therapies were considered. Five-year survival was 12% for patients who did not have surgical resection, 12% for those who had surgery with unknown margin status, 16% for those who had surgery with positive margins, and 27% for those who had surgery with negative margins. Multivariate analysis showed that

■ **Table 10.1** Studies of primary tumor resection in patients with metastatic breast cancer

Study	N	% Surgery	Patient Age (yrs)	Survival	Adjusted HR in Surgical Group (95% CI)
Khan et al. (Ref. 3)	16,023	57	62.5 (mean)	NS 19.3, PM 26.9, TM 31.9[a] NS 17.3%, PM 27.7%, TM 31.8%[c]	0.61 (0.58–0.65)[b]
Babiera et al. (Ref. 5)	224	37	52 (median)	NR	NR[d]
Rapiti et al. (Ref. 4)	300	42	67.4 (mean)	S– 27%, S+ 16%, NS 12%[e]	0.6 (0.4–1.0)
Gnerlich et al. (Ref. 7)	9,734	47	S 62; NS 66 (median)	S 36, NS 21; S 18, NS 7[f]	0.63 (0.6–0.66)
Fields et al. (Ref. 8)	409	46	57 (median)	S 26.8, NS 12.6[g]	0.53 (0.42–0.67)
Blanchard et al. (Ref. 9)	807	61	60.4 (mean)	S 27.1, MS 16.8[h]	0.71 (0.56–0.91)
Cady et al. (Ref. 11)	622	38	60 (median)	NR	NR
Bafford et al. (Ref. 10)	147	41	51 (mean)	S 42.2, SB 48.6, SA 28.9, NS 28.3[g]	0.47[h]

CI, confidence interval; HR, hazard ratio; NR, not reported; NS, no surgery; PM, partial mastectomy; S, surgery; S–, surgery with negative margins; S+, surgery with positive margins; SA, surgery after diagnosis of stage 4 disease; SB, surgery before diagnosis of stage 4 disease; TM, total mastectomy.

[a]Mean survival in months.
[b]Surgical resection with free margins.
[c]Three-year survival.
[d]HR for metastatic progression-free survival 0.54 (0.38 to 0.77).
[e]Five-year breast cancer–specific survival.
[f]Median survival in months in patients alive at the end of the study period and in those who died, respectively.
[g]Median survival in months.
[h]Surgery before or after stage 4 diagnosis compared with NS.

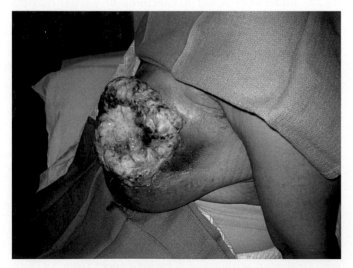

FIGURE 10.1 Symptomatic local disease in a patient with metastatic breast cancer.

surgery with negative margins was associated with prolonged overall survival compared with those who did not have surgery or who had surgery with positive margins. A subgroup analysis showed that this survival advantage was most strongly seen in patients who had metastatic disease limited to bone and those who had margin-negative surgical resection with an axillary lymph node dissection.

The MD Anderson Cancer Center (MDACC) identified all patients who presented with stage 4 breast cancer between 1997 and 2002 (5). Of these 224 patients, 37% underwent surgical resection of the primary breast cancer. Patients were included in the surgery group if they underwent breast surgery within 3 months of the diagnosis of stage 4 disease or at any point during follow-up. Patient and treatment characteristics including tumor size and grade, surgery type, use of chemotherapy, hormonal therapy, and radiation therapy were considered in the analysis. Margin status was not delineated. At median follow-up of 32.1 months, multivariate analysis showed that presence of one metastatic site and lack of HER2/neu amplification were the only variables statistically associated with improved overall survival. Surgery was not an independent predictor of improved survival, although there was a trend toward that conclusion ($P = 0.12$). This study also evaluated metastatic progression–free survival and found that patients with estrogen receptor–positive tumors and those having surgery had significantly improved progression-free survival ($P = 0.0012$ and $P = 0.007$, respectively).

A second publication by this institution examined the contributing factors to prolonged progression-free survival in the surgically treated group, with specific attention paid to timing of surgical intervention after diagnosis of stage 4 disease (6). Of 75 patients who had undergone surgery, Caucasian race, fewer metastatic sites, and negative surgical margins were all significantly associated with longer progression-free survival. With regards to timing of surgery, those patients who underwent their operation three months or later after diagnosis had superior metastatic progression–free survival to those who had their operation within 3 months of stage 4 diagnosis.

Gnerlich and colleague used the National Cancer Institute's Surveillance, Epidemiology and End Results (SEER) database to perform a retrospective population-based study of American breast cancer patients (7). From nine SEER registries from different regions of the United States, 9,734 patients were analyzed who were diagnosed with stage 4 breast cancer between 1988 and 2003. Primary site surgery was performed in 47% of patients. In an effort to account for biases owing to patient and tumor characteristics that may have influenced a patient's likelihood of being offered surgery, the statistical analysis of these data included creation of a propensity score covariate that was used in multiple Cox regression models. Overall survival of patients undergoing surgery was 24%, compared with 16% for those not having surgery (P <0.001). Of six different multivariate analyses performed to account for confounding variables, patients who underwent surgery had a 37% lower risk of death than those not having surgery. SEER data were not available to determine relationships of margin status, metastatic burden, and systemic therapies to survival.

These investigators also looked at their institutional experience with surgical resection of intact primary breast cancer at Washington University Medical Center (8). This was the first study to consider the impact of patient comorbidities on survival. Patient comorbidity was scored and categorized, ranging from none to severe. Of 409 patients presenting with stage 4 disease between 1996 and 2005, 46% underwent surgical resection of the primary tumor. After median follow-up of 142 months, median overall survival was 26.8 months in patients who underwent surgical resection and 12.6 months in those who did not (P <0.0001). As in the MDACC study, progression-free survival was also analyzed, but these investigators were unable to show a statistically significant difference between those undergoing surgery and those who did not (P = 0.3777). Multivariate analysis controlling for patient age, comorbidity, tumor grade, tumor size, histology, and metastatic sites consistently showed that surgical resection was associated with improved overall survival. Unlike in prior studies, tumor-free margins were not found to influence survival.

Blanchard and colleagues used data from a centralized lab in Texas that performs hormone receptor analysis from more than 250 institutions across the United States to create a database of patients with stage 4 disease (9).

Between 1973 and 1991, of 16,401 patients in this database, 807 had stage 4 disease at presentation. Surgical resection of the primary tumor was performed in 61% of patients. Median survival of patients undergoing surgery was 27.1 months, compared with 16.8 months for those who did not have surgery (P <0.0001).

These six studies opened the discussion about redefining the role of surgery in stage 4 breast cancer. However, bias is inherent to retrospective reviews, and in these studies this bias is further compounded by the selection bias of patients chosen for surgical resection. In the majority of studies, patients with younger age, smaller tumors, less nodal involvement, and fewer sites of metastasis were more likely to have undergone surgery. Patient demographics were also found to influence the likelihood of surgical resection, including Caucasian race, married marital status, and care received in the private sector. Given the strong selection bias acknowledged in each of these studies, it remains unclear whether the benefits seen in the surgically treated patients were because patients selected for operation had more indolent disease. To answer this question, two recent studies have attempted to isolate selection bias from their analysis.

Using a prospectively collected database from Brigham and Women's Hospital, Dana Farber Cancer Institute, and the Massachusetts General Hospital, Bafford and colleagues identified 147 patients who presented with stage 4 breast cancer from 1998 to 2005 (10). Of this cohort, 41% of patients underwent surgical resection of the primary breast cancer and 59% did not. To minimize the selection bias of surgical resection of "good responders" to adjuvant therapies, only patients who had surgery before or within 30 days of stage 4 diagnosis were allowed entry into the study. Patient and treatment characteristics including tumor stage, hormone receptor status, and adjuvant therapies were critically evaluated. After adjusting for age, number of metastatic sites, estrogen receptor positivity, HER2/neu status, and use of adjuvant therapies, including chemotherapy, trastuzumab, and endocrine therapy, survival in the surgery group was 4.13 years, compared with 2.36 years in the nonsurgery groups (P = 0.003). A second analysis was performed stratifying patients by timing of surgery in relationship to the diagnosis of stage 4 cancer. There were 36 patients who had surgery prior to being diagnosed with stage 4 disease, whereas 25 patients had surgery after. Interestingly, survival for those diagnosed with metastatic disease after primary breast surgery was 4.05 years, compared with 2.4 years for those diagnosed prior to surgery (P = 0.18). Moreover, survival in patients diagnosed with stage 4 disease prior to surgery was similar to that in patients not having surgery (2.4 years versus 2.36 years, P = not significant). The authors concluded that stage migration bias may account for the improved survival that had been previously reported in patients treated by surgical excision.

A second study used a matched-pair analysis to minimize selection bias. Cady and colleagues analyzed 622 patients from the Massachusetts General Hospital and Brigham and Women's Hospital diagnosed with stage 4 breast cancer between 1970 and 2002 (11). Patients in the surgical and nonsurgical groups were matched for age, date of diagnosis, location of metastatic disease, estrogen receptor status, and use of systemic therapy. In this study 38% of patients underwent surgery, whereas 62% did not. Sequence of surgery in relationship to chemotherapy was considered, and patients were classified into three groups: chemotherapy before surgery, surgery and chemotherapy concurrently, and chemotherapy after surgery. All three survival curves showed that patients having surgery had a survival advantage over those not having surgery. However, these curves demonstrated that survival of patients having surgery and chemotherapy concurrently was similar to survival of those having chemotherapy after surgery, whereas patients having chemotherapy first had a more slowly declining survival curve, suggesting that the benefits attributed to surgery were more likely due to selection bias for patients who had good responses to chemotherapy. This was also demonstrated in a subset analysis limited to patients with bone metastases. The case-matched analysis stratified patients by bone or visceral metastases and showed that case matching reduced or eliminated the survival advantage attributed to primary site surgery when compared with patients without surgery.

In the face of these studies, Morrogh and colleagues sought to investigate the decision-making process leading to surgical resection of patients with stage 4 disease over a 15-year period at Memorial Sloan-Kettering Cancer Center (12). To better delineate trends over time, practice patterns were compared between an early (1990 to 1995) and a more contemporary (1995 to 2005) period. Data from this single institution showed that in both early and more recent periods, mastectomy rates for patients with stage 4 disease remained stable and represented less than 2% of all mastectomies performed at that institution. However, the indications for mastectomy evolved over time. In the earlier period, symptom control was cited as the indication for 41% of mastectomies. This declined to 25% in the more recent period, whereas there was an increase in mastectomies for local control from 34% in the earlier period to 66% in the more recent period. The authors also analyzed data from all patients diagnosed with stage 4 disease from 1995 to 2005. Of these 12,529 patients, 256 (2%) underwent one or more surgical resections. There was a difference in presentation of these 256 patients because 33% presented with stage 4 disease at initial diagnosis, whereas 67% had been treated initially for stage 1 to 3 disease and progressed to stage 4 disease during their follow-up. For all operations performed on this cohort, palliation was cited as the indication in 19%, whereas optimizing local control in the setting of limited

distant disease was the indication in 50%. The authors conclude that over time, surgeons have broadened the indications for surgery in stage 4 patients.

Although the initial retrospective studies provided compelling evidence that surgical excision of an intact primary breast cancer may improve survival in patients with stage 4 disease, careful scrutiny of these data is warranted because the majority of these studies were not able to investigate timing of surgery in relationship to stage 4 diagnosis or adequately control for selection bias. Two studies, by Bafford and colleagues and Cady and colleagues, were better able to account for these biases, and both studies demonstrated that the survival advantage seen in the surgically treated patients could be attributable to patient selection bias or stage migration bias leading to a Will Rogers phenomenon (13). As such, routine surgical excision of an intact primary breast tumor is not currently recommended in patients with metastatic breast cancer.

Surgical resection of metastatic disease sites is generally indicated only for symptom palliation at specific anatomical locations. Resection of metastatic deposits may be considered for surgically accessible brain tumors because resection of both single and multiple tumors has been shown to improve survival and is not associated with undue risk in appropriately selected patients (14). Similarly, some small, nonrandomized studies suggest that resection or ablation of isolated hepatic and pulmonary metastases may increase median survival (15,16). However, all these trials are clouded by selection bias, and no prospective, randomized trials have been conducted to confirm these findings. Orthopedic stabilization followed by radiation of bony metastases is indicated for symptom palliation and prevention of pathologic fractures, particularly of the lower extremities (17).

The best way to approach the possibility of a survival benefit resulting from surgical resection of the intact primary tumor in stage 4 breast cancer patients is from prospectively designed trials, and two such trials are currently being planned. The Translational Breast Cancer Research Consortium is planning a trial that will prospectively collect patient data, including blood and tissue samples for molecular studies, from all patients presenting with stage 4 disease and intact primary tumors. In this study, patients will be stratified into two arms: (a) patients with stage 4 disease at diagnosis and (b) patients diagnosed with stage 4 disease within 3 months of resection of the primary breast cancer. Surgical resection of the intact primary breast cancer will be offered to patients in the first study arm after undergoing first-line systemic treatment. In the second study arm, patients will be treated with first-line systemic therapy and responders offered local radiation therapy. At all clinical decision points in the study, tumor sampling will be performed in order to allow for correlative molecular analysis before and after interventions.

A second study, proposed by the Eastern Cooperative Oncology Group, will randomize patients into two groups: early and delayed local therapy. Criteria for randomization in this study will be patients presenting with intact primary tumors and stage 4 disease who have responded to optimal systemic therapy. Early local therapy will consist of surgical treatment for all patients with or without radiation (on the basis of standards currently in place for nonmetastatic patients), whereas the second group will continue with appropriate systemic therapy with delayed surgical or radiation therapy only if required to provide symptomatic relief. Survival, time to progression, locoregional disease status, and quality of life will all be endpoints for this study. Together, these two studies will be able to offer more definitive clinical and biological evidence regarding the nature of stage 4 breast cancer and the impact of local control.

In view of all clinical data presently available, resection of an intact primary breast cancer in the setting of metastatic cancer remains appropriate for only a select group of patients, namely those with symptomatic local disease. For these patients, the multidisciplinary team may work together to identify which patients are appropriate candidates for resection. In addition, collaboration among multidisciplinary team members is important to determine the sequence of surgery in relationship to systemic therapy and radiation therapy to optimize the benefits and safety of surgical resection. Other members of the multidisciplinary team, including physical therapists, occupational therapists, and a pain service, may also work together to improve functional status and quality of life for patients with metastatic disease. Social work services can also provide the patient and the patient's family emotional support in dealing with a stage 4 diagnosis.

In conclusion, surgical resection of an intact primary breast cancer in the setting of stage 4 disease with the intent of prolonging survival is an intriguing, but yet unproven, approach and is presently not considered the standard of care. Prospective trials have been designed and may soon be under way to help better define the biological and clinical indications for surgery in patients with metastatic disease.

■ MULTIDISCIPLINARY CONSIDERATIONS

- Diagnosis and documentation of metastatic breast cancer is best completed by collaboration between medical oncology, surgery, and radiology.
- The multidisciplinary team can identify patients who may benefit from surgical resection for symptom palliation. The multidisciplinary team can optimize the timing of surgery in relation to other treatments, including chemotherapy and radiation.

- Collaboration with physical therapy and pain management teams is important for optimal symptom palliation. Social work services may also play a role for patient and family support.

■ REFERENCES

1. The American Cancer Society Cancer Facts & Figures 2008; available at www.cancer.org/docroot/STT/stt_0.asp; accessed October 6, 2008.
2. Bernard-Marty C, Cardoso F, Piccart MJ. Facts and controversies in systemic treatment of metastatic breast cancer. *Oncologist.* 2004;9:617–632.
3. Khan SA, Stewart AK, Morrow M. Does aggressive local therapy improve survival in metastatic breast cancer? *Surgery.* 2002; 132:620–627.
4. Rapiti E, Verkooijen HM, Vlastos G, et al. Complete excision of primary breast tumor improves survival of patients with metastatic breast cancer at diagnosis. *J Clin Oncol.* 2006;24:2743–2749.
5. Babiera GV, Rao R, Feng L, et al. Effect of primary tumor extirpation in breast cancer patients who present with stage IV disease and an intact primary tumor. *Ann Surg Oncol.* 2006;13:776–782.
6. Rao R, Feng L, Kuerer HM, et al. Timing of surgical intervention for the intact primary in stage IV breast cancer patients. *Ann Surg Oncol.* 2008;15:1696–1702.
7. Gnerlich J, Jeffe DB, Deshpande AD, Beers C, Zander C, Margenthaler JA. Surgical removal of the primary tumor increases overall survival in patients with metastatic breast cancer: analysis of the 1988–2003 SEER data. *Ann Surg Oncol.* 2007;14: 2187–2194.
8. Fields RC, Jeffe DB, Trinkaus K, et al. Surgical resection of the primary tumor is associated with increased long-term survival in patients with stage IV breast cancer after controlling for site of metastasis. *Ann Surg Oncol.* 2007;14:3345–3351.
9. Blanchard DK, Shetty PB, Hilsenbeck SG, Elledge RM. Association of surgery with improved survival in stage IV breast cancer patients. *Ann Surg.* 2008;247:732–738.
10. Bafford AC, Burstein HJ, Barkley CR, et al. Breast surgery in stage IV breast cancer: impact of staging and patient selection on overall survival. *Breast Cancer Res Treat.* 2009;115:7–12.
11. Cady B, Nathan NR, Michaelson JS, Golshan M, Smith BL. Matched pair analyses of Stage IV breast cancer with or without resection of primary breast site. *Ann Surg Oncol.* 2008;15: 3384–3395.
12. Morrogh M, Park A, Norton L, King TA. Changing indications for surgery in patients with stage IV breast cancer: a current perspective. *Cancer.* 2008;112:1445–1454.
13. Feinstein AR, Sosin DM, Wells CK. The Will Rogers phenomenon. Stage migration and new diagnostic techniques as a source of misleading statistics for survival in cancer. *New Engl J Med.* 1985;312:1604–1608.
14. Patchell RA, Tibbs PA, Walsh JW, et al. A randomized trial of surgery in the treatment of single metastases to the brain. *New Engl J Med.* 1990;322:494–500.
15. Staren ED, Sulerno C, Rongione A, et al. Pulmonary resection for metastatic breast cancer. *Arch Surg.* 1992;127:1282–1284.
16. Raab R, Nussbaum KT, Behrend M, et al. Liver metastases of breast cancer: results of liver resection. *Anticancer Res.* 1998; 18:2231–2233.
17. Townsend PW, Smalley SR, Cozad SC, et al. Role of postoperative radiation therapy after stabilization of fractures caused by metastatic disease. *Int J Radiat Oncol Biol Phys.* 1995;31:43–49.

Radiation Management of Metastatic Disease

JULIA S. WONG

The management of metastatic breast cancer continues to present challenges for the medical oncologist, radiation oncologist, and surgical oncologist. The diversity of presentations and clinical situations requires thoughtful consideration, and in many cases a multidisciplinary approach, to provide optimal and individualized palliation. Radiation therapy (RT) is often a component of the treatment plan, either alone or in conjunction with systemic therapy or surgery, or both.

■ PRINCIPLES OF METASTATIC DISEASE

A diagnosis of metastatic disease shifts the focus of treatment toward a palliative intent as opposed to a curative one. However, the biology of breast cancer is such that some metastatic cases have a long natural history; given this premise, some studies have examined a possible role for aggressive local therapy in the setting of oligometastatic disease in selected patients (1–5). The reader is directed to those studies for further discussion because this is beyond the scope of this chapter. In general, however, the treatment of metastatic breast cancer is geared toward minimizing symptoms and slowing or preventing symptomatic progression. RT is used for some sites of metastatic involvement, most commonly bone and brain.

■ GOALS OF TREATMENT

Symptom management to improve quality of life is the main goal of RT for metastatic breast cancer. This needs to be accomplished in a way that (a) minimizes treatment-related toxicity, (b) dovetails with other treatment modalities such as chemotherapy and surgery, and (c) has acceptable logistics for the patient. The risks and benefits of RT must be carefully weighed, with attention given to variables such as the status of other sites of metastatic disease, the need to interrupt systemic therapy in order to deliver RT, performance status, and patient preferences. These decisions can be complex because the subtleties of the selection of fields, total dose, and fraction size can be less defined than in curative cases.

This chapter discusses the use of RT for metastatic breast cancer in the settings most often seen by radiation oncologists: bone metastases, spinal cord compression, brain metastases, leptomeningeal metastases, and ocular metastases.

■ BONE METASTASES

Bone is one of the most common sites of metastatic involvement in breast cancer. Fortunately, many are asymptomatic and do not require RT. However, as some breast cancer patients with disease limited to bone can expect a long survival, long-term pain control is an important part of the management of bone metastases. The areas that cause symptoms typically present with persistent, focal pain. More serious presentations include pain with neurological symptoms and signs secondary to impingement of bone disease on nerves. The most urgent of these presentations is spinal cord compression (discussed below).

In addition to pain, other presentations can include minimally symptomatic, radiographic ones, such as a lytic lesion with or without impending fracture. Pathological fracture or impending pathological fracture of a weight-bearing bone is usually an indication for RT, sometimes preceded by surgical stabilization. Review of the imaging, including bone scan, plain films, and computed tomography (CT) scans with bone windows or magnetic resonance imaging (MRI), accompanied by a discussion with the orthopedic surgeon, can be helpful in determining the need for surgical intervention prior to RT. The decision as to whether to intervene surgically before RT may depend on the severity and location of the impending fracture, as well as the patient's overall disease burden and performance status.

RT is used routinely to palliate painful bone metastases and is effective in reducing or eliminating pain in more than 50% of cases (6). When pain control is the primary goal, the first step is optimization of pain medications, as the beginning of RT-induced relief of pain can be variable and may take months for maximum effect (7). If standard narcotic regimens are inadequate or not optimized, a consultation with the pain service is often helpful. Studies assessing the time frame and magnitude of pain reduction with radiotherapy are limited by the subjective quality of pain intensity, the concurrent usage of analgesics, and the timing of the assessments of pain response.

The selection of total dose and fraction size is often biased toward shorter courses, typically 10 fractions of

300 cGy delivered over 2 weeks, but ranging from 1 to 4 weeks in most situations. Larger and fewer fractions to a lower total dose generally are considered biologically equivalent to a greater number of smaller fractions taken to a higher dose, but clinicians may elect the longer courses in settings where there is concern for more long-term toxicity and less durable local control. These shorter regimens with larger fractions (as opposed to longer courses with smaller fractions and a higher total dose) are chosen in order to maximize pain relief, minimize patient inconvenience, and minimize delays in the reinitiation of systemic therapy in some cases. Different regimens have been compared prospectively, and meta-analyses have suggested similar rates of pain relief between single-fraction and multiple-fraction regimens, with a higher rate of retreatment in patients receiving a single fraction (8,9). The choice of total dose and fraction size is influenced by the patient's performance status and life expectancy and by the status of other sites of metastatic involvement (location, symptoms, and likelihood of progression during RT). Since metastatic breast cancer may have a lengthy natural history, some patients may be best treated with longer, slower fractionation to a higher dose. Often a discussion with the medical oncologist regarding proposed length of the RT course is helpful because chemotherapy may need to be interrupted in order to deliver RT. Finally, the field arrangement and field size and the attendant acute toxicity (gastrointestinal, bone marrow) can also influence decisions about fraction size. These toxicities can influence the ability to give chemotherapy after RT, as well as delay its initiation or reinitiation, and therefore must be taken into consideration when planning a course of RT.

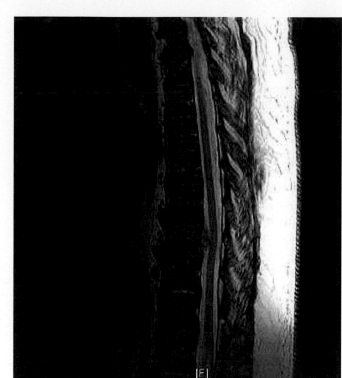

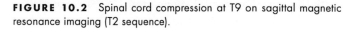

FIGURE 10.2 Spinal cord compression at T9 on sagittal magnetic resonance imaging (T2 sequence).

■ SPINAL CORD COMPRESSION

Spinal cord compression from epidural disease, typically arising from an adjacent vertebral body metastasis, requires prompt diagnosis and treatment, as the resulting neurological deficits can be permanent. The presentation can include back pain with a slow or rapid onset of weakness, incontinence, and sensory changes corresponding to the level of involvement along the spinal cord. MRI with gadolinium is the gold standard for imaging. An example of thoracic spinal cord compression on a sagittal MRI image is shown in Figure 10.2. If MRI is not feasible and information from a CT scan is not definitive enough for diagnosis and treatment, in rare occasions a myelogram is indicated. RT is the most standard treatment modality employed for spinal cord compression. Treatment is usually started quickly, although the timing may be less critical if asymptomatic. Dexamethasone is often used in conjunction with RT to decrease swelling/edema.

In the setting of minimal or modest neurological deficits, RT often preserves or improves function (10–12). The optimal radiation schedule for spinal cord compression remains unclear. Patients with a short life expectancy probably do not gain much from more protracted courses of RT. Patients with a longer life expectancy, however, may benefit from higher doses in smaller fractions. Rades and colleagues retrospectively compared five RT schedules ranging from 8 Gy in a single dose to 40 Gy divided into 20 doses over 4 weeks (13). Patients had similar posttreatment motor function and ambulation, but the in-field recurrence rates at 2 years were significantly lower with the protracted regimens (24% for the 8 Gy group and 7% for the 40 Gy group). In the setting of recurrent disease, re-irradiation is usually not recommended owing to the risk of radiation-induced myelopathy. However, when there is progressive loss of neurological function, few treatment options are available after consultation with medical oncology and neurosurgery, and when there is a reasonable interval since prior radiation, re-irradiation is sometimes considered and in some reports has been effective and safe (14,15), but it is not standard of care. Newer RT techniques such as intensity-modulated RT (IMRT), image-guided RT (IGRT), and stereotactic body approaches are being studied and may offer improvements in the ability to deliver precise radiation in this setting.

Rapidly progressive symptoms and paralysis are indications for an emergent neurosurgical consultation because RT is unlikely to reverse such severe deficits, especially when they occur in a short time frame, and in those situations, surgery offers the best likelihood of reversal of severe neurologic deficits (16). Deciding whether a patient is a good candidate for surgery can require input from the surgeon, medical oncologist, and radiation oncologist because variables such as life expectancy and likelihood that RT alone will suffice will affect the decision. If surgery is performed, RT is given postoperatively. Results of a randomized, multi-institutional trial comparing surgery and RT with RT alone were published in 2005 (17). RT in both groups consisted of 30 Gy in 10 fractions. The primary endpoint was ability to walk. An interim analysis showed a difference in favor of the surgery group, leading to early closure of the study with 101 patients randomized. Patients in the surgery plus RT group were more likely to walk than the RT-alone patients (84% versus 57%, $P = 0.001$) and retained the ability longer than the RT-alone patients (median 122 days versus 13 days, $P = 0.003$). Patients in the surgery group who had been unable to walk were more likely to regain the ability to walk than those in the RT-alone group (62% versus 19%, $P = 0.01$). It is important to note that the patients had different primary tumors, were good surgical candidates, and were required to have an expected survival of at least 3 months. While these randomized data support the efficacy of surgery, the optimal choice of therapy for spinal cord compression depends on the individual tumor and patient characteristics.

■ BRAIN METASTASES

The success of breast cancer treatment has led to more long-term survivors and therefore more interest in the dilemma presented by the identification of brain metastases, which in the modern era may be asymptomatic and may be detected solely by improved imaging (MRI) or as a result of improved systemic therapy that controls non–central nervous system (CNS) disease but is unable to penetrate the blood-brain barrier. Breast cancer metastasizes to the brain in 5% to 15% of cases in older series (18,19), with a higher incidence seen in autopsy series (20). The incidence of brain metastases is higher in patients with HER2/neu-positive disease treated with trastuzumab (21,22).

Patients typically present with symptoms such as headache, nausea and vomiting, and other symptoms or signs that are indicative of the affected area, such as focal weakness, numbness, balance or gait problems, or visual changes. Head CT scans, especially if done with contrast, can make the diagnosis; however, brain MRI is more sensitive and is often used to fully characterize the lesion(s)

and determine their number because the number of foci and their location can affect management decisions.

RT is standard in the treatment of brain metastases, with or without surgery. Symptomatic multiple brain metastases are typically treated with steroids and whole brain RT (WBRT), which provides a clinical response in 75% of patients (23). When WBRT is recommended, the dose and fractionation depend on the patient's life expectancy and the desire to avoid delays in restarting systemic therapy. Various RT schedules have been evaluated in randomized studies, with no clear superiority of any particular regimen (24). However, in breast cancer patients, it is not uncommon to use a more protracted course in patients with a longer life expectancy in order to maximize local control and minimize long-term toxicity. If a patient presents with hydrocephalus, a surgical opinion is useful to determine the need for a shunt prior to initiating RT. Radiographic findings suggestive of impending herniation are also indicators for a surgical opinion. If the onset of neurologic symptoms and signs is fairly acute and the findings significant, there may be a role for resection of a large, symptomatic metastasis, especially in a young patient with a good performance status and otherwise a minimal disease burden. Such surgery, if deemed appropriate, can provide the quickest improvement in symptoms.

The optimal management of a solitary brain metastasis continues to generate debate. The two most standard options are WBRT [with or without a stereotactic radiosurgery (SRS) boost when there are limited foci] and resection followed by WBRT. SRS delivers external-beam RT in a more focused way than standard RT and gives less RT to surrounding normal tissue. Two randomized trials of RT plus surgery or RT alone have demonstrated an improvement in median survival with the use of surgery in addition to RT (25,26) in patients with solitary brain metastases. The use of SRS after WBRT in patients with solitary brain metastases has been evaluated by the Radiation Therapy Oncology Group (RTOG) (27). The study randomized 333 patients with one to three new brain metastases to receive either WBRT or WBRT followed by SRS. Univariate analysis showed a survival benefit in the WBRT plus SRS group with a single brain metastasis compared with those with two or three metastases. Patients with a single brain metastasis who received SRS had an overall survival advantage over the patients who received WBRT alone (6.5 months versus 4.9 months, $P = 0.0393$). Patients in the SRS group were more likely to have a stable or improved Karnofsky performance status (KPS) at 6 months than patients who received WBRT alone (43% versus 27%, $P = 0.03$). The authors used a recursive partitioning analysis (RPA) classification system based on KPS, age, primary disease status, and extracranial disease status. Class 1 patients were younger than age 65 and had a KPS of 70 or greater, a controlled primary tumor, and brain-only disease. Class 2 patients were age 65 or older and had a KPS of 70 or greater, an uncontrolled primary tumor, and other sites of disease. Class 3 patients had a KPS of less than 70. On multivariate analysis, survival improved in patients with an RPA class 1 or favorable histological status. The authors concluded that WBRT plus SRS improved functional autonomy for all patients in the study and survival for patients with a single unresected brain metastasis.

Other approaches, such as SRS alone, are being investigated, and it remains to be seen which clinical settings may be most appropriate for this approach. This approach is appealing in that it may confer less morbidity from RT, but it may undertreat subclinical disease that manifests itself later, requiring further treatment with either additional SRS or whole brain RT. Conceptually, it is appealing to consider SRS alone in the setting of a small, asymptomatic brain metastasis when other systemic disease and its treatment are the priority clinically. In such a situation, SRS alone can minimize the interruption of systemic therapy and spare the patient the short-term morbidity of WBRT, which theoretically could compromise the ability to deliver systemic therapy in a timely fashion. Data on the use of SRS alone are emerging (28,29), but the use of SRS alone remains nonstandard at present. The long-term effects of WBRT are of concern, especially in breast cancer patients who may live many years with metastatic disease, which makes SRS as an alternative particularly appealing.

Studies using systemic therapies such as temozolomide (which crosses the blood-brain barrier) and targeted therapies such as lapatinib (a tyrosine kinase inhibitor) are ongoing and may improve the results of WBRT. A multidisciplinary approach with review of the patient's brain MRI and clinical situation with the neurosurgeon and medical oncologist, if appropriate, is extremely valuable in determining the best recommendation for each patient.

■ LEPTOMENINGEAL METASTASES

Breast cancer metastatic to the leptomeninges, otherwise known as carcinomatous meningitis, is an ominous presentation, often with a poor clinical response to treatment. Neurological symptoms and signs can be similar to those seen with parenchymal brain metastases and can include headache, nausea and vomiting, seizures, and cranial nerve palsies. Other presentations can reflect involvement lower in the neuraxis along the spinal cord. An MRI of the brain and entire spine with gadolinium can be useful in finding metastatic deposits, but these foci can be small and sometimes are not well visualized. Lumbar puncture can also establish the diagnosis, but cytology may be persistently negative in about 10% of patients. Establishing a diagnosis is not always straightforward. Patients may

have one or more of these three factors: positive cytology, clinical findings, and radiographic findings. Many do not have all three. The median survival is about 4 to 6 weeks without treatment, which increases to 3 to 6 months with treatment (30).

Once the diagnosis is established and treatment is felt to be indicated (which in many cases may mean having two of the three factors above, sometimes all three, and rarely one), RT to limited areas is often the first-line treatment recommendation. Full craniospinal RT is not recommended owing to the toxicity of such an approach. Focal areas, such as whole brain or limited segments of the spinal cord, are often considered for palliative RT. Intrathecal chemotherapy via an Ommaya reservoir or lumbar puncture may also be considered. Intravenous chemotherapy is also considered, but treatment results with any of these approaches are poor; breast cancer patients may have a slightly better outcome than patients with other solid tumors (31).

■ OCULAR METASTASES

Of malignant lesions that appear in or near the eye, breast cancer is one of the more common sources. The prevalence of asymptomatic ocular metastases in patients with known metastatic breast cancer is estimated to be between 5% and 30% (32–35).

Metastatic lesions may be intraocular or extraocular. With intraocular presentations, the uveal tract is most commonly affected, likely because it is highly vascularized. The most common location is the choroid, which is affected in 81% of ocular metastases, with lower rates of involvement of the iris, retina, and ciliary body (36). Extraocular presentations are often characterized by orbital involvement.

Symptoms and signs at presentation depend on the area affected. Choroidal involvement may be manifested by visual changes such as blurred vision or pain; orbital metastases may be accompanied by diplopia, pain, or proptosis. A detailed ophthalmologic examination with vision assessment, as well as imaging with CT or MRI, is useful for establishing the diagnosis. Synchronous bilateral presentations are seen not infrequently; bilateral choroidal metastases were seen in 38% in one series (37).

Treatment most commonly consists of local therapy, the mainstay being external beam RT, with either conventional or stereotactic approaches. RT was effective in 79% (34 of 43 eyes) in one series with a median dose of 40 Gy (38). Vision can be improved or preserved in the vast majority of patients (38,39). A prospective study of 65 eyes treated with 40 Gy in 20 fractions via standardized techniques found a median survival of 10 months for patients with breast cancer, with stabilization or improvement in

visual acuity in 50% and 36%, respectively, of all evaluable patients (40).

■ SUMMARY

- Metastatic disease presents many unique challenges
  and often requires multidisciplinary input to develop
  the best treatment plan for a given patient.
- Bone metastases are commonly treated with RT but
  may benefit from surgical intervention in some settings, such as impending fracture of a weight-bearing
  bone.
- Spinal cord compression typically is treated with
  RT, with or without preceding surgery; functional
  outcome is often tied to the severity of neurological
  deficits and the timing of their development.
- Brain metastases often require palliative whole-
  brain radiation, sometimes in conjunction with
  surgical resection. SRS is sometimes used to boost
  small lesions. The role of SRS alone remains to be
  defined, but it may be appropriate in selected clinical
  situations.
- Leptomeningeal carcinomatosis is associated with a
  poor prognosis. RT to whole brain and RT to focal
  areas along the neuraxis are common approaches.
  Intrathecal chemotherapy is sometimes used. The
  efficacy of all these approaches is limited.
- Ocular metastases can occur in various locations but
  often occur in the choroid. RT is well tolerated and
  often successful in improving or preventing progressive vision loss.

■ REFERENCES

1. Babiera GV, Rao R, Feng L, et al. Effect of primary tumor extirpa-
    tion in breast cancer patients who present with stage IV disease and
    an intact primary tumor. *Ann Surg Oncol*. 2006;13(6):776–782.
2. Khan SA, Stewart AK, Morrow M. Does aggressive local ther-
    apy improve survival in metastatic breast cancer? *Surgery*. 2002;
    132(4):620–626; discussion 626–627.
3. Rapiti E, Verkooijen HM, Vlastos G, et al. Complete excision of
    primary breast tumor improves survival of patients with metastatic
    breast cancer at diagnosis. *J Clin Oncol*. 2006;24(18):2743–2749.
4. Fields RC, Jeffe DB, Trinkaus K, et al. Surgical resection of the
    primary tumor is associated with increased long-term survival in
    patients with stage IV breast cancer after controlling for site of
    metastasis. *Ann Surg Oncol*. 2007;14(12):3345–3351.
5. Gnerlich J, Jeffe DB, Deshpande AD, Beers C, Zander C,
    Margenthaler JA. Surgical removal of the primary tumor increases
    overall survival in patients with metastatic breast cancer: analy-
    sis of the 1988–2003 SEER data. *Ann Surg Oncol*. 2007;14(8):
    2187–2194.
6. McQuay HJ, Collins SL, Carroll D, Moore RA. Radiotherapy for
    the palliation of painful bone metastases. *Cochrane Database Syst
    Rev*. 2000(2):CD001793.

7. Li KK, Hadi S, Kirou-Mauro A, Chow E. When should we define
    the response rates in the treatment of bone metastases by palliative
    radiotherapy? *Clin Oncol (R Coll Radiol)*. 2008;20(1):83–89.
8. Wu JS, Wong R, Johnston M, Bezjak A, Whelan T. Meta-
    analysis of dose-fractionation radiotherapy trials for the pallia-
    tion of painful bone metastases. *Int J Radiat Oncol Biol Phys*.
    2003;55(3):594–605.
9. Sze WM, Shelley MD, Held I, Wilt TJ, Mason MD. Palliation of
    metastatic bone pain: single fraction versus multifraction radio-
    therapy—a systematic review of randomised trials. *Clin Oncol
    (R Coll Radiol)*. 2003;15(6):345–352.
10. Helweg-Larsen S. Clinical outcome in metastatic spinal cord com-
    pression. A prospective study of 153 patients. *Acta Neurol Scand*.
    1996;94(4):269–275.
11. Helweg-Larsen S, Sorensen PS, Kreiner S. Prognostic factors in
    metastatic spinal cord compression: a prospective study using
    multivariate analysis of variables influencing survival and gait
    function in 153 patients. *Int J Radiat Oncol Biol Phys*. 2000;
    46(5):1163–1169.
12. Maranzano E, Latini P. Effectiveness of radiation therapy with-
    out surgery in metastatic spinal cord compression: final results
    from a prospective trial. *Int J Radiat Oncol Biol Phys*. 1995;
    32(4):959–967.
13. Rades D, Stalpers LJ, Veninga T, et al. Evaluation of five radiation
    schedules and prognostic factors for metastatic spinal cord com-
    pression. *J Clin Oncol*. 2005;23(15):3366–3375.
14. Rades D, Stalpers LJ, Veninga T, Hoskin PJ. Spinal reirradiation
    after short-course RT for metastatic spinal cord compression. *Int
    J Radiat Oncol Biol Phys*. 2005;63(3):872–875.
15. Rades D, Rudat V, Veninga T, Stalpers LJ, Hoskin PJ, Schild SE.
    Prognostic factors for functional outcome and survival after reir-
    radiation for in-field recurrences of metastatic spinal cord com-
    pression. *Cancer*. 2008;113(5):1090–1096.
16. Rades D, Rudat V, Veninga T, et al. A score predicting post-
    treatment ambulatory status in patients irradiated for metastatic
    spinal cord compression. *Int J Radiat Oncol Biol Phys*. 2008;
    72(3):905–908.
17. Patchell RA, Tibbs PA, Regine WF, et al. Direct decompressive
    surgical resection in the treatment of spinal cord compression
    caused by metastatic cancer: a randomised trial. *Lancet*. 2005;
    366(9486):643–648.
18. Miller KD, Weathers T, Haney LG, et al. Occult central nervous
    system involvement in patients with metastatic breast cancer:
    prevalence, predictive factors and impact on overall survival. *Ann
    Oncol*. 2003;14(7):1072–1077.
19. Schouten LJ, Rutten J, Huveneers HA, Twijnstra A. Incidence of
    brain metastases in a cohort of patients with carcinoma of the
    breast, colon, kidney, and lung and melanoma. *Cancer*. 2002;
    94(10):2698–2705.
20. Tsukada Y, Fouad A, Pickren JW, Lane WW. Central nervous
    system metastasis from breast carcinoma. Autopsy study. *Cancer*.
    1983;52(12):2349–2354.
21. Montagna E, Cancello G, D'Agostino D, et al. Central nervous
    system metastases in a cohort of metastatic breast cancer patients
    treated with trastuzumab. *Cancer Chemother Pharmacol*. 2009;
    63(2):275–280.
22. Bendell JC, Domchek SM, Burstein HJ, et al. Central nervous system
    metastases in women who receive trastuzumab-based therapy for
    metastatic breast carcinoma. *Cancer*. 2003;97(12):2972–2977.
23. Lin NU, Bellon JR, Winer EP. CNS metastases in breast cancer.
    J Clin Oncol. 2004;22(17):3608–3617.
24. Gaspar L, Scott C, Rotman M, et al. Recursive partitioning
    analysis (RPA) of prognostic factors in three Radiation Therapy
    Oncology Group (RTOG) brain metastases trials. *Int J Radiat
    Oncol Biol Phys*. 1997;37(4):745–751.
25. Patchell RA, Tibbs PA, Walsh JW, et al. A randomized trial of
    surgery in the treatment of single metastases to the brain. *New
    Engl J Med*. 1990;322(8):494–500.

26. Vecht CJ, Haaxma-Reiche H, Noordijk EM, et al. Treatment of single brain metastasis: radiotherapy alone or combined with neurosurgery? *Ann Neurol.* 1993;33(6):583–590.

27. Andrews DW, Scott CB, Sperduto PW, et al. Whole brain radiation therapy with or without stereotactic radiosurgery boost for patients with one to three brain metastases: phase III results of the RTOG 9508 randomised trial. *Lancet.* 2004;363(9422):1665–1672.

28. Aoyama H, Shirato H, Tago M, et al. Stereotactic radiosurgery plus whole-brain radiation therapy vs stereotactic radiosurgery alone for treatment of brain metastases: a randomized controlled trial. *JAMA.* 2006;295(21):2483–2491.

29. Chang EL, Shiu AS, Grossman P, et al. Stereotactic body radiosurgery for 121 cases of spinal metastases treated at M.D. Anderson Cancer Center [abstract]. *Int J Radiat Oncol Biol Phys.* 2008;72(1 Suppl):S51–S52.

30. Grossman SA, Krabak MJ. Leptomeningeal carcinomatosis. *Cancer Treat Rev.* 1999;25(2):103–119.

31. Grant R, Naylor B, Greenberg HS, Junck L. Clinical outcome in aggressively treated meningeal carcinomatosis. *Arch Neurol.* 1994;51(5):457–461.

32. Font RL, Ferry AP. Carcinoma metastatic to the eye and orbit: III. A clinicopathologic study of 28 cases metastatic to the orbit. *Cancer.* 1976;38(3):1326–1335.

33. Mewis L, Young SE. Breast carcinoma metastatic to the choroid: analysis of 67 patients. *Ophthalmology.* 1982;89(2):147–151.

34. Nelson CC, Hertzberg BS, Klintworth GK. A histopathologic study of 716 unselected eyes in patients with cancer at the time of death. *Am J Ophthalmol.* 1983;95(6):788–793.

35. Kreusel KM, Wiegel T, Stange M, Bornfeld N, Foerster MH. [Intraocular metastases of metastatic breast carcinoma in the woman. Incidence, risk factors and therapy]. *Ophthalmologe.* 2000; 97(5):342–346.

36. Shields JA, Shields CL. Metastatic tumours to the intraocular structures. In: Shields JA, Shields CL, eds. *Intraocular Tumours.* Philadelphia: Saunders; 1992:207–238.

37. Rosset A, Zografos L, Coucke P, Monney M, Mirimanoff RO. Radiotherapy of choroidal metastases. *Radiother Oncol.* 1998; 46(3):263–268.

38. Amichetti M, Caffo O, Minatel E, et al. Ocular metastases from breast carcinoma: a multicentric retrospective study. *Oncol Rep.* 2000;7(4):761–765.

39. Ratanatharathorn V, Powers WE, Grimm J, et al. Eye metastasis from carcinoma of the breast: diagnosis, radiation treatment and results. *Cancer Treat Rev.* 1991;18(4):261–276.

40. Wiegel T, Bottke D, Kreusel KM, et al. External beam radiotherapy of choroidal metastases—final results of a prospective study of the German Cancer Society (ARO 95–08). *Radiother Oncol.* 2002;64(1):13–18.

Medical Oncology Management of Metastatic Disease

NAGEATTE IBRAHIM

JOHN K. ERBAN

The decrease in breast cancer mortality rates in recent years can be attributed, in part, to the adoption of multidisciplinary approaches to the management of breast disease (1). On initial diagnosis of metastatic breast cancer (MBC), ideal management often involves a team composed of breast imagers and surgical, radiation, and medical oncologists to assess each patient's extent of disease, in consideration of surgical resection, local radiation, and chemotherapy and hormonal therapy options. In addition, comprehensive assessment requires nutritional and vitamin assessments as well as an understanding of the patient's physical capacity and exercise tolerance. Even though a majority of women diagnosed with breast cancer in the United States today will not experience a systemic recurrence, it is estimated that in the year 2008, 40,930 women died of metastatic disease (2). Thus comprehensive multimodality approaches to the management of MBC are still necessary for a large number of women each year.

It is of historical interest that the discovery of the first therapeutic molecular target, the estrogen receptor (ER), has presaged the field of drug discovery for breast cancer and the search for other useful molecular targets. Increasingly, the multidisciplinary interactions between pathologists, medical oncologists, and radiation oncologists are enhancing the considerations of effective treatment options for MBC. Examples are immunochemical and molecular approaches to measuring expression of the ER and analysis of *HER2/neu* gene amplification in tumor specimens, which will dictate the choice of treatment. Moreover, radiotherapy plays a pivotal role in palliation, and timely intervention will avoid not only patient discomfort but also associated morbidity.

■ HORMONAL THERAPY IN MBC: ESTROGEN DEPRIVATION STRATEGIES

Surgical Ovarian Ablation

The recognition that hormonal factors may influence breast cancer growth kinetics was made by surgeon Sir George Beatson in 1896, who documented tumor regression in women with inoperable breast cancer following oophorectomy (3,4). Both adrenalectomy and hypophysectomy may also lead to tumor regression, but these interventions are associated with considerable morbidity (5–7). These observations not only demonstrated the worth of estrogen withdrawal therapy (the basis for induction of menopause in premenopausal women and aromatase inhibition in postmenopausal women) but encouraged investigation of estrogen binding, ERs, and receptor blockade as well as downregulation. The ER signaling paradigm is an ideal example of the potential of a multidisciplinary approach to treatment, for estrogen suppression may include such options as radiation, surgery, and medical manipulation (3,8).

Medical Approaches for Estrogen-Responsive Breast Cancer

Selective Estrogen Receptor Modulators

Treatment of hormone receptor–positive (HR+) MBC with agents that reduce estradiol binding to the ER via several mechanisms (ER blockade, decrease in ligand concentration, or downregulation of the ER) has proven effective in both premenopausal and postmenopausal women (9). As a single intervention, the selective estrogen response modulator (SERM) tamoxifen remains the treatment of choice in premenopausal women with ER+ MBC who have never received hormonal therapy. Tamoxifen has demonstrated equal efficacy to bilateral oophorectomy in a randomized trial of premenopausal women with MBC (10). However, the combination of tamoxifen and ovarian suppression appears superior to tamoxifen alone in MBC (11) and should be considered standard practice in premenopausal females with ER+ MBC who are starting hormonal treatment. Tamoxifen's partial agonistic activities account for its accompanying increased risk of developing thromboembolic events and endometrial carcinoma and its potential for a positive effect on bone density and cholesterol in postmenopausal women.

Aromatase Inhibitors

At present, while aromatase inhibitors (AIs) have been shown to be superior to tamoxifen as initial therapy for HR+ metastatic disease in postmenopausal women (12), their use in premenopausal women must be accompanied by obligate ovarian suppression. An initial approach to the premenopausal patient with HR+ MBC may involve immediate introduction of tamoxifen plus either a luteinizing hormone–releasing hormone (LHRH) agonist, oophorectomy, or irradiation of the ovaries. Radiation for ovarian suppression is proven but not widely practiced in the United States (13). The use of AIs in premenopausal women then may be reserved for patients progressing on tamoxifen who have experienced effective ovarian suppression as primary therapy.

More than 80% of breast cancers occur in women over the age of 50 years, and while SERMs are effective, other agents are preferred as initial therapy for postmenopausal women only. Third-generation AIs of both steroidal and nonsteroidal chemistry have been developed with acceptably low side-effect profiles. Since the 1970s, inhibition of the cytochrome P450 enzyme aromatase, important in estrogen synthesis, has been known to induce regression of HR+ tumors (14). Earlier-generation AIs were associated with incomplete endocrine suppression as well as more frequent toxicities. Third-generation AIs, including anastrozole (Arimidex), letrozole (Femara), and exemestane (Aromasin), are nonsteroidal and steroidal inhibitors with improved toxicity profiles. These AIs have demonstrated efficacy in both locally advanced breast cancer and MBC in postmenopausal women. Anastrozole demonstrated better activity than tamoxifen as first-line therapy for advanced, ER+ breast cancer in postmenopausal women (15). The median time to progression (TTP) was 5.5 months longer in the anastrozole arm ($P = 0.005$), with an estimated progression hazards ratio for tamoxifen compared with anastrozole, after adjustment for patient characteristics, of 1.44 (lower one-sided 95% confidence limit 1.16). Furthermore, combined analysis of two randomized trials confirmed the benefit of anastrozole over tamoxifen, with improvement in TTP (10.7 months versus 6.4 months, $P = 0.022$) (16).

Letrozole was also compared head to head with tamoxifen for treatment of advanced breast cancer in postmenopausal women in an international phase III trial that showed an improved response rate (RR) favoring letrozole over tamoxifen when used as initial therapy (32% versus 21%, $P = 0.0002$) (17). TTP in this study was significantly longer in the letrozole arm than in the tamoxifen arm (41 weeks versus 26 weeks, $P < 0.0001$). Treatment with letrozole reduced the risk of progression by 30% [hazard ratio 0.70, 95% confidence interval (CI) 0.60 to 0.81, $P = 0.0001$]. In addition, in an unplanned analysis, for patients who did not cross over to the alternative agent at progression, letrozole was associated with improved survival over tamoxifen. In addition, exemestane, an irreversible inhibitor of aromatase, has also demonstrated superior efficacy to tamoxifen, with both a significantly higher RR (46% versus 31%, $P = 0.005$) and TTP (9.9 months versus 5.8 months) as first-line treatment in ER+ MBC in postmenopausal women (18). Exemestane has also demonstrated clinical efficacy in MBC refractory to anastrozole or letrozole (13,19).

It is premature to state with certainty that there is a preferred agent when introducing AI therapy. Selection of a first-line agent is based on many factors, including accessibility, cost, expectation of patient tolerability,

and efficacy. Development of an intolerable side effect prompting a need to discontinue the AI occurs in approximately 10% to 15% of patients (20); however, switching to anotheragent in the same class alleviates symptoms as often as half the time (21) and overcomes acquired resistance (22).

Fulvestrant, an agent that downregulates the ER, is approved as second-line therapy for ER+ advanced breast cancer in postmenopausal patients. Fulvestrant was shown to possess similar efficacy to anastrozole in patients with MBC refractory to tamoxifen, with similar median overall survival (OS) in the two arms (27.4 months versus 27.7 months in fulvestrant-treated and anastrozole-treated patients, respectively, $P = 0.809$). Fulvestrant was comparable with exemestane in MBC refractory to letrozole or anastrozole, demonstrating an objective tumor RR of 20% (95% CI 9.6 to 30.4), with an overall clinical benefit of 38.3% (95% CI 21.2 to 49.3) and a median duration of response of 20 months (range 9 to 26 months) (19,23).

Related to optimal timing of endocrine therapy, investigations seeking to understand whether intentional interruption of therapy with these agents may restore hormone responsiveness are under way.

When there is evidence of hormone therapy resistance, good performance status, and no medical contraindication to chemotherapy, hormonal therapy is discontinued, and palliative chemotherapy is initiated (discussed below). In the case of HR+ disease, reversion of sensitivity to hormonal agents following chemotherapy and withdrawal of antiestrogen therapy have been described (24–28).

The optimal duration of hormonal therapy has not been finally determined for all patients in the adjuvant setting. However, in the treatment of MBC outside of a clinical trial, hormonal therapy is usually continued until failure of response is demonstrated by disease progression. Fundamentally important questions regarding the worth of intermittent treatment as opposed to continual treatment and the role of AI withdrawal in inducing response mirror those raised in the past for tamoxifen and other effective therapeutics.

Finally, the complexity of endocrine response pathways is highlighted by recent data redemonstrating that estradiol may effectively treat metastatic disease resistant to AI therapy, with toxicity dependent upon dose (29).

■ CHEMOTHERAPY IN MBC

Triple-Negative Disease

The role of chemotherapy in MBC is to prolong survival or palliate symptoms or both. In hormone receptor negative (HR–) MBC patients, particularly those whose tumors are HER2-nonamplified, chemotherapy is the mainstay of therapy. Patients whose tumors express neither hormone receptors nor HER2 overexpression reflect a heterogeneous group that requires further molecular characterization. For example, recent evidence in triple-negative breast cancer (ER–, progesterone receptor–negative, *HER2/neu*-negative) indicates that only a subset of these tumors responds to platinum-based therapy (cisplatin). Studies are ongoing to identify predictive markers of response in these patients. Among the more promising predictors are the proteins p63 and p73, which are important in DNA repair. A subset of triple-negative breast tumor cell lines that coexpress the isoforms ΔNp63 and TAp73 exhibits sensitivity to cisplatin via phosphorylation-dependent dissociation of TAp73 from ΔNp63α, resulting in transcription of proapoptotic effectors (30). Furthermore, tumors derived from these lines are resistant to the common chemotherapy drugs used in breast cancer therapy (e.g., doxorubicin, paclitaxel). Ongoing clinical trials are evaluating the worth of first-line cisplatin therapy alone or in combination with other agents in triple-negative breast cancers. A recent trial employing neoadjuvant chemotherapy in breast cancer patients achieved a higher rate of pathological complete response in p63-positive tumors than in p63-negative tumors (23% versus 0%, *P* = 0.048) when regimens including cisplatin without anthracyclines were administered (31). Although no specific algorithm or regimen currently defines treatment of recurrent triple-negative breast cancer, it is likely that molecular profiling with predictive instruments such as p63/p73 analysis will lead to classifications that will influence therapeutic decisions, much as ER now does for ER+ breast cancer.

Combination Chemotherapy: Anthracycline-based and Taxane-based Therapy

Many drugs are effective in treating breast cancer, and the choice depends partly on patients' prior exposure to agents in the adjuvant setting and their performance status. Agents are shown by category in Table 10.2. Combination and sequential strategies have been evaluated, along with alterations in dose density and intensity. Hundreds of phase II and III studies have been completed comparing different combinations, doses, durations, and sequences in an attempt to prolong TTP and improve OS. Despite all the available clinical trial data, drawing conclusions regarding the choice and sequencing of agents poses a challenge, especially because the number of available drugs continues to increase. In general, the ability of a phase III study to demonstrate a survival advantage is severely limited by the availability of the more effective agent and other options for the patient at the time of progression. Thus a true survival advantage from assignment to one agent over another in a phase III trial is an important signal of activity. Recent examples include: doxorubicin and docetaxel versus FAC (fluorouracil, doxorubicin, and cyclophosphamide) as first-line therapy (32), single-agent docetaxel versus paclitaxel

■ Table 10.2 Agents with demonstrated efficacy in metastatic breast cancer

Drug Class	Agent
Anthracyclines or anthracenedione	Doxorubicin Epirubicin Mitoxantrone
Taxanes	Paclitaxel Docetaxel Nab-paclitaxel
Pyrimidine analogues	5-Fluorouracil[a] Capecitabine
Antimetabolites	Methotrexate[a]
Alkylating agents	Cyclophosphamide[a]
Nucleoside analogs	Gemcitabine
Epipodophyllotoxins	Etoposide
Epothilones	Ixabepilone
Vinca alkaloids	Vinblastine Vinorelbine

[a]Cyclophosphamide, methotrexate, and 5-fluorouracil are used in combination (CMF).

given every 3 weeks (33), epirubicin versus gemcitabine in postmenopausal women over age 60 (34), and combination capecitabine and docetaxel versus single-agent docetaxel in anthracycline-pretreated patients (35). Table 10.3 highlights several phase III trials of active agents showing a survival advantage favoring one arm in MBC.

Decisions for optimal treatment have been further confounded by the addition of novel targeted agents to chemotherapy (discussed below). The Cochrane Breast Cancer Group has published several meta-analyses of chemotherapy in MBC (36). In summary, taxanes demonstrated a modest survival benefit when compared with non-taxane-containing regimens. Increased RR and TTP also were associated with taxane-based chemotherapy. When anthracycline and nonanthracycline regimens were compared, improved TTP and RR were associated with the anthracyclines at the cost of increased toxicity and without a survival advantage. In terms of platinum-based therapy, for unselected patients with MBC, increased RR was observed, but as for the anthracycline-containing regimens, platinum regimens were associated with significant toxicity and did not result in an improved survival. To determine whether administration schedule influenced outcome, Sledge and colleagues tested combination doxorubicin and paclitaxel versus single-agent doxorubicin or paclitaxel in front-line treatment of MBC. The combination arm demonstrated an improved RR and TTP compared with either single arm, but the sequential administration of doxorubicin before or after paclitaxel did not affect OS when compared with the combination arm (37).

■ Table 10.3 Trials with an overall survival benefit (P < 0.05) in metastatic breast cancer

Author (Reference)	Number of Patients	Arm A	OS Arm A (months)	Arm B	OS Arm B (months)	P Value	Adverse Events
Feher (34)	410	Epirubicin	19.1	Gemcitabine	11.8	0.0004	Similar toxicity
O'Shaughnessy (35)	511	Docetaxel and capecitabine	14.5	Capecitabine	11.5	0.0126	Increased toxicity in arm A
Jassem (126)	267	Doxorubicin and paclitaxel	23.3	FAC	18.3	0.013	Arm A neutropenia; arm B emesis
Albain (42)	529	Paclitaxel and gemcitabine	18.5	Paclitaxel	15.8	0.018	Arm A increased toxicity
Bontenbal (32)	216	Docetaxel and doxorubicin	22.6	FAC	16.2	0.019	Increased febrile neutropenia in arm A
Stockler (49)	325	Intermittent or continuous capecitabine	22.0	CMF	18.0	0.02	Arm A hand and foot syndrome; arm B febrile neutropenia
Jones (33)	449	Docetaxel	15.4	Paclitaxel	12.7	0.03	Increased toxicity in arm A
Icli (144)	201	Oral etoposide and cisplatin	14.0	Paclitaxel	9.5	0.039	Similar toxicity

CMF, cyclophosphamide, methotrexate, and 5-fluorouracil used in combination; FAC, 5-fluorouracil, doxorubicin, and cyclophosphamide; OS, overall survival.

For patients who are anthracycline-naive, combination regimens have been explored in randomized trials. Combination doxorubicin and cyclophosphamide (AC) showed no clinical benefit in progression-free survival (PFS), RR, or OS over doxorubicin and paclitaxel (AT) (38). However, an increase in toxicity in the paclitaxel-based regimen was observed and compromised dose-intensity delivery of doxorubicin. In a separate study, cyclophosphamide and docetaxel (AD) was compared with AC, with the AD arm exhibiting a significantly improved TTP, time to treatment failure (TTF), and RR but with increased toxicity and no improvement in OS (39). The benefits of anthracycline and taxane–based therapy were supported by a phase III trial of docetaxel, doxorubicin, and cyclophosphamide (TAC) versus 5-fluorouracil, doxorubicin, and cyclophosphamide (FAC) that showed an improvement in the TAC arm in terms of RR, but again at the cost of higher toxicity and with no advantage in terms of survival (40).

In a recent meta-analysis, comparison of taxane-based single and combination regimens with anthracycline-based regimens in first-line treatment of MBC revealed a significantly higher RR in taxane-based combination arms than in the nontaxane arms (57% versus 46%, P <0.001) (41). However, this improved RR did not translate into an improved OS (hazard ratio 0.95, 95% CI 0.88 to 1.03) and showed only a marginal improvement in PFS (hazard ratio 0.92, 95% CI 0.85 to 0.99) for the taxane-based therapy compared with the anthracycline-containing regimens. For the single-agent trials, there was no difference in RR or OS between taxanes and anthracyclines, but a trend for a worse PFS in the taxane arm was observed (hazard ratio 1.19, 95% CI 1.04 to 1.36, P = 0.011). Therefore, in MBC, taxanes did not improve survival as single agents or in combination compared with anthracycline-based therapy.

In MBC patients with anthracycline-resistant disease, single-agent taxane therapy yields an RR of 19% to 42% and a TTP of 3.5 to 6.5 months, with docetaxel demonstrating superiority over paclitaxel across different trials in a meta-analysis (39). In a head-to-head comparison—a large randomized study comparing docetaxel and paclitaxel administered every 3 weeks—docetaxel demonstrated a significantly increased RR (5.7 months versus 3.6 months, P <0.001) and OS (15.4 months versus 12.7 months, P = 0.03) (33). Paclitaxel with and without gemcitabine was compared in a randomized phase III trial in MBC patients with prior anthracycline exposure in the adjuvant setting (42). The combination arm had a significantly improved TTP (6.14 months versus 3.98 months, P = 0.0002) and response (41.4% versus 26.2%, P = 0.0002). More toxicity, particularly neutropenia, fatigue, and neuropathy, were documented in the paclitaxel and gemcitabine combination arm. In general, combination chemotherapy may be reserved for patients with a good performance status and a large tumor burden, particularly in visceral organs, or with rapidly progressive disease.

Other Single-agent Chemotherapy Options

Nab-paclitaxel

Nab-paclitaxel (Abraxane) is a nanoparticle albumin-bound chemotherapeutic agent that is soluble in water, eliminating the need for Cremophor, and therefore is associated with fewer hypersensitivity reactions. Initial trials demonstrated the efficacy of nab-paclitaxel in taxane-naive MBC patients (43). Nab-paclitaxel was approved after a randomized trial in MBC patients compared an every-3-week administration of paclitaxel with nab-paclitaxel (44). Prior taxane therapy was allowed if the patient had a disease-free interval longer than 1 year following adjuvant treatment. No difference in OS was noted; however, nab-paclitaxel significantly improved RR (33% versus 19%, P <0.001) and TTP (by 6 weeks). Comparing nab-paclitaxel with docetaxel with varying regimens of nab-paclitaxel revealed weekly nab-paclitaxel to have a higher RR and improved PFS than every-3-week administration of docetaxel or nab-paclitaxel (45). This and other studies clearly demonstrate that both the choice of taxane and the schedule of administration have influenced the effectiveness of agents in this class of drugs.

Capecitabine

Over recent years, the development of capecitabine, an oral prodrug of 5-florouracil, with RRs of 20% to 35% and a median OS of approximately 1 year in MBC patients who received prior taxane therapy, has expanded the role of chemotherapy in heretofore chemotherapy-refractory MBC patients. Capecitabine demonstrated comparable results in terms of RR, TTP, and OS to paclitaxel in MBC patients progressing after prior anthracycline treatment (46). Capecitabine has been used singly and in combination with other agents and has demonstrated superiority in two trials in combination with docetaxel over docetaxel alone and CMF, respectively (35,47–49). Whether combination therapy with capecitabine is superior or inferior to sequential administration of identical agents remains uncertain.

Epothilones

Epothilones exert cytotoxic effects by binding to and stabilizing microtubules, much like the taxanes; however, unlike the taxanes, they preferentially inhibit the βIII-tubulin isotype (50) and do not succumb to the same mechanisms of acquired cellular resistance. There are three potential mechanisms of developing resistance to taxanes. The best-characterized mechanism is overexpression of the MDR-1 gene (multidrug resistance), which encodes the efflux pump, P-glycoprotein, and prevents the retention of taxanes and other cationic drugs (51). Two

other mechanisms are mutations in tubulin at the paclitaxel-binding site and overexpression of β-tubulin (52). The epothilones have demonstrated clinical activity in anthracycline-resistant or pretreated and taxane-resistant MBC (53–55). Ixabepilone (Ixempra) is an analogue of epothilone B with increased in vitro antineoplastic activity over paclitaxel (56). At a dose of 40 mg/m² every 3 weeks, ixabepilone (Ixempra) achieved an RR of 12% to 18% in patients with advanced breast cancer refractory to anthracycline or taxane therapy. When it was given as a first-line agent in MBC, the RR was 57%. Trials are under way to establish the role of epothilones in the adjuvant setting as well as in combination with biological agents. Other epothilones, including patupilone, KOS-862, and ZK-EPO, are being investigated (57).

■ BIOLOGICAL THERAPY

The era of targeted therapy has brought to the forefront selective active agents that singly or in combination with chemotherapy have demonstrated efficacy. MBC patients frequently respond to their first treatment with endocrine or chemotherapy agents, only to then progress. Tamoxifen remains the prototypical targeted therapy, and with better understanding of proliferative and apoptotic pathways, novel targeted therapies are consistently being developed and evaluated in MBC. Some, such as trastuzumab (Herceptin), have successfully demonstrated enough activity to make an important impact in the adjuvant setting as well.

Trastuzumab

Approximately one-quarter of breast cancer cases will exhibit amplification of the epidermal growth factor receptor 2 (HER2/neu), which is associated with a more aggressive disease course, increased likelihood of recurrence, and an overall poorer prognosis (58,59). A recombinant, humanized monoclonal antibody, traztuzumab, directed against the product of the HER2/neu gene improves survival and quality of life in front-line treatment of MBC in combination with taxanes and non-taxane-based chemotherapy (60–62) and is also efficacious as a single agent (RR 25% to 40%) (63,64). These positive results stimulated the initiation of four clinical trials evaluating the worth of trastuzumab in the adjuvant setting (reviewed in Ref. 65). While a slightly higher rate of congestive heart failure (CHF) was noted in the trastuzumab-containing arms of these trials (0.6% to 3.3%), the consistent result was a major reduction in recurrence of breast cancer of approximately 50%, independent of whether trastuzumab was combined with or used after chemotherapy. Trastuzumab is now recommended in the adjuvant setting for women with early breast cancer, although the optimal duration of therapy is not known. Trials in progress are seeking to evaluate the worth of a second anti-*HER2/neu* small-molecule kinase inhibitor lapatinib (discussed below) compared with trastuzumab or the combination of the two agents. For patients with *HER2/neu*-amplified tumors who have never received anti-HER2 therapy in the adjuvant setting for a *HER2/neu*-amplified tumor, the TEACH (Tykerb Evaluation After Chemotherapy) trial has assessed the worth of delayed anti-*HER2/neu* therapy in preventing recurrence.

On recurrence or presentation with stage 4 disease, tissue obtained from a diagnostic biopsy of the metastasis should be evaluated for hormone receptors and *HER2/neu* amplification. Studies of synchronous metastasis to bone or other organs have suggested a small but finite number of cases where primary tumor and metastasis are discordant. Similarly, *HER2/neu*-nonamplified recurrences have been documented in patients treated in the adjuvant setting with anti-*HER2/neu* therapy (66). If *HER2/neu* amplification in the metastasis is demonstrated, then the patient should be evaluated for initial or further treatment with trastuzumab or another anti-*HER2/neu* therapy in combination with one of several chemotherapies. Cardiac toxicity is a concern, with documented rates ranging from 2% to 9% in clinical trials for MBC (64,67). However, the risk of trastuzumab-associated contractile dysfunction appears to be lower in anthracycline-naive patients (68). Concurrent use with cardiotoxic agents such as anthracyclines is not advised owing to the increased rate of cardiac dysfunction (New York Heart Association classes III to IV), reported as 27% in the anthracycline-trastuzumab arm of the pivotal trial in *HER2/neu*-amplified MBC (62). Several studies have been conducted using liposomal doxorubicin in combination with trastuzumab in MBC because liposome encapsulation alters the safety profile of anthracyclines and results in the drug being preferentially directed away from sites of toxicity and toward the site of action. In an early phase I/II trial of combination nonpegylated liposomal doxorubicin with trastuzumab ($n = 37$), the overall response rate was 58%, with one patient developing CHF and a second developing asymptomatic cardiotoxicity (69). The rate of symptomatic cardiotoxicity was decreased dramatically; however, asymptomatic cardiotoxicity during and after treatment ranged from 11% to 67% across the pegylated liposomal doxorubicin trials (70–73). Periodic cardiac monitoring is advised during treatment.

Once initiated, it is not clear whether the best strategy for ongoing treatment involves continued combination of chemotherapeutic agents with trastuzumab or whether the drug should be interrupted periodically.

In an effort to deliver trastuzumab specifically to antigen-expressing tumors, modifications of the antibody by linking it to cytotoxic agents such as maytansinoids, derivatives of the antimitotic drug maytansine, or by modification of the affinity of the Fc (constant fragment) portion of the molecule have yielded new agents with different activities. Preclinical studies of trastuzumab linked to drug moiety 1 (DM1) demonstrated efficacy in trastuzumab-sensitive and trastuzumab-insensitive in vitro and in vivo models of *HER2/neu*-overexpressing cancer (74). Phase I and II studies of DM1 have yielded promising responses in trastuzumab-refractory patients (75,76), demonstrating the feasibility of this approach.

An inverse relationship between ER and *HER2/neu* expression has been established clinically (77). Reversion of ER– *HER2/neu*-overexpressing breast cancer to ER+ has been documented and was observed to occur anywhere from 9 to 37 weeks following treatment with trastuzumab with or without chemotherapy (78). Furthermore, these tumors were subsequently found to be responsive to endocrine therapy.

Lapatinib

An oral potent tyrosine kinase inhibitor of *HER1* and *HER2/neu*, lapatinib (Tykerb) has demonstrated modest efficacy as a single agent (RR 6%) and in combination with trastuzumab (RR 26%) (79,80). Lapatinib in combination with capecitabine compared with capecitabine alone was investigated in patients with *HER2/neu*-amplified MBC, where prior therapy with taxanes, anthracyclines, or trastuzumab was allowed. In this phase III trial, the combination of capecitabine and lapatinib was superior to capecitabine alone at a planned interim analysis, with an RR of 22% versus 14% and a TTP of 8.4 months versus 4.4 months (hazard ratio 0.49, 95% CI 0.34 to 30.71, $P < 0.001$) (81). Lapatinib has also demonstrated activity both singly and in combination with paclitaxel in inflammatory breast cancer (IBC) (46,82). Coexpression of *HER2/neu* and *HER3* (EGFR3) in tumors seemed to predict a favorable response to lapatinib as a single agent in a phase II trial of heavily pretreated *HER2/neu*-amplified IBC patients (46). Phase III trials are evaluating the combination of lapatinib with paclitaxel and trastuzumab as first-line therapy for MBC patients. In addition, lapatinib has shown activity in trastuzumab-resistant breast cancer (83), and combination with trastuzumab appears to enhance its activity.

Of particular interest is the treatment of metastases to the central nervous system (CNS). Lapatinib has demonstrated activity in patients with metastasis to brain from *HER2/neu*-amplified breast cancer. Fewer women treated with combination lapatinib and capecitabine than with capecitabine monotherapy developed new or progressive CNS metastases (4 versus 11), although the difference was not statistically significant ($P = 0.1$) (81). A phase II trial evaluating lapatinib in women who had developed brain metastases on trastuzumab therapy demonstrated a decline in tumor volume of more than 30% in 5 of 20 patients and a 15% to 30% decrease in 3 of 20 patients (84). In a larger phase II trial ($n = 238$) evaluating lapatinib after trastuzumab and radiotherapy in patients with *HER2/neu*-amplified breast cancer and brain metastases, one patient achieved a partial response in the CNS by RECIST (response evaluation criteria in solid tumors) for an RR of 2.6%, with 15.4% of patients exhibiting stable disease for 16 weeks or more in both CNS and non-CNS sites (85). This study did not meet its primary efficacy goal (at least four responses), but volumetric reductions in CNS target lesions were observed in some patients. This has prompted a large international study to further evaluate lapatinib in *HER2/neu*-amplified breast cancer with progressive CNS metastases following radiotherapy, and volumetric changes will be used as the primary end point.

Antiangiogeneic Agents

The vascular endothelial growth factor (VEGF) family of small molecules is important in angiogenesis (86). There is significant redundancy inherent in the angiogenic switch. The humanized recombinant anti-VEGF-A antibody bevacizumab (Avastin) has been the most extensively studied agent to date. Phase I/II trials in previously treated MBC patients reported a 6.7% to 17% RR as a single agent (87). Initial investigations in prospective, randomized trials comparing capecitabine with and without bevacizumab in anthracycline and taxane–pretreated MBC failed to meet the primary endpoint, improved PFS, although a significant improvement in RR with the combination arm was observed (88). A second randomized, prospective clinical trial by the Eastern Oncology Cooperative Group (E 2100) comparing combination paclitaxel and bevacizumab with paclitaxel alone as first-line therapy in MBC was initiated in 2001. Patients who received combination paclitaxel and bevacizumab had a highly statistically significant increase in RR (36.9% versus 21.2%, $P <0.001$) and TTP (11.8 months versus 5.9 months, hazard ratio 0.60, $P <0.001$) (89). No difference in median OS was observed between the two groups (26.7 months versus 25.2 months, hazard ratio 0.88, $P = 0.16$). A third trial (AVADO) demonstrated a superior RR and TTP for the combination of docetaxel every 3 weeks with bevacizumab compared with docetaxel alone. Again, survival was not different between the two groups (90).

The side-effect profile of bevacizumab has been found to be manageable, with combined data from trials in all metastatic disease revealing grade 3 hypertension in 15% to 20% of treated patients with rare grade 4 hypertension responsive to standard management (91). Major hemorrhage and wound-healing problems have been reported in trials for colon and lung cancers, but these complications appear to be less common in breast cancer. Of particular concern, however, in the multidisciplinary treatment of breast cancer patients is the use of this agent in a neoadjuvant setting where the potential for an effect on wound healing may increase mastectomy and reconstruction complications. Concerns in the metastatic setting of rare complications such as fatal hemoptysis (92) and osteonecrosis of the jaw (93) will require further experience and highlight the enormous complexity of predicting complication rates as agents approved for use enter the general practice of breast oncology.

Two randomized phase III trials investigating the role of bevacizumab with multiple chemotherapy agents in first-line (RiBBON 1) and second-line (RiBBON 2) treatment of MBC compared with chemotherapy plus placebo are ongoing (94). Phase I/II trials are ongoing with other angiogenesis inhibitors in combination with chemotherapy. Only with rigorous studies that increase combinations of classes of agents will principles emerge that help to inform future decisions.

PARP Inhibitors

PolyADP-ribose polymerase 1 (PARP-1) is an important enzyme in DNA repair. PARP-1 activation occurs in response to DNA damage as a result of chemotherapy and radiotherapy, as well as in stroke, head trauma, and heart ischemia. In addition, recent reports have documented the upregulation of PARP in patients with hereditary breast cancer, *BRCA1,* because loss of *BRCA1* contributes to impaired DNA repair mechanisms. Inhibiting PARP-1 has many clinical implications because it may potentiate the benefits of chemotherapy or radiotherapy. Furthermore, in *BRCA1/2* mutation carriers with breast cancer, there is preclinical evidence that inhibition of PARP-1 may reverse acquired chemoresistance, particularly in combination with platinum agents (95,96). An oral PARP inhibitor, AG-014699, has been developed and is currently in clinical phase I/II trials. A phase I trial was completed with AG-014699 in combination with temozolomide (Temodar) in advanced solid malignancies to determine the maximal safe tolerated dose (97).

Other PARP inhibitors are further along in clinical trials. British investigators evaluated the oral PARP inhibitor AZD2281 (olaparib) in patients with chemotherapy-refractory *BRCA*-deficient advanced breast cancer using two doses (400 mg or 100 mg) given twice daily in 54 patients (98). One complete response and 10 partial responses were achieved with the higher dosing, for an overall RR of 41%, compared with an overall RR of 22% (six partial responses) with the lower dose. The most exciting finding, however, has been the significant improvement in RR (48% versus 16%, $P = 0.002$) and OS (9.2 months versus 5.7 months, $P = 0.0005$) when the PARP inhibitor BSI-201 was added to gemcitabine and carboplatin compared chemotherapy alone in patients with triple-negative MBC in a randomized phase II trial (99). There was also a significant improvement in PFS from 3.3 months to 6.9 months ($P <0.0001$) favoring the PARP arm. These findings have spurred excitement in the field, and more studies are anxiously awaited to confirm these results and refine the dosing and chemotherapy combination regimens.

■ SUPPORTIVE INTERVENTIONS

Bone Metastases

Bone is a common site of metastasis in breast cancer, and bone metastases can lead to skeletal complications and decreased quality of life. Skeletal-related events include pain, hypercalcemia, pathological fracture, and spinal cord compression. Historically, the goals of therapy have been to prevent fracture, neurological complications, and further metastases emanating from the site(s). Recent investigations have presented intriguing data that early intervention with bisphosphonates may alter the natural history of developing metastases (100) as well as treatment of established metastases (101).

In addition, bisphosphonates, which inhibit osteoclast-mediated bone resorption, are the standard of care for treatment of cancer-induced hypercalcemia and were demonstrated to reduce the risk of skeletal-related events by approximately 17% (102). The second-generation bisphosphonates pamidronate (Aredia), ibandronate (Boniva), and zoledronic acid (Zometa) prevent protein prenylation of osteoclasts in vitro and have enhanced clinical activity compared with first-generation bisphosphonates. Evidence for antiangiogenic properties of these agents, in particular zoledronic acid, is now emerging (103). These agents are generally well tolerated but do have potential for serious side effects such as renal failure and osteonecrosis of the jaw (104–106). The dosing frequency and optimal or maximal duration of treatment have not been established for intravenous bisphosphonates for the treatment of metastatic bone lesions. Relative to complications, completed studies that have evaluated the benefits of bisphosphonates have not evaluated the maximum duration of use or the complication rates past 24 consecutive months of administration. Thus their prolonged use should be employed with caution, particularly as other targeted agents are being used concurrently with increasing frequency and survival is being extended.

Once a bone metastasis has been diagnosed, a decision must be made as to whether the treatment is primarily medical or multidisciplinary. Often pain or structural considerations make evaluation by radiation oncology for palliative radiotherapy, by orthopedics for stability of a long bone, and by neurosurgery for surgical spinal cord decompression necessary. Radiotherapy has the advantage of rapid alleviation of pain but does not obviate the use of analgesics and steroids as part of pain management because the early use of corticosteroids can be remarkably effective. With the advent of modern neurosurgical techniques, surgical intervention for painful spinal metastasis with radiation has resulted in superior functional outcomes and survival over radiotherapy alone (107). Vertebral collapse, when significant and associated with pain, should prompt referral to interventional radiology for consideration of

■ **Table 10.4** Regimens with reported activity in central nervous system metastases from breast cancer

Regimen	Reference
Combination chemotherapy	
Cyclophosphamide, 5-fluorouracil and prednisone	127
Cyclophosphamide, 5-fluorouracil, prednisone, methotrexate, and vincristine	127
Methotrexate, vincristine, and prednisone	127
Cyclophosphamide, methotrexate, and 5-fluorouracil	128
Cyclophosphamide, doxorubicin, and 5-fluorouracil	128
Single-agent or combination chemotherapy	
Bendamustine	129
Capecitabine alone or in combination with temozolomide	130–132
Temozolomide alone or in combination with radiotherapy, capecitabine, cisplatin, or vinorelbine	132–137
Targeted therapy: Anti-HER2/neu	
Lapatinib	85
Trastuzumab	138
Hormonal agents	
Tamoxifen	139, 140
Anastrazole	141
Letrozole	142
Megestrol acetate	143

vertebroplasty, which can be remarkably effective in ameliorating pain and improving mobility.

Brain Metastases

Brain metastases also contribute to the high morbidity from breast cancer and are of growing concern as systemic therapy becomes increasingly effective. Initial neurosurgical and radiation oncology opinions regarding the optimal treatment of a patient with isolated brain lesions are critical. Therapeutic options include surgical resection, stereotactic radiosurgery, and whole brain external-beam radiation, depending on the number of lesions and location. Systemic therapy should not be discounted on diagnosis of CNS metastases because partial CNS activity is seen on a case-by-case basis. There is evidence of long-term clinical response in patients with breast cancer metastases to the brain who were treated with capecitabine

(108,109). Table 10.4 lists agents with reported activity in MBC patients with CNS disease.

Locoregional Disease Control: The Role of Radiofrequency Ablation

With the advent of active chemotherapy, targeted agents, and newer modalities such as radiofrequency ablation (RFA), patients with solitary lung and liver metastases can have an improved prognosis. A subset of MBC patients with disease confined to the liver appear to have an improved outcome following surgical resection (110,111). Three-year survival rates range from 35% to 71%; however, the disease-free survival (DFS) rates are reportedly much lower (112–114). RFA is a relatively simple, safe, and well-tolerated percutaneous procedure that has demonstrated efficacy as a cytoreductive strategy in hepatic carcinomas (115,116). Case reports of RFA for hepatic metastases in MBC patients have demonstrated encouraging survival, with one series of 19 patients documenting a 41.6% survival at 30 months (117). Another series treated 24 patients, with 10 (41.6%) being disease-free at a median of 10 months' follow-up (118,119). RFA to other sites of oligometastases such as the lung and bone are plausible options for tumor control in a selected group of patients with limited or stable disease (120).

For patients presenting with de novo stage 4 breast cancer, locoregional management of the primary tumor is controversial. Traditional management has been systemic therapy, with locoregional breast treatment (surgery and radiation) reserved for palliation of symptomatic disease. The effect of local therapy of the primary tumor on outcomes and survival is the subject of investigation. A recent retrospective study to investigate the role of surgical resection in the control of chest wall disease among women with MBC demonstrated a significant decrease in symptomatic chest wall disease as well as a significant increase in time to first progression (TTFP) in patients who underwent resection of their primary tumor (121). A trend toward improved OS was also observed but did not reach statistical significance. The goal of locoregional control to achieve negative surgical margins and to consolidate therapy with radiation should be considered where regional considerations may become paramount prior to systemic progression.

■ NOVEL THERAPEUTIC STRATEGIES

The future of rationally designed, targeted therapy in breast cancer is bright, and laboratory investigations are bringing many novel compounds and combinations of treatments to the forefront. Much attention is being focused on the mitogen activated protein kinase (MAPK) pathway, which is involved in cellular proliferation and survival. Farnesyl transferase inhibitors, which inhibit the

posttranslational modification of the tyrosine kinase, Ras, necessary for its membrane localization and activation of downstream effectors of the MAPK pathway, have demonstrated activity in advanced breast cancer (122,123). In addition, inhibition of the mammalian target of rapamycin (mTOR), a downstream effector in the MAPK pathway, with temsirolimus (Torisel) has demonstrated an RR of 9.2% in heavily pretreated patients (124). Combination of temsirolimus with letrozole has led to an improvement in PFS compared with single-agent letrozole in a phase II study, but this benefit was not replicated in a large phase III trial. Ongoing trials are investigating the combination of everolimus (Certican), another mTOR inhibitor, with chemotherapy or trastuzumab in MBC. Other investigational targeted agents include inhibitors of type I insulin-like growth factor receptor (IGFR), *BRAF*, aurora kinases, *Src*, platelet-derived growth factor (PDGF), and nuclear factor kappa-light-chain-enhancer of activated B cells (NFκB). The IGFR pathway is of particular interest and induces cellular proliferation and inhibits apoptosis in preclinical models. It is postulated to modulate resistance to other targeted therapies such as trastuzumab. Denosumab, an NFκB inhibitor, is another agent being investigated for prevention of skeletal-related events in patients with bone metastases. Denosumab resulted in significant bone density increase in non-MBC patients on an AI compared with placebo (125).

■ CONCLUSION

The treatment of MBC very frequently necessitates a multidisciplinary approach. A thorough evaluation of the extent of disease and sites of disease dictates the therapeutic approach, in combination with the age and health of the patient. Although the goals of surgery and radiotherapy in the metastatic setting remain palliative, they serve to improve the quality of life and treat foci of disease to reduce the tumor burden or prevent relapse, or both. The interplay of conventional chemotherapy and hormonal treatments remains instrumental in achieving disease control. Combining these modalities with targeted therapy is currently under active investigation for many agents and has proven beneficial with agents such as trastuzumab and bevacizumab. Furthermore, many novel agents are currently in clinical trials, and patients should be evaluated for enrollment in such trials throughout their treatment course. Finally, combining novel active agents with effective minimally invasive interventional procedures provides the most elegant care for many patients with extended survivals.

As patients live longer free of debilitating complications of metastatic disease, it will be increasingly important to maximize efficacy while minimizing toxicity of therapy. Thus, careful longitudinal follow-up of patients treated with novel combinations of agents will require renewed vigilance and dedication to track the effectiveness and particularly the toxicity of treatments, even after agents are released for general use. The judicious use of surgery, radiation, and minimally invasive procedures such as RFA will continue to expand the many options available to patients with MBC in a continual effort to improve their quality of life.

■ SUMMARY

- The treatment of MBC involves a multidisciplinary team to coordinate the administration of effective chemotherapy, radiotherapy, and surgical interventions when needed.
- New advances in understanding the biology of breast cancer have yielded effective targeted and biological therapies that can either be added to more traditional chemotherapy for an enhanced effect or used singly to overcome resistance. Long-term studies are needed to fully understand potential for toxicity.
- The molecular characterization of breast cancer is critical in selecting appropriate treatment for each patient on the basis of ER, progesterone receptor, and *HER2/neu* status.
- Newer modalities such as RFA make it possible to control localized oligometastatic disease in an attempt to improve progression-free survival.

■ REFERENCES

1. Berry DA, Cronin KA, Plevritis SK, et al. Effect of screening and adjuvant therapy on mortality from breast cancer. *New Engl J Med.* 2005;353(17):1784–1792.
2. Jemal A, Siegel R, Ward E, et al. Cancer statistics, 2008. *CA Cancer J Clin.* 2008;58(2):71–96.
3. Higgins MJ, Davidson NE. What is the current status of ovarian suppression/ablation in women with premenopausal early-stage breast cancer? *Curr Oncol Rep.* 2009;11(1):45–50.
4. Beatson G. On the treatment of inoperable cases of carcinoma of the mamma: suggestions for a new method of treatment, with illustrative cases. *Lancet.* 1896;2:104–107,62–65.
5. Moulder S, Hortobagyi GN. Advances in the treatment of breast cancer. *Clin Pharmacol Ther.* 2008;83(1):26–36.
6. Talalay P, Takano GM, Huggins C. Studies on the Walker tumor. II. Effects of adrenalectomy and hypophysectomy on tumor growth in tube-fed rats. *Cancer Res.* 1952;12(11):838–843.
7. Pearson OH, Ray BS. Hypophysectomy in the treatment of advanced cancer of breast. *Ann Surg.* 1956;144(3):394–406.
8. Ovarian ablation in early breast cancer: overview of the randomised trials. Early Breast Cancer Trialists' Collaborative Group. *Lancet.* 1996;348(9036):1189–1196.
9. Rodriguez Lajusticia L, Martin Jimenez M, Lopez-Tarruella Cobo S. Endocrine therapy of metastatic breast cancer. *Clin Transl Oncol.* 2008;10(8):462–467.
10. Ingle JN, Krook JE, Green SJ, et al. Randomized trial of bilateral oophorectomy versus tamoxifen in premenopausal women with metastatic breast cancer. *J Clin Oncol.* 1986;4(2):178–185.
11. Klijn JG, Blamey RW, Boccardo F, Tominaga T, Duchateau L, Sylvester R. Combined tamoxifen and luteinizing hormone-releasing hormone (LHRH) agonist versus LHRH agonist alone in premenopausal advanced breast cancer: a meta-analysis of four randomized trials. *J Clin Oncol.* 2001;19(2):343–353.
12. Goss PE, Ingle JN, Martino S, et al. A randomized trial of letrozole in postmenopausal women after five years of tamoxifen therapy for early-stage breast cancer. *New Engl J Med.* 2003; 349(19):1793–1802.
13. Lees AW, Giuffre C, Burns PE, Hurlburt ME, Jenkins HJ. Oophorectomy versus radiation ablation of ovarian function in patients with metastatic carcinoma of the breast. *Surg Gynecol Obstet.* 1980;151(6):721–724.
14. Schwarzel WC, Kruggel WG, Brodie HJ. Studies on the mechanism of estrogen biosynthesis. 8. The development of inhibitors of the enzyme system in human placenta. *Endocrinology.* 1973;92(3):866–880.
15. Nabholtz JM, Buzdar A, Pollak M, et al. Anastrozole is superior to tamoxifen as first-line therapy for advanced breast cancer in postmenopausal women: results of a North American multicenter randomized trial. Arimidex Study Group. *J Clin Oncol.* 2000;18(22):3758–3767.
16. Bonneterre J, Buzdar A, Nabholtz JM, et al. Anastrozole is superior to tamoxifen as first-line therapy in hormone receptor positive advanced breast carcinoma. *Cancer.* 2001;92(9):2247–2258.
17. Mouridsen H, Gershanovich M, Sun Y, et al. Superior efficacy of letrozole versus tamoxifen as first-line therapy for postmenopausal women with advanced breast cancer: results of a phase III study of the International Letrozole Breast Cancer Group. *J Clin Oncol.* 2001;19(10):2596–2606.
18. Paridaens RJ, Dirix LY, Beex LV, et al. Phase III study comparing exemestane with tamoxifen as first-line hormonal treatment of metastatic breast cancer in postmenopausal women: the European Organisation for Research and Treatment of Cancer Breast Cancer Cooperative Group. *J Clin Oncol.* 2008;26(30):4883–4890.
19. Gennatas C, Michalaki V, Carvounis E, et al. Third-line hormonal treatment with exemestane in postmenopausal patients with advanced breast cancer progressing on letrozole or anastrozole. A phase II trial conducted by the Hellenic Group of Oncology (HELGO). *Tumori.* 2006;92(1):13–17.
20. Henry NL, Giles JT, Ang D, et al. Prospective characterization of musculoskeletal symptoms in early stage breast cancer patients treated with aromatase inhibitors. *Breast Cancer Res Treat.* 2008; 111(2):365–372.
21. Cella D, Fallowfield LJ. Recognition and management of treatment-related side effects for breast cancer patients receiving adjuvant endocrine therapy. *Breast Cancer Res Treat.* 2008;107(2): 167–180.
22. Lonning PE. Lack of complete cross-resistance between different aromatase inhibitors; a real finding in search for an explanation? *Eur J Cancer.* 2009;45(4):527–535.
23. Howell A, Pippen J, Elledge RM, et al. Fulvestrant versus anastrozole for the treatment of advanced breast carcinoma: a prospectively planned combined survival analysis of two multicenter trials. *Cancer.* 2005;104(2):236–239.
24. Bhide SA, Rea DW. Metastatic breast cancer response after Exemestane withdrawal: a case report. *Breast.* 2004;13(1):66–68.
25. Legault-Poisson S, Jolivet J, Poisson R, Beretta-Piccoli M, Band PR. Tamoxifen-induced tumor stimulation and withdrawal response. *Cancer Treat Rep.* 1979;63(11–12):1839–1841.
26. Stein W, 3rd, Hortobagyi GN, Blumenschein GR. Response of metastatic breast cancer to tamoxifen withdrawal: report of a case. *J Surg Oncol.* 1983;22(1):45–46.
27. Belani CP, Pearl P, Whitley NO, Aisner J. Tamoxifen withdrawal response. Report of a case. *Arch Intern Med.* 1989;149(2):449–450.
28. Cigler T, Goss PE. Aromatase inhibitor withdrawal response in metastatic breast cancer. *J Clin Oncol.* 2006;24(12):1955–1956.
29. Ellis MJDF, Kommareddy A, Jamalabadi-Majidi S, et al. A randomized phase 2 trial of low dose (6 mg daily) versus high dose (30 mg daily) estradiol for patients with estrogen receptor positive aromatase inhibitor resistant advanced breast cancer. San Antonio Breast Conference, San Antonio, Texas, 2008 (Abstract 16).

30. Leong CO, Vidnovic N, DeYoung MP, Sgroi D, Ellisen LW. The p63/p73 network mediates chemosensitivity to cisplatin in a biologically defined subset of primary breast cancers. *J Clin Invest.* 2007;117(5):1370–1380.

31. Rocca A, Viale G, Gelber RD, et al. Pathologic complete remission rate after cisplatin-based primary chemotherapy in breast cancer: correlation with p63 expression. *Cancer Chemother Pharmacol.* 2008;61(6):965–971.

32. Bontenbal M, Creemers GJ, Braun HJ, et al. Phase II to III study comparing doxorubicin and docetaxel with fluorouracil, doxorubicin, and cyclophosphamide as first-line chemotherapy in patients with metastatic breast cancer: results of a Dutch Community Setting Trial for the Clinical Trial Group of the Comprehensive Cancer Centre. *J Clin Oncol.* 2005;23(28):7081–7088.

33. Jones SE, Erban J, Overmoyer B, et al. Randomized phase III study of docetaxel compared with paclitaxel in metastatic breast cancer. *J Clin Oncol.* 2005;23(24):5542–5551.

34. Feher O, Vodvarka P, Jassem J, et al. First-line gemcitabine versus epirubicin in postmenopausal women aged 60 or older with metastatic breast cancer: a multicenter, randomized, phase III study. *Ann Oncol.* 2005;16(6):899–908.

35. O'Shaughnessy J, Miles D, Vukelja S, et al. Superior survival with capecitabine plus docetaxel combination therapy in anthracycline-pretreated patients with advanced breast cancer: phase III trial results. *J Clin Oncol.* 2002;20(12):2812–2823.

36. Wilcken N, Dear R. Chemotherapy in metastatic breast cancer: A summary of all randomised trials reported 2000–2007. *Eur J Cancer.* 2008;44(15):2218–2225.

37. Sledge GW, Neuberg D, Bernardo P, et al. Phase III trial of doxorubicin, paclitaxel, and the combination of doxorubicin and paclitaxel as front-line chemotherapy for metastatic breast cancer: an intergroup trial (E1193). *J Clin Oncol.* 2003;21(4):588–592.

38. Biganzoli L, Cufer T, Bruning P, et al. Doxorubicin and paclitaxel versus doxorubicin and cyclophosphamide as first-line chemotherapy in metastatic breast cancer: The European Organization for Research and Treatment of Cancer 10961 Multicenter Phase III Trial. *J Clin Oncol.* 2002;20(14):3114–3121.

39. Sparano JA. Taxanes for breast cancer: an evidence-based review of randomized phase II and phase III trials. *Clin Breast Cancer.* 2000;1(1):32–40; discussion 1–2.

40. Mackey PA Jr, Dirix L, et al. Final results of the phase III randomized trial comparing docetaxel (T), doxorubicin (A) and cyclophosphamide (C) to FAC as first line chemotherapy (CT) for patients (pts) with metastatic breast cancer (MBC). *Proc Am Soc Clin Oncol.* 2002;21:35a (abstract 137).

41. Piccart-Gebhart MJ, Burzykowski T, Buyse M, et al. Taxanes alone or in combination with anthracyclines as first-line therapy of patients with metastatic breast cancer. *J Clin Oncol.* 2008; 26(12):1980–1986.

42. Albain KS, Nag SM, Calderillo-Ruiz G, et al. Gemcitabine plus paclitaxel versus paclitaxel monotherapy in patients with metastatic breast cancer and prior anthracycline treatment. *J Clin Oncol.* 2008;26(24):3950–3957.

43. Henderson IC, Bhatia V. Nab-paclitaxel for breast cancer: a new formulation with an improved safety profile and greater efficacy. *Exp Rev Anticancer Ther.* 2007;7(7):919–943.

44. Gradishar WJ, Tjulandin S, Davidson N, et al. Phase III trial of nanoparticle albumin-bound paclitaxel compared with polyethylated castor oil-based paclitaxel in women with breast cancer. *J Clin Oncol.* 2005;23(31):7794–7803.

45. Mieog JS, van der Hage JA, van de Velde CJ. Neoadjuvant chemotherapy for operable breast cancer. *Br J Surg.* 2007;94(10):1189–1200.

46. Johnston S, Trudeau M, Kaufman B, et al. Phase II study of predictive biomarker profiles for response targeting human epidermal growth factor receptor 2 (HER2) in advanced inflammatory breast cancer with lapatinib monotherapy. *J Clin Oncol.* 2008;26(7):1066–1072.

47. Oshaughnessy JA, Blum J, Moiseyenko V, et al. Randomized, open-label, phase II trial of oral capecitabine (Xeloda) vs. a reference arm of intravenous CMF (cyclophosphamide, methotrexate, and 5-fluorouracil) as first-line therapy for advanced/metastatic breast cancer. *Ann Oncol.* 2001;12(9):1247–1254.

48. Verma S, Maraninchi D, O'Shaughnessy J, et al. Capecitabine plus docetaxel combination therapy. *Cancer.* 2005;103(12):2455–2465.

49. Stockler M ST, Grimison P, et al. A randomized trial of capecitabine given intermittently rather than continuously compared to classical CMF as first-line chemotherapy for advanced breast cancer. ASCO Annual Meeting Proceedings Part I. *J Clin Oncol.* 2007;25(8S):1031.

50. Jordan MA, Miller H, Ray A et al. The Pat-21 breast cancer model derived from a patient with primary Taxol resistance recapitulates the phenotype of its origin has altered b-tubulin expression and is sensitive to ixabepilone. AACR Annual Meeting, Washington, DC, April 1–5, 2006 (Abstract LB-280).

51. Horwitz SB, Lothstein L, Manfredi JJ, et al. Taxol: mechanisms of action and resistance. *Ann NY Acad Sci.* 1986;466:733–744.

52. Dumontet C, Jordan MA, Lee FF. Ixabepilone: targeting betaIII-tubulin expression in taxane-resistant malignancies. *Mol Cancer Ther.* 2009;8(1):17–25.

53. Perez EA, Lerzo G, Pivot X, et al. Efficacy and safety of ixabepilone (BMS-247550) in a phase II study of patients with advanced breast cancer resistant to an anthracycline, a taxane, and capecitabine. *J Clin Oncol.* 2007;25(23):3407–3414.

54. Thomas E, Tabernero J, Fornier M, et al. Phase II clinical trial of ixabepilone (BMS-247550), an epothilone B analog, in patients with taxane-resistant metastatic breast cancer. *J Clin Oncol.* 2007;25(23):3399–3406.

55. Thomas ES, Gomez HL, Li RK, et al. Ixabepilone plus capecitabine for metastatic breast cancer progressing after anthracycline and taxane treatment. *J Clin Oncol.* 2007;25(33):5210–5217.

56. Lee FY, Borzilleri R, Fairchild CR, et al. BMS-247550: a novel epothilone analog with a mode of action similar to paclitaxel but possessing superior antitumor efficacy. *Clin Cancer Res.* 2001;7(5):1429–1437.

57. Cortes J, Baselga J. Targeting the microtubules in breast cancer beyond taxanes: the epothilones. *Oncologist.* 2007;12(3):271–280.

58. Slamon DJ, Godolphin W, Jones LA, et al. Studies of the *HER2/neu* proto-oncogene in human breast and ovarian cancer. *Science* 1989;244(4905):707–712.

59. Slamon DJ, Clark GM, Wong SG, Levin WJ, Ullrich A, McGuire WL. Human breast cancer: correlation of relapse and survival with amplification of the *HER2/neu* oncogene. *Science* 1987; 235(4785):177–182.

60. Marty M, Cognetti F, Maraninchi D, et al. Randomized phase II trial of the efficacy and safety of trastuzumab combined with docetaxel in patients with human epidermal growth factor receptor 2-positive metastatic breast cancer administered as first-line treatment: the M77001 study group. *J Clin Oncol.* 2005;23(19):4265–4274.

61. Osoba D, Slamon DJ, Burchmore M, Murphy M. Effects on quality of life of combined trastuzumab and chemotherapy in women with metastatic breast cancer. *J Clin Oncol.* 2002;20(14):3106–3113.

62. Slamon DJ, Leyland-Jones B, Shak S, et al. Use of chemotherapy plus a monoclonal antibody against HER2 for metastatic breast cancer that overexpresses HER2. *New Engl J Med.* 2001; 344(11):783–792.

63. Baselga J, Carbonell X, Castaneda-Soto NJ, et al. Phase II study of efficacy, safety, and pharmacokinetics of trastuzumab monotherapy administered on a 3-weekly schedule. *J Clin Oncol.* 2005; 23(10):2162–2171.

64. Vogel CL, Cobleigh MA, Tripathy D, et al. Efficacy and safety of trastuzumab as a single agent in first-line treatment of HER2-overexpressing metastatic breast cancer. *J Clin Oncol.* 2002;20(3):719–726.

65. Baselga J, Perez EA, Pienkowski T, Bell R. Adjuvant trastuzumab: a milestone in the treatment of HER-2-positive early breast cancer. *Oncologist.* 2006;11(Suppl 1):4–12.

66. Dawood S, Resetkova E, Gonzalez-Angulo AM. Trastuzumab administration associated with change in HER2 status. *Clin Breast Cancer.* 2008;8(4):366–369.

67. Rayson D, Richel D, Chia S, Jackisch C, van der Vegt S, Suter T. Anthracycline-trastuzumab regimens for HER2/neu-overexpressing breast cancer: current experience and future strategies. *Ann Oncol.* 2008;19(9):1530–1539.

68. Tan-Chiu E, Yothers G, Romond E, et al. Assessment of cardiac dysfunction in a randomized trial comparing doxorubicin and cyclophosphamide followed by paclitaxel, with or without tras-tuzumab as adjuvant therapy in node-positive, human epidermal growth factor receptor 2-overexpressing breast cancer: NSABP B-31. *J Clin Oncol.* 2005;23(31):7811–7819.

69. Theodoulou M CS, Batist G. TLC D99 (D, Myocet) and Herceptin (H) is safe in advanced breast cancer (ABC): final cardiac safety and efficacy analysis. *Proc Am Soc Clin Oncol.* 2002;21:55a.

70. Andreopoulou E, Gaiotti D, Kim E, et al. Feasibility and cardiac safety of pegylated liposomal doxorubicin plus trastuzumab in heav-ily pretreated patients with recurrent HER2-overexpressing meta-static breast cancer. *Clin Breast Cancer.* 2007;7(9):690–696.

71. Wolff AC. Liposomal anthracyclines and new treatment approaches for breast cancer. *Oncologist.* 2003;8(Suppl 2):25–30.

72. Chia S, Clemons M, Martin LA, et al. Pegylated liposomal doxo-rubicin and trastuzumab in HER-2 overexpressing metastatic breast cancer: a multicenter phase II trial. *J Clin Oncol.* 2006;24(18):2773–2778.

73. Stickeler E WD, Woll J et al. Cardiac safety of pegylated lipo-somal doxorubicin (PLD) in combination with trastuzumab (T) in patients with metastatic breast cancer (MBC): results from a mul-ticenter phase II study. ASCO Meeting Proceedings Part I. *J Clin Oncol.* 2007;25(18S):1106.

74. Lewis Phillips GD, Li G, Dugger DL, et al. Targeting HER2-positive breast cancer with trastuzumab-DM1, an antibody-cytotoxic drug conjugate. *Cancer Res.* 2008;68(22):9280–9290.

75. Vukelja S RH, Vogel C, Borson R, Tan-Chiu E, Birkner M, Holden SN, Klencke B, O'Shaughnessy J, Burris HA. A phase II study of trastuzumab-DM1, a first-in-class HER2 antibody-drug conjugate, in patients with HER2+ metastatic breast cancer. San Antonio Breast Cancer Symposium, San Antonio, Texas, 2008 (Abstract 33).

76. Beeram M BHI, Modi S, Birkner M, Girish S, Tibbitts J, Holdne SN, Lutzker SG, Krop IE. A phase I study fo trastuzumab-DM1 (T-DM1), a first-in-class HER2 antibody conjugate (ADC), in patients (pts) with advanced HER2+ breast cancer (BC). *J Clin Oncol.* 2008;26(Suppl):26 (Abstract 1028).

77. Jones A. Combining trastuzumab (Herceptin) with hormonal therapy in breast cancer: what can be expected and why? *Ann Oncol.* 2003;14(12):1697–1704.

78. Munzone E, Curigliano G, Rocca A, et al. Reverting estrogen-receptor-negative phenotype in HER-2-overexpressing advanced breast cancer patients exposed to trastuzumab plus chemother-apy. *Breast Cancer Res.* 2006;8(1):R4.

79. Burris HA 3rd, Hurwitz HI, Dees EC, et al. Phase I safety, phar-macokinetics, and clinical activity study of lapatinib (GW572016), a reversible dual inhibitor of epidermal growth factor receptor tyrosine kinases, in heavily pretreated patients with metastatic carcinomas. *J Clin Oncol.* 2005;23(23):5305–5313.

80. Storniolo AM, Pegram MD, Overmoyer B, et al. Phase I dose escalation and pharmacokinetic study of lapatinib in combination with trastuzumab in patients with advanced ErbB2-positive breast cancer. *J Clin Oncol.* 2008;26(20):3317–3323.

81. Geyer CE, Forster J, Lindquist D, et al. Lapatinib plus capecit-abine for HER2-positive advanced breast cancer. *New Engl J Med.* 2006;355(26):2733–2743.

82. Cristofanilli Mea. A phase II combination study of lapatinib and paclitaxel as a neoadjuvant therapy in patients with newly diagnosed inflammatory breast cancer (IBC). *Breast Cancer Res Treat.* 2006;100(Suppl 1).

83. Bilancia D, Rosati G, Dinota A, Germano D, Romano R, Manzione L. Lapatinib in breast cancer. *Ann Oncol.* 2007;18(Suppl 6):vi, 26–30.

84. Lin NU. Phase II trial of lapatinib for brain metastases in patients with HER2+ breast cancer. *J Clin Oncol.* 2007;25(Suppl):1012.

85. Lin NU, Carey LA, Liu MC, et al. Phase II trial of lapatinib for brain metastases in patients with human epidermal growth factor receptor 2-positive breast cancer. *J Clin Oncol.* 2008;26(12):1993–1999.

86. Hayes DF, Miller K, Sledge G. Angiogenesis as targeted breast cancer therapy. *Breast.* 2007;16(Suppl 2):S17–S19.

87. Cobleigh MA, Langmuir VK, Sledge GW, et al. A phase I/II dose-escalation trial of bevacizumab in previously treated metastatic breast cancer. *Semin Oncol.* 2003;30(5 Suppl 16):117–124.

88. Miller KD, Chap LI, Holmes FA, et al. Randomized phase III trial of capecitabine compared with bevacizumab plus capecitabine in patients with previously treated metastatic breast cancer. *J Clin Oncol.* 2005;23(4):792–799.

89. Miller K, Wang M, Gralow J, et al. Paclitaxel plus bevacizumab versus paclitaxel alone for metastatic breast cancer. *New Engl J Med.* 2007;357(26):2666–2676.

90. Miles D, Chan A, Romiew G, Dirix LY, Cortes J, Pivot X, Tomczak P, Taran T, Harbeck N, Steger GG. Randomized, dou-ble-blind, placebo-controlled, phase III study of bevacizumab with docetaxel with placebo as first-line therapy for patients with locally recurrent or metastatic breast cancer (mBC): AVADO. *J Clin Oncol.* 2008;26(Suppl) (Abstract LBA1011).

91. Shih T, Lindley C. Bevacizumab: an angiogenesis inhibitor for the treatment of solid malignancies. *Clin Ther.* 2006;28(11):1779–1802.

92. Philippin-Lauridant G, Thureau S, Ouvrier MJ, Blot E. Fatal hemoptysis in a patient with breast cancer treated with bevaci-zumab and paclitaxel. *Ann Oncol.* 2008;19(11):1977–1978.

93. Estilo CL, Fornier M, Farooki A, Carlson D, Bohle G 3rd, Huryn JM. Osteonecrosis of the jaw related to bevacizumab. *J Clin Oncol.* 2008;26(24):4037–4038.

94. O'Shaughnessy JA, Brufsky AM. RiBBON 1 and RiBBON 2: phase III trials of bevacizumab with standard chemotherapy for metastatic breast cancer. *Clin Breast Cancer.* 2008;8(4):370–373.

95. Bryant HE, Schultz N, Thomas HD, et al. Specific killing of BRCA2-deficient tumours with inhibitors of poly(ADP-ribose) polymerase. *Nature.* 2005;434(7035):913–917.

96. Farmer H, McCabe N, Lord CJ, et al. Targeting the DNA repair defect in BRCA mutant cells as a therapeutic strategy. *Nature.* 2005;434(7035):917–921.

97. Plummer R, Jones C, Middleton M, et al. Phase I study of the poly(ADP-ribose) polymerase inhibitor, AG014699, in combina-tion with temozolomide in patients with advanced solid tumors. *Clin Cancer Res.* 2008;14(23):7917–7923.

98. Tutt A, Robson M, Garber JE, et al. Phase II trial of the oral PARP inhibitor olaparib in BRCA-deficient advanced breast can-cer. *J Clin Oncol.* 2009;27(Suppl 15) (Abstract CRA501).

99. O'Shaughnessy J, Osborne C, Pippen J, Efficacy of BSI-201, a poly (ADP-ribose) polymerase-1 (PARP1) inhibitor, in combina-tion with gemcitabine/carboplatin in patients with metastatic triple-negative breast cancer: results of a randomized phase II trail. *J Clin Oncol.* 2009;27 (Suppl 15) (Abstract 3).

100. Gnant M, Mlineritsch B, Schippinger W, et al. Endocrine therapy plus zoledronic acid in premenopausal breast cancer. *New Engl J Med.* 2009;360(7):679–691.

101. Pecherstorfer M. Treatment options for breast cancer and bone metastases. *Womens Health.* 2009;5(2):149–163.

102. Coleman RE. Bisphosphonates in breast cancer. *Ann Oncol.* 2005;16(5):687–695.

103. Yamada J, Tsuno NH, Kitayama J, et al. Anti-angiogenic property of zoledronic acid by inhibition of endothelial progenitor cell dif-ferentiation. *J Surg Res.* 2009;151(1):115–120.

104. Kuehn BM. Long-term risks of bisphosphonates probed. *JAMA.* 2009;301(7):710–711.

105. Durie BG, Katz M, Crowley J. Osteonecrosis of the jaw and bisphosphonates. *New Engl J Med.* 2005;353(1):99–102; discus-sion 99.

106. Diel IJ, Bergner R, Grotz KA. Adverse effects of bisphosphonates: current issues. *J Support Oncol.* 2007;5(10):475–482.

107. Feiz-Erfan I, Rhines LD, Weinberg JS. The role of surgery in the management of metastatic spinal tumors. *Semin Oncol.* 2008;35(2):108–117.

108. Tham YL, Hinckley L, Teh BS, Elledge R. Long-term clinical response in leptomeningeal metastases from breast cancer treated with capecitabine monotherapy: a case report. *Clin Breast Cancer.* 2006;7(2):164–166.

109. Carmona-Bayonas A. Concurrent radiotherapy and capecitabine, followed by high-dose methotrexate consolidation, provided effective palliation in a patient with leptomeningeal metastases from breast cancer. *Ann Oncol.* 2007;18(1):199–200.

110. Hoe AL, Royle GT, Taylor I. Breast liver metastases—incidence, diagnosis and outcome. *J R Soc Med.* 1991;84(12):714–716.

111. Solbiati L, Ierace T, Goldberg SN, et al. Percutaneous US-guided radio-frequency tissue ablation of liver metastases: treatment and follow-up in 16 patients. *Radiology.* 1997;202(1):195–203.

112. Amersi FF, McElrath-Garza A, Ahmad A, et al. Long-term survival after radiofrequency ablation of complex unresectable liver tumors. *Arch Surg.* 2006;141(6):581–587; discussion 7–8.

113. Selzner M, Morse MA, Vredenburgh JJ, Meyers WC, Clavien PA. Liver metastases from breast cancer: long-term survival after curative resection. *Surgery.* 2000;127(4):383–389.

114. Yoshimoto M, Tada T, Saito M, Takahashi K, Uchida Y, Kasumi F. Surgical treatment of hepatic metastases from breast cancer. *Breast Cancer Res Treat.* 2000;59(2):177–184.

115. Curley SA, Izzo F, Delrio P, et al. Radiofrequency ablation of unresectable primary and metastatic hepatic malignancies: results in 123 patients. *Ann Surg.* 1999;230(1):1–8.

116. Solbiati L, Goldberg SN, Ierace T, et al. Hepatic metastases: percutaneous radio-frequency ablation with cooled-tip electrodes. *Radiology.* 1997;205(2):367–373.

117. Lawes D, Chopada A, Gillams A, Lees W, Taylor I. Radiofrequency ablation (RFA) as a cytoreductive strategy for hepatic metastasis from breast cancer. *Ann R Coll Surg Engl.* 2006;88(7):639–642.

118. Livraghi T, Solbiati L, Meloni MF, Gazelle GS, Halpern EF, Goldberg SN, eds. *Treatment of Focal Liver Tumors With Percutaneous Radio-Frequency Ablation: Complications Encountered in a Multicenter Study*; 2003.

119. Livraghi T, Solbiati L. [Percutaneous treatment: radiofrequency ablation of hepatic metastases in colorectal cancer]. *Tumori.* 2001;87(1 Suppl 1):S69.

120. Majerovic M, Augustin G, Jelincic Z, et al. Endomedullary radiofrequency ablation of metastatic lesion of the right femur 5 years after primary breast carcinoma: a case report. *Coll Antropol.* 2008;32(4):1267–1269.

121. Hazard HW, Gorla SR, Scholtens D, Kiel K, Gradishar WJ, Khan SA. Surgical resection of the primary tumor, chest wall control, and survival in women with metastatic breast cancer. *Cancer.* 2008;113(8):2011–2019.

122. Sparano JA, Moulder S, Kazi A, et al. Targeted inhibition of farnesyltransferase in locally advanced breast cancer: a phase I and II trial of tipifarnib plus dose-dense doxorubicin and cyclophosphamide. *J Clin Oncol.* 2006;24(19):3013–3018.

123. Johnston SR, Hickish T, Ellis P, et al. Phase II study of the efficacy and tolerability of two dosing regimens of the farnesyl transferase inhibitor, R115777, in advanced breast cancer. *J Clin Oncol.* 2003;21(13):2492–2499.

124. Chan S, Scheulen ME, Johnston S, et al. Phase II study of temsirolimus (CCI-779), a novel inhibitor of mTOR, in heavily pretreated patients with locally advanced or metastatic breast cancer. *J Clin Oncol.* 2005;23(23):5314–5322.

125. Ellis GK, Bone HG, Chlebowski R, et al. Randomized trial of denosumab in patients receiving adjuvant aromatase inhibitors for nonmetastatic breast cancer. *J Clin Oncol.* 2008;26(30):4875–4882.

126. Jassem J, Pienkowski T, Pluzanska A, et al. Doxorubicin and paclitaxel versus fluorouracil, doxorubicin, and cyclophosphamide as first-line therapy for women with metastatic breast cancer: final results of a randomized phase III multicenter trial. *J Clin Oncol.* 2001;19(6):1707–1715.

127. Rosner D, Nemoto T, Lane WW. Chemotherapy induces regression of brain metastases in breast carcinoma. *Cancer.* 1986;58(4):832–839.

128. Boogerd W, Dalesio O, Bais EM, van der Sande JJ. Response of brain metastases from breast cancer to systemic chemotherapy. *Cancer.* 1992;69(4):972–980.

129. Zulkowski K, Kath R, Semrau R, Merkle K, Hoffken K. Regression of brain metastases from breast carcinoma after chemotherapy with bendamustine. *J Cancer Res Clin Oncol.* 2002;128(2):111–113.

130. Wang ML, Yung WK, Royce ME, Schomer DF, Theriault RL. Capecitabine for 5-fluorouracil-resistant brain metastases from breast cancer. *Am J Clin Oncol.* 2001;24(4):421–424.

131. Siegelmann-Danieli N, Stein M, Bar-Ziv J. Complete response of brain metastases originating in breast cancer to capecitabine therapy. *Isr Med Assoc J.* 2003;5(11):833–834.

132. Rivera E, Meyers C, Groves M, et al. Phase I study of capecitabine in combination with temozolomide in the treatment of patients with brain metastases from breast carcinoma. *Cancer.* 2006;107(6):1348–1354.

133. Abrey LE, Olson JD, Raizer JJ, et al. A phase II trial of temozolomide for patients with recurrent or progressive brain metastases. *J Neurooncol.* 2001;53(3):259–265.

134. Martinez-Cedillo J AA, Lara F, et al. Temozolomide (TMZ) in metastatic breast cancer (BC) to central nervous system (CNS). *Proc Am Soc Clin Oncol.* 2003;22:88.

135. Christodoulou C, Bafaloukos D, Linardou H, et al. Temozolomide (TMZ) combined with cisplatin (CDDP) in patients with brain metastases from solid tumors: a Hellenic Cooperative Oncology Group (HeCOG) Phase II study. *J Neurooncol.* 2005;71(1):61–65.

136. Iwamoto FM, Omuro AM, Raizer JJ, et al. A phase II trial of vinorelbine and intensive temozolomide for patients with recurrent or progressive brain metastases. *J Neurooncol.* 2008;87(1):85–90.

137. Antonadou D, Paraskevaidis M, Sarris G, et al. Phase II randomized trial of temozolomide and concurrent radiotherapy in patients with brain metastases. *J Clin Oncol.* 2002;20(17):3644–3650.

138. Mir O, Ropert S, Alexandre J, Lemare F, Goldwasser F. High-dose intrathecal trastuzumab for leptomeningeal metastases secondary to HER-2 overexpressing breast cancer. *Ann Oncol.* 2008;19(11):1978–1980.

139. Pors H, von Eyben FE, Sorensen OS, Larsen M. Longterm remission of multiple brain metastases with tamoxifen. *J Neurooncol.* 1991;10(2):173–177.

140. Salvati M, Cervoni L, Innocenzi G, Bardella L. Prolonged stabilization of multiple and single brain metastases from breast cancer with tamoxifen. Report of three cases. *Tumori.* 1993;79(5):359–362.

141. Boogerd W, Dorresteijn LD, van Der Sande JJ, de Gast GC, Bruning PF. Response of leptomeningeal metastases from breast cancer to hormonal therapy. *Neurology.* 2000;55(1):117–119.

142. Goyal S, Puri T, Julka PK, Rath GK. Excellent response to letrozole in brain metastases from breast cancer. *Acta Neurochir.* 2008;150(6):613–614; discussion 4–5.

143. Stewart DJ, Dahrouge S. Response of brain metastases from breast cancer to megestrol acetate: a case report. *J Neurooncol.* 1995;24(3):299–301.

144. Icli F, Akbulut H, Uner A, et al. Cisplatin plus oral etoposide (EoP) combination is more effective than paclitaxel in patients with advanced breast cancer pretreated with anthracyclines : a randomised phase III trial of Turkish Oncology Group. *Br J Cancer.* 2005;92(4);639–644.

Palliative Care for Metastatic Disease

MARYBETH SINGER

CATHERINE FURLANI

The advent of better treatment has shifted the paradigm of advanced breast cancer from a terminal diagnosis to a chronic life-limiting disease. While some patients live many years with advanced breast cancer, the median survival for patients with metastatic breast cancer is 2 to 3 years (1,2). While the focus of care is on controlling the disease and associated symptoms, optimizing the patient's functional status and quality of life is paramount. In this chapter we will discuss the challenges of integrating a palliative perspective of care into the support of patients and their families as they cope with advanced breast cancer. The role of the interdisciplinary team in achieving optimal care will be detailed. Timing and discussion of goals of care, advanced care planning, and shifting goals of treatment require open communication between clinicians, patients, and their families. Attention to preventing and treating symptoms associated with advancing disease and end of life are critical to the primary goal of alleviating suffering. It takes a team of dedicated clinicians to provide comprehensive palliative care. Oncology clinicians caring for patients with advanced breast cancer must possess basic palliative care skills and knowledge. Quite simply, it is a necessary component of good medical practice.

■ OVERVIEW OF PALLIATIVE CARE

Brief Historical Perspective

The origins of early hospice or end-of-life care can be traced to the Middle Ages and use of monastic hospices as places to find care and comfort for pilgrims seeking respite, cures, and care at religious sites (3). Modern-day hospice and palliative care is credited to the life's work of Dame Cicely Saunders. She began her work as a nurse and sought training as a social worker and then physician. Her work in the care of terminally ill cancer patients led her to establish, with her colleagues, the first modern hospice, St. Christopher's Hospice in London, in 1967 (4). Over the past 40 years, end-of-life care has become increasingly recognized as a neglected aspect of care. With support from such endeavors as the Robert Wood Johnson's Foundation Last Acts organization and the Open Society's Project on Death in America, modern healthcare has begun to recognize the need to integrate palliative care into the mainstream delivery of care (3–5). Specialty organizations such as the American Medical Association (AMA), the Institute of Medicine (IOM), the American Society of Clinical Oncology (ASCO), the Oncology Nursing Society (ONS), the Hospice and Palliative Nurses Association (HPNA), and the American Academy of Hospice and Palliative Medicine (AAHPM) have worked to increase awareness among and education of healthcare providers. The Center to Advance Palliative Care (CAPC) has provided tangible tools and assistance with access to centers of excellence for mentoring organizations striving to develop palliative care programs (www.capc.org). Hospice and palliative medicine was recognized as a medical specialty in 2006 by the American Board of Specialty Medicine (ABSM). Specialty certification is available for nurses at the generalist and advanced-practice levels through the National Board for Certification in Hospice and Palliative Care Nursing (www.nbchpn.org), and since 2008, physicians have been able to obtain ABSM certification in hospice and palliative medicine (6).

Disease Trajectory in Advanced Breast Cancer

Many patients with advanced breast cancer are living full and active lives despite numerous symptoms and treatment (7). Patients and their families cope with the chronic nature of the disease and incorporate the rigors into their day-to-day life. The disease trajectory is one that can be characterized by periods of relative stability, with progressive decline over the last 8 to 12 weeks of life (8). As a result, advanced breast cancer is often characterized by a pattern of recurrent chronic treatment. The chronic need for medical treatment and the ongoing assessment and treatment of symptoms relating to disease or complications present repeated opportunities for discussion with the healthcare team about goals of care. When everything "appears" to be stable, both patients and providers often avoid having discussions about goals of care. Many patients seek reassurance about what the next treatment plan may be without considering discussions regarding shifting goals of care. Active palliative care recognizes the need for continued effective disease treatment while maximizing symptom control and quality of life. Opportunities for discussion about decision making regarding end-of-life care exist but are often delayed until a crisis occurs. Palliative care can be integrated into cancer treatment from diagnosis along the entire disease trajectory. Palliative care is not just care directed at the end of life; it also involves incorporating attention to symptoms, function, and psychosocial and spiritual care throughout the treatment of this chronic, life-limiting illness.

Palliative Care and Hospice Care

The World Health Organization (WHO) defines palliative care as care that is directed toward improving the quality of life of patients and families who face life-threatening illness by providing pain and symptom relief and spiritual and psychosocial support from diagnosis to the end of life and bereavement (9). It is appropriate to apply the principles of palliative care along the entire disease continuum. This does not reflect a dichotomous belief of cure or care (10); rather, it integrates excellence in symptom control regardless of treatment goals. Hospice care, largely defined by the Medicare benefit, applies the need for a defined prognosis of 6 months and has been limited by the need to forgo life-extending therapy. Hospice referrals are often made late in the disease process, and in 37% of cases, death occurs within 1 week of enrollment (11).

Interdisciplinary Team

Although all healthcare providers should have basic knowledge of palliative care, unfortunately, this is not always the case. Access to palliative care specialists can help to bridge this gap in care, though frequently they are underutilized or consulted late in the treatment course (11).

Figure 10.3 illustrates conceptually an integrated vision of how palliative care crosses all spheres of care along the disease continuum of advanced breast cancer. One could state that it is a central component to care along the disease continuum. Screening for palliative care needs as outlined by National Comprehensive Cancer Network (NCCN) guidelines includes (a) uncontrolled symptoms, (b) moderate or severe distress related to cancer diagnosis and treatment, (c) severe comorbid illness, (d) life expectancy of less than 12 months, (e) patient's or family's concerns about course of disease or decision making, and (f) patient's or family's request for a palliative care consult (12).

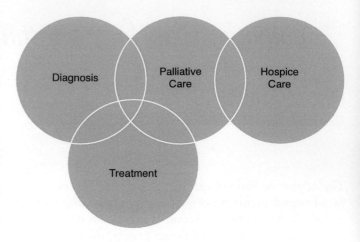

FIGURE 10.3 Palliative care along advanced breast cancer disease trajectory.

Care for patients with advanced breast cancer requires a coordinated team approach, led by the medical oncologist. Medical oncologists should have basic knowledge of palliative care. They work closely with their nursing colleagues, both advanced-practice nurses (nurse practitioners and clinical nurse specialists) and staff nurses, to provide for the care of patients with metastatic breast cancer and their families. Because of the myriad complications from metastatic disease that can require intervention for symptom control and improved functional status, referrals to interventional radiology, orthopedics, radiation oncology, rehabilitation specialists, and surgical oncology may be necessary. Palliative care and pain specialists should be available for consultation. In addition, advanced-practice nurses and both inpatient and outpatient nursing staff are integral to the assessment and management of disease-related symptoms, patient and family education, and coordination of care. Medical social workers and mental health clinicians can provide much needed support for psychosocial concerns, as well as financial

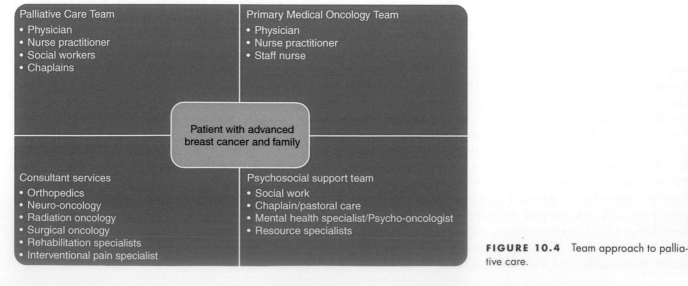

FIGURE 10.4 Team approach to palliative care.

and community support. Rehabilitation specialists such as physical therapists and occupational therapists can be pivotal in supporting patients' strength and function. For many patients and their families access to pastoral care or chaplains is critical to coping with the challenges posed by ever-changing disease. Figure 10.4 illustrates a conceptual model of interdisciplinary palliative care.

■ PSYCHOSOCIAL AND SPIRITUAL NEEDS OF PATIENTS AND THEIR FAMILIES DURING ADVANCED DISEASE

Developmental Stages and Impact of Living With Advanced Breast Cancer

The impact of breast cancer on the family depends on the developmental stage of the family and individual. As mentioned earlier, advanced breast cancer presents a chronicity of illness that requires some aspect of life-long treatment. With novel therapies and individualized treatment contributing to current 10-year survival of 27%, most patients eventually will die of their disease (13). It is not uncommon for patients to receive on average four different regimens for the treatment of metastatic breast cancer, and many may receive up to 10 regimes (14). As a result, when there are limited or no further active treatment options, the transition to end-of-life care can become extremely difficult for both the patient and the family to grasp. Erikson's developmental stages/psychosocial crises (15) can be used to appreciate the impact of metastatic breast cancer and impending death on both the individual and the family. Kemp (15) suggested that regardless of the patient's age or developmental stage, it is Erikson's last stage—integrity versus despair—that is applicable to terminal-stage illness (Table 10.5).

Chronic Versus Terminal Disease Model of Care

Despite a patient having lived with advanced breast cancer, the terminal phase of illness often feels like a "shock" to the patient and family. With successful treatment, both symptoms and quality of life are maintained or optimized

■ Table 10.5 Erikson's adult stages of development

Stage/Age (yrs)	Psychosocial Crises
Late adolescence (18–22)	Individual identity versus role diffusion
Young adult (23–30)	Intimacy versus isolation
Middle adult (31–50)	Generativity versus stagnation
Later adult (50 to death)	Integrity versus despair

for so long that the last phase of illness is typically weeks to 2 to 3 months. As a result, patients and their families can feel unprepared for the sudden change in events. The clinicians involved in caring for patients are charged with the delicate balance of providing realistic hope. A recent study using focus-group methodology to evaluate dying patients' and their families' need for emotional support and personalized care from physicians found that it was critical to "leave on a positive note, even though something dreadful was happening" (16). The delicate balancing of realistic hope and honest communication is a skill that is at the heart of care for patients and their families during the crisis of terminal-phase disease.

In caring for women with breast cancer, it is important for clinicians to have an accurate assessment of the multiple roles within their families that patients may serve. These include but are not limited to mother, daughter, sister, and friend. For mothers, the concern is always for the well-being of the children, with the caveat that age is critical to planning for the future. Single mothers are particularly vulnerable to crises if there has not been open discussion about prognosis, advanced-care planning, and custody of minor children. Consultation with social workers, family specialists, and resource specialists is critical to preparing both patient and family for the future. Is the middle-aged woman with breast cancer also the primary caregiver of aging parents as well as teenage children or young adults? Lack of attention to these sometimes hidden stressors can be at the heart of poorly controlled symptoms, both physical and psychological.

Impact of Culture

Family kinship, resources, and culture play an important role in communication and planning of care. The medical oncology team has often had an opportunity over many months to years to develop relationships with patient and family. Ongoing assessment of cultural norms for the patient and family is important during all phases of the clinician's relationship with patient and family. It is critical during discussion of bad news and transitioning from active treatment to end of life care. The family system and its coping style and function will influence the types of resources and supports available. Helping family and friends to organize help at home is crucial to day-to-day living in the last weeks and months of life. The primary caregiver for women with breast cancer may be a spouse, mother, sister, daughter, other family member, or friend. In a study of patients' and families' need for emotional support during terminal illness, several components of emotional support were identified using focus group methodology with over 130 subjects (16). Emotional support components identified were compassion, responsiveness to emotional needs, maintaining hope and a positive attitude, and providing comfort through touch (16). The concept of personalization was defined by patients as treating the whole person not the disease, making the patient feel unique and special, and considering the patient's social situation.

Existential and Spiritual Distress

The concept of hope and realistic guidance for patients and their families becomes a very difficult "gray zone" for many clinicians. It is the delicate balance of hope for effective treatment and quality of life along with planning for the uncertainty of the future. It involves planning for the "what ifs?": What if the latest treatment doesn't have the desired effect? What if the cancer no longer responds to treatment? Honest dialogue about the uncertainties of illness requires sensitivity, compassion, and support for patients, families, and clinicians alike. Nurses provide the backbone of care for patients both within institutions and at home. It is critical for nurses to assess values and assumptions that may impact care. Nursing is charged with providing competent care in managing symptoms, preparing and teaching family members for their role in providing care, and supporting patients and their families through the process of impending death and grief (17). Byock has suggested that there are five tasks needing completion at the end of life for patients and families (18): Forgive me; I forgive you; Thank you; I love you; Goodbye (18). Spiritual distress faced by patients and families often is grounded in trying to understand and find meaning in their circumstances. Values, religious beliefs, past losses, and coping with those losses contribute to the ability of the patient and family to cope with current realities. The patient's and family's experience with loss and suffering impacts how they will cope with a life-threatening illness within the family (17). An integrated team approach to caring for the patient with metastatic breast cancer can help make this difficult and sad time more bearable for families.

■ COMMUNICATION WITH PATIENTS AND FAMILIES

Breaking Bad News

Open communication and ongoing discussion with patients and families is critical to facilitate coping with the changes as they evolve over time, yet the language used, the environment, and the personal support offered during the interaction can have dramatic effects on the patient and family. The ability to balance hope and information regarding prognosis requires knowledge of the patient's and family's needs. Information desires may change over the course of illness and vary from the individual's and the family's perspective (19). Knowing the patient and taking cues from the patient and family involves development of an empathic relationship built on active listening and constantly checking in with them about their desires for how information is shared and with whom information is shared. Poor communication can become a major obstacle in providing comprehensive, compassionate care. One of the most useful protocols for breaking bad news is the SPIKES protocol (20). How bad news is communicated has implications for how patients understand information, their satisfaction with care, and their hopefulness and coping (Table 10.6) (2).

It should be emphasized that communication is a continuous process. Within an interdisciplinary team, communication among team members is crucial to patient and family communication. Using clear communication in documentation can assist greatly in helping the team to be consistent when defining goals of care. When there is conflict or miscommunication, particularly around truth telling or do not resuscitate orders, consultation with the institutional ethics committee can be very helpful. In fact, end-of-life issues are the most frequent reason for ethics committee consultation (3).

Advance Care Planning

Advance care planning for patients with advanced breast cancer should include more than just discussion of advance directives. Opportunities to discuss advance care planning exist throughout treatment. Discussion of patients' wishes, their values, and their beliefs is an essential component of care. Because of the taboo associated with death and dying in our culture, frank discussions surrounding death and the tasks associated with decision making are too often avoided until they become the elephant in the room. As a result, these discussions often are left until a medical crisis occurs. Many clinicians find it helpful to take their cues from patients. When a patient or family member opens the door for such discussions, it is important for clinicians to be able to listen and give guidance based on realistic assessment of the patient's current status. The NCCN offers objective prognostic criteria to help assist clinicians (Table 10.7).

Family Meetings

For many patients with advanced breast cancer, the chronicity of their illness may have limited the clinician's exposure to family as a result of the general overall health and function of the patient. As the disease progresses and symptoms and function are affected, the need for active caregiving from family and friends may increase. Planning with patients to have a meeting to which they can invite family to discuss disease progression and end-of-life care can assist patients and their families with clarifying information, establishing realistic goals of care, and planning for care as the patient declines. The medical social worker

■ **Table 10.6** SPIKES protocol for delivering bad news	
Setting up the interview	Ensure privacy
	Have the patient choose who should be there
	Sit down; have the patient dress if you have recently examined her
	Manage any time constraints
	Silence beepers
Assessing patient's Perception	Ask the patient what she understands about current situation/why a test was done, how she thinks treatment has been going
	Correct any misinformation/misunderstanding
Obtaining the patient's Invitation	Prior to ordering tests, ask how the patient would like to receive information, how detailed; would she like brief information with more time for treatment discussion?
	Offer to answer any questions or give more detail at later date, or perhaps patient would like you to discuss with a family member or friend
Giving Knowledge and information to the patient	Give a warning that the news is not what you expected
	Give information in clear, non–medical jargon terms
	Avoid undue bluntness; give information in pieces that can be digested, and check understanding
	Focus on what can be done (i.e., symptom control)
Addressing emotions with Empathic responses	Responses can be variable and difficult
	Observe response, identify emotion and reason for emotion, be comfortable with silence and ask patient after time what she is thinking; respond with empathy
Strategy and summary	Discussion of goals of care, and what will happen next
	Focus on care, nonabandonment
	Time to think and revisit issues later in day or next day depending on status (e.g., for a hospitalized patient making end-of-life decisions, offer to give patient and family some time alone to discuss with clear plan of when to return)
	Focus on patient's hopes and goals

Source: Adapted from Ref. 20.

■ **Table 10.7** Evaluation of life expectancy
Potential Indicators of Life Expectancy <12 months
Eastern Cooperative Oncology Group performance status ≥3 or Karnofsky performance score ≤50
Hypercalcemia
Brain or cerebrospinal fluid metastases
Delirium
Spinal cord compression
Superior vena cava syndrome
Cachexia
Malignant effusions
Bilirubin ≥2.5 mg/dL
Creatinine ≥3.0 mg/dL

Source: Adapted from Ref. 12.

can be instrumental in planning the meeting and facilitating the discussion with both nursing and medical providers. The SPIKES protocol mentioned earlier can offer some guidance on how to utilize an effective communication strategy for family meetings (20).

Both nursing and social work need to assess family caregivers for their ability to manage complex medical tasks in the setting of coping with the emotional and psychological stressors of care (21). Case managers offer invaluable information about home care resources and hospice and palliative care programs within the community that can serve to bolster family caregivers. In the last weeks of life, caregiving demands may be exhausting. Helping families to create realistic goals and planning support and resources are crucial to providing the best possible situation for a difficult transition from life to death. Under the best of circumstances, it is difficult for families. In the case of intractable symptoms or inability of family to continue care at home, inpatient hospice or hospital admission may be an alternative. Financial burdens owing to caregiving can be variable, with younger caregivers at higher risk for financial hardship (22).

■ SYMPTOM MANAGEMENT

Evidence-based Approaches

Evidence-based symptom management is presented in numerous guidelines that can be found on readily accessible websites. It behooves clinicians working with patients with advanced cancer to become familiar with commonly occurring symptoms and treatment strategies. Treatment of reversible causes of pain, nausea, delirium, dyspnea, and so on is always indicated when death is not imminent. For patients with advanced breast cancer effective treatment can often palliate symptoms effectively for some time. Patients with bone metastases benefit from use of focal radiotherapy, effective systemic treatment, and chronic use of analgesics. The advent of bisphosphonates has greatly improved the control of pain due to bone metastases for women with breast cancer (11,12). Complications that commonly occur in patients with metastatic breast cancer and their associated symptoms are listed in Table 10.8. Resources for evidence-based practice guidelines and treatment algorithms appear in the last column of the table.

Symptom Clusters

The emergence of interest in symptom clusters has stimulated interest in evaluating how symptoms might be interrelated in specific cancers and how they may change over time. Difficulty in methodology and the need to validate

■ Table 10.8 Selected metastatic sites and associated symptoms			
Metastatic Site	**Symptom**	**Consultant/Palliative Procedures**	**Treatment Resources**
Bone	Pain Impaired mobility Risk of pathologic fracture Risk of spinal cord compression Risk of hypercalcemia Insomnia Risk of bone marrow infiltration → pancytopenia Nausea and vomiting Constipation Fatigue	Radiation oncologist → palliative radiation therapy Orthopedic consult for fracture or risk of fracture Pain and palliative care consult if symptoms are not controlled Systemic anticancer therapy if appropriate Rehab consult → physical therapy Bisphosphonates	Opioid and nonsteroidal as indicated using established clinical practice guidelines National Comprehensive Cancer Network Pain Guidelines National Comprehensive Cancer Network Palliative Care Guidelines for symptom management algorithms Oncology Nursing Society "Putting Evidence Into Practice" cards for specific symptoms Home care/hospice, per patient preferences
Pleural effusions Lymphagitic pulmonary metastases	Dyspnea Breathlessness Air hunger Pain Cough Impaired functional status Fatigue Anxiety/agitation	Therapeutic thoracenteses CT surgery consult for pleurodesis if appropriate Anticancer therapy as appropriate	National Comprehensive Cancer Network Palliative Care Guidelines for treatment algorithms Fan Oxygen, if subjectively better Opioids to control dyspnea Antitussives Oncology Nursing Society "Putting Evidence Into Practice" cards Home care services as above
Abdominal carcinomatosis	Nausea and vomiting Constipation Diarrhea Bloating Pain Cachexia Anorexia Weakness Fatigue	Paracentesis if ascites present Nutritional consult for conservative measures Surgical consult if indicated to relief obstruction	National Comprehensive Cancer Network Palliative Care Guidelines Oncology Nursing Society "Putting Evidence Into Practice" cards End of Life/Palliative Education Resource Center Fast Facts Home care services as above
Leptomeningeal disease/CNS disease	Headaches Nausea and vomiting Confusion Memory/cognitive dysfunction Weakness Fatigue	Radiation oncology Neurosurgery/neuro-oncology consults Physical therapy/occupational therapy Home care services	National Comprehensive Cancer Network Palliative Care Symptom algorithms Attention to acute and poorly controlled symptoms at end of life (i.e., delirium/agitation) Caregiver strain Home care services as above

■ **Table 10.9** Resources
Center to Advance Care: www.capc.org
Growth House: www.growthhouse.org
EPERC (End of Life/Palliative Education Resource Center): www.eperc.mcw.edu
National Comprehensive Cancer Network, Palliative and Supportive Care Guidelines: www.nccn.org
Oncology Nursing Society, Putting Evidence Into Practice resources: www.ons.org

observations regarding symptom clusters limits their use in clinical care (23–25). That said, it has long been observed that patients with advanced cancer often experience numerous symptoms simultaneously with varying levels of intensity. Use of symptom inventories to adequately assess the presence and intensity of certain commonly occurring symptoms is strongly recommended in order to address the symptoms affecting patients' quality of life. Symptom distress and inability to manage those symptoms in the home are a major source of caregiver distress (21). Additional Internet resources are listed in Table 10.9.

Last Weeks of Life

The last weeks of life for patients with advanced breast cancer are marked by rapidly declining functional status as a result of disease progression. Common sites of disease include bone, liver, lung, and central nervous system. Exquisite attention to symptom management can maximize comfort, allow for time with family and friends, and avoid hospitalization. Hospice care is ideally suited to provide for the holistic care of the patient and family during this time. While early referral to a hospice can provide continuity and relationship building, very often referrals happen in the last weeks to days of life. In a study evaluating hospice utilization in the United States, the average length of time in hospice was 23 days in 2003, with death occurring for 37% of patients within 1 week of enrollment (26). A recent review of determinants of place of end-of-life care for patients with advanced cancer revealed several factors that influence place of death (27). Patients in this review were more apt to die at home if they had less complex care needs, higher functional status, past experiences with death, perceived good quality of life, multidisciplinary team support and visits, home care support, and a caregiver or spouse living with them (27).

Case Vignette

Ms. Y presented with stage IIA left breast cancer at age 38 in 1987. She underwent left modified radical mastectomy and three cycles of standard cyclophosphamide, methotrexate, and 5-fluorouracil (CMF), stopped owing to difficulty with intractable nausea. She subsequently presented with solitary metastasis at T4–5 two years later.

She underwent radiotherapy followed by anthracycline-based chemotherapy, followed by tamoxifen and bilateral salpingo-oophorectomy. She had quiescent disease until 2002 (13-year interval), when she was noted to have a new right adrenal mass and numerous new sclerotic bone metastases. Her endocrine therapy was changed to letrozole, with improvement in adrenal mass and stable bone disease until late 2004, when she was noted to have an increasing adrenal mass and retroperitoneal adenopathy. She began weekly docetaxel treatment with stable disease. She had evidence of progression 6 months later and began capecitabine for the next 13 months, with good improvement and tolerability. At best response, she underwent intensity-modulated radiation therapy to the right adrenal mass and began exemestane. Six months later, she presented with bone pain at left midfemur requiring palliative radiation. She began vinorelbine and continued on it for 5 months. She was switched to toremifene in an effort to maintain response with an effective endocrine therapy approach. Unfortunately, 5 months later, she presented with headaches, nausea, and weight loss and was found to have a large cerebellar mass. She underwent craniotomy for resection and completed whole brain radiation. In addition, at the time of staging, she had extensive hepatic metastases. She had a rapid decline in functional status over the next several months and elected to enroll in hospice care. She had a peaceful death at home with her family, cared for by home hospice, family, and friends. She had, over the course of her illness, been able to pursue graduate studies, obtaining a master's degree, and had become active in local politics and advocacy programs. She was beloved by family, friends, and caregivers. She had expert care from a team led by her medical oncologist and nurse practitioner. Her hospice team at home was outstanding and provided necessary attention to symptoms.

■ CONCLUSIONS

Oncology clinicians from the interdisciplinary team make major contributions to caring for patients with advanced breast cancer as they approach the end of life. Good communication, evidence-based symptom management, and exquisite compassion and care can help patients and their families cope with this end-of-life transition.

■ SUMMARY

To provide exceptional palliative care requires

- Honest and respectful communication among team members and with patients and family
- Exquisite attention to symptom management

- Individualized care that supports the whole person, with attention to physical, developmental, psychosocial, and spiritual needs of the patient and family

■ REFERENCES

1. Giordano SH, Budzar AU, Smith TL, Kau SW, Yang Y, Hortobagyi GN. Is breast cancer survival improving? *Cancer.* 2004;100: 44–52.

2. Greenberg PA, Hortobagyi GN, Smith TL, Ziegler LD, Frye DK, Budzar AU. Long term follow-up of patients with complete remission following combination chemotherapy for metastatic breast cancer. *J Clin Oncol.* 1996;14(8):2197–2205.

3. Fins JJ. *Palliative Ethic of Care.* Boston: Jones and Bartlett; 2006.

4. Clark D. From margins to centre: a review of the history of palliative care in cancer. *Lancet Oncol.* 2007;8:430–438.

5. National Consensus Project. Clinical Practice Guidelines for Quality Palliative Care. Pittsburgh, PA: National Consensus Project; 2004. Available at www.nationalconsensusproject.org.

6. American Academy of Hospice and Palliative Medicine. 2008 ABMS statement on specialty certification in palliative medicine. Available at www.aahpm.org.

7. Santos-Madeya S, Bauer-Wu S, Gross A. Activities of daily living in women with advanced breast cancer. *Oncol Nurs Forum.* 2007;34(4):841–846.

8. Dy S, Lynn J. Getting services right for those sick enough to die. *Br Med J.* 2007;334:551–513.

9. World Health Organization. Palliative care definition. Available at www.who.int/cancer/palliative/en.

10. Krammer LM, Martinez J, Ring EA, Williams MB, Jacobs MJ. The nurse's role as a member of the interdisciplinary palliative care team. In: Matzo ML, Sherman DW, eds. *Palliative Care Nursing.* 2nd ed. New York: Springer; 2006:133.

11. Brunnhuber K, Nash S, Meier D, Weissman D, Woodcock J. Putting evidence into practice: palliative care spring 2008. A report commissioned by the United Health Foundation, published by BMJ Group.

12. NCCN Clinical Practice Guidelines: Palliative Care. Available at www.nccn.org.

13. Mahon S, Palmieri F. Metastatic breast cancer: the individualization of therapy. *Clin J Oncol Nurs.* 2009;13(1):S19–S28.

14. Seidman AD. Systemic treatment of breast cancer: two decades of progress. *Oncology.* 2006;20:983–990.

15. Kemp C. *Terminal Illness.* Philadelphia: JB Lippincott; 1995.

16. Wenrich MD, Curtis JR, Ambrozy DA, Carline JD, Shannon SE, Ramsey PG. Dying patients need for emotional support and personalized care from physicians: perspectives of patients with terminal illness, families and health care providers. *J Pain Sympt Manag.* 2003;25(3):236–246.

17. Goetschius SK, Matzo ML. Caring for families: the other patient in palliative care. In: Matzo ML, Sherman DW, eds. *Palliative Care Nursing.* 2nd ed. New York: Springer; 2006:247–272.

18. Byock I. *Dying Well: The Prospects for Growth at the End of Life.* New York: Riverhead; 1997.

19. Curtis JR, Engelberg R, Young J, et al. An approach to understanding the interaction of hope and desire for explicit prognostic information among individuals with severe obstructive pulmonary disease or advanced cancer. *J Pall Med.* 2008;11(4):610–620.

20. Baile WF, Buckman R, Lenzl R, Glober G, Beale EL, Kudelka AF. SPIKES—a six step protocol for delivering bad news: application to the patient with cancer. *Oncologist.* 2000;5:302–311.

21. Given B, Sherwood PR, Given CW. What knowledge and skills do caregivers need? *Am J Nursing.* 2008;108(9):28–34.

22. Moore CD. Caregiver issues. In: Esper P, Kuebler KK, eds., *Palliative Practices From A–Z for the Bedside Clinician.* 2nd ed. Pittsburgh: ONS; 2008:55.

23. Fan G, Hadi S, Chow E. Symptom clusters in patients with advanced stage cancer referred for palliative radiation therapy in an outpatient setting. *Support Cancer Ther.* 2007;4(3):157–162.

24. Hadi S, Zhang L, Hird A, daSa Z, Chow E. Validation of symptom clusters in patients with metastatic bone pain. *Curr Oncol.* 2008; 15(5):211–218.

25. Barsevick AM. The elusive concept of symptom cluster. *Oncol Nurs Forum.* 2007;34(5):971–988.

26. Plonk WM, Arnold RM. Terminal care in the last weeks of life. *J Pall Med.* 2005;8:1042–1054.

27. Murray MA, Fiset V, Young S, Kryworuchko J. Where the dying live: a systematic review of determinants of place of end of life cancer care. *Oncol Nurs Forum.* 2009;36(1):69–77.

II Multidisciplinary Approach in the Management of Locally Recurrent Disease

Surgical and Radiation Management of Locally Recurrent Disease

LAURIE KIRSTEIN

MOHAMED A. ALM EL-DIN

ALPHONSE G. TAGHIAN

Multiple studies (1–10) have shown survival equivalence for stage 1 and 2 breast cancer treated with mastectomy or breast-conserving therapy (BCT), which is defined as lumpectomy followed by whole breast irradiation. This knowledge has changed the local treatment for breast cancer from radical surgery to a more conservative approach. While there does not appear to be a survival difference between these treatment strategies, there is a difference in locoregional recurrence with respect to overall rate, time to recurrence, and detection of recurrence. Traditionally, there have been few options available to treat locally recurrent breast cancer. But in the past few years, novel strategies have been developed that are once again challenging the status quo.

The current guidelines from the National Comprehensive Cancer Network (NCCN) recommend a mammogram every 6 months and clinical breast examination every 3 months for the first 2 years following a breast cancer and mammograms once a year with clinical breast examination twice a year for the following 3 years (11). This ensures close follow-up and early detection of recurrence. The rate of 10-year postmastectomy locoregional recurrence has been shown to be 5% to 10% (4,6,7,12–15), compared with 10% to 15% after BCT (3,16–18). The median time to recurrence after mastectomy is 2 to 3 years, whereas, after BCT, recurrences appear after a median of 3 to 4 years (7,19–22) or even longer (5 to 7 years) with the use of adjuvant tamoxifen or chemotherapy or both (23,24). Recurrence after mastectomy usually reflects true recurrent disease, whereas reappearance of disease in an ipsilateral preserved breast can represent either a local recurrence of the initial cancer or a second primary tumor. Finally, the recurrences after mastectomy are usually diagnosed by physical examination, whereas many ipsilateral breast tumor recurrences (IBTRs) after BCT are typically detected by mammography. This reinforces the need to comply with NCCN guidelines in the follow-up of the breast cancer patient, which recommend both mammogram and clinical breast examination.

It is important to distinguish between a true recurrence, which is usually located within the primary tumor site or the boost volume of the treated breast, and a new primary. This can sometimes be accomplished with a pathological comparison between the primary tumor and the new disease, but not always. Locally recurrent beast cancer after BCT may be either invasive or in situ, irrespective of pathology of the primary tumor. For those patients initially treated for in situ carcinoma, approximately one half will recur with invasive disease (25), whereas among patients initially treated for a primary invasive cancer, more than 80% of locoregional recurrences are also invasive.

In addition, while some patients may present with an isolated local recurrence, others may have concurrent distant metastasis. The majority (75%) of recurrences in patients with primary invasive disease are isolated to the breast, whereas 5% to 15% present with a simultaneous regional nodal recurrence, and another 5% to 15% have distant metastases at diagnosis (7,22,26–29). While the local recurrence in and of itself is easily treated, it is viewed as a harbinger of things to come, namely, distant metastases. Data supporting this hypothesis have shown that differences in local treatment that substantially affect the rates of locoregional recurrence would avoid one cancer death over 15 years for every four recurrences avoided and consequently should reduce the 15-year mortality (30). It is this association with distant metastases, diagnosed either concurrently or at a later date, that accounts for the decrease in overall survival associated with local recurrence (31). It is important to distinguish between these two groups of patients because management of the isolated recurrence begins with surgery, whereas patients with stage 4 distant disease should be referred to a medical oncologist for systemic treatment. Therefore, the first step in evaluating a patient with local recurrence should be to rule out distant disease with staging studies, consisting of a computed tomography scan of the chest, abdomen, and pelvis and a bone scan.

The management of patients at the time of recurrence is complex because several factors are considered. These include the type of primary surgery, receptor status of the tumor, adjuvant treatment of the primary tumor, age of the patient, and mutation carrier status. With the introduction of novel treatment strategies such as targeted therapies and recent radiation techniques, patients with local recurrence need to be managed by a multidisciplinary team consisting of surgical, medical, and radiation oncologists because the treatment plan for each patient needs to be individualized. The guiding surgical principle in all cases, however, is to achieve clear margins, thereby reducing the risk of future recurrence.

Finally, in this chapter, breast conservation and mastectomy will be discussed as the two surgical options currently available to manage a local breast cancer recurrence. It is generally recommended that a patient undergoing mastectomy be referred to a plastic surgeon to discuss reconstructive options, as is done for a patient with a primary breast cancer who is undergoing mastectomy. While this recommendation will not be mentioned in each section in the chapter, it should be an integral part of the multidisciplinary discussion and treatment plan for this population. There are patients for whom immediate reconstruction is not appropriate, but this should be decided by consultation among a group of surgical, medical, and radiation oncologists with input from a plastic surgeon.

■ LOCAL RECURRENCE IN THE PREVIOUSLY NONIRRADIATED BREAST

For those patients whose primary breast cancer was surgically treated with a local excision, without adjuvant radiation, there are a variety of options available to manage a local recurrence. The options for surgical management of recurrence in this group of patients are exactly the same as in managing a primary breast cancer. When choosing between a lumpectomy and mastectomy, it is important to consider both oncologic and cosmetic factors. Just as with a primary breast cancer, one must consider multicentric disease and the ability to obtain clear margins as factors in the surgical outcome.

If the patient desires another attempt at breast conservation, it is important to determine whether another lumpectomy will leave a cosmetically acceptable result, taking into consideration the size of the recurrence compared with the size of the breast. In some cases, oncoplastic reconstructive techniques will need to be employed to achieve this end.

Adjuvant treatment in the management of recurrence in this patient population should be similar to that for primary breast cancer. Generally, the patient should receive postoperative radiation following lumpectomy, while the results of surgical pathology will define those patients who would benefit from postmastectomy radiation. In addition, adjuvant systemic or hormone therapy, or both, should be employed as appropriate, taking into account the prior exposure, if any, to cardiotoxic drugs.

■ LOCAL RECURRENCE IN THE PREVIOUSLY IRRADIATED BREAST

Surgical Treatment

Mastectomy remains the standard of care for IBTR following BCT. The risk of chest wall recurrence after mastectomy for IBTR depends on the type of recurrence (invasive or noninvasive) (29,32). At a median follow-up of 39 months, Abner and colleagues reported no chest wall recurrences observed in patients with noninvasive or focally invasive recurrent tumors treated by mastectomy (29). For invasive recurrences, rates of chest wall recurrence after salvage mastectomy for IBTR from several large series varied between 2% and 32% (33), strongly suggesting that mastectomy after IBTR does not necessarily eliminate the risk of subsequent secondary local recurrences at the chest wall. It should be noted that initial treatment of primary breast cancer with lumpectomy and radiation was shown to be a determinant factor with regards to the risk of chest wall recurrence following salvage mastectomy, with those who received adjuvant radiation shown to be at a lower risk.

The patient's acceptance of mastectomy as a treatment decision should be considered. Some women are reluctant or refuse to undergo mastectomy. The appropriate treatment in this scenario is not known. The available treatment options would be the following: lumpectomy alone, lumpectomy with whole breast irradiation, or lumpectomy with partial breast irradiation.

Data regarding the outcome of patients treated with conservative surgery alone for IBTR are rare. The local failure rate after breast-conserving surgery alone for IBTR varied between 19% and 50% (22,29,34–36). It should be noted that in the series by Voogd and colleagues, the local recurrence rate after local excision was not found to be significantly different from that reported after mastectomy (38% versus 25%, respectively; $P = 0.27$) (34).

Kurtz and colleagues demonstrated that 5-year local control rates were higher in patients who had negative margins of resection compared with patients with positive margins of resection (73% vs 36%, respectively) and were higher in patients with a local recurrence occurring after 5 years than in patients with shorter intervals to recurrence (92% versus 49%, respectively) (35).

It is difficulty to interpret the abovementioned studies because numerous patients were treated before modern-day standard mammography and sonography were available to rule out diffuse tumors or multicentricity and to select appropriate patients for whom breast-conserving approaches are reasonable options.

Regarding survival, investigators at the European Institute of Oncology in Milan, Italy, at a median follow-up of 73 months after the second surgery, found a 5-year overall survival rate of 70% in the 134 patients who had undergone a mastectomy, compared with 85% in patients who underwent local excision (36). No difference was noted with respect to the disease-free survival between the two groups of patients. Approximately 19% of patients treated with local excision developed a second in-breast local recurrence. In comparison, 4% of patients in the mastectomy group developed a chest wall recurrence. These studies indicate that local recurrence rates with conservative surgery alone for IBTR appear to be 35% on average, which is similar to the rate encountered in patients initially treated with breast-conserving surgery without postoperative radiation therapy. Therefore, the addition of radiation to local excision of IBTR is crucial because it would reduce the risk of subsequent recurrence.

Re-irradiation of the Breast

There are many concerns about the potential for severe tissue morbidity arising after re-irradiation of the whole breast after repeat lumpectomy. These include tissue necrosis, rib and lung damage, and for left-sided lesions, potential cardiac toxicity. Therefore, a second whole breast irradiation following local excision of IBTR is not generally recommended (11). Yet without radiation after resection of a recurrence, the risk of future recurrence is markedly increased. Therefore, mastectomy remains the preferred surgical option in this setting.

Partial breast irradiation has been in the forefront as a potential alternative to standard whole breast irradiation after initial breast-conserving surgery and may be emerging as an option for the management of local recurrence. While it is still investigational, there are centers currently exploring nonaccelerated partial breast irradiation after lumpectomy for a recurrence in a breast previously treated with whole breast irradiation (22,33,35–42). The method of delivery of partial breast irradiation varies from interstitial brachytherapy to three-dimensional conformal external beam dosing (38–45).

Investigators from France reported their experience with resection followed by brachytherapy in 15 patients with IBTR (39). All patients had invasive tumors (mean dimension of 2.4 cm), and resection margin status was not reported. After local resection, patients received interstitial brachytherapy with a total dose of 30 Gy (dose rate not mentioned). At a mean follow-up of 4 years, four patients (26%) had developed a second local recurrence. Cosmetic outcomes were reported for eight patients: five had minor or no sequelae, and three patients had major sequelae. One patient had skin necrosis that was treated successfully with local wound care, and one patient had extensive erythema and underwent mastectomy (no tumor was evident on pathological examination).

Another study using interstitial brachytherapy with a dose ranging from 30 to 50 Gy following second lumpectomy for local recurrence on 69 patients was also reported from France (40). The rate of complications was as follows: fibrosis in 16 cases (23.2%), breast retraction in 6 cases (8.7%), telangiectasia in 5 cases (7.3%), necrosis requiring surgery in 2 cases (2.9%), association of the preceding complications in 15 cases (21.7.%), and other complications in 6 cases (8.7%). A second local recurrence occurred in 11 cases after a median interval of 24.3 months (range 6 to 58 months). Five-year freedom from second local recurrence was 77.4%.

The study from Vienna University included nine patients with IBTR who were treated prospectively with partial breast irradiation using interstitial pulse dose rate brachytherapy with 40.2 to 50 Gy, and eight patients were treated with repeat whole breast irradiation with 30 Gy combined with an additional pulse dose rate interstitial brachytherapy boost dose of 12.5 Gy to the surgical bed (41). All the recurrent tumors were infiltrating ductal carcinomas, with tumor size ranging from 0.5 to 2.5 cm. The authors did not indicate whether preoperative mammography or sonography was performed to determine patient eligibility. All patients underwent resection of the recurrence to obtain negative margins. At 5 years of follow-up, four patients developed a second local recurrence, with a median time to recurrence of 8 months. All local recurrences occurred in the patients who received combined whole breast radiation with a brachytherapy boost. Two of the patients with local recurrence developed a concomitant distant recurrence and died of disease. In this study, cosmetic outcome as rated by a physician and the patient was good to excellent in approximately one third of the patients and moderate or acceptable in the remaining patients. The cosmetic outcome was not rated as unacceptable in any patient. Nevertheless, longer-term follow-up might alter these results.

The best example of re-irradiation using external beam comes from the University of Pittsburgh Medical Center. Deutsch reported his experience with repeat external beam irradiation for IBTR after prior lumpec-tomy and whole breast irradiation in 39 patients [31 had invasive cancer and 8 had ductal carcinoma in situ (DCIS)] treated since 1985 (38). The author did not report eligibility and selection criteria with respect to lesion size or whether diagnostic mammography or sonography was used to exclude multicentric disease. Patients underwent repeat resection of the recurrence, and 15% of patients had positive margins of resection. Patients were re-treated with electron therapy to the sur-gical bed with 50 Gy in 25 fractions at a median of 63 months (range 16 to 291 months) after their initial radia-tion treatment. The repeat course of radiotherapy to the new operative area was well tolerated in all patients, and no late sequelae were reported other than skin pigmen-tation changes. At a median follow-up of 52 months, 21% of patients had developed an in-breast local recur-rence. Four of these patients (44%) also developed dis-tant metastases. Thus 30 women (76.9%) had an intact breast free of tumor at death or at last follow-up of 1 to 180 months (median 51.5 months) after re-irradiation. The 5-year overall and disease-free survival rates were 78% and 69%, respectively. These survival rates are similar to survival rates reported in women treated with mastectomy for an in-breast local recurrence. Although this was not a prospective study with strict criteria for reporting the side effects and cosmesis, there were no reports of radiation-induced necrosis, and the cosmesis was reported as excellent or good in 69% of patients. The remaining patients had an obvious deformity, a marked difference in the size of the breast, or excessive skin pigmentation. This study did not specifically report problems with wound healing. The author suggested that excision of the IBTR followed by repeat external-beam radiotherapy to the operative area may be an acceptable alternative to mastectomy in selected patients. These reports indicate that approximately 75% of women who underwent breast-conserving surgery and re-irradiation of the surgical bed for the treatment of IBTR ultimately avoided mastectomy for their local recurrence and had no need for further local therapy.

The feasibility of repeat breast irradiation has also been explored in the setting of breast cancer following irradia-tion for lymphoma. Deutsch and colleagues reported good to excellent cosmetic results in 12 patients with breast can-cer previously irradiated for lymphoma who underwent lumpectomy followed by radiotherapy to a dose of 50 Gy in 25 to 30 fractions to the whole breast, and 9 to 10 Gy boost to the operative area, with a follow-up of 46 months (46). Aref and Cross also reported favorable outcomes in two patients with breast cancer after Hodgkin's lymphoma treated with lumpectomy and whole breast radiotherapy (47). One of the two patients received 48 Gy, whereas the other was treated with 46 Gy followed by a 14 Gy boost to the tumor bed. No complications were observed at

follow-up of 27 and 30 months, respectively. Conversely, Wolden and colleagues reported severe soft tissue necrosis 6 years after lumpectomy and radiation for a breast cancer patient with a history of mantle radiotherapy. The patient was treated with tangential whole breast fields of 45.6 Gy and a boost of 15 Gy to the upper inner quadrant, and the breast irradiation fields overlapped with the prior mantle field in some regions (48).

Partial breast irradiation using intraoperative elec-tron beam radiotherapy (ELIOT) or three-dimensional conformal external beam radiation has been also tried in the same patient population. In the study by Intra and colleagues from Milan, six breast cancer patients pre-viously irradiated for Hodgkin's lymphoma received a single fraction of 21 Gy in five cases and 17 Gy in one case delivered directly to the tumor bed. No acute com-plications were reported, and cosmetic results were good after follow-up of 30 months (49). Sanna and colleagues also suggested breast-conserving surgery and ELIOT as a valid alternative to radical surgery for early breast cancer in patients previously irradiated for Hodgkin's lymphoma (50). They reported breast cancer local relapse rate under 5% at a median follow-up of 41 months in 53 lymphoma patients. It should be noted that only 18 patients in this study cohort were treated by breast con-servation and ELIOT.

At Massachusetts General Hospital, Alm El-Din and colleagues reported excellent cosmetic results 27 months after irradiation for a patient previously irradiated for Hodgkin's lymphoma who was treated for breast cancer using three-dimensional conformal fractionated partial breast irradiation following lumpectomy delivering 50 Gy in 25 fractions (Figure 11.1) (51). Although the above-mentioned studies have suggested the feasibility of partial breast irradiation (using ELIOT or three-dimensional con-formal technique) following lumpectomy for patients with history of irradiation for lymphoma, longer follow-up is warranted to better evaluate the late effects that may arise after repeat irradiation.

Since the inception of the National Surgical Adjuvant Breast and Bowel Project (NSABP) B-39 trial in 2005 (52), there has been increasing use of accelerated partial breast irradiation following lumpectomy in the management of primary breast cancer. It is possible that in the near future, these techniques could be prospectively evaluated in the treatment of IBTR after whole breast or initial par-tial breast irradiation.

Although, partial breast irradiation in the manage-ment of local recurrence is promising, it remains investiga-tional, and there are as of yet no long-term data on safety or efficacy. Proper selection of the patients by a multidis-ciplinary team is crucial. Negative margins after resection of breast recurrence and exclusion of multicentricity, using sonography or breast magnetic resonance imaging or both, have a key role in success of breast preservation and

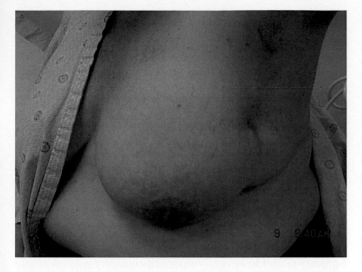

FIGURE 11.1 Patient with a history of mantle radiation for Hodgkin's lymphoma who presented with early breast cancer. She refused mastectomy and underwent lumpectomy and fractionated partial breast irradiation at a dose of 50 Gy in 25 fractions over 5 weeks. (From Ref. 51.)

repeat irradiation. It is also possible that the time interval between original treatment and local failure might play a role in the selection for a second chance for conservative treatment for patients with IBTR. Prospective studies evaluating a conservative approach with lumpectomy and partial breast irradiation are needed.

■ CHEST WALL RECURRENCE

After distant metastatic disease has been ruled out in the patient with a chest wall recurrence, the standard of care is wide local excision (11). The challenge in this patient is closure of the wound. If the area of excision is small, local tissue flaps can be raised and the wound can be closed primarily. If the patient has received postmastectomy radiation, or if the size of the recurrence is large, it may not be possible to close the wound primarily. In these instances, plastic surgery consultation should be obtained for closure with tissue transfer, in the form of either a skin graft or a myocutaneous flap. Because of the increasing use of postmastectomy chest wall irradiation, many chest wall recurrences will be in previously irradiated women. However, if the patient has not previously received radiation, then referral to a radiation oncologist is recommended to consider radiation to maximize local control and reduce the risk of future recurrence (53,54). Sometimes a prior breast reconstruction will need to be removed before the patient undergoes radiation. Again, consultation with both a plastic surgeon and radiation oncologist is necessary for optimal care.

■ AXILLARY RECURRENCE

Historically, between 1% and 10% of patients present with disease in the axilla as the initial site of recurrence (55,56), with recurrence risk dependent on the number of nodes previously dissected, nodal status, and adjuvant treatment delivered at initial diagnosis. Risk of local failure has changed since the inception of the sentinel node biopsy (57–59), and with improvements in adjuvant therapy. Axillary recurrence can present as a mass palpated in the axilla or seen on imaging studies. Sometimes it presents symptomatically with edema of the extremity or pain from brachial plexus involvement.

It is important to confirm first that the patient indeed has an axillary recurrence. This is best accomplished with a fine-needle aspiration or core needle biopsy, with or without ultrasound guidance. If a percutaneous biopsy of the lymph node is not an option or is nondiagnostic, an excisional biopsy can be performed. If the node is seen on imaging but totally inaccessible to biopsy by any means, then a positron emission tomography (PET) scan can be performed to see whether the node is PET-avid. If so, it should be assumed that there is disease in the lymph node, and the patient should be referred to a medical oncologist.

Once metastatic disease in the axilla is confirmed, surgical management consists of completion axillary dissection with excision of palpable disease. If the location of the axillary recurrence or involvement of critical axillary structures precludes surgical resection, referral for consideration of systemic therapy and radiation is appropriate. The goal of treatment in this setting is to avoid development of symptoms from bulky axillary disease such as lymphedema, axillary vein thrombosis, or brachial plexopathy.

■ SENTINEL NODE BIOPSY IN LOCAL RECURRENCE

Several factors must be considered in determining appropriate axillary evaluation of the patient with local recurrence. It is important to note whether prior axillary evaluation or dissection was performed in the treatment of the primary tumor, and whether the recurrence is invasive or in situ.

Until recently, all patients with a local recurrence underwent completion axillary dissection, if it had not already been performed with the treatment of the primary tumor. As sentinel node biopsy has become the standard of care for initial axillary staging of clinically node-negative breast cancer, fewer patients have undergone full axillary dissection in the treatment of their primary breast cancer. Initially there was speculation as to whether a repeat sentinel node biopsy would be technically possible and whether it would accurately reflect axillary node status in the setting of an invasive recurrence. There are now numerous studies demonstrating the success of performing a reoperative sentinel node biopsy after prior axillary surgery (Table 11.1) (60–71). The success rate of finding an ipsilateral sentinel node in the setting of local recurrence is higher when fewer than 10 nodes were previously dissected (62,70). While the success rate of finding a sentinel node is 95% or higher in the setting of a primary tumor, it is generally lower for recurrent disease, ranging from 63% to 100% (see Table 11.1). This success rate is high enough to justify an attempt at reoperative sentinel node biopsy for local recurrence and may spare some patients a full axillary dissection. With respect to the reoperative sentinel node biopsy, there are currently no data on the axillary recurrence rate or on the false negative rate, since there is not yet long-term follow-up after this procedure. Thus successful mapping has been interpreted as accurately reflecting axillary node status in recurrent disease as in primary disease, and clinical management is based on sentinel node status in recurrent disease if mapping is successful.

During initial development of the sentinel node biopsy technique, most patients underwent preoperative lymphoscintigraphy to demonstrate the pattern of lymphatic drainage and identify the location of the sentinel node. This was initially helpful to document success of the mapping and number of sentinel nodes. It also helped establish that the sentinel node was located in the ipsilateral axilla and not in an internal mammary or supraclavicular location. Preoperative lymphoscintigraphy has largely been abandoned as subsequent studies have demonstrated the identification of the sentinel node(s) more than 95% of the time with blue dye and radioactive tracer, without lymphoscintigraphy (72). However, lymphoscintigraphy was routinely performed in studies of reoperative sentinel node biopsy in the setting of recurrent disease, to check for new drainage patterns.

■ Table 11.1 Reoperative sentinel node biopsy

Study (Ref.)	Number of Patients	Number of Positive Identifications of Sentinel Node	Previous Axillary Surgery	Number of Positive Sentinel Nodes	Number of Alternate Site of Drainage
Intra et al. (60)	18	18/18	SNB	2/18	
Intra et al. (61)	65	63/65	65 SNB	2/63	5/63
Port et al. (62)	32	24/32	12 SNB 10 ALND 2 Lymph node biopsy	3/24	
Taback et al. (63)	15	11/15	SNB	3/15	8/11
Agarwal (64)	2	2/2	ALND		2/2
Roumen et al. (65)	12	10/12	8 SNB 2 ALND	2/10	7/10
Dinan et al. (66)	16	11/16	2 SNB 14 ALND	0/11	7/11
Newman et al. (67)	10	9/10	1 SNB 7 ALND 2 None	0/9	7/9
Barone et al. (68)	19	16/19	7 SNB 12 ALND	2/16	
Koizumi et al. (69)	31	29/31	3 SNB 16 ALND 12 None	4/28	12/29
Schrenk et al. (70)	30	19/30	13 SNB 13 ALND 2 Node sampling 2 None	4/19	6/19
Cox et al. (71)	56	45/56	56 SNB	5/45	1/45

ALND, axillary lymph node dissection; SNB, sentinel node biopsy.

These studies of repeat sentinel node mapping have demonstrated that new lymphatic drainage patterns to a place other than the ipsilateral axilla are observed. New drainage patterns as identified on lymphoscintigraphy showed the sentinel node might be found in the contralateral axilla, internal mammary, supraclavicular, and even abdominal node basin (61,63–67,69,71). These results confirm that lymphoscintigraphy should be performed in the setting of a reoperative sentinel node biopsy to document sentinel node location prior to surgery.

This aberrant drainage also poses a treatment challenge as to whether to remove these nonaxillary sentinel nodes and examine them for metastatic disease. In the absence of clinical trial data to answer this question, most clinicians would likely forgo dissection in places that would both pose an operative challenge and increase morbidity with little benefit to the patient.

Knowing when to perform a sentinel node biopsy for axillary evaluation in the setting of local recurrence is paramount. For patients with an invasive recurrence, it appears the sentinel node biopsy should be attempted when a prior sentinel node biopsy has been performed. When a previous axillary dissection has been performed, it is important to obtain the pathology report to see how many nodes were removed. If fewer than 10 nodes were removed, then it appears that a reoperative sentinel node biopsy may be recommended. If a prior axillary dissection consisted of more than 10 nodes, the success rate of a reoperative sentinel node mapping is likely to be low, but it could be considered with particular attention to evaluating nonaxillary node locations.

When a local recurrence of breast cancer presents as DCIS, the role of sentinel node biopsy remains controversial. In general the guidelines for performing a sentinel node biopsy for local recurrence of DCIS are similar to those for a primary diagnosis of DCIS, namely, (a) when there is a palpable mass, (b) when there is multicentric disease, (c) when there is suspicion of microinvasion, or (d) when a mastectomy is performed (73,74). When a patient presents with a palpable mass and a diagnosis of DCIS preoperatively on core biopsy, this correlates with a high suspicion for invasive cancer on final pathology, and a sentinel node biopsy should be performed. This will spare some patients a second surgery for axillary staging if final pathology demonstrates invasive disease. This is particularly important with mastectomy, since the opportunity to perform a sentinel node biopsy after a mastectomy is lost, and a full axillary dissection would be required.

Just as the sentinel lymph node biopsy approach revolutionized axillary management in the treatment of primary breast cancer, it is now having a similar effect in the management of locally recurrent breast cancer. It is important to consider the sentinel node biopsy approach as a viable alternative to full axillary node dissection in patients with locally recurrent breast cancer.

■ LOCAL RECURRENCE IN THE ELDERLY

There are many challenges in the surgical management of local recurrence that apply to the elderly population and to other patients with significant comorbidities. These issues revolve around (a) the definition of what is considered an elderly patient or one with significant comorbidity, (b) the challenge of balancing risk of treatment with risk of mortality from other causes, (c) whether it is safe to omit some aspects of treatment normally offered to younger, healthier patients, and (d) whether an individual patient can safely undergo surgery. These same issues apply to the management of a primary breast cancer in the elderly and medically frail populations, and there is no consensus as to the optimum treatment approach. In addition, the elderly have been underrepresented in many clinical trials, making evidence-based decisions difficult.

The first challenge one encounters in the reviewing the literature pertains to the definition of what is elderly. Some studies use an age cutoff of 65 years, whereas others use 70 or 80 years (75–77). Yet, even within particular age groups, individual patient conditions vary widely. There are healthy, active octogenarians who could tolerate surgery and have a relatively long life expectancy. On the other hand, there are frail 60-year-olds who would have difficulty tolerating general anesthesia and likely succumb from comorbidities other than breast cancer. Formulating an individualized treatment plan for each patient is paramount.

The treatment options to consider in an elderly patient are slightly different than in any other population and take into account that the great majority of tumors will be estrogen receptor–positive (ER+). They consist of (a) surgery alone, (b) surgery followed by radiation, whole or partial breast, plus or minus endocrine therapy, and for ER+ tumors, (c) surgery with endocrine therapy without radiation or (d) endocrine therapy alone without surgery. Chemotherapy may also be considered for ER– tumors or for advanced ER+ tumors in patients fit enough for treatment. It is important to determine the safest course of treatment for each individual patient with respect to both her breast cancer recurrence and her overall functional status.

Surgical excision of a breast cancer recurrence should be considered for all but the most elderly or medically frail patients. Studies have shown that the surgical mortality of an elderly breast cancer patient is around 2% (78) and that surgical excision is associated with improved survival (77). However, for that small group of patients who cannot undergo surgery, endocrine therapy, in lieu of surgery, can halt the growth of the tumor and is likely to cause near-complete tumor regression (79,80). This is appropriate for patients who are unable to tolerate anesthesia (78) or for patients with larger tumors who require neoadjuvant hormonal therapy to allow surgical excision. It is important to reach a consensus among the patient's primary care physician, surgeon, and medical oncologist in assessing fitness for surgery and choosing among systemic therapy options.

The use of adjuvant radiation therapy in the management of recurrent breast cancer in the elderly is controversial, with arguments similar to those surrounding the use of radiation at the time of initial diagnosis. As the goals of radiation are local control and reduction in risk of recurrence, the life expectancy of the elderly patient with breast cancer must be considered when deciding whether radiation therapy is indicated.

Since most primary breast cancers are managed with lumpectomy and whole breast radiation, a recurrence should be treated with a mastectomy if the patient can tolerate anesthesia, or with hormone therapy for endocrine-positive tumors if the patient cannot tolerate surgery. For the elderly patient who presents with an in-breast recurrence without prior radiation, the risk of future recurrence is weighed against life expectancy when considering adjuvant radiation therapy. Several studies support omission of radiation in elderly patients, with most studies advocating adjuvant hormonal therapy for ER+ tumors. (75,81,82). Cancer and Leukemia Study Group B (CALGB) study 9343 in women 70 and older with ER+ tumors reported an acceptable recurrence rate of 4% in elderly patients who underwent lumpectomy followed by tamoxifen without adjuvant radiation, compared with a recurrence rate of 1% when adjuvant radiation was added (75). However, other studies did not find age to be an independent risk factor for recurrence and advocated adjuvant radiation in this population (78). Some of these studies have found a statistically significant increase in disease-free survival when radiation was administered.

As discussed earlier, radiation options now include both whole breast radiation and partial breast irradiation. Some clinicians see partial breast irradiation as particularly beneficial in the elderly population, with the option for risk reduction and local control, and a less burdensome time course for treatment (78). Consultation among all treating specialists is important in deciding whether adjuvant radiation is appropriate.

■ LOCAL RECURRENCE IN *BRCA* GENE MUTATION CARRIERS

The management of local recurrence in the *BRCA1* and *BRCA2* gene mutation carriers is more straightforward than in the general population, with adherence to NCCN guidelines for mastectomy (11). While the risk of recurrence of the initial tumor after lumpectomy and radiation in the mutation carrier is no higher than for nonmutation carriers (83), the risk of multicentric breast cancer and risk of future primary breast cancers are markedly increased

(37). One must question whether a recurrence in a mutation carrier is a true recurrence or a new primary breast cancer or evidence of initially untreated multicentric disease. These factors support mastectomy as the standard of care for an in-breast recurrence in a *BRCA* gene mutation carrier. Partial breast irradiation is not considered an appropriate option in these patients.

At the time of surgery, the axillary status should be addressed in the same way as discussed earlier in this chapter, with sentinel node biopsy if feasible and axillary dissection for an invasive recurrence if mapping is not successful.

BRCA gene mutation carriers are also at increased risk for chest wall recurrence in retained breast tissue after mastectomy. Such chest wall tumor recurrences are treated with local excision with consideration of systemic therapy and radiation, as discussed earlier in this chapter.

The other issue to be addressed in the *BRCA* gene mutation carrier is whether to address contralateral breast cancer risk at the time of mastectomy. Since the patient will already be undergoing anesthesia, with loss of one breast and with possible reconstruction, it is an opportune time to discuss risk reduction with a contralateral prophylactic mastectomy. Prophylactic contralateral mastectomy is generally reserved for patients with a good prognosis/recurrence risk, such as DCIS or a small invasive recurrence, where the risk of a new contralateral primary remains significant relative to the mortality risk posed by the initial primary and by the recurrent tumor itself.

■ CONCLUSIONS

As our knowledge about breast cancer increases and our armamentarium of treatment options grows, management options for locally recurrent breast cancer have increased, often requiring multidisciplinary input in decision making. While mastectomy and axillary dissection remain valuable options, many patients may be offered smaller surgical procedures. Many patients may have reoperative sentinel node biopsy, thereby sparing the morbidity associated with an axillary dissection. Other patients may be eligible for partial breast irradiation after whole breast irradiation, thereby avoiding mastectomy. Use of these newer treatment options requires discussion of treatment plans with a multidisciplinary team to ensure consensus and to optimize the treatment plan for the individual patient.

■ MULTIDISCIPLINARY APPROACH IN THE TREATMENT OF IBTR

With the complexities of choices for managing the patient with locally recurrent breast cancer, it is important to seek counsel from the various specialties involved in the care of the patient. Without communication between services, there is risk of undertreatment, overtreatment, or misunderstanding regarding the individualized plan. Services involved should include surgical, medical, and radiation oncology, and plastic surgery if necessary. In addition, it can be valuable to review the imaging and pathology slides as a group. This helps to ensure that all aspects of the diagnostic workup and details of the treatment plan have been adequately addressed. Since many of these treatment plans are different from the known standard of care, it important to document the reason for the deviation and that the case has been discussed and agreed on as acceptable to all members of the treatment team. With this team approach, ultimately, each patient would receive the best individualized care for her breast cancer recurrence.

■ SUMMARY

- Management of local recurrence is complex and requires a multidisciplinary approach.
- Preoperative workup for metastatic disease is crucial.
- The standard of care for a previously irradiated breast is mastectomy.
- All patients having mastectomy should be considered for reconstruction.
- Partial breast irradiation on a clinical trial may be a possible alternative for breast conservation in local recurrence.
- There are many options to deliver partial breast irradiation.
- A sentinel node biopsy to evaluate the axilla may be possible, even in a previously operated axilla.
- Management of chest wall recurrence should involve a consultation with a plastic surgeon if closure of the wound is an issue.
- Management of local recurrence in the elderly should be multidisciplinary because standard therapies such as surgery or radiation may be omitted.
- Management of recurrence in *BRCA1* and *BRCA2* mutation carriers should include a discussion of bilateral mastectomies, with a consult for reconstruction.

■ REFERENCES

1. Blichert-Toft M, Rose C, Andersen JA, et al. Danish randomized trial comparing breast conservation therapy with mastectomy: six years of life-table analysis. Danish Breast Cancer Cooperative Group. *J Natl Cancer Inst Monogr*. 1992;11:19–25.
2. Fisher B, Anderson S, Bryant J, et al. Twenty-year follow-up of a randomized trial comparing total mastectomy, lumpectomy, and lumpectomy plus irradiation for the treatment of invasive breast cancer. *New Engl J Med*. 2002;347(16):1233–1241.
3. Fisher B, Anderson S, Redmond CK, Wolmark N, Wickerham DL, Cronin WM. Reanalysis and results after 12 years of follow-up in a randomized clinical trial comparing total mastectomy with lumpectomy with or without irradiation in the treatment of breast cancer. *New Engl J Med*. 1995;333(22):1456–1461.
4. Jacobson JA, Danforth DN, Cowan KH, et al. Ten-year results of a comparison of conservation with mastectomy in the treatment of stage I and II breast cancer. *New Engl J Med*. 1995;332(14): 907–911.
5. Poggi MM, Danforth DN, Sciuto LC, et al. Eighteen-year results in the treatment of early breast carcinoma with mastectomy versus breast conservation therapy: the National Cancer Institute Randomized Trial. *Cancer*. 2003;98(4):697–702.
6. Thomas F, Arriagada R, Spielmann M, et al. Pattern of failure in patients with inflammatory breast cancer treated by alternating radiotherapy and chemotherapy. *Cancer*. 1995;76(11): 2286–2290.
7. van Dongen JA, Voogd AC, Fentiman IS, et al. Long-term results of a randomized trial comparing breast-conserving therapy with mastectomy: European Organization for Research and Treatment of Cancer 10801 trial. *J Natl Cancer Inst*. 2000;92(14):1143–1150.
8. Veronesi U, Cascinelli N, Mariani L, et al. Twenty-year follow-up of a randomized study comparing breast-conserving surgery with radical mastectomy for early breast cancer. *New Engl J Med*. 2002; 347(16):1227–1232.
9. Veronesi U, Salvadori B, Luini A, et al. Breast conservation is a safe method in patients with small cancer of the breast. Long-term results of three randomised trials on 1,973 patients. *Eur J Cancer*. 1995;31A(10):1574–1579.
10. Effects of radiotherapy and surgery in early breast cancer. An overview of the randomized trials. Early Breast Cancer Trialists' Collaborative Group. *New Engl J Med*. 1995;333(22): 1444–1455.
11. National Comprehensive Cancer Network Practice Guidelines in Oncology: Breast Cancer v.1, 2009. Available at www.nccn.org.
12. Buchanan CL, Dorn PL, Fey J, et al. Locoregional recurrence after mastectomy: incidence and outcomes. *J Am Coll Surg*. 2006; 203(4):469–474.
13. Jatoi I, Tsimelzon A, Weiss H, Clark GM, Hilsenbeck SG. Hazard rates of recurrence following diagnosis of primary breast cancer. *Breast Cancer Res Treat*. 2005;89(2):173–178.
14. Schmoor C, Sauerbrei W, Bastert G, Schumacher M. Role of isolated locoregional recurrence of breast cancer: results of four prospective studies. *J Clin Oncol*. 2000;18(8):1696–1708.
15. Stefanik D, Goldberg R, Byrne P, et al. Local-regional failure in patients treated with adjuvant chemotherapy for breast cancer. *J Clin Oncol*. 1985;3(5):660–665.
16. Delouche G, Bachelot F, Premont M, Kurtz JM. Conservation treatment of early breast cancer: long term results and complications. *Int J Radiat Oncol Biol Phys*. 1987;13(1):29–34.
17. Veronesi U, Saccozzi R, Del Vecchio M, et al. Comparing radical mastectomy with quadrantectomy, axillary dissection, and radiotherapy in patients with small cancers of the breast. *New Engl J Med*. 1981;305(1):6–11.
18. Wapnir IL, Anderson SJ, Mamounas EP, et al. Prognosis after ipsilateral breast tumor recurrence and locoregional recurrences in five National Surgical Adjuvant Breast and Bowel Project node-positive adjuvant breast cancer trials. *J Clin Oncol*. 2006;24(13): 2028–2037.
19. van Tienhoven G, Voogd AC, Peterse JL, et al. Prognosis after treatment for loco-regional recurrence after mastectomy or breast conserving therapy in two randomised trials (EORTC 10801 and DBCG-82TM). EORTC Breast Cancer Cooperative Group and the Danish Breast Cancer Cooperative Group. *Eur J Cancer*. 1999; 35(1):32–38.
20. Haffty BG, Carter D, Flynn SD, et al. Local recurrence versus new primary: clinical analysis of 82 breast relapses and potential applications for genetic fingerprinting. *Int J Radiat Oncol Biol Phys*. 1993;27(3):575–583.

21. Carstens PH, Greenberg RA, Francis D, Lyon H. Tubular carcinoma of the breast. A long term follow-up. *Histopathology.* 1985; 9(3):271–280.

22. Dalberg K, Mattsson A, Sandelin K, Rutqvist LE. Outcome of treatment for ipsilateral breast tumor recurrence in early-stage breast cancer. *Breast Cancer Res Treat.* 1998;49(1):69–78.

23. Pisansky TM, Ingle JN, Schaid DJ, et al. Patterns of tumor relapse following mastectomy and adjuvant systemic therapy in patients with axillary lymph node-positive breast cancer. Impact of clinical, histopathologic, and flow cytometric factors. *Cancer.* 1993;72(4):1247–1260.

24. Hsi RA, Antell A, Schultz DJ, Solin LJ. Radiation therapy for chest wall recurrence of breast cancer after mastectomy in a favorable subgroup of patients. *Int J Radiat Oncol Biol Phys.* 1998;42(3): 495–499.

25. Fisher B, Costantino JP, Wickerham DL, et al. Tamoxifen for prevention of breast cancer: report of the National Surgical Adjuvant Breast and Bowel Project P-1 Study. *J Natl Cancer Inst.* 1998; 90(18):1371–1388.

26. de la Rochefordiere A, Mouret-Fourme E, Asselain B, et al. Metachronous contralateral breast cancer as first event of relapse. *Int J Radiat Oncol Biol Phys.* 1996;36(3):615–621.

27. Chauvet B, Reynaud-Bougnoux A, Calais G, et al. Prognostic significance of breast relapse after conservative treatment in node-negative early breast cancer. *Int J Radiat Oncol Biol Phys.* 1990; 19(5):1125–1130.

28. Fowble B, Solin LJ, Schultz DJ, Rubenstein J, Goodman RL. Breast recurrence following conservative surgery and radiation: patterns of failure, prognosis, and pathologic findings from mastectomy specimens with implications for treatment. *Int J Radiat Oncol Biol Phys.* 1990;19(4):833–842.

29. Abner AL, Recht A, Eberlein T, et al. Prognosis following salvage mastectomy for recurrence in the breast after conservative surgery and radiation therapy for early-stage breast cancer. *J Clin Oncol.* 1993;11(1):44–48.

30. Clarke M, Collins R, Darby S, et al. Effects of radiotherapy and of differences in the extent of surgery for early breast cancer on local recurrence and 15-year survival: an overview of the randomised trials. *Lancet.* 2005;366(9503):2087–2106.

31. Fisher B, Anderson S, Fisher ER, et al. Significance of ipsilateral breast tumour recurrence after lumpectomy. *Lancet.* 1991; 338(8763):327–331.

32. Recht A, Schnitt SJ, Connolly JL, et al. Prognosis following local or regional recurrence after conservative surgery and radiotherapy for early stage breast carcinoma. *Int J Radiat Oncol Biol Phys.* 1989;16(1):3–9.

33. Kuerer HM, Arthur DW, Haffty BG. Repeat breast-conserving surgery for in-breast local breast carcinoma recurrence: the potential role of partial breast irradiation. *Cancer.* 2004;100(11):2269–2280.

34. Voogd AC, Peterse JL, Crommelin MA, et al. Histological determinants for different types of local recurrence after breast-conserving therapy of invasive breast cancer. Dutch Study Group on local Recurrence after Breast Conservation (BORST). *Eur J Cancer.* 1999;35(13):1828–1837.

35. Kurtz JM, Jacquemier J, Amalric R, et al. Is breast conservation after local recurrence feasible? *Eur J Cancer.* 1991;27(3): 240–244.

36. Salvadori B, Marubini E, Miceli R, et al. Reoperation for locally recurrent breast cancer in patients previously treated with conservative surgery. *Br J Surg.* 1999;86(1):84–87.

37. Alpert TE, Kuerer HM, Arthur DW, Lannin DR, Haffty BG. Ipsilateral breast tumor recurrence after breast conservation therapy: outcomes of salvage mastectomy vs. salvage breast-conserving surgery and prognostic factors for salvage breast preservation. *Int J Radiat Oncol Biol Phys.* 2005;63(3):845–851.

38. Deutsch M. Repeat high-dose external beam irradiation for in-breast tumor recurrence after previous lumpectomy and whole breast irradiation. *Int J Radiat Oncol Biol Phys.* 2002;53(3): 687–691.

39. Maulard C, Housset M, Brunel P, Delanian S, Taurelle R, Baillet F. Use of perioperative or split-course interstitial brachytherapy techniques for salvage irradiation of isolated local recurrences after conservative management of breast cancer. *Am J Clin Oncol.* 1995;18(4):348–352.

40. Hannoun-Levi JM, Houvenaeghel G, Ellis S, et al. Partial breast irradiation as second conservative treatment for local breast cancer recurrence. *Int J Radiat Oncol Biol Phys.* 2004;60(5): 1385–1392.

41. Resch A, Fellner C, Mock U, et al. Locally recurrent breast cancer: pulse dose rate brachytherapy for repeat irradiation following lumpectomy—a second chance to preserve the breast. *Radiology.* 2002;225(3):713–718.

42. Chadha M, Feldman S, Brus C, Harrison L. Phase I/II study for partial breast brachytherapy in patients who have previously received external beam radiation therapy to the breast. In: *Proceedings of the American Society of Radiation Oncology, Biology and Physics,* Abstract 53. Philadelphia, PA; 2006.

43. Formenti SC, Truong MT, Goldberg JD, et al. Prone accelerated partial breast irradiation after breast-conserving surgery: preliminary clinical results and dose-volume histogram analysis. *Int J Radiat Oncol Biol Phys.* 2004;60(2):493–504.

44. Taghian AG, Kozak KR, Doppke KP, et al. Initial dosimetric experience using simple three-dimensional conformal external-beam accelerated partial-breast irradiation. *Int J Radiat Oncol Biol Phys.* 2006;64(4):1092–1099.

45. Vicini FA, Remouchamps V, Wallace M, et al. Ongoing clinical experience utilizing 3D conformal external beam radiotherapy to deliver partial-breast irradiation in patients with early-stage breast cancer treated with breast-conserving therapy. *Int J Radiat Oncol Biol Phys.* 2003;57(5):1247–1253.

46. Deutsch M, Gerszten K, Bloomer WD, Avisar E. Lumpectomy and breast irradiation for breast cancer arising after previous radiotherapy for Hodgkin's disease or lymphoma. *Am J Clin Oncol.* 2001;24(1):33–34.

47. Aref I, Cross P. Conservative surgery and radiation therapy for early stage breast cancer after previous mantle radiation for Hodgkin's disease. *Br J Radiol.* 2000;73(872):905–906.

48. Wolden SL, Hancock SL, Carlson RW, Goffinet DR, Jeffrey SS, Hoppe RT. Management of breast cancer after Hodgkin's disease. *J Clin Oncol.* 2000;18(4):765–772.

49. Intra M, Gentilini O, Veronesi P, et al. A new option for early breast cancer patients previously irradiated for Hodgkin's disease: intraoperative radiotherapy with electrons (ELIOT). *Breast Cancer Res.* 2005;7(5):R828–R832.

50. Sanna G, Lorizzo K, Rotmensz N, et al. Breast cancer in Hodgkin's disease and non-Hodgkin's lymphoma survivors. *Ann Oncol.* 2007; 18(2):288–292.

51. Alm El-Din MA, Feng JK, Taghian AG. Lumpectomy and partial breast irradiation for early-stage breast cancer following mantle irradiation for Hodgkin's lymphoma. *Natl Clin Pract Oncol.* 2008;5(7):426–429.

52. National Surgical Adjuvant Breast and Bowel Project B-39 Protocol. A randomized phase III study of conventional whole breast irradiation (WBI) versus partial breast irradiation (PBI) for women with stage 0, I, or II breast cancer. Available at www.rtog.org/members/protocols/0413/0413.pdf.

53. Recht A, Edge SB, Solin LJ, et al. Postmastectomy radiotherapy: clinical practice guidelines of the American Society of Clinical Oncology. *J Clin Oncol.* 2001;19(5):1539–1569.

54. Truong PT, Olivotto IA, Whelan TJ, Levine M. Clinical practice guidelines for the care and treatment of breast cancer: 16. Locoregional post-mastectomy radiotherapy. *CMAJ.* 2004;170(8):1263–1273.

55. Carpenter R, Royle GT, Cross M, Hamilton C, Buchanan R, Taylor I. Loco-regional recurrence and survival after wide local excision, radiotherapy and axillary clearance for early breast cancer. *J R Soc Med.* 1992;85(8):454–456.

56. Graversen HP, Blichert-Toft M, Andersen JA, Zedeler K. Breast cancer: risk of axillary recurrence in node-negative patients

following partial dissection of the axilla. *Eur J Surg Oncol.* 1988; 14(5):407–412.

57. Heuts EM, van der Ent FW, Hulsewe KW, Heeren PA, Hoofwijk AG. Incidence of axillary recurrence in 344 sentinel node negative breast cancer patients after intermediate follow-up: a prospective study into the accuracy of sentinel node biopsy in breast cancer patients. *Acta Chir Belg.* 2008;108(2):203–207.

58. Palesty JA, Foster JM, Hurd TC, Watroba N, Rezaishiraz H, Edge SB. Axillary recurrence in women with a negative sentinel lymph node and no axillary dissection in breast cancer. *J Surg Oncol.* 2006;93(2):129–132.

59. Takei H, Suemasu K, Kurosumi M, et al. Recurrence after sentinel lymph node biopsy with or without axillary lymph node dissection in patients with breast cancer. *Breast Cancer.* 2007;14(1):16–24.

60. Intra M, Trifiro G, Viale G, et al. Second biopsy of axillary sentinel lymph node for reappearing breast cancer after previous sentinel lymph node biopsy. *Ann Surg Oncol.* 2005;12(11):895–899.

61. Intra M, Trifiro G, Galimberti V, Gentilini O, Rotmensz N, Veronesi P. Second axillary sentinel node biopsy for ipsilateral breast tumour recurrence. *Br J Surg.* 2007;94(10):1216–1219.

62. Port ER, Fey J, Gemignani ML, et al. Reoperative sentinel lymph node biopsy: a new option for patients with primary or locally recurrent breast carcinoma. *J Am Coll Surg.* 2002;195(2): 167–172.

63. Taback B, Nguyen P, Hansen N, Edwards GK, Conway K, Giuliano AE. Sentinel lymph node biopsy for local recurrence of breast cancer after breast-conserving therapy. *Ann Surg Oncol.* 2006;13(8):1099–1104.

64. Agarwal A, Heron DE, Sumkin J, Falk J. Contralateral uptake and metastases in sentinel lymph node mapping for recurrent breast cancer. *J Surg Oncol.* 2005;92(1):4–8.

65. Roumen RM, Kuijt GP, Liem IH. Lymphatic mapping and sentinel node harvesting in patients with recurrent breast cancer. *Eur J Surg Oncol.* 2006;32(10):1076–1081.

66. Dinan D, Nagle CE, Pettinga J. Lymphatic mapping and sentinel node biopsy in women with an ipsilateral second breast carcinoma and a history of breast and axillary surgery. *Am J Surg.* 2005;190(4):614–617.

67. Newman EA, Cimmino VM, Sabel MS, et al. Lymphatic mapping and sentinel lymph node biopsy for patients with local recurrence after breast-conservation therapy. *Ann Surg Oncol.* 2006; 13(1):52–57.

68. Barone JL, Feldman SM, Estabrook A, Tartter PI, Rosenbaum Smith SM, Boolbol SK. Reoperative sentinel lymph node biopsy in patients with locally recurrent breast cancer. *Am J Surg.* 2007; 194(4):491–493.

69. Koizumi M, Koyama M, Tada K, et al. The feasibility of sentinel node biopsy in the previously treated breast. *Eur J Surg Oncol.* 2008;34(4):365–368.

70. Schrenk P, Tausch C, Wayand W. Lymphatic mapping in patients with primary or recurrent breast cancer following previous axillary surgery. *Eur J Surg Oncol.* 2008;34(8):851–856.

71. Cox CE, Furman BT, Kiluk JV, et al. Use of reoperative sentinel lymph node biopsy in breast cancer patients. *J Am Coll Surg.* 2008; 207(1):57–61.

72. Krag DN, Anderson SJ, Julian TB, et al. Technical outcomes of sentinel-lymph-node resection and conventional axillary-lymph-node dissection in patients with clinically node-negative breast cancer: results from the NSABP B-32 randomised phase III trial. *Lancet Oncol.* 2007;8(10):881–888.

73. Lyman GH, Giuliano AE, Somerfield MR, et al. American Society of Clinical Oncology guideline recommendations for sentinel lymph node biopsy in early-stage breast cancer. *J Clin Oncol.* 2005; 23(30):7703–7720.

74. O'Sullivan MJ, Morrow M. Ductal carcinoma in situ—current management. *Surg Clin North Am.* 2007;87(2):333–351, viii.

75. Hughes KS, Schnaper LA, Berry D, et al. Lumpectomy plus tamoxifen with or without irradiation in women 70 years of age or older with early breast cancer. *New Engl J Med.* 2004;351(10): 971–977.

76. Mustacchi G, Cazzaniga ME, Pronzato P, De Matteis A, Di Costanzo F, Floriani I. Breast cancer in elderly women: a different reality? Results from the NORA study. *Ann Oncol.* 2007;18(6): 991–996.

77. Rao VS, Jameel JK, Mahapatra TK, McManus PL, Fox JN, Drew PJ. Surgery is associated with lower morbidity and longer survival in elderly breast cancer patients over 80. *Breast J.* 2007; 13(4):368–373.

78. Wildiers H, Kunkler I, Biganzoli L, et al. Management of breast cancer in elderly individuals: recommendations of the International Society of Geriatric Oncology. *Lancet Oncol.* 2007;8(12):1101–1115.

79. Ellis MJ, Coop A, Singh B, et al. Letrozole is more effective neoadjuvant endocrine therapy than tamoxifen for *ErbB-1-* and/or *ErbB-2*-positive, estrogen receptor-positive primary breast cancer: evidence from a phase III randomized trial. *J Clin Oncol.* 2001;19(18):3808–3816.

80. Sivasubramaniam V. Compared to tamoxifen, letrozole increases tumor response in post-menopausal women with estrogen-receptor-positive primary breast cancer. *Evidence-Based Oncol.* 2002;3(1):29–30.

81. Martelli G, Miceli R, Costa A, et al. Elderly breast cancer patients treated by conservative surgery alone plus adjuvant tamoxifen: fifteen-year results of a prospective study. *Cancer.* 2008;112(3):481–488.

82. Hughes KS, Schnaper LA, Berry D, et al. Lumpectomy plus tamoxifen with or without irradiation in women 70 years of age or older with early breast cancer. *Breast Cancer Res Treat.* 2006;100S (Abstract 11).

83. Kirova YM, Stoppa-Lyonnet D, Savignoni A, Sigal-Zafrani B, Fabre N, Fourquet A. Risk of breast cancer recurrence and contralateral breast cancer in relation to BRCA1 and BRCA2 mutation status following breast-conserving surgery and radiotherapy. *Eur J Cancer.* 2005;41(15):2304–2311.

Medical Oncology Management of Locally Recurrent Disease

IRENE KUTER

Locoregional recurrence of breast cancer, in the absence of overt metastatic disease, has traditionally been treated primarily with more surgery, radiation, or both, as it is widely accepted that medical therapy alone is unlikely to be curative for patients with gross disease (1,2). Medical oncologists are generally consulted regarding systemic therapy options, but the heterogeneity of locoregionally recurrent disease makes generalizations about the role of systemic therapy challenging. In this chapter, we will discuss how and when to incorporate systemic medical therapy into the multidisciplinary treatment of locoregionally recurrent breast cancer.

■ PROGNOSTIC SIGNIFICANCE OF LOCOREGIONAL RECURRENCE

The prognostic significance of locoregionally recurrent disease has been much debated, but the discussion has been heavily influenced by the outcomes of the National Surgical Adjuvant Breast and Bowel Project (NSABP) B-04 and B-06 trials. The 25-year results of the B-04 trial (3) showed that breast cancer patients treated with simple mastectomy without an axillary lymph node dissection had no different distant disease-free survival or overall survival than those who underwent a radical mastectomy, despite the fact that 19% of women in the former group had subsequent axillary recurrences requiring a delayed axillary dissection. The 20-year results of the B-06 study (4) suggested that women treated with lumpectomy alone, or with lumpectomy plus radiation, experienced disease-free and overall survival rates similar to those of women treated with total mastectomy, despite an ipsilateral breast tumor recurrence (IBTR) of 39% in the lumpectomy group and 14% in the lumpectomy plus radiation group. On the basis of these results, strong arguments have been made that IBTR is a marker of risk of distant recurrence but not a cause of it (5), although debate on this issue continues. (6,7). In a review of five NSABP trials involving women with positive lymph nodes, Wapnir and colleagues (8) reported an overall distant disease-free survival at five years of 85%; however, in women with IBTR the comparable number was 51%, and in women with other

locoregional recurrence only 18.8%. Locoregional recurrence is clearly a marker of poor prognosis, even if not a direct cause of it.

■ ROLE OF SYSTEMIC THERAPY IN LOCOREGIONALLY RECURRENT DISEASE: LITERATURE REVIEW

There are two reasons to consider systemic therapy for patients with locoregionally recurrent disease: to attempt to eradicate microscopic metastases systemically and to assist in the control of the locoregional disease and its associated morbidity. It is disappointing that there have not, to date, been many clinical trials addressing the efficacy of systemic therapy for either of these indications. Although a number of studies have suggested a benefit from systemic therapy as part of multimodality treatment of locoregional recurrence, most of these studies are retrospective reviews, and it is likely that there is significant selection bias with regard to which patients received systemic therapy (9–11). Even prospective studies have generally been flawed for one reason or another, usually because the studies have been small and the patients were not randomized. A recent systematic literature search (11) identified only three prospective studies, with a total of only four randomized comparisons of systemic therapy to observation alone for women who were treated with radiation therapy for locoregional recurrence of breast cancer. A trial by Olson and colleagues (12) included 32 women with recurrence in the chest wall or regional lymph nodes who were treated with radiation therapy with or without actinomycin-D. This study reported better local control with the addition of chemotherapy but no effect on survival. A second trial of 32 women, reported by Fentiman (13), had a similar design, randomizing women with chest wall or nodal recurrences to radiation with or without a year of alpha-interferon. This trial showed no benefit from the systemic therapy. Finally, the Swiss Group for Clinical Cancer Research SAKK trial (14) was started in 1982 and originally planned to enroll 300 patients, but closed in 1991 due to poor accrual. There were 228 patients enrolled with "locoregional recurrence" in the absence of distant metastatic disease, and they were divided into "poor risk" and "good risk" subgroups. The 178 good risk patients had either estrogen receptor–positive (ER+) recurrence or, if hormone receptors were unknown, a disease-free survival of longer than 12 months and three or fewer recurrent tumor nodules, each less than or equal to 3 cm in diameter. All women underwent surgical resection of the recurrent disease followed by radiation therapy (50 Gy); they were then randomized to observation or tamoxifen 20 mg per day until progression. Improvement in disease-free survival was seen with tamoxifen, but there was no benefit for overall survival. At a median follow-up of 11.6 years, median disease-free survival was 6.5 years with tamoxifen and 2.7 years with observation ($P = 0.053$); overall survival was 11.2 years in the observation group and 11.5 years in the tamoxifen group (15). An apparent deleterious effect of tamoxifen for the premenopausal subgroup (16) should be interpreted with caution: there was no adverse effect on disease-free survival and there were no major tamoxifen-induced adverse events. It is likely that the difference in overall survival was due simply to the small number ($n = 20$) of eligible premenopausal patients in the analysis. In addition to being small, this study was imperfect in that it included women with ipsilateral and contralateral cervical lymph node involvement, as well as those with skin involvement in the shoulder, neck, and upper arm. These patients in fact had stage 4 disease, not locoregional recurrence as generally defined.

The poor risk group in the SAKK trial (14) comprised those women deemed unsuitable for endocrine therapy. Only 50 women were randomized after excision of the recurrent disease and radiation therapy to either observation or chemotherapy with doxorubicin, cyclophosphamide, and vincristine. No results have been reported due to the poor accrual.

Clearly, it is difficult to draw any conclusions from these limited studies. With heterogeneous populations, small numbers of patients, and (in the Olson and Fentiman studies) treatments with no recognized benefit in breast cancer, one must conclude only that better trials are necessary to assess the role of systemic therapies for patients with locoregionally recurrent disease.

■ CONSIDERATIONS FOR THE MEDICAL ONCOLOGIST

Without the benefit of adequate clinical trial results, how should the medical oncologist decide whether to recommend systemic therapy to a particular patient with locoregionally recurrent disease? Most oncologists will approach the decision in much the same way they approach the question of systemic therapy in the adjuvant setting for treatment of a primary breast cancer. To assess the benefit of systemic therapy in decreasing the risk of systemic metastases, we take into consideration the likelihood of systemic recurrences, the likely magnitude of benefit from the various systemic therapies available, and the potential

side effects of treatment before a recommendation can be made.

The ideal candidate for systemic therapy based on these considerations would be the patient with a high risk of systemic recurrence whose cancer is likely to be responsive to an available systemic therapy with acceptable toxicity. Likewise, the patient who might benefit from systemic therapy for locoregional control would be one who is at high risk of further local recurrence despite surgery, radiation, or both (e.g., a patient who has recurrence in a previously irradiated field), or one who is not a good candidate for either surgery or radiation for a variety of reasons. A patient who is already experiencing bulky recurrent disease with local symptoms such as pain, lymphedema, bleeding, ulceration, or vascular or neurological compromise, where combined modality therapy incorporating medical therapy (concurrent or sequential) might offer better palliation than surgery or radiation alone, would also be an appropriate candidate.

Lack of data from randomized trials is only one of the factors complicating the care of patients with locoregionally recurrent breast cancer. Concern that occult metastases may have developed in the interval between treatment of the primary cancer and development of the recurrent disease also needs to be addressed. Prior surgeries (such as sentinel lymph node mapping) and radiation therapy may complicate management recommendations, and prior systemic therapies will generate concern about acquired resistance of the tumor to these therapies. Finally, one must take into account tolerability of the therapies to the patient, the patient's acceptance of the recommendations for systemic therapy when she has already experienced side effects from prior adjuvant treatment, and her disappointment at facing yet more potential side effects.

Before embarking on treatment, the patient with locoregionally recurrent disease should be evaluated for systemic metastases. A literature review (17) suggests that about one third of women with locoregional recurrence after mastectomy will have simultaneous or antecedent distant metastases, compared with 10% of women with IBTR. One large review of more than 6,000 patients treated with either mastectomy or breast conservation therapy found locoregional recurrence as an isolated recurrence in only 18% of patients (18). Of these, only 33% remained free of distant metastases in long-term follow-up. The usual studies to rule out distant metastases would be a bone scan and computed tomography (CT) scans of the chest, abdomen, and pelvis. There are advocates of positron emission tomography (PET)/CT scans, but the cost and the high false positive rates have limited general acceptance of this as a routine test by most oncologists. For triple-negative or HER2/neu-positive disease, a brain magnetic resonance imaging (MRI) scan might also be considered because of the high percentage of brain metastases in these patients (19–21).

■ HETEROGENEITY OF PROGNOSIS OF PATIENTS WITH LOCOREGIONAL RECURRENCE

If there is no evidence of distant metastases, the focus will be on eradicating the locoregional disease, but the high incidence of subsequent systemic metastases will also prompt the question of the need for systemic therapy. Various centers or cooperative groups have reported their experiences with locoregional recurrence (22–25), and it is apparent that some recurrences have a more favorable prognosis than others. Patients with the highest subsequent systemic recurrent risk after locoregional recurrence include those who had: large (T3 or T4) primary tumors, primary axillary lymph node involvement, high tumor grade, lymphatic or blood vessel invasion, tumor necrosis, negative ER and progesterone receptor (PR), nonaxillary lymph node involvement, recurrence within the first one to two years, nonscar chest wall recurrences, multiple tumor nodules, or tumor nodules larger than 5 cm.

Patients with locoregional recurrence who have a lower subsequent systemic recurrence risk include those with: recurrence confined to the treated breast after breast conservation therapy, a single involved axillary mass (especially if the patient is aged over 50), a small primary tumor, low initial stage, prolonged disease-free interval (more than one year in some studies, more than two to more than five years in others), few sites of involvement by the recurrent disease, and small size of the recurrence.

Clemons and colleagues conducted a survey polling medical, surgical, and radiation breast oncologists in Canada, the United Kingdom, and the United States on their current beliefs regarding the curability of different types of locoregional recurrence (26). There was broad consensus about which recurrences were potentially curable and which were not. Respondents were in broad agreement that "potentially curable" sites of locoregional recurrence included: IBTR, surgical scar after mastectomy, axilla, and chest wall. For recurrences at these sites, surgical excision was recommended. Sites of locoregional recurrence thought not to be curable by a majority of the oncologists included: infraclavicular, internal mammary, supraclavicular, and cervical lymph nodes, although it was pointed out that the difficulty of resecting disease at these sites might have influenced the oncologists' opinions. For locoregional recurrence, 57% of the oncologists recommended extended field radiation after surgery, and 85% recommended systemic therapy if no prior systemic therapy had been given. If locoregional recurrence occurred in a patient while on some form of systemic therapy, 97% recommended a change in systemic therapy. Interestingly, however, the oncologists appeared to be overly optimistic about long-term outcome after locoregional recurrence given the observed high rates of subsequent systemic relapse reported in the literature.

■ DEFINING THE ROLE OF SYSTEMIC THERAPY IN AN INDIVIDUAL PATIENT

Defining the likelihood of a cure with locoregional therapy alone is the important first step in approaching the decision on whether to add systemic therapy. The Clemons survey suggests that most oncologists will recommend a systemic therapy for most patients on the basis of perceived risk alone rather than on documented benefit. In addition to the likelihood of subsequent distant recurrence, the likelihood of failure of surgery, radiation, or both to control the locoregional recurrence can be another reason to add systemic therapy. It is well known that the efficacy of radiation depends on the amount of gross disease in the target; for example, breast radiation is highly successful in local control after lumpectomy with clean margins but less so if margins are involved (27). So too with locoregional recurrence: it is preferable to remove gross disease before radiating, but if this is impossible or too morbid, systemic therapy might be chosen to shrink the target to improve the efficacy of radiation.

The success of locoregional radiation after mastectomy in improving survival in the era of adjuvant systemic therapy, but not in the prior era when systemic therapy was not widely used (28,29), bolsters the hypothesis that systemic therapy and radiation combined would likely be more efficacious than radiation alone for treatment of locoregional recurrence. It is tempting to extrapolate from adjuvant trials that have shown improved locoregional control of disease after breast conservation (with or without radiation) in patients who receive systemic therapy also (4,30,31) and infer that systemic therapy would improve the success of surgery and radiation in controlling locally recurrent disease. There are indeed studies claiming benefit from systemic therapy as part of multimodality therapy for locoregional control of recurrent disease, but other studies report conflicting results. The heterogeneity of cases and lack of randomization make it difficult to generalize about the role of systemic agents for this indication (32).

If systemic therapy is to be considered for locoregional recurrent disease because of high risk of subsequent systemic recurrence, then the likely efficacy of the treatment should also be addressed. Given the lack of data from clinical trials, a logical approach is to consider each case on the basis of its intrinsic biology and the patient's prior history of systemic therapy. For example, triple-negative cancers (estrogen receptor–negative, progesterone receptor–negative, and HER2/neu-negative) are often very responsive to chemotherapy. Some of the highest rates of pathological complete responses to neoadjuvant chemotherapy can be seen in patients with this type of cancer (33). On the other hand, when triple-negative cancers recur after "standard chemotherapy," they tend to respond poorly to salvage chemotherapy (34). Thus, locoregional recurrence in a patient with triple-negative disease who has not received chemotherapy may be approached with an aggressive regimen such as Taxotere, Adriamycin, and Cytoxan (TAC) or adriamycin and cytoxan (AC) followed by a taxane, whereas a patient with recurrent disease after standard therapy might be better served by enrollment in a clinical trial specifically targeting triple-negative cancers. For example, there is currently a lot of interest in using platinum drugs for these patients (35) and in exploring the use of poly(ADP-ribose) polymerase (PARP) inhibitors (36). Since platinum is a radiation sensitizer, patients with triple-negative locoregional recurrence might be suitable for a protocol utilizing concurrent platinum and radiation therapy, as used in recurrent head and neck cancer.

Patients with locoregional recurrence of HER2/neu-positive disease who have not had prior systemic therapy would be excellent candidates for systemic therapy with both chemotherapy and HER2/neu-targeted therapy, with a realistic expectation of excellent benefit. If they had previously received anthracycline-based chemotherapy, trastuzumab and vinorelbine, or trastuzumab and a taxane with or without a platinum drug, or capecitabine plus lapatinib (which has shown activity in patients who have progressed on a trastuzumab-based regimen), would be reasonable choices. Patients with tumors that are strongly ER+ and PR+ and low grade, on the other hand, may not benefit significantly from systemic chemotherapy [by extrapolation from recent analysis of adjuvant trials (37)] but stand to benefit significantly from systemic hormonal therapy. A patient who has had only tamoxifen, or has had only an aromatase inhibitor, could be prescribed the other type of endocrine therapy. If these patients have recurred while on an aromatase inhibitor and have hormone-refractory disease, they may be candidates for chemotherapy. Chemotherapy that seems to work well for indolent ER+ disease includes well-tolerated drugs such as capecitabine or vinorelbine, but since treatment with these single agents is unlikely to be curative, it could be argued that outside of a clinical trial it makes more sense to watch and wait for observable evidence of metastatic disease before initiating therapy unless, as above, systemic therapy is to be used in an attempt to improve locoregional control. Clearly the treating oncologist and the patient need to discuss these options in an individualized way. Sometimes patients may find it difficult to choose to forgo systemic therapy when they feel threatened by the risk of another recurrence; other patients may be happy to avoid toxicity and adopt a "wait and see" approach.

As with systemic adjuvant therapy, the medical oncologist's zeal in prescribing systemic therapy for patients with locoregional recurrence needs to be counterbalanced by the anticipated morbidity, taking into account the patient's age, comorbid conditions, and motivation, as well as the likely toxicity of the proposed regimen.

The published literature on long-term outcomes from treatment of locoregional recurrence may be less relevant to today's patients, who are often the beneficiaries of earlier detection of primary disease (and frequently of their recurrent disease too) and of improvements in therapy for their primary cancers. In contrast to patients in past studies, today's patients are more likely to have had sentinel lymph node mapping rather than a full axillary dissection, so that the significance of an axillary recurrence may be different than previously reported. Patients are also more likely to have had postmastectomy chest wall and regional nodal radiation, adjuvant or neoadjuvant systemic therapy, extended adjuvant endocrine therapy, if appropriate, with an aromatase inhibitor, or targeted adjuvant therapy with trastuzumab for HER2/neu-positive disease. Thus, the patient with locoregional recurrence today may be even more challenging than in the past because of more intense primary therapy. It would be useful, from a medical oncologist's perspective, to simplify the complex literature on locoregional recurrence by categorizing the types of recurrences in the context of prior treatments.

■ DISTINGUISHING TRUE RECURRENCES FROM NEW PRIMARY CANCERS BY MOLECULAR CHARACTERIZATION OF TUMORS

Several recent studies have addressed the importance of distinguishing a true recurrence from a second primary cancer. Traditionally, pathologists looked at the location within the breast, the histology, and the hormone receptors to distinguish recurrent disease from a new primary cancer. More recently, HER2/neu status has been added, but it is well known that HER2/neu expression can be heterogeneous within a tumor. In recent years, studies have been reported using such techniques as flow cytometry (38), loss of heterozygosity of certain markers (39,40), and gene expression arrays (41). These studies have been helpful in distinguishing true recurrences (in the ipsilateral breast, contralateral breast, and contralateral lymph nodes) from new primaries, and this is important, as prognosis is considerably better for a new primary compared with recurrent disease. Interestingly, in a follow-up study (42) comparing the clonality of distant metastases with both the primary tumor and the locally recurrent disease, some cases were found in which the distant metastases seemed to have derived from the locoregional recurrence rather than from the primary tumor. It is, of course, important to recognize that parallel dissemination of a subclone not detected in the primary could populate the locoregional recurrence as well as the distant recurrence, so further work is necessary before this can be fully accepted as a common occurrence. However, if locoregionally recurrent disease can be implicated as a significant source of systemic dissemination, we need to modify our traditional thinking and pay even more attention to minimizing locoregional recurrences, detecting them as early as possible, and treating them aggressively (probably with triple-modality therapy where feasible) when they occur.

One of the most interesting areas of cancer biology is the search for a biological profile that determines metastatic behavior. Primary tumors undoubtedly also have biological attributes that promote locoregional recurrence, and it would be of great interest to know to what degree the genetic signatures for locoregional recurrence and for metastases overlap. Nuyten (43) has reported some data suggesting that a wound signature gene expression profile could distinguish patients with a high (29%) from those with a low (5%) risk of locoregional recurrence at 10 years. If this type of predictor could be validated, then more aggressive locoregional therapy could be attempted for patients with a high local recurrence risk indicated by tumor biology (rather than by traditional factors such as tumor size, close margins, number of involved lymph nodes, and lymphovascular invasion). These patients might benefit from more aggressive systemic therapy at the outset, from concurrent chemotherapy with radiation, or alternatively from a more aggressive surgery (mastectomy versus lumpectomy) or a higher dose of radiation therapy.

■ SUGGESTED GUIDELINES FOR SYSTEMIC THERAPY

To summarize general guidelines based on the published literature, taking into account prognosis, biology of the cancer, and the patient's health and motivation, it would seem reasonable to classify patients with locoregional recurrence as:

- Those likely to do well with surgery alone or surgery with radiation:
  - In-breast recurrence only
  - Isolated resectable axillary recurrence
  - Isolated small chest wall recurrence, especially if in mastectomy scar
  - Low initial stage
  - Recurrence more than two to five years after primary surgery
  - Small volume of recurrence
- Those for whom chemotherapy should be given greater consideration, especially if there was no prior adjuvant chemotherapy:
  - Recurrence in nonaxillary regional lymph nodes, skin of breast or chest wall outside of mastectomy scar

- Recurrence less than one to two years after treatment of the primary cancer
  - Primary tumor large, or with positive lymph nodes or tumor necrosis
  - Grade 3
  - Grade 2 but ER–
  - ER+ but relapsing after two prior hormonal therapies
  - Multiple recurrent nodules or any nodule larger than 5 cm
- Those who should be offered hormonal therapy:
  - ER+, PR+, or both
  - No, or only one, prior hormonal therapy
  - Recurrence after discontinuation of prior hormonal therapy
- Those for whom systemic therapy should be given prior to surgery or radiation, or in conjunction with radiation for symptoms from locoregional recurrence:
  - Bulky locoregional disease
  - Symptoms due to impingement on vascular or neural structures

■ ONGOING CLINICAL TRIALS OF SYSTEMIC THERAPY FOR LOCOREGIONAL RECURRENCE AND FUTURE DIRECTIONS

Several ongoing trials (listed in Cochrane) are trying to address in a prospective fashion the role of systemic therapy in locally recurrent disease. The German Breast Cancer Study Group-Gynecological Adjuvant Study Group Germany GBSG-GABGG trial aims to accrue 500 women with locoregional recurrence and randomize them to locoregional therapy followed by four cycles of doxorubicin 50/docetaxel 75 given once every three weeks or a control group given locoregional therapy only. The Breast International Group, International Breast Cancer Study Group and the National Surgical Adjuvant Breast and Bowel Project BIG 1-02/IBCSG 27-02/NSABP B-37 trial (44) initially planned to randomize 977 women with locoregional recurrence to chemotherapy of the oncologist's choice or no systemic therapy in addition to locoregional treatment; however, because of slow accrual the study has been revised and now aims to accrue only 270 patients, of whom 150 have already enrolled (S. Aebi, personal communication, May 2009). Finally, the Programme Adjuvant Cancer Sein (PACS-03) trial is randomizing 370 women with intramammary recurrence to FEC-100 given every 21 days for three cycles followed by docetaxel 100 mg/m^2 every 21 days for three cycles versus no systemic therapy. Clearly, if a patient with locoregional recurrence is eligible for one of these trials, it would be desirable to encourage participation to improve our understanding of the benefit of systemic therapy for these patients, since so little is currently known about this.

In the future, as the biology of metastases is elucidated, there is a hope that tumor dormancy may be understood and new drugs developed to target dormant cancer cells. Intriguing data already reported in a recent study (45) can be interpreted as suggesting that bisphosphonates may decrease visceral metastases by decreasing the ability of micrometastases in the bone marrow to grow and disseminate from there. In this study, only premenopausal women with hormone receptor–positive cancers were studied, but data from other trials suggest that this may be a more general phenomenon. If it can be proved that the bone marrow is a major site of dormancy and a source of future visceral metastases, then perhaps patients at increased risk of locoregional recurrence (or even with established locoregional recurrence) might also be candidates for bisphosphonates. Antiangiogenic agents or even tumor vaccines might also be useful in this setting. As suggested by Nuyten's work, perhaps prolonged anti-inflammatory treatment could also be a useful systemic treatment to decrease risk of systemic dissemination after locoregional recurrence. Other exciting prospects include the increased use of targeted agents and the possibility of restoring hormone sensitivity to ER+ cells that have become refractory to hormonal therapy.

■ SUMMARY

- Locoregional recurrence is an indicator of increased risk of systemic recurrence.
- Systemic therapy may be considered both to decrease the risk of subsequent systemic recurrence and to improve locoregional control.
- Prospective studies to date have been inadequate to address the benefit of systemic therapy in locoregionally recurrent disease.
- Heterogeneity of sites of locoregional recurrence, biological cancer subtypes, and prior therapies complicate recommendations for systemic therapy.
- Distant metastatic disease should be ruled out at the time locoregionally recurrent disease is found.
- Reported series in the literature suggest that some sites of locoregional recurrence are more favorable than others with respect to systemic recurrence risk.
- In a poll, breast oncologists considered some sites of recurrent disease potentially curable and others not; however, they recommended systemic medical therapy for most patients with recurrent disease.
- The likely efficacy of the systemic therapy, as well as a number of host factors, need to be considered in balancing the potential benefit against the likely toxicity of systemic treatment.

- Recurrent disease needs to be distinguished from new primary disease, and molecular techniques can be helpful in this effort.
- New molecular biological markers for locoregional recurrence are being sought.
- Guidelines for use of systemic therapy take into account site of recurrence, biology of the cancer, prior therapies, and time to recurrence.
- Ongoing, prospective trials are under way to clarify the role of chemotherapy in locally recurrent disease.

■ REFERENCES

1. Mundt AJ, Sibley GS, Williams S, et al. Patterns of failure of complete responders following high dose chemotherapy and autologous bone marrow transplantation for metastatic breast cancer: implications for use of adjuvant radiation therapy. *Int J Radiat Oncol Biol Phys.* 1994;30:151–160.
2. Buchholz TA, Tucker SL, Moore RA, et al. Importance of radiation therapy for breast cancer patients treated with high-dose chemotherapy and stem cell transplant. *Int J Radiat Oncol Biol Phys.* 2000;46:337–343.
3. Fisher B, Jeong J-H, Anderson S, Bryant J, Fisher ER, Wolmark N. Twenty-five-year follow-up of a randomized trial comparing radical mastectomy, total mastectomy, and total mastectomy followed by irradiation. *N Engl J Med.* 2002;347:567–575.
4. Fisher B, Anderson S, Bryant J, et al. Twenty-year follow-up on a randomized trial comparing total mastectomy, lumpectomy, and lumpectomy plus irradiation for the treatment of invasive breast cancer. *N Engl J Med.* 2002;347:1233–1241.
5. Fisher B, Anderson S, Fisher ER, et al. Significance of ipsilateral breast tumour recurrence after lumpectomy. *Lancet.* 1991;338: 327–331.
6. Haffty BG, Reiss M, Beinfield M, Fischer D, Ward B, McKhann C. Ipsilateral breast tumor recurrence as a predictor of distant disease: implications for systemic therapy at the time of local relapse. *J Clin Oncol.* 1996;14:52–57.
7. Fortin A, Larochelle M, Laverdiere J, Lavertu S, Tremblay D. Local failure is responsible for the decrease in survival for patients with breast cancer treated with conservative surgery and postoperative radiotherapy. *J Clin Oncol.* 1999;17:101–109.
8. Wapnir IL, Anderson SJ, Mamounas EP, et al. Prognosis after ipsilateral breast tumor recurrence and locoregional recurrences in five National Surgical Adjuvant Breast and Bowel Project node-positive adjuvant breast cancer trials. *J Clin Oncol.* 2006; 24:2028–2037.
9. Haylock BJ, Coppin CML, Jackson J, Basco VE, Wilson KS. Locoregional first recurrence after mastectomy: prospective cohort studies with and without immediate chemotherapy. *Int J Radiat Oncol Biol Phys.* 2000;46:355–362.
10. Kuo SH, Huang CS, Kuo WH, Cheng AL, Chang KJ, Chia-Hsien Cheng J. Comprehensive locoregional treatment and systemic therapy for postmastectomy isolated locoregional recurrence. *Int J Radiat Oncol Biol Phys.* 2008;72:1456–1464.
11. Rauschecker HHF, Clarke MJ, Gatzemeier W, Recht A. Systemic therapy for treating locoregional recurrence in women with breast cancer. *Cochrane Database Syst Rev.* 2009(2). CD002195.
12. Olson CE, Ansfield FJ, Richards MJ, Ramirez G, Davis HL. Review of local soft tissue recurrence of breast cancer irradiated with and without actinomycin D. *Cancer.* 1977;39:1981–1983.
13. Fentiman IS, Balkwill FR, Cuzick J, Hayward JL, Rubens RD. A trial of human alpha interferon as an adjuvant agent in breast

cancer after loco-regional recurrence. *Eur J Surg Oncol.* 1987;13:425–428.

14. Borner M, Bacchi M, Goldhirsch A, et al. First isolated locoregional recurrence following mastectomy for breast cancer: results of a phase III multicenter study comparing systemic treatment with observation after excision and radiation. *J Clin Oncol.* 1994;12:2071–2077.

15. Waeber M, Castiglione-Gertsch M, Dietrich D, et al. Adjuvant therapy after excision and radiation of isolated postmastectomy locoregional breast cancer: definitive results of a phase III randomized trial (SAKK 23/82) comparing tamoxifen with observation. *Ann Oncol.* 2003;14:1215–1221.

16. Borner MM, Bacchi M, Castiglione M. Possible deleterious effects of tamoxifen in premenopausal women with locoregional recurrence of breast cancer. *Eur J Cancer.* 1996;32A:2173–2176.

17. Clemons M, Danson S, Hamilton T, Goss P. Locoregionally recurrent breast cancer: incidence, risk factors and survival. *Cancer Treat Rev.* 2001;27:67–82.

18. Colleoni M, O'Neill A, Gelber RD, et al. Subsequent sites of recurrence in patients with local, regional and soft tissue relapse: an analysis on 1217 cases. *Proc ASCO.* 1999 (Abstract 300).

19. Nam B-H, Kim SY, Han H-S, et al. Breast cancer subtypes and survival in patients with brain metastases. *Breast Cancer Res.* 2008;10:R20.

20 Dawood S, Broglio K, Esteva FJ, et al. Survival among women with triple-negative breast cancer and brain metastases. *Ann Oncol.* 2009;20:621–627.

21. Lin NU, Winer EP. Brain metastases: the HER2 paradigm. *Clin Cancer Res.* 2007;13:1648–1655.

22. Buchanan CL, Dorn PL, Fey J, et al. Locoregional recurrence after mastectomy: incidence and outcomes. *J Am Coll Surg.* 2006;203:469–474.

23. Willner J, Kiricuta IC, Kolbl O. Locoregional recurrence of breast cancer following mastectomy: always a fatal event? Results of univariate and multivariate analysis. *Int J Radiat Oncol Biol Phys.* 1997;37:853–863.

24. Moran MS, Haffty BG. Local-regional breast cancer recurrence: prognostic groups based on patterns of failure. *Breast J.* 2002;8:81–87.

25. Schwaibold F, Fowble BL, Solin LJ, Schultz DJ, Goodman RL. The results of radiation therapy for isolated local regional recurrence after mastectomy. *Int J Radiat Oncol Biol Phys.* 1991; 21:299–310.

26. Clemons M, Hamilton T, Mansi J, Lockwood G, Goss P. Management of recurrent locoregional breast cancer: oncologist survey. *Breast.* 2003;328–337.

27. Schnitt SJ, Abner A, Gelman R, et al. The relationship between microscopic margins of resection and the risk of local recurrence in patients with breast cancer treated with breast-conserving surgery and radiation therapy. *Cancer.* 1994;74:1746–1751.

28. Overgaard M, Hansen PS, Overgaard J, et al. Postoperative radiotherapy in high-risk premenopausal women with breast cancer who receive adjuvant chemotherapy. *N Engl J Med.* 1997;337:949–955.

29. Ragaz J, Jackson SM, Le N, et al. Adjuvant radiotherapy and chemotherapy in node-positive premenopausal women with breast cancer. *N Engl J Med.* 1997;337:956–962.

30. Levine MN, Bramwell V, Abu-Zahra H, et al. The effect of systemic adjuvant chemotherapy on local breast recurrence in node positive breast cancer patients treated by lumpectomy without radiation. *Br J Cancer.* 1992;65:130–132.

31. Haffty BG, Wilmarth L, Wilson L, Fischer D, Beinfeld M, McKhann C. Adjuvant systemic chemotherapy and hormonal therapy. Effect on local recurrence in the conservatively treated breast cancer patient. *Cancer.* 1994;73:2543–2548.

32. Clemons M, Hamilton T, Goss P. Does treatment at the time of locoregional failure of breast cancer alter prognosis? *Cancer Treat Rev.* 2001;27:83–97.

33. Liedtke C, Mazouni C, Hess KR, et al. Response to neoadjuvant therapy and long-term survival in patients with triple-negative breast cancer. *J Clin Oncol.* 2008;26:1275–1281.

34. Dent R, Trudeau M, Pritchard KI, et al. Triple-negative breast cancer: clinical features and patterns of recurrence. *Clin Cancer Res.* 2007;13:4429–4434.

35. Sirohi B, Arnedos M, Popat S, et al. Platinum-based chemotherapy in triple-negative breast cancer. *Ann Oncol.* 2008;19:1847–1852.

36. Tan AR, Swain SM. Therapeutic strategies for triple-negative breast cancers. *Cancer J.* 2008;14:343–351.

37. Berry DA, Cirrincione C, Henderson IC, et al. Estrogen receptor status and outcomes of modern chemotherapy for patients with node-positive breast cancer. *JAMA.* 2006;295:1658–1667.

38. Smith TE, Lee D, Turner BC, Carter D, Haffty BG. True recurrence vs. new primary ipsilateral breast tumor relapse: an analysis of clinical and pathologic differences and their implications in natural history, prognoses, and therapeutic management. *Int J Radiat Oncol Biol Phys.* 2000;48:1281–1289.

39. Vicini FA, Antonucci JV, Goldstein N, et al. The use of molecular assays to establish definitively the clonality of ipsilateral breast tumor recurrences and patterns of in-breast failure in patients with early stage breast cancer treated with breast-conserving therapy. *Cancer.* 2007;109:1264–1272.

40. Goldstein NS, Vicini FA, Hunter S, et al. Molecular clonality determination of ipsilateral recurrence of invasive breast carcinomas after breast-conserving therapy: comparison with clinical and biologic factors. *Am J Clin Pathol.* 2005;123:679–689.

41. Schlechter BL, Yang Q, Larson PS, et al. Quantitative DNA fingerprinting may distinguish new primary breast cancer from disease recurrence. *J Clin Oncol.* 2004;22:1830–1838.

42. Vicini FA, Goldstein NS, Wallace M, Kestin L. Molecular evidence demonstrating local treatment failure is the source of distant metastases in some patients treated for breast cancer. *Int J Radiat Oncol Biol Phys.* 2008;71:689–694.

43. Nuyten DS, Kreike B, Hart AA, et al. Predicting a local recurrence after breast-conserving therapy by gene expression profiling. *Breast Cancer Res.* 2006;8:R62.

44. Wapnir IL, Aebi S, Gelber S, et al. Progress on BIG 1-02/IBCSG 27-02/NSABP B-37, a prospective randomized trial evaluating chemotherapy after local therapy for isolated locoregional recurrences of breast cancer. *Ann Surg Oncol.* 2008;15:3227–3231.

45. Gnant M, Mlineritsch B, Schippinger W, et al. Endocrine therapy plus zoledronic acid in premenopausal breast cancer. *N Engl J Med.* 2009;360:679–691.

12 Multidisciplinary Approach to the Patient's Quality of Life

Multidisciplinary Approach to Quality of Life

LIDIA SCHAPIRA

Health-related quality of life is an important determinant of outcome in the treatment of breast cancer. This chapter addresses definitions and measurements available for use in research trials and clinical settings. Special considerations when treating young and geriatric patients are addressed. The impact of physical symptoms is discussed, as well as the importance of screening for emotional distress and appropriate referral. Common concerns such as the effect of treatment on sexuality, fertility, and physical function are reviewed, as well as the challenges associated with parenting for women after a diagnosis of cancer. Finally, coping with the knowledge of increased genetic risk is explored, and practice recommendations are offered for follow-up of survivors and treatment of women living with advanced cancer.

■ DEFINITIONS AND MEASUREMENT

Early in the history of medicine, physicians recognized the importance of individual perceptions in shaping interpretations of a patient's state of health and quality of life. In a recent review of this topic, Bottomley (1) references the work of Rosser (2), who reminds us that ancient Greeks performed theatrical evening plays in hospital theatres and carefully "observed and recorded" the patients' expressions. The reactions to both comedy and tragedy were noted, as well as the range of emotions displayed. Centuries later, Karnofsky introduced a formal performance scale. This subsequently became the gold standard for measurement of a patient's general state of health (3). It allowed objective assessment of a patient's abilities, role functioning, and need for care. Easy to use, the Karnofsky score has enjoyed remarkable success, although it is not very precise, ignores the patient's emotions and feelings, and depends completely on the clinician's judgment. The brilliance of Karnofsky's contribution was in recognizing that researchers needed to include an assessment of the patient's quality of life as an independent outcome measure. This paved the way for the current emphasis placed on documenting the impact of new treatments on patient well-being. This is relevant and important to all cancer professionals irrespective of their specific disciplines. Surgeons and medical and radiation oncologists alike need to be mindful of a patient's symptoms and the impact of the disease and its treatment on her life and that of her family. Two of the earliest papers on quality of life in breast cancer date back to the mid to late 1970s and deserve special mention. In 1974, Moore and colleagues reported on the effects of adrenalectomy and chemotherapy with 5-fluorouracil on the treatment of advanced breast cancer (4). They asked the question "Does the achievement of a remission actually mean a longer and better life for the patient, or is it merely a transient medical improvement, of little actual worth in an otherwise downhill course?" Results showed that effective disease palliation was accompanied by a return to near-normal living (4). The second early paper was published by Priestman and Baum in 1976 and introduced a linear analog self-assessment to measure the subjective effects of treatment in women with advanced breast cancer (5). They suggested that assessment tools could be used to monitor and compare toxicities of various chemotherapeutic regimens, a concept that we now take for granted and that constitutes a requirement of clinical trial design.

A large body of research has been devoted to conceptualizing and measuring health-related quality of life. Montazeri published a bibliographic review of the literature on health-related quality of life in breast cancer for the period between 1947 and 2007 and identified 477 papers, which were examined in some detail (6). Broadly, quality of life measures can be classified as general, disease-specific, and site-specific. Instruments that have emerged provide valid tools to measure social, physical, psychological, and sexual function, symptoms of disease, and side effects of treatment. Medical, radiation, and surgical oncologists typically concentrate on assessments of physical functioning, symptoms, and side effects and inconsistently address psychological functioning. Yet it is now well established that psychological functioning, as well as social functioning (which refers to the ability to interact with family and friends, continue working, and enjoy recreational activities), is also integral to individual perceptions of quality of life.

The most commonly used instruments for measurement of health-related quality of life are the European Organisation for Research and Treatment of Cancer (EORTC) tool developed by Aronson, and Cella's functional assessment of cancer therapy (FACT). Both have been validated and translated into many languages (6–11). The EORTC core instrument, known as the Quality of Life Questionnaire, or QLQ-30, incorporates nine multi-item scales to assess physical, role, cognitive, emotional, and social function; three symptom scales to measure fatigue, pain, and nausea and vomiting; and one global health and quality of life scale. FACT-B is a 46-item self-report instrument designed to measure multidimensional quality of life (12) that has been administered as a research tool and also in clinical settings. Other instruments were developed specifically for the assessment of psychological function and are used to detect distress, anxiety, depression, mood disorders, and other common psychiatric conditions among patients with chronic illness or among the general population. Among these is the Hospital Anxiety and Depression Scale (HADS), which, although developed as a research tool, is also used as a screening tool and has the advantage of being brief (13–15). Another commonly used instrument is the Medical Outcomes Study Short Form (SF-36), which was designed for use in both clinical practice and research. This measures eight aspects of functional status, well-being, and self-perceived health (16). The SF-36 has been widely used in breast cancer studies, and a shorter version, the SF-12, is available as a quick screen for quality of life. The Brief Symptom Inventory (BSI) was used in an early multicenter study and measures changes in level of distress over time (17). For more than a decade the BSI has been used for psychosocial screening of patients seen at the Johns Hopkins Oncology Center (11,18). Using this approach clinicians then refer patients who are identified as showing distress to a mental health professional or trained social worker. The BSI is a 53-item measure written at a sixth grade reading level that requires – five to seven minutes to complete. A shorter, 18-item version has been developed by Zabora (19). The Cancer Rehabilitation Evaluation System (CARES) instrument was one of the first cancer-specific quality of life instruments and has helped identify special rehabilitation needs of cancer patients (20–23). CARES has been extensively used by Ganz and colleagues in studies of symptom management and quality of life (11,24).

Discussion, assessment, and incorporation of quality of life measures are now common parlance. However, some experts continue to argue that there is still no conceptual basis for quality of life measures (25). As described in preceding paragraphs, these assessments were initially developed to monitor more closely the outcome of medical interventions. The problem is that these determinations are increasingly patient driven and rely on self-reporting, and this, in turn, depends on the individual's psyche, value systems, and opinions. Moreover, some studies simply use a validated instrument because of its availability, and the information does not really contribute to our knowledge or understanding of the topic. Just how much "control" of measurements should be given to patients or participants in trials is still debated and influences the body of emerging knowledge. Current assessments do not accurately reflect individual or cultural values that impact self-perceived fulfillment and happiness, although this is another important locus of study for social scientists and those interested in comparing results among different populations.

■ SCREENING FOR DISTRESS

Distress is an unpleasant emotional experience of a psychological (cognitive, behavioral, emotional), social, or spiritual nature that may interfere with the ability to cope effectively with cancer (26). It extends along a continuum, from normal feelings of vulnerability, sadness, and fears to problems that can become disabling, such as anxiety, depression, panic, social isolation, and existential crisis (26). The National Comprehensive Cancer Network (NCCN) task force chose the term "distress" over any existing psychiatric terms in order to eliminate any embarrassment or stigma associated with the cancer diagnosis.

Published guidelines for the recognition and management of distress in clinical practice (27) are available online and include recommendations for routine screening using the NCCN Distress Thermometer and Problem List. Patients are asked to rate with measurements on a scale of 1 to 10 how distressed they have been over the preceding week. This is accompanied by a problem list in which patients see a list of common concerns and are asked to check off those that are personally relevant. These tools provide a visual and practical aid for identifying problems related to childcare, housing, insurance, transportation, work, and family issues. They also assess emotional problems and physical symptoms relating to the disease itself or its treatment. They are intended for use by the primary oncology team to determine the particular psychosocial services needed. Patients who score five or higher on the thermometer scale are identified as having a significant measure of distress. Following practice guidelines, they are then referred for supportive services according to both need and availability. This brief screen has been implemented in different settings and in many countries and is well suited for use in busy offices and clinics. The panel recommended that a multidisciplinary institutional committee should be formed to implement standards for distress management and that educational and training programs be developed to ensure that healthcare professionals and pastoral caregivers have knowledge and skills for the assessment of distress (26).

Patients and families should be informed that screening for distress is an integral aspect of the total medical care and provided with appropriate information about psychosocial services in the community and the treatment facility. Patients at increased risk for significant distress include those with a past history of psychiatric disease or substance abuse, those with a history of depression or prior suicidality, and those with cognitive impairment or communication barriers. Periods of increased vulnerabilities range from the first finding of suspicious symptoms to most medical transitions (26).

■ FROM RESEARCH TO PRACTICE

There is consensus among scientists and clinicians regarding the importance of assessing cancer patients' needs and function in objective ways, responding to individual concerns and remaining attentive to psychological well-being throughout the disease trajectory. The science of health-related quality of life has evolved considerably in the past three decades, and we now have an abundance of validated instruments and tools used in research. Controversial areas remain regarding the subjectivity of the data, occasional lack of concordance between professional grading by healthcare professionals and patient self-reports, and the validity of a patient's perspective (25–28).

Little is known about the dissemination and uptake of NCCN guidelines for psychosocial distress or the delivery of psychosocial services to women with breast cancer. A survey of oncologists published by Pirl and colleagues (29) showed that less than one third of responders were at least somewhat familiar with these guidelines. Although the majority replied that they routinely screened for distress, only a few used a validated screening instrument (28). A companion study reported that most oncologists actually deliver some level of psychosocial care, including initiating medical therapy for anxiety and depression, and that only half have affiliated mental health services (30). Despite the study limitations, these data suggest that there are currently no standardized practices in the United States, and indeed patients may not have access to proper screening and referral for psychological problems or assistance with practical issues. If basic needs such as transportation, child care, and loss of income or lack of affordability

of medications are not addressed, the consequence is that those with fewer resources or greater psychological morbidity will receive substandard care.

In 2002, the Institute of Medicine (IOM) held a comprehensive workshop and subsequently published a monograph to address the psychosocial needs of women with breast cancer (11). This was followed by the publication in 2007 of the IOM report, "Cancer Care for the Whole Patient" (31). The latter examines the psychosocial health services from the perspective of cancer survivors. The report indicates that attention to psychosocial health needs is the exception rather than the rule in oncology practice and puts forth a vision for a system of care that routinely integrates psychosocial services into the medical care of cancer patients (30). The IOM report notes that psychosocial obstacles can interfere with a patient's healthcare and diminish her health and functioning. Furthermore, the impact of emotional and social issues can be significantly reduced through effective communication between patients and healthcare professionals. Patients should be encouraged to take an active role in addressing any and all issues they are worried about by asking questions and volunteering information that may not be obvious to clinicians trained to focus on physical function and treatment of disease. Clinicians need to have some knowledge of the resources available to their patients in the community. These many include national or local volunteer societies, support groups, chaplains, financial counselors, and mental health professionals. It is now clear that appropriate services can provide an enormous benefit to the patient's overall care and contribute to her sense of well-being.

■ ADDRESSING THE NEEDS OF YOUNG WOMEN WITH BREAST CANCER

There is some evidence to suggest that women under the age of 50—nearly a quarter of all those diagnosed with breast cancer—are especially vulnerable to physical and psychosocial immediate and late effects of their treatment (32,33). This topic was addressed at a National Cancer Institute (NCI) conference, and a monograph was published in 1994 (32). Concerns expressed by young patients and survivors are related to all areas previously described as important determinants of self-reported quality of life. Certain issues deserve special mention and include changes in body image, sexuality, consequences of a premature menopause on physical and psychological function, preservation of fertility, and the effect of diagnosis and prognosis on a woman's ability to remain in her role as primary caregiver for her children. For women diagnosed during pregnancy, the added decisional conflict regarding treatment options poses special challenges to the medical team. For those diagnosed shortly after pregnancy, conflicting emotions, as well as the needs of the infant, require that oncology clinicians display great sensitivity and ideally include a mental health professional in the care team.

Studies of young breast cancer survivors show that the possible loss of fertility (which occurs as an unintended consequence of cancer treatment) can be as painful as the diagnosis of cancer itself (34–36). Qualitative studies and clinical experience indicate that women want to achieve their goal of motherhood (37). In many instances, the desire for a biological child becomes the vehicle for expression of hope for a normal future. A substantial proportion of young women do remain premenopausal after modern adjuvant chemotherapy for early-stage breast cancer (38). However, menstruation is a poor surrogate for fertility, especially as women age. Increased incidence of amenorrhea is associated with use of alkylators and older age (39). At present there are sparse data on actual fertility and pregnancy outcomes following chemotherapy in breast cancer survivors. Even in the absence of rigorously defined ovarian failure, women may experience varying degrees of short-term and long-term ovarian dysfunction after chemotherapy, presumably due to destruction of ovarian follicles or due to a natural decrease in ovarian function over the time required to take hormonal therapy. Ongoing research to find better estimates of ovarian reserve following chemotherapy will allow survivors to estimate their need for contraception and likelihood of future pregnancy (Partridge, personal communication).

Responding to patients' concerns and advances in reproductive technologies, the American Society of Clinical Oncology convened a panel of experts to develop guidelines for fertility preservation in cancer patients. Their recommendations, published in 2006, state that oncologists should address the possibility of infertility in patients treated during their reproductive years and be prepared to discuss possible fertility preservation options or refer appropriate and interested patients to reproductive specialists (40). In order for clinicians to discuss this aspect of care as early as possible during treatment planning, it is important for the multidisciplinary team to have a coordinated and consistent approach. Following these recommendations necessitates a quick referral mechanism to reproductive specialists who are willing to collaborate with the cancer team in providing guidance and specialized services. Many of the available techniques or strategies for fertility preservation have not been fully evaluated in terms of both efficacy and safety for breast cancer patients. These limitations complicate referrals and discussions and may dampen the enthusiasm of specialists and patients alike. Faced with a young woman recently diagnosed, the oncologist needs to provide personalized recommendations that are based on considerations of relapse risk, safety data, and personal preference (41–43). If initiation of systemic breast cancer treatment can be delayed for several weeks, it is possible to refer newly diagnosed patients to a reproductive specialist who can guide her and weigh pros and cons of available options. Ovarian stimulation and oocyte harvesting followed by in vitro fertilization (IVF) is the only widely available, effective procedure for fertility preservation, with an excellent track record among infertile couples. In women with breast cancer it has been hypothesized that the supraphysiological estradiol levels arising from conventional ovarian stimulation might increase a woman's risk of recurrence, particularly for women with hormone receptor–positive disease (41). Given this uncertainty, as well as the possibility that delay in the initiation of systemic therapy may negatively impact outcome, only a small proportion of young breast cancer patients utilize this option. Recent studies, nonrandomized and with short follow-ups, have reported favorable results regarding the use of assisted reproductive technologies for young breast cancer patients. However, the data do not yet allow us to routinely recommend these practices for all patients.

■ BODY IMAGE AND SEXUALITY

A woman's satisfaction with her body and her sexual function can be assessed by interviews or questionnaires. There is a vast literature that addresses personal satisfaction with cosmetic results following primary surgery and no simple formula for predicting or measuring personal satisfaction following breast conservation or mastectomy. Early studies showed, and clinicians have often observed, that women who are invited to participate in decision making regarding primary surgery, are given sufficient information, and feel heard and respected are more likely to cope better postoperatively. Whether women who preserve their breast have more positive feelings towards their bodies remains an area of some controversy.

In a review of the impact of breast cancer on sexuality and body image, Schover notes that a woman's overall psychological health, relationship satisfaction, and premorbid sexual life appear to be far stronger predictors of postcancer sexual satisfaction than is the extent of damage to her breast (44). Available studies unfortunately do not approach the level of specificity necessary to address the physiological basis for sexual problems, and most studies do not include any assessment of sexual function prior to diagnosis. Suffice it to say that sexual dysfunction is more likely a consequence of premature or severe menopausal symptoms secondary to chemotherapy and endocrine therapy (44). As increasing numbers of women are prescribed long courses of endocrine treatments, we will learn more about quality of life measures and sexual side effects associated with specific medications.

For premenopausal women who undergo chemotherapy, the likelihood of premature menopause is a real concern and increases with age at the time of treatment (44).

Some premenopausal women are also treated with ovarian ablation, thus exposing them to low levels of circulating estrogen for at least a few years, if not indefinitely. They typically experience symptoms of ovarian failure, which include hot flashes, loss of vaginal lubrication, and eventual atrophy of the vulva and vaginal walls. These cause dryness, itching, and dyspareunia. Treatment with local estrogen remains an effective option, although in practice many young women are reluctant to use these medications for fear of increasing their risk of relapse. Experts recommend that every woman with breast cancer should be asked about sexual function and concerns by a member of her primary oncology team. One or two brief questions are sufficient to at least identify the women who need more time for symptom assessment and possibly triage to an expert. It is important for clinicians to be alert to the fact that some women are at higher risk for sexual and relationship problems. These include younger women, those without a committed partner, and those in unhappy relationships or with a prior history of sexual problems or trauma (44). In addition to screening for possible sexual dysfunction, it is important to provide accurate information to all women and avoid making assumptions based on a woman's age or marital status. Elements of brief counseling or education may include specific advice about resuming an active sex life, asking about difficulties such as loss of libido, discussing use of lubricants, addressing pain related to arm edema or chest wall discomfort, talking about scars and consequences of reconstruction, and guiding a woman to better communicate with her partner. Finally, it is important for one designated member of the multidisciplinary team to be knowledgeable in this area or provide a referral to a sex therapist for those who need or request additional help. There are no data about the frequency of discussions between women and oncology professionals about sexual issues. It is likely that only a minority of patients receive guidance, information, and support in these matters, despite substantial evidence that they are an integral feature of health-related quality of life.

■ PARENTING

Parenting concerns are of paramount importance to women with breast cancer. Clinicians know that the desire to remain alive and well for the sake of minor children often influences a woman's choice of primary surgical and adjuvant therapy. Maternal distress and depression impact family function and may have lasting effects on the emotional life of a patient's children (45). Despite the overwhelming need to provide consistent advice, information, and support to women, there are no available guidelines. Experience with a parent guidance program at the Massachusetts General Hospital established by Rauch in

1995 offers clear recommendations for practice and has been well received by families and staff at our institution (46–48).

Physicians and nurses of various disciplines can provide helpful tips to their patients for coping with the disease. Mothers are typically eager to talk about their children and welcome expressions of concern from their doctors. Many mothers imagine that their children will experience a magnified version of their own reaction. They are often reassured to learn that children are typically resilient and will take cues from their parents. Helping patients requires an understanding of child development that is beyond the scope of most oncology clinicians. A child psychologist, psychiatrist, or trained social worker can help the multidisciplinary team and provide psycho-education and support to patients.

On the basis of the experience of the parenting program at the Massachusetts General Hospital, parents are encouraged to be honest and strive for frank communication with children (49). Learning about cancer indirectly, such as by overhearing a parent talking on the phone, is problematic and may lead to confusion and an exacerbation of fears. Euphemisms are more apt to cause fear than the word "cancer" and may contribute to future misunderstandings (46–49). A developmental approach allows clinicians to give tailored advice. Preschool children, who have magical thinking, may well imagine they are the cause of events and may need constant reminders of the fact that they are not responsible for their mother's illness. School-age children (7 to 12 years) are old enough to understand that the cancer is not caused by their actions. At this age they expect an orderly and fair world and may have rigid notions of causality that need to be explored and addressed. Adolescents can understand the full meaning of a cancer diagnosis, including uncertainty about prognosis and the absence of guarantees. They usually do better when parents offer empathy regarding the stress of uncertainty and provide hopeful strategies (47,49). Parenting adolescents is often stressful, and the added complication of maternal illness needs to be negotiated with wisdom and sensitivity. The challenge faced by patients is to allow the adolescent the necessary freedom while preserving and protecting family time.

Oncology teams can provide appropriate guidance for parents and steer them away from burdening their children with adult roles. In the course of typical medical office visits for patients receiving adjuvant therapy, returning for scheduled follow-ups, or living with advanced disease, doctors and nurses can provide models for open and respectful communication and address issues of family communication as well. By reminding patients that the best approach is to welcome questions even if they have no immediate answers, to link medical news to observable changes, to seek out opportunities to talk, and to connect their children with other adults who may provide guidance, we can assist our patients in coping with their disease.

■ MORBIDITY SECONDARY TO PHYSICAL AND COGNITIVE SYMPTOMS

Women living with breast cancer are likely to experience many uncomfortable physical symptoms. These range from postoperative pain and local complications of surgery and reconstruction to side effects of adjuvant chemotherapy and the more pervasive and chronic untoward effects associated with endocrine therapy. Certain physical and cognitive symptoms and side effects are commonly described and bear mentioning as they are likely to impact quality of life.

Pain deserves special mention and attention from healthcare professionals. With the widespread use of pain scales and the recognition and acceptance of pain's negative impact on function and well-being, there is no reason to withhold adequate pain relief. Cancer pain may result from direct invasion of tumor into nerves, bones, soft tissue, and fascia and may induce visceral pain through distension and obstruction. For patients with unusual pain syndromes, a consultation with a pain specialist or palliative care physician can help identify adequate strategies for pain control. Barriers to adequate pain relief include specific concerns of patients themselves or their family members and the reluctance of healthcare professionals to formulate appropriate treatment plans. After 20 years of use, the World Health Organization analgesic ladder still serves as the mainstay of treatment. Nonopioid analgesics are tried first for mild pain, and opioids are used for treatment of severe cancer-related pain. To maintain freedom from pain, drugs should be given "by the clock", that is every three to six hours, rather than on demand. Multidisciplinary approaches to pain management include the consideration of palliative radiation for skeletal complications in addition to bisphosphonates, surgical palliation for patients with bulky local masses, and psychological and physical rehabilitation for patients with an extensive symptomatic burden.

Fatigue is one of the most common symptoms experienced by cancer patients. The prevalence varies widely depending on how it is measured and which populations of patients are studied (50–52). Prevalence estimates vary as a result of the lack of systematic assessments, unknown physiological mechanism, and lack of rigorous longitudinal follow-up. Two of the most plausible mechanisms to explain this prevalent symptom are the release of physiological mediators as a result of an abnormal inflammatory response and disruption of the hypothalamic pituitary adrenal axis in patients with advanced disease (53). Most investigators refer to some variant of the definition proposed by the NCCN, which defines cancer-related fatigue as an "unusual, persistent, subjective sense of tiredness related to cancer or cancer treatment that interferes with usual functioning" (54). The definition fails to include two important distinguishing aspects, which are that it does not improve with rest and sleep and that the symptoms are disproportionate to the individual's level of physical exertion (55). In addition to tiredness, numerous descriptors have been applied in conceptualizing cancer-related fatigue, including lethargy, weariness and exhaustion (51). Cancer-related fatigue has also been described in terms of deficiency, such as lack of energy, vigor, or vitality. Numerous scales have been developed to obtain more precise assessments. The Profile of Mood States (POMS) Fatigue Scale is one of the most frequently used single-dimensional subscales (56).

A wide range of nonpharmacological and pharmacological interventions have been used. A general approach includes strategies for energy conservation such as setting priorities, pacing, delegating, scheduling activities at peak energy, labor-saving devices, postponing nonessential activities, limiting daytime naps, and structuring daily routines. Exercise programs, rehabilitation, and behavioral interventions such as cognitive behavioral therapy have been tried and may be helpful to individual patients. However, to date there are no firm data relating to effectiveness on which to base a recommendation for any of these interventions. Exercise is routinely recommended and widely assumed to have no ill effects. NCCN guidelines recommend treating any reversible causes of fatigue such as anemia, poor nutrition, or depression and attending to general supportive measures and psychological support. The only specific drug recommendation is for the use of the psychostimulant methylphenidate. The data upon which this is based were extrapolated from studies of patients with other chronic conditions and should therefore be viewed with caution when considering breast cancer survivors (50). A systematic review and meta-analysis of the pharmacological treatment of cancer-related fatigue found no evidence of efficacy for the antidepressant paroxetine, good evidence that treatment of anemia is helpful, and insufficient data to evaluate the possible role of psychostimulants (50).

Systematic approaches for assessing and intervening are recommended for implementation in outpatient cancer treatment centers. Fatigue is practically considered the sixth "vital sign" (57–59), routinely assessed (by self-report) at our institution at every visit, and documented in the medical record. At the Massachusetts General Hospital clinicians and patients have access to a formal fatigue program staffed by a psychiatrist with expertise in treatment of cancer-related fatigue and symptom management.

There is considerable interest among patients and clinicians as to the effects of chemotherapy on cognitive function. For some, the fear of this side effect enters into their decision regarding treatment. The range of reported deficits in function relate specifically to language skills, short-term memory, spatial abilities, and speed of information processing.

This area also suffers from a lack of rigorous definitions, prediagnostic assessment of functions, and proper longitudinal follow-up. Data are not strong enough at the moment to establish causality between treatment and cognitive decline. It is quite possible that subtle, but physiologically and personally meaningful functionality is diminished as a result of the diagnosis or its treatment. Until studies are better able to define the syndrome and provide specific interventions, it seems most appropriate to record each patient's symptoms and offer support and guidance as needed.

■ COPING

Several factors have been identified that help patients cope with the diagnosis and treatment of cancer. These include having a positive outlook, the ability to take things a day at a time, remaining optimistic, meeting a challenge head-on, having enough information about the treatment, its goals, and possible side-effects, and having a caring and supportive medical team and a belief system that gives meaning to life (60). In contrast, individuals who seem unable to make a decision, cannot prioritize their concerns or questions, appear excessively needy, or have a pessimistic outlook are quite likely having a very difficult time coping and require additional assistance (60).

Clinicians can assist patients by reminding them to live one day at a time, listening to expressed concerns without interrupting, helping patients to avoid blaming themselves for their diagnosis, and asking how they have effectively coped with other major crises in their lives. Creating a shame-free environment and helping patients feel safe during medical visits is a major aspect of good-quality care. Patients should be encouraged to discuss use of complementary and alternative therapies or their reluctance to take prescribed medication. Listening and responding in a nonjudgmental way will lead to more productive communication and the establishment of a collaborative relationship between doctors and patients. Other useful interventions include a recommendation to keep a journal, which can be used both to provide accurate information about symptoms and use of prescribed medications and as a venue for self-expression.

Peer support, defined as a relationship in which people with a shared condition provide emotional support to each other and share knowledge about dealing effectively with that condition, constitutes a valuable resource. It helps to bolster self-efficacy, which is increasingly viewed as a key predictor of how effectively an individual will persevere and cope in the face of adversity. Peer support programs can provide one-on-one support, as in the American Cancer Society's Reach to Recovery program, or support from groups. For patients living in remote areas who have access to the Internet, web-based support groups can provide this service. It is natural for patients and families to access the Internet hoping to find useful information and to be confused by the vast number of sites and claims. The American Society of Clinical Oncology's website for the public, Cancer.Net, provides up-to-date information that is vetted by experts and includes sections that are disease-specific as well as information about coping with cancer. Brochures and printed literature are also available free of charge from the society for members and are intended to provide a service to their patients.

A number of effective psychosocial interventions have been reported to help women deal with the stress of diagnosis and treatment. Goodwin reviewed 31 randomized trials in women with breast cancer and two meta-analyses and concluded they had beneficial effects in both early and metastatic breast cancer (61). She found evidence for benefit of relaxation/hypnosis/imagery interventions in early-stage disease, for group support interventions in both early and metastatic disease, and for individual interventions primarily in the early setting (61). Subsequent studies have added to the level of evidence suggesting that psychosocial interventions of many kinds can favorably impact quality of life for patients with breast cancer.

■ COPING WITH GENETIC RISK

As the number of women undergoing genetic testing increases, it becomes all the more important that clinicians understand the human factors influencing choices to proceed with testing, adhere to screening practices, undergo risk reduction surgery, and opt for chemoprevention or participation in clinical trials evaluating new interventions aimed at reducing risk. It is also important to consider these issues in the context of family and community and to recognize the key role of information and communication in shaping decisions and promoting healthy coping. Important challenges affecting individuals from high-risk families are how to bear the uncertainty associated with being a carrier of a known mutation, how to deal with inconclusive test results, and how and when to transmit sensitive information to family members and minor children (64).

It can take years before a positive test result is sometimes conveyed by the tested individual to sisters, brothers, adult children, stepchildren, or parents due to psychological hesitancies that take precedence over the perceived "duty" to inform (62–64). One aspect of genetic testing for *BRCA1/2* that has far-reaching implications but that has not been well studied is the impact of testing on the family unit. Policy statements have been issued by the ASCO (American Society of Clinical Oncology) and the ASHG (American Society of Human Genetics) discouraging the testing of minors. Little is known, however, of how and when children learn of their mothers' test results and their interpretation of them. Studies have shown that mothers' motivations for testing often revolve around their belief that the information gathered will be useful to their children (65).

Ongoing research is evaluating the effectiveness of decision aids to help individuals facing these situations. Future research will hopefully shed more light on the relationship between cultural expectations and personal beliefs in informing health-related choices and behaviors. Recommendations from physicians are powerful motivators for lifestyle and behavioral changes, and yet healthcare professionals receive little or no training in counseling. Multidisciplinary teams need to have a designated expert trained in genetic counseling and the longitudinal follow-up of women identified as being at high risk for developing breast cancer.

■ SPECIAL CONSIDERATIONS FOR THE MULTIDISCIPLINARY TREATMENT OF GERIATRIC PATIENTS

Breast cancer is common in older women, and the segment of the US population aged 65 years and older is growing rapidly. In both the geriatric and oncology literature, an individual's functional status is one of the strongest predictors of overall survival and resource requirement. However, the measures traditionally used in oncology practice to assess functional status in patients of all ages—and to determine the course of treatment—do not identify the subtle degrees of functional impairment that predict morbidity and mortality in the geriatric population. The International Society of Geriatric Oncology created a task force to assess the available evidence on breast cancer in elderly individuals and to provide evidence-based recommendations for clinicians. The panel published a review of the published work between 1990 and 2007 and of abstracts from key international conferences. Recommendations were offered on many topics, including screening, surgery, radiotherapy, (neo)adjuvant hormonal therapy, and treatment of metastatic disease (66). The NCCN Breast Cancer in the Older Woman Task Force was convened to provide a forum for framing relevant questions on topics that impact older women with breast cancer (67). These experts remarked on the sparse data available to guide clinical practice. This is a consequence of the fact that elderly women have been underrepresented in breast clinical trials, with the majority of studies being restricted to patients aged below 70. Since elderly patients frequently have comorbidities and impaired organ function, they are at risk from death from causes other than cancer, potentially nullifying the benefit of adjuvant treatment (67). Furthermore, they render extrapolation of standard treatment recommendations to the elderly potentially hazardous, particularly with respect to chemotherapy (67).

There is remarkable biological diversity among older individuals that makes chronological age a poor proxy for physiological function. In fact, labeling a patient as "old" is a matter of opinion. Fit individuals in their mid-sixties are likely to consider themselves middle aged and may well have a life expectancy of more than two decades. Aging is associated with a functional decline in many organ systems, which often becomes apparent at a time of stress. There is a greater prevalence of comorbid conditions and memory disorders, increased dependence, and decreased social and economic support. Estimates of life expectancy are useful to frame discussion of therapeutic options. Tools have been developed for use in the oncology clinic for estimating life expectancy and tolerance of treatment and for identifying reversible factors that may interfere with cancer treatment, including depression, polypharmacy, malnutrition, anemia, and lack of caregiver support (68,69). Shorter versions of these extensive assessments are being evaluated (70), and particular screening questions, such as the "mini-mental status" exam or the "timed-up-and-go" test, may be useful in busy clinical practices (67).

At the time of writing, there is growing interest in developing specific protocols for treatment of older women based on accurate health assessments and the biology of disease. Historically, older women have been underscreened and undertreated, leading to worse outcomes. It is important for multidisciplinary teams to work closely with referring physicians and to consider using available tools in order to obtain a more precise and comprehensive health assessment prior to making cancer-specific treatment recommendations.

■ LIVING WITH CANCER

Cancer survivors often describe the period following their initial diagnosis as a time of heightened awareness and worry (71). Many describe being unable to enjoy the present for fear of recurrence, while others see the period as a time of opportunity to reconfigure meaning in their lives (71). Many survivors experience the period following completion of the "active" phase of disease as one of increased anxiety. Frequent visits to clinics and hospitals following surgery and during radiation therapy or chemotherapy allow patients contact with dedicated and compassionate professionals. Suddenly finding themselves without this protective net may unmask deep worries and fears. The intensity of emotional distress is not necessarily related to disease stage or prognosis. Women with ductal carcinoma in situ (DCIS) are also vulnerable and may develop an anxiety disorder, depression, or posttraumatic stress and may benefit from a referral to a mental health professional.

Weisman and Worden's classic studies in the early 1980s showed that most cancer patients seem to cope surprisingly well with the emotional shock of recurrence (72). Some patients exhibit depressive symptoms, such as the loss of hope for recovery, anxieties and fear of death, resurfacing of unresolved issues, strong attempts to maintain control, and often the urgent need to adapt to living with increasing disabilities (72–74). Some may not fully grasp the prognostic significance of a recurrence and may fail to understand at first that the disease is no longer curable. They anticipate more, similar treatments (e.g., chemotherapy, targeted therapy, or endocrine manipulations) without recognizing that the intention of treatment has evolved from cure to palliation. This is best handled by repeated conversations over many days or weeks, thus allowing patients the necessary time to process the information and come to terms with their losses. In a prospective randomized clinical trial, Andersen and colleagues at Ohio State University studied patients with breast cancer who were followed for a number of years after the initial diagnosis and at the time of recurrent disease (75). They found that patients reported stress but that the news of recurrence was not accompanied by global distress or disruption of quality of life. The authors proposed that these women's previous experiences with a cancer diagnosis may have enabled them to be emotionally resilient upon hearing the news of relapse (75).

Metastatic breast cancer has become a model for advanced cancer as a "chronic illness." This is partly due to the slow progressive course of endocrine-sensitive metastatic disease, especially in older women. The heterogeneity of breast cancer requires detailed biological information in order to estimate life expectancy after diagnosis of distant metastases. The outlook for a young woman with triple-negative breast cancer that is widely metastatic may be quite grim, in sharp contrast with that of an older woman with endocrine-sensitive recurrence limited to bone. Detailed prognostic information is required to provide appropriate recommendations for treatment. When cure is not an option, patients' preferences for treatment should be carefully discussed. It may be most appropriate to focus on reduction of unpleasant symptoms and minimize the toxicity and added burden of cancer-specific therapies. However, with the development of endocrine therapies, targeted therapies, and more "friendly" chemotherapeutic drugs with better tolerability and better supportive measures, it is now possible to continue to treat patients for long periods of time. Care of patients with advanced cancer requires meticulous attention to symptom management. Models for comanagement with palliative care clinicians allow patients to derive the benefits of both disciplines. Alternative models call for the integration of palliative care principles into oncology practice, with timely referral to hospice care and coordination of home services as needed. There is no single best practice to meet the needs of patients; thus the multidisciplinary team should include a professional with expertise in symptom management and end of life care.

■ LONGITUDINAL CARE OF CANCER SURVIVORS

Not all patients are comfortable identifying themselves as cancer "survivors." This term is used in the medical literature to denote any individual diagnosed with cancer and encompasses those newly diagnosed, in remission, likely cured, and living with advanced disease. With early detection of breast cancer and the aging of the general population, it is estimated that the number of breast cancer survivors needing routine care is likely to grow and may well exceed the capacity of the oncology workforce (76–78). Oncologists are well aware of the fact that a substantial number of women treated for breast cancer continue to experience late effects from treatment and require specialized attention. Many patients receive their initial treatment in multidisciplinary care units. Teams of specialists provide consultation and recommendations for treatment, and ancillary personnel are available to help navigate the healthcare system and obtain necessary referrals and services. It is rare to find similar models for delivery of care at the end of "active" treatment. Coordination of care is a new challenge. The ASCO and leading experts in care of survivors recommend that all cancer patients be given a treatment summary upon completion of the active phase of treatment. This records the cancer type, stage, use of primary therapies, complications, and recommendations for screening and surveillance and lists the names of the treating cancer specialists. This portable document allows a patient to establish care with subsequent healthcare professionals with a clear roadmap for testing and follow-up (76).

With the growing interest in the need for coordinated survivorship care, investment in specialized survivorship centers of excellence is growing. The Lance Armstrong Foundation awarded grants to seven centers of excellence (76). These innovative centers are conducting research and pilot projects to identify and evaluate best practices for longitudinal follow-up and coordination of care with primary care physicians. Some of these units also provide comprehensive consultations to cancer survivors with complex needs (76,79). Efforts to provide guidance, education, and state-of-the-art medical care for breast cancer survivors will require both ingenuity from and cooperation between members of the multidisciplinary team.

■ CONCLUSION

Health-related quality of life estimates are now prevalent in the oncology literature and considered important prognostic determinants. There is ample documentation of the physical and emotional burdens associated with a diagnosis of breast cancer and the chronicity of side effects. Careful evaluation and attention to minimizing the unpleasant effects of treatment or diminishing the burden of symptoms of the disease is the challenge for multidisciplinary teams. Emotional, psychological, and social concerns impact the experience of women treated for breast cancer, with possible serious consequences for their adherence to treatment and ability to remain active in multiple roles. There are many effective psychosocial interventions available in cancer centers and in the community to assist patients and families. Timely recommendations from healthcare professionals will impact adjustment and facilitate coping for women diagnosed and living with breast cancer.

■ SUMMARY

- Cancer care involves more than disease-specific technical interventions. Surgeons and medical and radiation oncologists need assessment tools to document and treat a variety of symptoms and conditions that result from the diagnosis and treatment of breast cancer.
- Distress management is essential to maintain a patient's sense of well-being and ensure adherence to cancer treatment. NCCN guidelines include quick and effective screening tools.
- Clinicians need to be familiar with common concerns affecting women with breast cancer, such as changes in body image and sexuality, parenting concerns, and the multiple physical symptoms and medical consequences of premature menopause. Caring for survivors requires a multidisciplinary approach and knowledge of long-term effects of all treatment modalities.

■ REFERENCES

1. Bottomley A. The journey of health-related quality of life assessment. *Lancet Oncol.* 2008;9(9):906.
2. Rosser R. The history of health related quality of life in 10½ paragraphs. *J R Soc Med.* 1003;86:315–318.
3. Karnofsky D, Abelmann W, Craver L, Burchenal J. The use of nitrogen mustard in the palliative treatment of cancer. *Cancer.* 1948;1:634–656.
4. Moore FD, Van Devanter SB, Boyden CM, Lokich J, Wilson RE. Adrenalectomy with chemotherapy in the treatment of advanced breast cancer: objective and subjective response rates; duration and quality of life. *Surgery.* 1974;76(3):376–388.
5. Priestman TJ, Baum M. Evaluation of quality of life in patients receiving treatment for advanced breast cancer. *Lancet.* 1976;1:899–900.
6. Montazeri A. Health- related quality of life in breast cancer patients: a bibliographic review of the literature from 1974 to 2007. *J Exp Clin Cancer Res.* 2008;27:32.
7. Aaronson Nk, Ahmedzai S, Bergman B, et al. The European Organization for Research and Treatment of Cancer QLQ-C30; a quality of life instrument for use in international clinical trials in oncology. *J Natl Cancer Inst.* 1993;85(5):365–376.
8. Cella DF. Methods and problems in measuring quality of life. *Support Care Cancer.* 1995;3(1):11–22.

9. Mandelblatt JS, Eisenberg JM . Historical and methodological perspectives on cancer outcomes research. *Oncology.* 1995;9 (11 Suppl):23–32.
10. Montazeri A, Gillis CR, McEwen J. Measuring quality of life in oncology: is it worthwhile? I. Meaning, purposes and controversies. *Eur J Cancer Care.* 1996;5(3):159–167.
11. Hewitt M, Herdman R, Holland J, eds. *Meeting Psychosocial Needs of Women with Breast Cancer.* Washington, DC: National Academies Press; 2004.
12. Brady MJ, Cella DF, Mo F, Bonomi AE, et al. Reliability and validity of the Functional Assessment of Cancer Therapy-Breast quality of life instrument. *J Clin Oncol.* 1997;15(3):974–986.
13. Bjelland I, Dahl AA, Haug TT, Neckelman D. The validity of the Hospital Anxiety and Depression Scale. An updated literature review. *J Psychosom Res.* 2002;52(2):69–77.
14. Hopwood P, Howell A, Maguire P. Psychiatric morbidity in patients with advanced cancer of the breast: prevalence measured by two self-rating questionnaires. *Br J Cancer.* 1991;64(2):349–352.
15. Hopwood P, Howell A, Maguire P. Screening for psychiatric morbidity in patients with advanced cancer: validation of two self-report questionnaires. *Br J Cancer.* 1991;64(2):353–356.
16. Ware JE Jr, Sherbourne CD. The MOS 36-item short-form health survey (SF-36). I. Conceptual framework and item selection. *Med Care.* 1992;30(6):473–483.
17. Bloom JR, Cook M, Flamer DP, et al. Psychological response to mastectomy. *Cancer.* 1987;59(1):189–196.
18. Derogatis LR, Morrow GR, Fetting J, et al. The prevalence of psychiatric disorders among cancer patients. *JAMA.* 1983;288(23):3027–3034.
19. Zabora J, BrintzenhorferSzoc K, Jacobsen P, et al. A new psychosocial screening instrument for use with cancer patients. *Psychosomatics.* 2001;42(3):241–246.
20. Heinrich RL, Schag CA, Ganz PA. Living with cancer: the Cancer Inventory of Problem Situations. *J Clin Psychol.* 1984;40(4):972–980.
21. Schag CA, Heinrich RL. Development of a comprehensive quality of life measurement tool: CARES. *Oncology.* 1990;4(5):135–138.
22. Schag CA, Ganz PA, Heinrich RL. Cancer Rehabilitation Evaluation System–short form (CARES-SF). A cancer specific quality of life and rehabilitation instrument. *Cancer.* 1991;68(6): 1406–1413.
23. Schag CC, Heinrich RL, Ganz PA. Karnofsky performance status revisited: reliability, validity, and guidelines. *J Clin Oncol.* 1984;2:187–193.
24. Ganz PA, Greendale GA, Petersen L, Ziebecchi L, Kahn B, Belin TR. Managing menopausal symptoms in breast cancer survivors: results of a randomized, controlled trial. *J Natl Cancer Inst.* 2000;92(13):1054–1064.
25. Leplege A, Hunt S. The problem of quality of life in medicine. *JAMA.* 1997;278(1):47–50.
26. Holland JC, Andersen B, Breitbart WS, et al. Distress management. *J Natl Compr Canc Netw.* 2007;5(1):66–98.
27. www.nccn.org/professionals/physician_gls/PDF/distress.pdf.
28. Bahrami M, Parker S, Blackman I. Patients' quality of life: a comparison of patient and nurse perceptions. *Contemp Nurse.* 2008; 29(1):67–79.
29. Fallowfield L. Acceptance of adjuvant therapy and quality of life issues. *Breast.* 2005;14:612–616.
30. Pirl WF, Muriel A, Hwang V, et al. Screening for psychosocial distress: a national survey of oncologists. *J Support Oncol.* 2007;5(10): 499–504.
31. Muriel AC, Hwang VS, Kornblith A, et al. Management of psychosocial distress by oncologists. *Psychiatr Serv.* 2009;60(8):1132–1134.
32. Adler NE, Page AEK, eds. *Cancer Care for the Whole Patient: Meeting Psychosocial Needs.* Washington, DC: National Academies Press; 2007.
33. Bloom JR, Kessler L. Risk, timing of counseling and support interventions for younger women with breast cancer. *J Natl Cancer Inst Monogr.* 1994;16:199–206.

34. Fobair P, Stewart SL, Chang S, D'Onofrio C, Banks PJ, Bloom JR. Body image and sexual problems in young women with breast cancer. *Psychooncology.* 2006;15(7):579–594.

35. Surbone A, Petrek JA. Pregnancy after breast cancer. The relationship of pregnancy to breast cancer development and profession. *Crit Rev Oncol Hematol.* 1998;27(3):169–178.

36. Surbone A, Petrek JA. Childbearing issues in breast carcinoma survivors. *Cancer.* 1997;79(7):1271–1278.

37. Dow KH, Harris JR, Roy C. Pregnancy after breast-conserving surgery and radiation therapy for breast cancer. *J Natl Cancer Inst Monogr.* 1994;16:131–137.

38. Schover LR. Motivation for parenthood after cancer: a review. *J Natl Cancer Inst Monogr.* 2005;34:2–5.

39. Partridge A, Gelber S, Peppercorn J, et al. Fertility and menopausal outcomes in young breast cancer survivors. *Clin Breast Cancer.* 2008;8:65–69.

40. Walshe JM, Denduluri N, Swain SM. Amenorrhea in premenopausal women after adjuvant chemotherapy for breast cancer. *J Clin Oncol.* 2006;24:5769–5779.

41. Lee SJ, Schover LR, Partridge AH, et al. American Society of Clinical Oncology recommendations on fertility preservation in cancer patients. *J Clin Oncol.* 2006;24(18):2917–2931.

42. Partridge AH, Ruddy KJ. Fertility and adjuvant treatment in young women with breast cancer. *Breast.* 2007;16(Suppl 2):S175–S181.

43. Partridge AH. Fertility preservation: a vital survivorship issue for young women with breast cancer. *J Clin Oncol.* 2008;26(16):2612–2613.

44. Dow KH, Kuhn D. Fertility options in young breast cancer survivors: a review of the literature. *Oncol Nurs Forum.* 2004;31(3):E46–E53.

45. Schover LR. The impact of breast cancer on sexuality, body image, and intimate relationships. *CA Cancer J Clin.* 1991;41:112–120.

46. Watson M, St. James-Roberts I, Ashley S, et al. Factors associated with emotional and behavioral problems among school age children of breast cancer patients. *Br J Cancer.* 2006;94:43–50.

47. Swick SD, Rauch PK. Children facing the death of a parent: the experiences of a parent guidance program at the Massachusetts general hospital cancer center. *Child Adolesc Psychiatr Clin North Am.* 2006;15(3):779–794. [Review]

48. Muriel AC, Rauch PK. Suggestions for patients on how to talk with children about a parent's cancer. *J Supportive Oncol.* 2003;1(2):143–145.

49. Rauch PK, Muriel AC. The importance of parenting concerns among patients with cancer. *Crit Rev Oncol Hematol.* 2004;49(1):37–42.

50. Rauch P, Muriel A. *Raising an Emotionally Healthy Child When a Parent Is Sick.* New York: McGraw-Hill; 2006.

51. Minton O, Richardson A, Sharpe M, Hotopf M, Stone P. A systematic review and meta-analysis of the pharmacological treatment of cancer-related fatigue. *J Natl Cancer Inst.* 2008;100(16):1155–1166.

52. Kangas M, Bovbjerg DH, Montgomery GH. Cancer-related fatigue: a systematic and meta-analytic review of non-pharmacologic therapies for cancer patients. *Psychol Bull.* 2008;134(5):700–741.

53. Butt Z, Rosenbloom SK, Abernethy AP, et al. Fatigue is the most important symptom for advanced cancer patients who have had chemotherapy. *J Natl Compr Canc Netw.* 2008;6(5):448–455.

54. Ryan JL, Carroll J, Ryan EP, Mustian KM, Fiscella K, Morrow G. Cancer-related fatigue and sleep disorders. *Oncologist.* 2007;12(Suppl 1):35–42.

55. Mock V, Atkinson A, Barsevick A, et al.; National Comprehensive Cancer Network. NCCN practice guidelines for cancer-related fatigue. *Oncology.* 2000;14(11A):151–161.

56. Jean-Pierre P, Figueroa-Moseley C, Kohli S, Fiscella K, Palesh O, Morrow GR. Assessment of cancer-related fatigue: implications for clinical diagnosis and treatment. *Oncologist.* 2007;12:11–21.

57. Wu HS, McSweeny M. Measurement of fatigue in people with cancer. *Oncol Nurs Forum.* 2001;28(9):1371–1384.

58. Amen K. Cancer-related fatigue: the sixth vital sign? *ONS Connect.* 2007;22(8 Suppl):17–18.

59. Biedrzycki BA. Could fatigue become the sixth vital sign? *ONS News.* 2003;18(4):1,4–5.

60. Given B. Cancer-related fatigue: a brief overview of current nursing perspectives and experiences. *Clin J Oncol Nurs.* 2008;12(5 Suppl):7–9.

61. Holland JC, Lewis S. *The Human Side of Cancer. Living With Hope, Coping With Uncertainty.* New York: HarperCollins; 2000.

62. Ormondroyd E, Moynihan C, Ardern-Jones A, et al. Communicating genetics research results to families: problems arising when the patient participant is deceased. *Psychooncology.* 2008;17:804–811.

63. Hewitt M, Herdman R, Holland J, eds. *Meeting Psychosocial Needs of Women With Breast Cancer.* Washington, DC: National Academies Press; 2004.

64. Clarke S, Esplen MJ, Butler K. The phases of disclosing BRCA 1.2 genetic information to offspring. *Psychooncology.* 2008;17:797–803.

65. Farkas-Patenaude A, Julian-Reynier C. Cancer genetic testing: current and emerging issues. *Psychooncology.* 2008;17:733–736.

66. Tercyak KP, Peshkin BN, DeMarco T, et al. Information needs of mothers regarding communicating BRCA I/II cancer genetic test results to their children. *Genet Test.* 2007;11(3):249–255.

67. Wildiers H, Kunkler I, Biganzoli L, et al.; International Society of Geriatric Oncology. Management of breast cancer in elderly individuals: recommendations of the International Society of Geriatric Oncology. *Lancet Oncol.* 2007;8(12):1101–1115.

68. Carlson RW, Moench S, Hurria A, et al. NCCN Task Force report: breast cancer in the older woman. *J Natl Compr Canc Netw.* 2008;6(Suppl 4):S1–S25.

69. Balducci L. New paradigms for treating elderly patients with cancer: the comprehensive geriatric assessment and guidelines for supportive care. *J Support Oncol.* 2003;1(4 Suppl 2):30–37.

70. Hurria A. We need a geriatric assessment for oncologists. *Natl Clin Pract Oncol.* 2006;3(12):642–643.

71. Hurria A, Gupta S, Zaudere M, et al. Developing a cancer-specific geriatric assessment: a feasibility study. *Cancer.* 2005;104(9):1998–2005.

72. Kissane D, Bultz B, Butow P, Finlay I, eds. *Handbook of Communication in Oncology and Palliative Care.* Oxford, England: Oxford University Press; 2009.

73. Weisman AD, Worden JW. The emotional impact of recurrent cancer. *J Psychosocial Oncol.* 1985;3:5–16.

74. Mahon SM, Casperson DM. Exploring the psychosocial meaning of recurrent cancer: a descriptive study. *Cancer Nurs.* 1997;20:178–186.

75. Ekwall E, Ternestedt. Recurrence of ovarian cancer—living in limbo. *Cancer Nurs.* 2007;30(4):270–277.

76. Andersen BL, Shapiro CL, Farrar WB, Crespin T, Wells-Digregorio S. Psychological responses to cancer recurrence. *Cancer.* 2005;104:1540–1547.

77. Ganz PA, Hahn EE. Implementing a survivorship care plan for patients with breast cancer. *J Clin Oncol.* 2008;26(5):759–767.

78. Earle CC. Failing to plan is planning to fail. *J Clin Oncol.* 2006;24:5112–5116.

79. Erikson C, Salsberg E, Forte G, et al. Future supply and demand for oncologists: challenges to assuring access to oncology services. *J Oncol Pract.* doi:10.1200/JOP.0723601.

Lymphedema: A Modern Approach to Evaluation and Treatment

JEAN O'TOOLE

TARA A. RUSSELL

As survival from breast cancer continues to improve, it is our responsibility as healthcare providers to collaborate as a team and proactively address the quality of life challenges that result from the management of breast cancer (1). Lymphedema following treatment for breast cancer is a major challenge for the patients who experience this complication, as well as for those who fear developing this condition (2,3). Our patients deserve an aggressive collegial approach from a multidisciplinary team willing to work with them to address this problem (2,3).

Lymphedema is swelling that occurs in the interstitial tissues when the lymphatic system is unable to transport the amount of fluid for which it has capacity (4). The enormously negative impact on quality of life due to lymphedema secondary to treatment for breast cancer is well documented (5–7). For breast cancer patients, lymphedema can present not only in the arm or hand but also in the trunk and breast (1,8,9). Discomfort, alteration of body image, functional problems, decreased physical activity, fatigue, emotional distress, anxiety, loss of confidence in one's body, and depression have all been associated with the presence of lymphedema (3–6). In addition, even the threat of developing edema results in a compromised quality of life for many patients, as they often alter their lifestyle in the hope of preventing lymphedema from occurring (6,10–23). A comprehensive multidisciplinary approach that includes team awareness, patient education, ongoing surveillance, and a network of available resources for treatment provides substantial support to patients who are at risk and who have already experienced lymphedema (5).

A well-coordinated team includes patients and their support system, medical caregivers, certified lymphedema therapists, physical and occupational therapists, social workers, dieticians, durable medical equipment (DME) providers, and community resources. Each team member plays an important role in the education and management of lymphedema. The patient is the centering point for the team, and the needs and goals of the patient should be the focus of the group effort. All team members must be willing to openly discuss lymphedema with patients during the course of breast cancer treatment and throughout the years of follow-up. It is the intention of this chapter

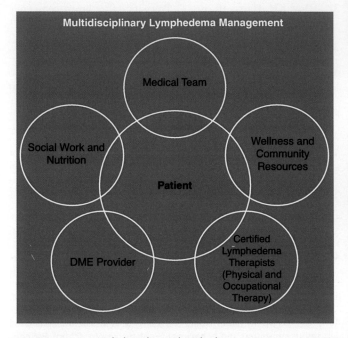

FIGURE 12.1 Multidisciplinary lymphedema management. (DME, durable medical equipment.)

to demonstrate the benefit and necessity of a committed and proactive team approach to this troubling side effect of treatment. This chapter will address the current state of knowledge regarding lymphedema risk factors and incidence and provide a practical approach to surveillance for early identification of lymphedema. It will outline strategies for intervention, and highlight the important contributions of all team members as they work together to minimize the extraordinary burden of breast cancer–related lymphedema (Figure 12.1).

■ LYMPHEDEMA: CURRENT STATE OF KNOWLEDGE

Definition and Measurement

The true incidence of breast cancer–related lymphedema is difficult to state with accuracy because of the lack of uniformity regarding measurement and definition (24,25). Throughout the literature, there is currently no consensus on how much edema is clinically significant. Variations in definition depend on the method of measurement utilized and what volumetric threshold constitutes edema worthy of attention (26–35). These discrepancies have led to the

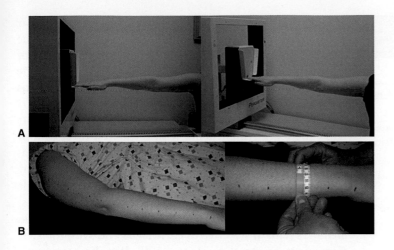

FIGURE 12.2 Two forms of arm volume measurement. (A) Perometer (Juzo Systems). Infrared light receiver pairs located within the frame are passed over the arm. Pero-Plus, the coordinating computer system, calculates circumferential and volumetric measurements. (B) Circumferential arm measurements. The arm is marked at 4 cm intervals from the ulnar styloid to the axillary fold. Circumferential measurements are then taken with a tape measure at each interval. The equation for a truncated cone (frustrum) can be used to calculate volume.

reporting of a broad range of incidence values between 11% and 56% (24,36–38).

The first step in establishing a threshold for clinically significant edema is to select a method for measuring the limb. Within the literature the techniques used to quantify lymphedema vary. Instruments commonly used for quantification of lymphedema include: circumferential tape measurement, water displacement (39), bioimpedance spectroscopy (40), and infrared light perometry. Tape measurement was the clinical standard for many years and continues to be utilized (27,41). Water displacement, although accurate and reliable, is burdensome and time-consuming for both the practitioner and the patient (39,41). Currently, there are other measurement tools that are more technologically advanced, reliable, and efficient. Assessment with bioimpedance spectroscopy quantifies extracellular fluid rather than arm volume (35,42). The modern gold standard for limb volume measurement is the Perometer (Juzo Systems) (39). Utilizing paired infrared light receivers to calculate volume and circumference, the Perometer, although expensive, is efficient and reliable within 1% (Figure 12.2) (43–45).

Once a method for measurement has been selected, the next step is to determine a threshold that justifies the diagnosis of lymphedema. In clinical research investigating lymphedema secondary to breast cancer, it is not uncommon for edema to be defined as a 2 cm difference

in limb girth or a volumetric change of 20% or greater (4,23,46–50). Alternatively, some authors have highlighted that even lower volume or subclinical edemas can be symptomatic and warrant intervention (51–53). Armer defines a 10% volume change of the involved arm over the uninvolved arm as a "conservative" threshold for diagnosing a limb as edematous, which is more useful than using a circumferential difference. Francis's trial considered a 5% difference above baseline as a meaningful definition of lymphedema (54). As volume increases, the upper limb undergoes physical changes (Figure 12.3).

The International Society of Lymphology has graded lymphedema in stages (see below) (27). This framework goes beyond the common adjectives of "mild," "moderate," and "severe," as it describes the condition of the limb and considers the fibrosis present, which Cheville and McGarvey also report as an important consideration (24). The International Staging model is also helpful, as it recognizes the stage of edema (preclinical) when fluid is accumulating and symptoms may be present but edema is not visible and volume changes are not yet apparent (5,40). The International Society of Lymphology and lymphedema researchers recognize that this system is still not a complete definition, as it does not encompass the functional or emotional toll on the patient; therefore patient reports or symptom questionnaires are also useful tools to determine a definition of clinically significant lymphedema (Table 12.1) (27,35,55,56).

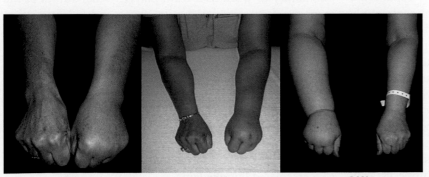

| 9% | 19% | 31% |

FIGURE 12.3 Varying levels of lymphedema.

■ Table 12.1 International Society of Lymphology lymphedema staging

Stage	Definition
0	Latent, subclinical condition, swelling is not evident despite impaired lymph transport
I	Early accumulation of fluid relatively high in protein content, subsides with limb elevation, some pitting may occur
II	Limb elevation does not reduce swelling, pitting, tissue fibrosis increases
III	Lymphostatic elephantiasis: pitting absent, trophic skin changes (acanthosis, fat deposits, warty outgrowth)

Risk Factors and Incidence

In light of the disparities in the measurement and definition of lymphedema, the most commonly reported and conservatively estimated incidence of breast cancer–related lymphedema is 20% to 30% (4,11,26,38,57–60). It is well documented that the risk of developing lymphedema is related to axillary surgery and lymph node radiation (14,24,25,31,34,61). Axillary lymph node dissection is a well-supported risk factor, with increased vulnerability as the number of nodes excised increases (62). Sentinel lymph node biopsy (SLNB) is reported to impart a much lower risk of lymphedema (46). Recent research has reported an incidence rate among those receiving only SLNB and no further axillary surgery at 6.9% (63). Postoperative wound infection has been cited as an additional risk factor (46). Strong evidence supports regional lymph node radiation as a contributor to the risk of edema development (4,28,30,47,61,62,64–66). A serious side effect of having a challenged lymphatic system is the vulnerability for developing cellulitis, and an episode of cellulitis typically increases the volume of edema (2,50,67).

Unlike clinical and treatment risk factors, lifestyle-associated risks have yet to be evaluated with a high degree of scientific rigor (1). Current research focusing on this aspect of risk assessment has identified only increased body mass index (BMI) as increasing the risk of lymphedema development (4,27,36,62,68–71). Avoiding venipuncture within the quadrant has been the subject of some study (1,4); otherwise, cautionary warnings regarding repetitive activity, weight lifting, air flight, and avoiding blood pressure reading lack the evidence to support them. The data emerging from post–breast cancer exercise trials are very encouraging and seem to suggest that activity and exercise introduced gradually do not incite the development of lymphedema and may be beneficial in managing swelling (38,61,72–75). This information is exciting because the health benefits of exercise are so rich that women who have been treated for breast cancer should not be unnecessarily

denied the enjoyment or the positive rewards of regular exercise (76–78). Educating patients on risk factors and the positive impact of physical activity is the responsibility of the entire team, and the conversation should begin in the early postoperative period. Methods for approaching this topic are discussed in the following sections.

In summary, it is estimated that at least 25% of patients will experience lymphedema within the first three to four years following treatment (6,36). Lymphedema can continue to develop over subsequent years and is a lifetime risk (1,6,36). Axillary dissection, regional lymph node radiation, and high BMI carry the greatest risk for breast cancer–related lymphedema. It is imperative that all team members remain sensitive to early signs and symptoms, as there is often a preclinical stage (79). Regular assessment beginning at diagnosis, with ongoing long-term follow-up that includes assessment of arm volume, symptoms, functional compromise, and quality of life, are integral components of surveillance that will identify lymphedema in a timely manner (1). To accomplish this goal, creating your team is a first step.

■ COLLABORATIVE MULTIDISCIPLINARY NETWORK

Optimal management of breast cancer–related lymphedema begins with establishing a multidisciplinary team committed to a proactive approach. Ideally, team members should include:

- Representatives from the medical team (surgery, radiation, medical oncology, nursing, physician assistants, etc.)
- Physical/occupational therapists
- Certified lymphedema therapists
- Social workers
- Nutritionists
- Wellness community leaders

These colleagues should be chosen on the basis of their interest in and knowledge regarding lymphedema, their commitment to serving patient-centered goals, demonstrated dependability, effective communication skills, and ability to work as a team player. Other values of the team are a sustained commitment to early identification of lymphedema and the willingness to openly discuss lymphedema with patients. The team should agree on the roles and responsibilities of all members and establish mechanisms for regular and ongoing communication. Goals and plans should be decided by the group, with realistic consideration to the time and resources available. The group should determine methods to evaluate the efficacy of their program and stay abreast of new developments in the etiology and identification of, and interventions for, breast cancer–related lymphedema.

■ MONITORING FOR LYMPHEDEMA DEVELOPMENT

One of the cornerstones to a comprehensive team approach is the ability to provide patients with ongoing access to a screening system that will identify early changes in the involved upper quadrant. With early identification as a primary goal of this effort, the group should establish a screening protocol that is realistic given the resources available in their setting. The screening protocol should include: (a) tools of assessment, (b) screening timeline, (c) individuals' or team members' responsibilities, (d) patient education materials, and (e) communication strategies.

Tools of Assessment

The measurement tool you choose for your program (tape measure, water displacement, bioimpedance, or perometry) should be practical for your clinical setting. In determining an instrument for measurement, it is important to note that measurement methods should not be used interchangeably, as results are not comparable (80,81).

In addition to the quantification of edema, questionnaires for monitoring symptoms, quality of life, and functional problems are important methods to utilize in screening. Patients with early lymphedema often report symptoms of heaviness, tightness, warmth, numbness, and difficulty wearing rings or watches (52,71). For this reason, individual patient reports may be among the most useful tools in evaluating early signs of lymphedema, in conjunction with monitoring limb volume or fluid (5,56). Furthermore, patients should be encouraged from the beginning of their treatment to report any perceived changes in their trunk, breast, or arm to any of the team members, with assurance that their report will be evaluated and taken seriously.

Screening Timeline

Developing a consistent timeline for evaluation will ensure patients are evaluated and monitored during and after their treatment for breast cancer. The literature clearly demonstrates that measuring patients at diagnosis (prior to definitive surgery) is essential (4,29,37,82). This preoperative assessment of arm volume will establish a baseline that provides a framework for meaningful interpretation of postoperative changes (29,37,46,82). In the first year and during the active phase of treatment, it is recommended that screening is performed every three months. Following the conclusion of active treatment, screening at six-month intervals is appropriate. Because the risk of developing lymphedema remains for a lifetime, surveillance should continue throughout follow-up.

Team Member Responsibilities

All team members must play an active role in promoting lymphedema screening. The primary responsibility for screening for lymphedema should be assigned to at least two members of your team. This will ensure consistency and reliability and will provide some depth of coverage. This duty may be accomplished by scheduling the screening at the time follow-up appointments are made. This ensures that screening is as much a part of the protocol for visits as monitoring weight and vital signs.

Patient Education

Educating patients about lymphedema is of primary importance and should be a collective effort and shared responsibility of all team members. However, it may be useful to assign the dissemination of educational materials to two of the members so that it will be consistently included as a part of routine examination. This education material should include information regarding risk factors, signs and symptoms, identification of cellulitis, activity progression, and when to contact the team (33). This information can be available in a teaching sheet or booklet (1,83). These are inexpensive to create and can be available to your patients either on paper or on your website. They should be available in languages appropriate to you patient population. See Figure 12.4 for examples. Although many external websites and pamphlets are available that provide lymphedema information, many are not evidence based (48). You may want to customize one appropriate for your patient population.

Communication Strategies

As with any team, communication between members is a determinant of success (84). As a team you should agree on modes of communication to apprise each other of a change in the status of the patient. Methods will vary from center to center, but seamless and timely communication among the team is essential for successful implementation of your program.

■ MANAGEMENT OF LYMPHEDEMA

Beyond screening, a multidisciplinary approach to lymphedema must include a plan for management for those patients who experience lymphedema. At the point that edema becomes apparent, the patient should be evaluated by the medical team to determine the etiology of the new swelling (85). Once vascular occlusion or recurrent disease have been ruled out, treatment for breast cancer–related lymphedema can be initiated. The goal of intervention should be control of the edema, while also attempting to minimize the burden that management can impose on the patient with respect to time and cost. It has been our experience that it is essential to allow the patient to drive the decision-making process by providing a safe and

LYMPHEDEMA AND BREAST CANCER

What is lymphedema?

Lymphedema is a type of swelling or edema. It happens when lymphatic fluid builds up in tissue under the skin. Lymphatic fluid is made of water, protein, and waste products. Normally, your organs produce lymphatic fluid and it is circulated throughout your body by the lymphatic system. When the fluid cannot flow freely, lymphedema can occur. Lymphedema sometimes happens when lymph nodes are removed during surgery. It can also happen after radiation treatment.

After surgery, it is normal to have some swelling, and it usually goes away as you heal. Lymphedema is a type of swelling that remains longer than expected. It happens in the chest, breast, or arm. It can happen soon after breast surgery or radiation treatment; or it may happen weeks, months or even years later.

Can I prevent lymphedema?

We are not sure how to prevent lymphedema. However, we do know that being overweight can increase your risk of lymphedema.

How will I know if I have lymphedema?

Lymphedema can begin anywhere on the side where you were treated. For example, if you had surgery on your right breast, the area from the center of your chest to your right shoulder and from your belly button to hip could all develop lymphedema. The most common site for lymphedema is in the arm. The lymphatic fluid can collect in your hand alone, only at your elbow, or in your whole arm. Call your doctor or nurse if you see any puffiness or swelling.

Some early signs of lymphedema can be:
- A sensation of heaviness or fatigue in the arm.
- Your sleeves, bra or jewelry feeling tighter than usual.
- Any red or warm area.
- Any visible puffiness or swelling.

Should I avoid certain activities?

There is no research that shows that avoiding certain activities will prevent lymphedema. The following are only suggestions.

However, if you HAVE lymphedema, you may want to take this advice.

1. Be careful lifting heavy objects
   - The amount of weight that is safe to lift is different for each person. It is best to start lifting lightweight objects. Starting with 2–3 pounds is a good idea.
   - Gradually increase the weight of what you lift when you see how your body reacts. Let your arm tell you how much weight you can lift.

2. Try not to carry bags or luggage over your shoulder

3. Be careful doing tasks with forceful arm movements that you repeat many times
   - Some patients have reported that activities with forceful arm movements, like mopping, vacuuming, painting, weight lifting and using machines at the gym, have triggered their lymphedema.
   - As you start doing these activities, watch your arm for symptoms. If your arm does not swell, you can gradually continue doing these activities.
   - Ask your doctor, nurse or therapist about your work and exercise activities.

4. Avoid putting anything tight around your arm, hands or fingers
   - Avoid wearing tight jewelry or elastics around your fingers or arms. For example, tight rings, bracelets, rubber bands and tight sleeves.
   - Avoid having your blood pressure taken, or injections placed, on the arm or side of surgery.

5. Avoid getting cuts, insect bites and injuries to your arm
   - These can lead to infections if you have had lymph nodes removed or sampled.

   To avoid cuts, bites and injuries you can:
   - Wear gloves when you garden, wash dishes or do other work with your hands.
   - Do not cut your cuticles.
   - Use an electric razor when you shave to minimize skin cuts.

If you notice a red or warm area, call your doctor or nurse. This may be a sign of infection.

Can lymphedema be treated?

Yes, lymphedema can be treated. There are therapists with special training in this area, and your doctor or nurse will refer you for treatment if needed. Treatment can include:
- Helping you learn ways that you can exercise or massage your arm to relieve the swelling.
- Seeing the therapist for a special massage (called manual lymph drainage). This is done before a sleeve is prescribed.
- Using a compression sleeve to contain the swelling during the day.
- If you have lymphedema, use your sleeve when flying in an airplane.
- If you do not have lymphedema, talk with your doctor or nurse before flying.

If you notice any of the signs of lymphedema, call your doctor or nurse. You should do this before consulting a lymphedema therapist.

© Massachusetts General Hospital Cancer Center • The General Hospital Corporation

FIGURE 12.4 Avon Foundation Comprehensive Breast Evaluation Center information sheet.

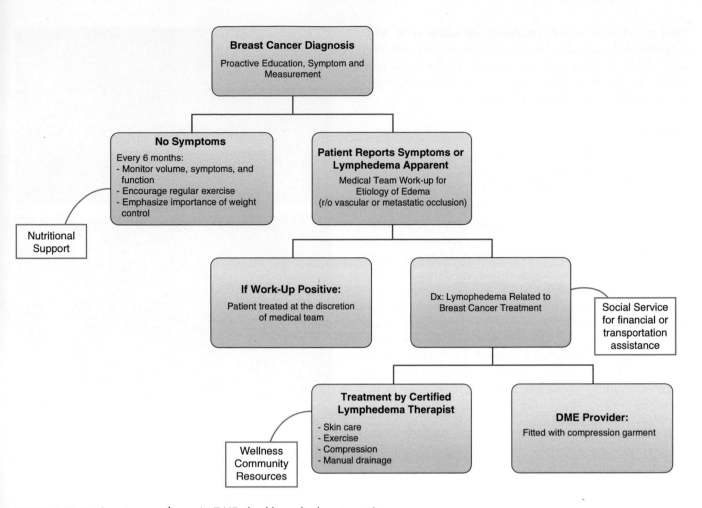

FIGURE 12.5 Breast cancer diagnosis. (DME, durable medical equipment.)

nonjudgmental environment that enables patients to honestly express what commitment they feel they can make to the care of their lymphedema. If the management plan is created with patients' goals and expectations fully considered and respected, successful follow-through may be more reasonably anticipated (Figure 12.5).

Intervention for lymphedema is commonly referred to as complex decongestive therapy (CDT). The components of CDT are skin care, compression, exercise, and manual lymph drainage (23,31,38,82,86–88). While small studies have demonstrated the efficacy of a full CDT approach, to date sample sizes have been small and lack a strong case-control format (31,33,75,86,89–92). Thus, a full CDT program has yet to be examined with a high degree of scientific rigor, which makes it difficult to unconditionally endorse for all patients (38,82,87,88). Given this lack of evidence, the complexity of your interventions should be determined by the tenacity of the edema, the patient's goals, and available resources (93). If your community has certified lymphedema therapists (typically physical or occupational therapists) available, they would be the practitioners of choice to treat these patients. A computer search can help you locate these practitioners, and

the Lymphedema Association of North America webpage provides a quick link to identifying local therapists. Although many disciplines are eligible for certification (including massage therapists and nurses), third-party payers will usually reimburse for this therapy only if it is billed as a skilled physical or occupational therapy. There is an important role for social work in the management of lymphedema. Funding for treatment and garments or transportation may be a problem for patients, and our colleagues in social service are often pivotal in obtaining available resources for the patient, as well as providing emotional support.

Within the CDT treatment scheme, many or all of the components can be utilized for the management of lymphedema. Management options include some combination of the following.

Skin Care

Instructions on vigilant skin care are always important. Well-moisturized skin can inhibit the need to scratch or itch frequently, which are habits that might increase the risk of cellulitis (8,68). Helping the patient understand signs of cellulitis is also necessary. In addition to well-hydrated skin, use of a sun block with a sun protection factor (SPF) of 35 or higher and insect repellant and protecting the quadrant from unnecessary cuts or punctures are recommendations for good skin care.

Exercise

The role of exercise is to stimulate the muscular pumps that assist in drainage and to encourage deep breathing as another strategy to assist lymphatic transport (24). Typically, stretching and aerobic exercises are strongly encouraged. Your Wellness Community may offer exercise classes for breast cancer survivors, and it would benefit the team to become familiar with what resources are available in your community. You may choose to invite the instructors to come and speak with your team or provide you with information about their services so that you can evaluate the appropriateness of the classes available in your area. Exercise will also assist the patient in maintaining ideal weight. Because high BMI is associated with lymphedema, having patients consult with your team's nutritionist if needed would be a positive contribution to the multidisciplinary care of this problem. The physical or occupational therapist on the team can also screen patients for any musculoskeletal or neuromuscular impairments that should be considered when designing an exercise regimen.

Compression

Compression utilized over the edematous area, with a garment or bandaging, or both, can be an extremely efficacious tool in the management of lymphedema (32,69,82,85,87). Medical contraindications to the use of compression include renal and cardiac disease, so if these conditions exist, clearance by the medical team is crucial prior to implementing compression strategies. If a compression garment is desired to control the edema, a sleeve for the arm and a glove or gauntlet for the hand are used. Compression garments are for day use only (82,88). The rationale for not using them overnight is that the elastic composition of the garments could create a tourniquet effect and constrict circulatory flow, depending upon sleeping positions. All garments should be washed by hand on a daily basis and allowed to dry overnight. The choices for compression sleeves are "ready to wear" garments that are available off the shelf and custom garments. Ready to wear sleeves come presized; the ranges of arm measurements are provided on each box and serve as a guide to fitting the patient properly. Custom garments are more costly than the ready to wear sleeves but may be necessary, depending on the size and shape of the arm. Custom garments are made in Germany with specific measurements of the patient and can be tailored to the patient's need (Figure 12.6) (94). If the edema is located in the breast or trunk, a long line bra, tank top,

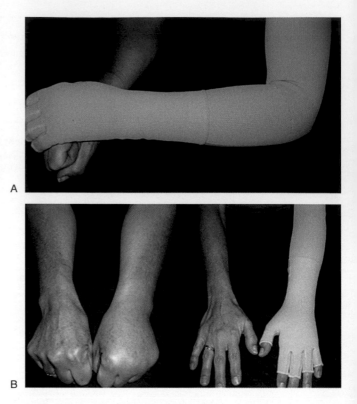

FIGURE 12.6 (A and B) Examples of class 1 custom compression sleeve and glove.

or T-shirt made from Lycra or spandex can be helpful in providing compression to those areas (82).

Compression garments are also available in different grades of pressure. In the United States, class 1 typically indicates 20 to 30 mg Hg, and class 2 30 to 40 mg Hg. A certified lymphedema therapist or your DME provider is typically very skilled in helping to make these decisions and can measure patients for the appropriate garment. It is important to ensure that whoever is providing the garments for patients is licensed to bill insurances for these garments. At this time, most private insurance companies have a DME benefit, and each patient should contact the carrier to learn the dollar amount of the benefit. Social services can be very useful in assisting patients with this step. In addition, it is important to note that currently Medicare does not cover the cost of compression garments.

If the patient's edema requires more control than is provided by the compression sleeve, all-cotton, short-stretch (inelastic) bandages are utilized (82,87). Ace bandages are not recommended for lymphedema, because of the high resting pressure they exert on the limb (24,94). Your team can purchase these to provide for the patient or obtain them through DME providers, or the patient can purchase them from one of the many online vendors. They are not manufactured in the United States and are not typically available at drug stores. Certified lymphedema therapists are trained in this type of bandaging and about the variety of bandaging strategies that can be employed.

Patients often use these bandages at night and apply the compression sleeve in the morning for day use (67).

The physical or occupational therapist on your team can evaluate the patient for physical or cognitive impairments that would inhibit the patient from applying compression garments or bandaging independently or safely. Often, adaptive devices for donning and doffing a garment are available, and adaptations in bandage applications can be made. A family member can be instructed as to how to help with bandaging. Providing the patient with written instructions, even with diagrams, is suggested.

Manual Lymphatic Drainage

Manual lymphatic drainage refers to the use of the hands as a pump in an attempt to mobilize the lymph fluid (24,95). It is recommended that a certified lymphedema therapist be utilized for this step. The treatment could be carried out two to five times a week for two to four weeks, or longer (82). Although this technique is often reported as useful, large, well-controlled, randomized trials are yet to be done, and systematic reviews have not found strong evidence supporting the technique (3,87,89).

Another mode of mobilizing the fluid is to use a pneumatic compression pump. The use of these devices in breast cancer–related lymphedema remains somewhat controversial (96,97). However, there are newer devices on the market today that have a different design from the older models but have yet to be tested in well-controlled, randomized studies with large sample sizes (96,98). The use of a pneumatic pump requires the patient to use the device once or twice a day for one or more hours. There is no solid evidence to guide the prescription of how much time a patient will need to use the pump for. They are costly and often not covered by third-party payers. If your team is interested, it would be worthwhile investigating what devices are available in your area and determining whether the cost of rental or purchase of a unit is realistic for the patient before a pneumatic compression pump is given to a patient as a trial, as it presently not standard practice for breast cancer–related lymphedema.

Patients who are treated for lymphedema by your team should be reevaluated at regular intervals to assess the efficacy of intervention. Frequency may vary, depending upon how well the patient is able to follow through with the treatment scheme and how well the plan is succeeding in controlling the edema. It may be necessary to check with the patient within the first week and follow up at least within the first month. Managing lymphedema can be a burden for a patient (99). Wearing compression garments, bandaging at night, controlling weight, and exercising regularly requires a diligent commitment, and we have found that ongoing surveillance and support from the team is important.

Once the active phase of intervention is completed and patients are on their own to manage their swelling with whatever strategies have been recommended for their situation, reevaluating volume and symptoms at three-month intervals during the first six months of treatment is important. After 6 to 12 months of garment use, the patient should be evaluated to determine whether there should be any changes in the management plan (94). Garments typically need to be replaced after between six and nine months, depending on use as fabric stretches, and may not be as effective if not replaced regularly.

■ PRACTICAL APPLICATION OF THE TEAM APPROACH

A multidisciplinary network is created from a shared recognition that breast cancer–related lymphedema is a serious quality-of-life problem for patients. It is the result of the passionate resolve of colleagues willing to put together a structured approach to screening and intervention. As resources vary at every facility, programs will differ, but the core value of addressing this side effect as a team should be universal.

Implementation of a lymphedema program includes three major steps: basic awareness, network development, and clinical implementation (Figure 12.7). Basic awareness begins with the joint effort of a few colleagues to motivate and develop a proactive approach to lymphedema. Implementation of this program includes the recruitment of other practitioners and team members to collaborate in a similar cause. Network development is initiated once awareness has been established within the clinic, and the team mobilized with a plan of action. Finally, clinical implementation includes a protocol for education, screening, and management.

In summary, as documented in this chapter, breast cancer–related lymphedema can be a devastating side effect of treatment, not only for patients who experience it but also for the patients who fear that they will develop it. The modern and ideal management of this condition is accomplished by developing and implementing a

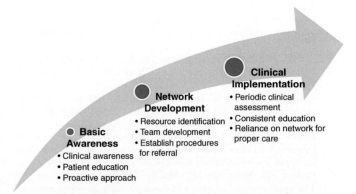

FIGURE 12.7 This arrow illustrates the three major steps of implementation of a lymphedema program.

comprehensive multidisciplinary team approach. Proactive and early identification of lymphedema accompanied by intervention strategies based on the goals of the patient are cornerstones of successfully confronting this problem. The responsibilities of this multidisciplinary group effort include ensuring that preoperative volume measurements are taken, that patients are provided with information regarding risk factors, signs and symptoms, and that discussion of lymphedema is encouraged. The plan of care that is developed is tailored to meet the individual needs of the patient and often includes contributions from many different colleagues. Regular screening for volume changes and symptoms must continue over the entire length of follow-up for the patient, because of the lifetime risk of developing lymphedema.

Your team can begin with only a few dedicated colleagues and limited resources and can evolve and grow over time. All centers should be able to provide some level of lymphedema education, screening, and management. With this level of commitment, perhaps together we can change the experience for women in the generations to come.

■ SUMMARY

- The presence or fear of developing lymphedema is a serious quality of life concern for breast cancer patients.
- Modern management of lymphedema requires a proactive and multidisciplinary approach.
- Lymphedema management should be guided by patient-centered goals.
- Regardless of the resources available, all centers should be able to provide patients with lymphedema education, screening, and management.

■ REFERENCES

1. Nielsen I, Gordon S, Selby A. Breast cancer-related lymphoedema risk reduction advice: a challenge for health professionals. *Cancer Treat Rev.* 2008;34:621–628.
2. Lewis M, Morgan K. Managing chronic oedema: a collaborative community approach. *Br J Community Nurs.* 2008;13:S25–S26,S8–S32.
3. Erickson VS, Pearson ML, Ganz PA, Adams J, Kahn KL. Arm edema in breast cancer patients. *J Natl Cancer Inst.* 2001;93:96–111.
4. Clark B. SJ, Harlow W. Incidence and risk of arm oedema following treatment for breast cancer: a three-year follow-up study. *Q J Med.* 2005;98:343–348.
5. Hayes SC, Janda M, Cornish B, Battistutta D, Newman B. Lymphedema after breast cancer: incidence, risk factors, and effect on upper body function. *J Clin Oncol.* 2008;26:3536–3542.
6. Paskett ED, Naughton MJ, McCoy TP, Case LD, Abbott JM. The epidemiology of arm and hand swelling in premenopausal breast cancer survivors. *Cancer Epidemiol Biomarkers Prev.* 2007;16:775–782.
7. Oliveri JM, Day JM, Alfano CM, et al. Arm/hand swelling and perceived functioning among breast cancer survivors 12 years post-diagnosis: CALGB 79804. *J Cancer Surviv.* 2008 Dec 2(4) 233–42.
8. Honnor A. Classification, aetiology and nursing management of lymphoedema. *Br J Nurs.* 2008;17:576–586.
9. Stanton AW, Modi S, Mellor RH, et al. A quantitative lymphoscintigraphic evaluation of lymphatic function in the swollen hands of women with lymphoedema following breast cancer treatment. *Clin Sci (Lond).* 2006;110:553–561.
10. Engel J, Kerr J, Schlesinger-Raab A, Sauer H, Holzel D. Axilla surgery severely affects quality of life: results of a 5-year prospective study in breast cancer patients. *Breast Cancer Res Treat.* 2003;79:47–57.
11. Beaulac SM, McNair LA, Scott TE, LaMorte WW, Kavanah MT. Lymphedema and quality of life in survivors of early-stage breast cancer. *Arch Surg.* 2002;137:1253–1257.
12. Armer JM, Heckathorn PW. Post-breast cancer lymphedema in aging women: self-management and implications for nursing. *J Gerontol Nurs.* 2005;31:29–39.
13. Ridner SH. Breast cancer lymphedema: pathophysiology and risk reduction guidelines. *Oncol Nurs Forum.* 2002;29:1285–1293.
14. Ververs JM, Roumen RM, Vingerhoets AJ, et al. Risk, severity and predictors of physical and psychological morbidity after axillary lymph node dissection for breast cancer. *Eur J Cancer.* 2001;37:991–999.
15. Coster S, Poole K, Fallowfield LJ. The validation of a quality of life scale to assess the impact of arm morbidity in breast cancer patients post-operatively. *Breast Cancer Res Treat.* 2001;68:273–282.
16. Courneya KS, Mackey JR, Bell GJ, Jones LW, Field CJ, Fairey AS. Randomized controlled trial of exercise training in postmenopausal breast cancer survivors: cardiopulmonary and quality of life outcomes. *J Clin Oncol.* 2003;21:1660–1668.
17. Hack TF, Cohen L, Katz J, Robson LS, Goss P. Physical and psychological morbidity after axillary lymph node dissection for breast cancer. *J Clin Oncol.* 1999;17:143–149.
18. Heiney SP, McWayne J, Cunningham JE, et al. Quality of life and lymphedema following breast cancer. *Lymphology.* 2007;40:177–184.
19. Janz NK, Mujahid M, Chung LK, et al. Symptom experience and quality of life of women following breast cancer treatment. *J Womens Health (Larchmt).* 2007;16:1348–1361.
20. Mirolo BR, Bunce IH, Chapman M, et al. Psychosocial benefits of postmastectomy lymphedema therapy. *Cancer Nurs.* 1995;18:197–205.
21. Poole K, Fallowfield LJ. The psychological impact of postoperative arm morbidity following axillary surgery for breast cancer: a critical review. *Breast.* 2002;11:81–87.
22. Lee TS, Kilbreath SL, Sullivan G, Refshauge KM, Beith JM. The development of an arm activity survey for breast cancer survivors using the Protection Motivation Theory. *BMC Cancer.* 2007;7:75.
23. Karadibak D, Yavuzsen T, Saydam S. Prospective trial of intensive decongestive physiotherapy for upper extremity lymphedema. *J Surg Oncol.* 2008;97:572–577.
24. Cheville AL, McGarvey CL, Petrek JA, Russo SA, Thiadens SR, Taylor ME. The grading of lymphedema in oncology clinical trials. *Semin Radiat Oncol.* 2003;13:214–225.
25. Rietman JS, Dijkstra PU, Hoekstra HJ, et al. Late morbidity after treatment of breast cancer in relation to daily activities and quality of life: a systematic review. *Eur J Surg Oncol.* 2003;29:229–238.
26. Rampaul RS, Mullinger K, Macmillan RD, et al. Incidence of clinically significant lymphoedema as a complication following surgery for primary operable breast cancer. *Eur J Cancer.* 2003;39:2165–2167.
27. The diagnosis and treatment of peripheral lymphedema. Consensus document of the International Society of Lymphology. *Lymphology.* 2009;42:51–6-;36:84–91.

28. Hinrichs CS, Watroba NL, Rezaishiraz H, et al. Lymphedema secondary to postmastectomy radiation: incidence and risk factors. *Ann Surg Oncol.* 2004;11:573–580.

29. Gergich N, Pfalzer LA, McGarvey C, Springer B, Gerber LH, Soballe P. Preoperative assessment enables the early diagnosis and successful treatment of lymphedema. *Cancer.* 2008;112(12): 2809–2819.

30. Herd-Smith A, Russo A, Muraca MG, Del Turco MR, Cardona G. Prognostic factors for lymphedema after primary treatment of breast carcinoma. *Cancer.* 2001;92:1783–1787.

31. Mondry TE, Riffenburgh RH, Johnstone PA. Prospective trial of complete decongestive therapy for upper extremity lymphedema after breast cancer therapy. *Cancer J.* 2004;10:42–48; discussion 17–19.

32. McNeely ML, Magee DJ, Lees AW, Bagnall KM, Haykowsky M, Hanson J. The addition of manual lymph drainage to compression therapy for breast cancer related lymphedema: a randomized controlled trial. *Breast Cancer Res Treat.* 2004;86:95–106.

33. Box RC, Reul-Hirche HM, Bullock-Saxton JE, Furnival CM. Physiotherapy after breast cancer surgery: results of a randomised controlled study to minimise lymphoedema. *Breast Cancer Res Treat.* 2002;75:51–64.

34. Morrell RM, Halyard MY, Schild SE, Ali MS, Gunderson LL, Pockaj BA. Breast cancer-related lymphedema. *Mayo Clin Proc.* 2005;80:1480–1484.

35. Hayes S, Cornish B, Newman B. Comparison of methods to diagnose lymphoedema among breast cancer survivors: 6-month follow-up. *Breast Cancer Res Treat.* 2005;89:221–226.

36. Petrek JA, Senie RT, Peters M, Rosen PP. Lymphedema in a cohort of breast carcinoma survivors 20 years after diagnosis. *Cancer.* 2001;92:1368–1377.

37. Armer JM, Stewart BR. A comparison of four diagnostic criteria for lymphedema in a post-breast cancer population. *Lymphat Res Biol.* 2005;3:208–217.

38. Bicego D, Brown K, Ruddick M, Storey D, Wong C, Harris SR. Exercise for women with or at risk for breast cancer-related lymphedema. *Phys Ther.* 2006;86:1398–1405.

39. Deltombe T, Jamart J, Recloux S, et al. Reliability and limits of agreement of circumferential, water displacement, and optoelectronic volumetry in the measurement of upper limb lymphedema. *Lymphology.* 2007;40:26–34.

40. Warren AG, Janz BA, Slavin SA, Borud LJ. The use of bioimpedance analysis to evaluate lymphedema. *Ann Plast Surg.* 2007;58:541–543.

41. Tewari N, Gill PG, Bochner MA, Kollias J. Comparison of volume displacement versus circumferential arm measurements for lymphoedema; implications for the SNAC trial. *ANZ J Surg.* 2008;78:889–893.

42. Ward LC. Bioelectrical impedance analysis: proven utility in lymphedema risk assessment and therapeutic monitoring. *Lymphat Res Biol.* 2006;4:51–56.

43. Petlund C. Lymph stasis: Pathophysiology, diagnosis and treatment. In: *Volumetry of Limbs.* Boston: Olszewski & Waldeman; 1991:443–451.

44. Stanton AW, Northfield JW, Holroyd B, Mortimer PS, Levick JR. Validation of an optoelectronic limb volumeter (Perometer). *Lymphology.* 1997;30:77–97.

45. Tierney S, Aslam M, Rennie K, Grace P. Infrared optoelectronic volumetry, the ideal way to measure limb volume. *Eur J Vasc Endovasc Surg.* 1996;12:412–417.

46. McLaughlin SA, Wright MJ, Morris KT, et al. Prevalence of lymphedema in women with breast cancer 5 years after sentinel lymph node biopsy or axillary dissection: objective measurements. *J Clin Oncol.* 2008 Nov 10;26(32):5213–9.

47. van der Veen P, De Voogdt N, Lievens P, Duquet W, Lamote J, Sacre R. Lymphedema development following breast cancer surgery with full axillary resection. *Lymphology.* 2004;37:206–208.

48. McLaughlin SA, Wright MJ, Morris KT, et al. Prevalence of lymphedema in women with breast cancer 5 years after sentinel lymph node biopsy or axillary dissection: patient perceptions and precautionary behaviors. *J Clin Oncol.* 2008 Nov 10:26(32):5220–6.

49. Andersen L, Hojris I, Erlandsen M, Andersen J. Treatment of breast-cancer-related lymphedema with or without manual lymphatic drainage—a randomized study. *Acta Oncol.* 2000; 39:399–405.

50. Ozaslan C, Kuru B. Lymphedema after treatment of breast cancer. *Am J Surg.* 2004;187:69–72.

51. Radina ME, Armer J, Daunt D, Dusold J, Culbertson S. Self-reported management of breast cancer-related lymphoedema. *J Lymphoedema.* 2007;2:12–21.

52. Armer JM, Radina ME, Porock D, Culbertson SD. Predicting breast cancer-related lymphedema using self-reported symptoms. *Nurs Res.* 2003;52:370–379.

53. Haid A, Kuehn T, Konstantiniuk P, et al. Shoulder-arm morbidity following axillary dissection and sentinel node only biopsy for breast cancer. *Eur J Surg Oncol.* 2002;28:705–710.

54. Francis WP, Abghari P, Du W, Rymal C, Suna M, Kosir MA. Improving surgical outcomes: standardizing the reporting of incidence and severity of acute lymphedema after sentinel lymph node biopsy and axillary lymph node dissection. *Am J Surg.* 2006;192:636–639.

55. American Physical Therapy Association; *Guide to Physical Therapy Practice. Phys Ther.* 2001;81.

56. Pain SJ, Vowler SL, Purushotham AD. Is physical function a more appropriate measure than volume excess in the assessment of breast cancer-related lymphoedema (BCRL)? *Eur J Cancer.* 2003;39:2168–2172.

57. Johansson K, Ohlsson K, Ingvar C, Albertsson M, Ekdahl C. Factors associated with the development of arm lymphedema following breast cancer treatment: a match pair case-control study. *Lymphology.* 2002;35:59–71.

58. Meek AG. Breast radiotherapy and lymphedema. *Cancer.* 1998; 83:2788–2797.

59. Querci della Rovere G, Ahmad I, Singh P, Ashley S, Daniels IR, Mortimer P. An audit of the incidence of arm lymphoedema after prophylactic level I/II axillary dissection without division of the pectoralis minor muscle. *Ann R Coll Surg Engl.* 2003;85:158–161.

60. Williams AF, Franks PJ, Moffatt CJ. Lymphoedema: estimating the size of the problem. *Palliat Med.* 2005;19:300–313.

61. Park JH, Lee WH, Chung HS. Incidence and risk factors of breast cancer lymphoedema. *J Clin Nurs.* 2008;17:1450–1459.

62. Geller BM, Vacek PM, O'Brien P, Secker-Walker RH. Factors associated with arm swelling after breast cancer surgery. *J Womens Health (Larchmt).* 2003;12:921–930.

63. Wilke LG, McCall LM, Posther KE, et al. Surgical complications associated with sentinel lymph node biopsy: results from a prospective international cooperative group trial. *Ann Surg Oncol.* 2006;13:491–500.

64. Coen JJ, Taghian AG, Kachnic LA, Assaad SI, Powell SN. Risk of lymphedema after regional nodal irradiation with breast conservation therapy. *Int J Radiat Oncol Biol Phys.* 2003;55:1209–1215.

65. Golshan M, Martin WJ, Dowlatshahi K. Sentinel lymph node biopsy lowers the rate of lymphedema when compared with standard axillary lymph node dissection. *Am Surg.* 2003;69:209–211; discussion 12.

66. Silberman AW, McVay C, Cohen JS, et al. Comparative morbidity of axillary lymph node dissection and the sentinel lymph node technique: implications for patients with breast cancer. *Ann Surg.* 2004;240:1–6.

67. Vignes S, Porcher R, Arrault M, Dupuy A. Long-term management of breast cancer-related lymphedema after intensive decongestive physiotherapy. *Breast Cancer Res Treat.* 2007;101: 285–290.

68. Vignes S, Arrault M, Dupuy A. Factors associated with increased breast cancer-related lymphedema volume. *Acta Oncol.* 2007;46:1138–1142.

69. Karki A, Simonen R, Malkia E, Selfe J. Efficacy of physical therapy methods and exercise after a breast cancer operation: a systematic review. *Crit Rev Phys Rehab Med.* 2001;13:159–190.

70. Rockson SG. Lymphedema therapy in the vascular anomaly patient: therapeutics for the forgotten circulation. *Lymphat Res Biol.* 2005;3:253–255.

71. Ridner SH. Quality of life and a symptom cluster associated with breast cancer treatment-related lymphedema. *Support Care Cancer.* 2005;13:904–911.

72. Ahmed RL, Thomas W, Yee D, Schmitz KH. Randomized controlled trial of weight training and lymphedema in breast cancer survivors. *J Clin Oncol.* 2006;24:2765–2772.

73. Cheema BS, Gaul CA. Full-body exercise training improves fitness and quality of life in survivors of breast cancer. *J Strength Cond Res.* 2006;20:14–21.

74. Cheema B, Gaul CA, Lane K, Fiatarone Singh MA. Progressive resistance training in breast cancer: a systematic review of clinical trials. *Breast Cancer Res Treat.* 2008;109:9–26.

75. Leduc O, Leduc A. Rehabilitation protocol in upper limb lymphedema. *Ann Ital Chir.* 2002;73:479–484.

76. Knobf MT, Insogna K, DiPietro L, Fennie C, Thompson AS. An aerobic weight-loaded pilot exercise intervention for breast cancer survivors: bone remodeling and body composition outcomes. *Biol Res Nurs.* 2008;10:34–43.

77. Johansson K, Tibe K, Weibull A, Newton RC. Low intensity resistance exercise for breast cancer patients with arm lymphedema with or without compression sleeve. *Lymphology.* 2005;38:167–180.

78. Payne JK, Held J, Thorpe J, Shaw H. Effect of exercise on biomarkers, fatigue, sleep disturbances, and depressive symptoms in older women with breast cancer receiving hormonal therapy. *Oncol Nurs Forum.* 2008;35:635–642.

79. Langbecker D, Hayes SC, Newman B, Janda M. Treatment for upper-limb and lower-limb lymphedema by professionals specializing in lymphedema care. *Eur J Cancer Care (Engl).* 2008:;17(6):557–64.

80. Meijer RS, Rietman JS, Geertzen JH, Bosmans JC, Dijkstra PU. Validity and intra- and interobserver reliability of an indirect volume measurements in patients with upper extremity lymphedema. *Lymphology.* 2004;37:127–133.

81. Sander AP, Hajer NM, Hemenway K, Miller AC. Upper-extremity volume measurements in women with lymphedema: a comparison of measurements obtained via water displacement with geometrically determined volume. *Phys Ther.* 2002;82:1201–1212.

82. Harris SR, Hugi MR, Olivotto IA, Levine M. Clinical practice guidelines for the care and treatment of breast cancer: 11. Lymphedema. *CMAJ.* 2001;164:191–199.

83. Vallance JK, Courneya KS, Taylor LM, Plotnikoff RC, Mackey JR. Development and evaluation of a theory-based physical activity guidebook for breast cancer survivors. *Health Educ Behav.* 2008;35:174–189.

84. Salas E, Wilson KA, Murphy CE, King H, Salisbury M. Communicating, coordinating, and cooperating when lives depend on it: tips for teamwork. *Jt Comm J Qual Patient Saf.* 2008;34:333–341.

85. Garfein ES, Borud LJ, Warren AG, Slavin SA. Learning from a lymphedema clinic: an algorithm for the management of localized swelling. *Plast Reconstr Surg.* 2008;121:521–528.

86. Koul R, Dufan T, Russell C, et al. Efficacy of complete decongestive therapy and manual lymphatic drainage on treatment-related lymphedema in breast cancer. *Int J Radiat Oncol Biol Phys.* 2007;67:841–846.

87. Badger C, Preston N, Seers K, Mortimer P. Physical therapies for reducing and controlling lymphedema of the limbs. The Cochrane Database of Systemic Reviews; 2006:3.

88. Kligman L, Wong RK, Johnston M, Laetsch NS. The treatment of lymphedema related to breast cancer: a systematic review and evidence summary. *Support Care Cancer.* 2004;12:421–431.

89. Didem K, Ufuk YS, Serdar S, Zumre A. The comparison of two different physiotherapy methods in treatment of lymphedema after breast surgery. *Breast Cancer Res Treat.* 2005;93:49–54.

90. Ko DS, Lerner R, Klose G, Cosimi AB. Effective treatment of lymphedema of the extremities. *Arch Surg.* 1998;133:452–458.

91. Casley-Smith JR, Boris M, Weindorf S, Lasinski B. Treatment for lymphedema of the arm—the Casley-Smith method: a noninvasive method produces continued reduction. *Cancer.* 1998;83:2843–2860.

92. Szuba A, Cooke JP, Yousuf S, Rockson SG. Decongestive lymphatic therapy for patients with cancer-related or primary lymphedema. *Am J Med.* 2000;109:296–300.

93. Morgan P, Moffatt C. The National Lymphoedema Framework project. *Br J Community Nurs.* 2006;11:S19–S22.

94. Foldi M, Foldi E, Kubik S (Eds). *Textbook of Lymphology for Physicians and Lymphedema Therapists.* Munich: Urban & Fischer; 2003.

95. Howell D, Watson M. Evaluation of a pilot nurse-led, community-based treatment programme for lymphoedema. *Int J Palliat Nurs.* 2005;11:62–69.

96. Ridner SH, McMahon E, Dietrich MS, Hoy S. Home-based lymphedema treatment in patients with cancer-related lymphedema or noncancer-related lymphedema. *Oncol Nurs Forum.* 2008;35:671–680.

97. Cheville AL, McGarvey CL, Petrek JA, Russo SA, Taylor ME, Thiadens SR. Lymphedema management. *Semin Radiat Oncol.* 2003;13:290–301.

98. Wilburn O, Wilburn P, Rockson SG. A pilot, prospective evaluation of a novel alternative for maintenance therapy of breast cancer-associated lymphedema [ISRCTN76522412]. *BMC Cancer.* 2006;6:84.

99. Armer J, Fu MR, Wainstock JM, Zagar E, Jacobs LK. Lymphedema following breast cancer treatment, including sentinel lymph node biopsy. *Lymphology.* 2004;37:73–91.

13 Psychiatric Issues in Breast Cancer

ILANA MONICA BRAUN

DONNA BETH GREENBERG

Breast cancer diagnosis, treatment, and surveillance frequently lead to distress. Reactions to the disease can include feelings of vulnerability, sadness, fear, denial, and anger. When circumscribed and time-limited, such emotions constitute normal coping mechanisms, allowing individuals to come to terms with the implications of their disease gradually and organically.

Some patients remain extremely depressed or anxious, become preoccupied with physical symptoms, persistently think about death, or, rarely, develop psychosis. While many of these symptoms may also represent expected grieving, they raise the specter of primary psychiatric illness or pathophysiological changes resulting from cancer and its treatment (e.g., those stemming from brain metastases or steroid use). Presentations such as these are worthy of psychiatric evaluation and, likely, management. This chapter reviews the phenomenology and treatment of two varieties of psychiatric syndromes commonly encountered in the breast cancer setting: depression and anxiety.

■ DEPRESSION AND ANXIETY

The challenges that may face a breast cancer patient include existential fear; shifting roles within the family, community, and workplace; threat of disfigurement; economic hardship; social isolation; guilt; loss of independence; pain; fatigue; menopausal symptoms; a marathon treatment regimen; in the surveillance stage of treatment, a sense that "the other shoe might drop" at any moment; and particularly for those with known genetic risk factors, concern for the health of loved ones. Sadness, irritability, and fear can occur as isolated emotions, in the context of larger psychiatric syndromes such as major depressive disorder and generalized anxiety disorder, or as biological consequences of cancer and its treatment. Teasing out psychiatric syndromes from constellations of symptoms,

as well as differentiating the psychiatric from the medical, can be challenging, and these are tasks best attempted with a firm grounding in the diagnostic criteria for depression and anxiety.

Diagnosis and Workup

Depressive Disorders

While the vast majority of breast cancer patients experience some degree of dysphoria, not all patients with sadness meet the criteria for a major depressive disorder. A diagnosis of depression rests on at least two weeks of dysphoric mood or diminished interest in daily activities, as well as on the presence of an array of neurovegetative symptoms including change in appetite or weight; change in sleep pattern; fatigue; appearance of either psychomotor agitation (including fidgetiness, pacing, wide gesticulating) or retardation; feelings of worthlessness or excessive guilt; poor concentration or indecisiveness; and recurrent thoughts of death that are more extreme than simply a fear of dying. A breast cancer patient qualifying for a diagnosis of depression manifests at least five such symptoms, including depressed mood or anhedonia as a keystone. Often an individual will report some symptoms of depression but not enough to meet all the criteria for the disorder. In the context of breast cancer, one can describe such a person as having an adjustment disorder. Rarely, a breast cancer patient develops such severe depression that she experiences hallucinations, delusions, or paranoia. Such a patient can be described as having depression with psychotic features. Treatment of this serious illness is beyond the scope of this chapter and should be managed by a professional with psychiatric expertise.

Anxiety Disorders

Like depressed mood, anxiety is quite common in the context of breast cancer and does not always occur as part of a larger psychiatric syndrome. That said, anxiety disorders can present in many forms. Generalized anxiety is a pervasive sense of nervousness characterized by at least half a year of several of the following symptoms: edginess or restlessness, fatigue, distractibility, irritability, muscle tension, and insomnia. More days than not, a person with generalized anxiety disorder appears and feels anxious. In contrast, patients with panic disorder may seem relatively calm between episodes (even if their subjective experience is otherwise). Panic attacks are discrete, unexpected, and extremely distressing periods of intense fear. Developing suddenly, they typically peak within 10 minutes and are accompanied by a sense of impending doom and symptoms of autonomic arousal, including palpitations, sweating, nausea, and tingling in extremities. Isolated panic attacks are usually not worrisome. However, when such events begin to interfere with everyday life and an individual becomes preoccupied with fear of their recurrence, panic attacks are elevated to the status of a syndrome, termed panic disorder. Posttraumatic stress disorder describes a constellation of symptoms, including intrusive thoughts, flashbacks, avoidance behaviors, emotional numbness, and autonomic arousal following a real or perceived threat to one's life, such as receiving a cancer diagnosis.

Diagnostic Challenges in the Setting of Medical Illness

For the most part, diagnostic criteria for psychiatric syndromes were developed in medically healthy patients and present challenges in those with physical illnesses such as breast cancer. Several of the abovementioned symptoms occur commonly in breast cancer patients, independent of depression and anxiety. Examples are changes in appetite and weight, sleep disturbance, fatigue, and autonomic arousal. For this reason, suspicions of psychiatric diagnoses in cancer patients rest more heavily on psychological symptoms, including anhedonia, dysphoria, anxiety, edginess, social withdrawal, hopelessness, helplessness, worthlessness, guilt, low self-esteem, and suicidality. In short, psychiatric diagnosis in the medically ill remains an art, not a science.

Prevalence and Risk Factors

Prevalence estimates for depression among breast cancer patients range from 10% to 25%, higher than for patients with most other cancers (1). Prevalence estimates for a diagnosable anxiety disorder among breast cancer patients range from 16% to 38% (2,3). A clinical rule of thumb is that one fourth of cancer patients will be depressed or anxious enough during the course of their illness to necessitate evaluation and treatment (4). Risk factors in general cancer populations include poor physical condition, advanced stage, inadequately controlled pain, a history of depressive episodes, a history of other significant losses, and premature menopause triggered either by chemotherapeutics or estrogen-depleting endocrine therapies (5,6).

Somatic Etiologies

Several reversible medical conditions and their treatments can biologically induce depression or anxiety syndromes. Differentiating a psychiatric condition triggered by emotional stress from one brought on as a direct pathophysiological result of illness or substance use can prove challenging and requires a high level of suspicion. Table 13.1 details some of the possible medical underpinnings of depression and anxiety. Several occur commonly in the context of breast cancer and its treatment. These include poor appetite, menopausal estrogen decline, low vitamin B_{12}, hypothyroidism, anemia, sleep apnea, brain metastases, steroid use, pain, and, particularly in the setting of new-onset anxiety, congestive heart failure and pulmonary embolism. For this reason, careful medical history and workup can prove crucial in the psychiatric

■ **Table 13.1** Medical conditions triggering or exacerbating depressive or anxiety syndromes in patients with breast cancer

Vitamin and dietary deficiencies	Low vitamin B_{12} Low folate Anorexia
Endocrine abnormalities	Menopausal estrogen decline Thyroid dysfunction Parathyroid dysfunction Adrenal dysfunction
Blood disorders	Anemia Electrolyte abnormalities (i.e., hypercalcemia)
Sleep disorders	Sleep apnea (central or obstructive) Restless legs syndrome
Infections	Mononucleosis Lyme disease Syphilis
Neurological disorders	Brain mass Stroke Traumatic brain injury Epilepsy Parkinson's disease Multiple sclerosis
Medications and other substances	Corticosteroids Selective estrogen receptor modulators Interferon Alcohol Narcotics Withdrawal syndromes
Other	Pain syndromes Pulmonary embolism Congestive heart failure

evaluation of breast cancer patients. Medications and supplements should be reviewed in detail. Routine laboratory assessment might include a complete blood count, folate level, vitamin B_{12} level, thyroid-stimulating hormone level, and if there is concern about substance abuse, urine toxicology and blood alcohol level. If there is a suggestion of focal neurological deficits, computed tomography or magnetic resonance imaging of the brain should be performed.

Suicidal Thinking

One of the most dreaded outcomes of depression and anxiety is suicide. Thoughts of dying span a continuum from the desire for a hastened death on one end of the spectrum to suicidal plan, intent, and attempt on the other. Thoughts of suicide without clear plan or intent are quite common in cancer patients and provide a sense of control in those overwhelmed by suffering, uncertainty, and helplessness. Thankfully, few cancer patients actually attempt suicide. There is evidence, however, that they are at mildly higher risk than the general population, particularly in the months following diagnosis (7–9). For this reason, it is of utmost importance that patients intimating suicidal thoughts or hopelessness be asked specifically and directly about suicidal intentions, precipitants, plan, and means. Those who endorse a suicidal plan or intent should be assessed further by a provider with psychiatric expertise, often in the setting of an emergency department.

Treatment

Despite the high prevalence of depression and anxiety in breast cancer patients, few studies have examined treatment options in this population (1). By convention, comprehensive treatment of depression and anxiety involves a multimodal approach that includes addressing all reversible medical etiologies, individual and group counseling, and psychotropic medications.

Addressing Medical Etiologies

Medical factors exacerbating psychiatric syndromes should, if possible, be minimized or neutralized. Treating clinicians should screen for and address dietary deficiencies such as low vitamin B_{12} or folate, endocrine dysfunctions such as hypothyroidism, pain syndromes, menopausal symptoms, anemia, and substance abuse. Agents with appetite-stimulating properties (e.g., the antidepressant mirtazapine) can be offered to anorectic patients. Nonessential steroid use (e.g., for an antinausea indication) should be limited as much as is possible. When sleep disturbances and fatigue present as part of depressive or anxiety syndromes, healthcare providers should consider medical etiologies in the differential. Obstructive

sleep apnea, diagnosed via sleep study, is best managed with a positive airway pressure machine; restless legs syndrome with the removal of exacerbating agents or with the addition of medications such as gabapentin or both.

Psychotherapy

One modality that is effective, alone or in combination with psychotropic medication, is psychotherapy. Several clinical trials in breast cancer patients have demonstrated improvements in both quality of life and perception of physical symptoms with both group and individual talk therapies (10,11). A variety of models of one-on-one and group talk therapy exist. Brief interventions commonly employed in the cancer setting include supportive psychotherapy, cognitive behavioral therapy (CBT), and supportive-expressive psychotherapy. Supportive psychotherapists encourage patients to vent their distress within the safety of the therapeutic relationship and aim to bolster patients' defense mechanisms through the offering of advice, support, and empathy. CBT therapists operate within the following theoretical framework: Negative beliefs promote feelings of depression and anxiety that, in turn, lead to avoidant or compulsive behaviors. These deleterious behaviors help to cement negative cognitions and perpetuate a maladaptive cycle. Through homework exercises and structured sessions with clearly defined goals, CBT therapists encourage patients to examine the automatic thoughts that underlie both deleterious behaviors (e.g., medical noncompliance) and negative emotions. A growing literature demonstrates the efficacy of supportive-expressive group therapy in improving mood symptoms among breast cancer patients. Supportive-expressive psychotherapists offer cancer survivors unstructured, existentially based psychotherapy focused on concerns of death, meaning making, freedom, and isolation (12,13). At this time, there is no evidence to suggest that one therapeutic modality is better than another for patients with breast cancer.

Antidepressants

The Food and Drug Administration (FDA) has approved antidepressants as a treatment for a variety of depressive and anxiety disorders in the general public. However, there has been a paucity of positive randomized, placebo-controlled trials assessing the risks and benefits of these medications in cancer patients (14). Antidepressants commonly employed in the breast cancer setting are listed in Table 13.2.

These medications exert their primary effects by modulating one or both of the serotonin and norepinephrine neurotransmitter systems. For poorly understood reasons, antidepressants have a pronounced latency, on the order of weeks, in the onset of their effect. Thus, treatment failure

■ Table 13.2   Antidepressants used in patients with breast cancer

Drug	Dose (mg/d PO)	Possible Unique Benefits	Possible Side Effects
Bupropion/ Bupropion ER	75–450	May be helpful for concentration and low energy; fewer sexual side effects	Seizures, headache, nausea, likely impedes tamoxifen's efficacy
Citalopram	10–40	Few P450 interactions (including with tamoxifen)	Headache, diarrhea, constipation, restlessness, sexual dysfunction
Duloxetine	20–60	Management of neuropathic pain	Worsening of narrow angle glaucoma, possible worsening of liver disease in those with liver injury, nausea, dizziness, fatigue, sexual dysfunction
Escitalopram	10–20	Few P450 interactions (including with tamoxifen)	Headache, constipation, restlessness, sexual dysfunction
Fluoxetine	10–80	Long-acting so (a) may be dosed once weekly in a special 90 mg preparation and (b) least likely to trigger discontinuation syndrome	Nausea, nervousness, weight gain, headache, insomnia, strong inhibition of tamoxifen and other CYP2D6 substrates
Mirtazapine	15–45	Sleep aid at low doses; appetite stimulant; antiemetic; fewer gastrointestinal side effects than others; minimal sexual dysfunction	Dry mouth, sedating at low doses, weight gain
Paroxetine/ Paroxetine CR	5–60 (62.5 for CR)	Management of hot flashes	Headache, somnolence, dizziness, sexual dysfunction, gastrointestinal upset, dry mouth, prominent discontinuation syndrome, strong inhibition of tamoxifen and other 2D6 substrates
Sertraline	25–200		Headache, diarrhea, constipation, restlessness, sexual dysfunction
Trazodone	25–250	Sleep aid	Sedation, orthostasis, priapism, sexual dysfunction
Venlafaxine/ Venlafaxine SR	37.5–300	Management of hot flashes and neuropathic pain; least interaction with tamoxifen and few P450 interactions in general	Blood pressure increases, sexual dysfunction, prominent discontinuation syndrome

for depression and anxiety should not be declared until four to six weeks after initiation of an adequate dose of a particular antidepressant.

In addition to ameliorating depression and anxiety, antidepressants boast a wide variety of secondary effects that can sometimes be harnessed to advantage in the management of nonpsychiatric symptoms. In general, these uses are off-label and not FDA approved. Providers can offer sedating antidepressants such as mirtazapine and trazodone to patients with insomnia and appetite-stimulating ones such as mirtazapine to patients with unintended weight loss or cachexia. Duloxetine and venlafaxine may help to manage chemotherapy-triggered neuropathic pain syndromes;

hot flashes often improve with nonhormonal treatments such as paroxetine and venlafaxine.

Antidepressant side effects are usually quite tolerable but can include headache, gastrointestinal disturbances, sedation, weight gain (particularly with paroxetine), sexual dysfunction, blood pressure increases (particularly with venlafaxine), lowering of the seizure threshold (particularly with bupropion), restlessness, and, in individuals with underlying bipolar disorder, mania.

Long-term antidepressant use may be associated with increased risk of fracture in the elderly and of gastrointestinal bleeding. These vulnerabilities probably arise through antidepressants' serotonergic effects on bone and platelets, respectively. Risks of long-term use should be weighed against potential benefits.

Abrupt antidepressant withdrawal (particularly of short-acting antidepressants such as duloxetine, paroxetine, and venlafaxine) may be associated with a discontinuation syndrome characterized by malaise, light-headedness, dizziness, and lightning-like pains in extremities. To avoid this outcome, discontinuation of any antidepressant should be gradual over the course of several weeks to months.

Benzodiazepines

Because antidepressants take weeks to exert their full antidepressant and anxiolytic effects, other, more rapidly acting agents can serve as stop-gap measures. Benzodiazepines act through the inhibitory gamma-aminobutyric acid (GABA) neurotransmitter system to quell anxiety and are useful adjuncts to antidepressants as sleep aids. They are frequently used to manage anticipatory anxiety (e.g., prior to first chemotherapy infusion or magnetic resonance imaging). Because they do little to prevent future episodes of anxiety, however, they are rarely used in place of antidepressants in the setting of major depression or an enduring anxiety disorder. In addition to treating acute psychiatric distress, benzodiazepines have far-reaching medical utility in the cancer setting as skeletal muscle relaxants, antiemetics, and anticonvulsants and in the management of the potentially life threatening syndrome of alcohol withdrawal. Benzodiazepines commonly employed in breast cancer patients are listed in Table 13.3.

Benzodiazepines can trigger central nervous system side effects, including sedation, dizziness, ataxia and frequent falling, anterograde amnesia, irritability, and disorientation. As a sleep aid, they can have adverse effects on respiration and on sleep architecture, with diminution in both slow-wave sleep and rapid eye movements.

■ **Table 13.3** Benzodiazepines used in patients with breast cancer				
Drug	Dose (mg/d)	Half-Life (h)	Possible Unique Benefits	Possible Side Effects and Risks
Alprazolam	0.125–2 PO	6–20	Helpful in the management of anxiety, higher potential for dependence and abuse than others	Sedation, dizziness, ataxia (or other psychomotor impairment), memory impairment, irritability, sexual dysfunction, disorientation, abuse, tolerance, dependence, withdrawal on abrupt discontinuation; bradycardia and respiratory depression with diazepam and lorazepam; CYP3A4–based drug-drug interactions with alprazolam
Clonazepam	0.25–4 PO	20–50	Helpful in the management of anxiety, seizure disorders, nocturnal sleep disorders, neuralgia, mania; may have less abuse liability than shorter-onset agents	
Diazepam	1–20 PO, IV, IM	30–60	Helpful in the management of anxiety, alcohol withdrawal, muscle spasm, seizure disorders	
Lorazepam	0.5–5 PO, IV, IM	10–18	Helpful in the management of anxiety, depression, seizure disorders, alcohol withdrawal, and as an antiemetic; preferable in those with liver disease as not subject to phase I metabolism	
Oxazepam	5–30 PO	6–12	Helpful in the management of anxiety and alcohol withdrawal; preferable in those with liver disease as not subject to phase I metabolism; may have less abuse liability than shorter-onset agents	
Temazepam	7.5–15 PO	10–12	Helpful in the management of anxiety, depression, insomnia; preferable in those with liver disease as not subject to phase I metabolism; may have less abuse liability than shorter-onset agents	

The abovementioned side effects may be particularly pronounced in the elderly and in those with central nervous system fragility (e.g., as a result of brain metastases). Benzodiazepines carry abuse liability and should be used with caution in individuals with histories of substance abuse. Following prolonged use, these medications should be tapered very gradually over the course of weeks to months. Abrupt cessation may lead to a powerful and potentially life-threatening withdrawal reaction characterized by hyperthermia, autonomic arousal, sweating, neuromuscular irritability, paranoia, and hallucinations.

Hypnotics

Hypnotic drugs aid in sleep induction and maintenance. Sleep is often disrupted, not only in the setting of depression and anxiety but during breast cancer therapy in the absence of these psychiatric entities. Hypnotics commonly used in the breast cancer setting are listed in Table 13.4.

Like sedatives, these medication act on the GABAergic system, but they tend to have much more benign side effect profiles. A breast cancer patient may experience a mild hangover following their use. Eszopiclone has gained notoriety for a metallic taste following its ingestion. Zolpidem has received attention for its uncommon association with sleep-related disorders such as sleep walking, eating, and even driving. It has also been associated with hallucinations. Although hypnotics have low potential for tolerance and withdrawal, abrupt cessation following prolonged use may lead to a brief period of rebound insomnia. Unlike anxiolytics, they are not dependency forming; however, they do carry some abuse liability. For this reason, hypnotics are best avoided in individuals with strong histories of substance abuse or dependence. Finally, in a delirious patient with sleep difficulties, a sedating antipsychotic such as olanzapine or quetiapine is probably preferable to a hypnotic that might exacerbate a confusional state.

Drug Interactions

Because the majority of breast cancer patients rely on polypharmacy, attention to possible pharmacokinetic and pharmacodynamic drug-drug interactions is essential when considering the addition of a psychotropic medication. Pharmacokinetic interactions are those that alter the amount and duration of a drug's availability; pharmacodynamic interactions are the antagonistic, additive, or synergistic clinical effects exerted by concomitantly administered agents. A single agent can disrupt the balance of an established pharmaceutical regimen.

In general, antidepressants and anxiolytics have few drug-drug interactions. There are, however, some exceptions. These include antidepressants such as bupropion, fluoxetine, paroxetine, and duloxetine, and the benzodiazepine alprazolam. Fluoxetine and paroxetine, and to a lesser extent bupropion and duloxetine, are inhibitors of the cytochrome 2D6 (CYP2D6) pathway, which is responsible for metabolism of many antidepressants, antipsychotics, beta-blockers, and narcotics, including codeine, oxycodone, and methadone. Administration of these antidepressants along with 2D6 substrates can theoretically lead to accumulation of the latter in the body.

Duloxetine should be used with caution in the medically ill. In addition to inhibiting cytochrome CYP2D6, the agent is metabolized along a cytochrome 1A2 (CYP1A2) pathway. Fluoroquinolones and other drugs that inhibit this pathway can significantly increase duloxetine levels.

Alprazolam is metabolized along a cytochrome 3A (CYP3A) pathway, rendering it sensitive to a wide array of CYP3A inhibitors that raise its level, including macrolide

■ **Table 13.4** Hypnotics used in patients with breast cancer			
Drug	**Dose (mg/d)**	**Possible Unique Benefits**	**Possible Side Effects**
Eszopiclone	1–3	Low potential for tolerance and withdrawal; short half-life (~1 h) renders it ideal for patients with sleep initiation difficulties	Headache, dry mouth, somnolence, dizziness, hallucinations, rash, unpleasant metallic taste after ingestion
Zaleplon	5–20	Low potential for tolerance and withdrawal; short half-life (~1 h) renders it ideal for patients with sleep initiation difficulties	Headache, somnolence, amnesia, photosensitivity, edema; should be used with caution in patients with hepatic or renal insufficiency
Zolpidem/Zolpidem CR	2.5–10 (6.25–12.5 for CR)	Helpful in the short-term management of insomnia; low potential for tolerance and withdrawal; tends not to impair nocturnal respiratory and sleep architecture	Headache, dizziness, drowsiness, nausea, myalgia, sleep eating syndrome, hallucination, addiction

antibiotics, several antifungals, fluoxetine, and grapefruit juice. Cytochrome 3A inducers that lower its levels and can induce unwanted benzodiazepine withdrawal symptoms include several antiepileptic medications and, central to the practice of oncology, dexamethasone.

The interaction of many antidepressants and tamoxifen is worthy of special focus. Antidepressants are frequently prescribed in the setting of tamoxifen for their effectiveness both in treating psychiatric side effects and in ameliorating menopausal symptoms exacerbated by the hormone antagonist. Fluoxetine, paroxetine, and, to a lesser extent, other antidepressants are metabolized along a shared cytochrome P450 pathway with tamoxifen. This pathway is of the 2D6 isoenzyme. Antidepressants may decrease tamoxifen's efficacy by impeding the latter's conversion to active metabolites. When co-administration of tamoxifen and an antidepressant is indicated, the ideal antidepressant to select is venlafaxine, followed closely by escitalopram and citalopram.

■ CONCLUSION

Psychic distress in the context of breast cancer necessitates intervention when it is protracted, extreme, or accompanied by significant somatization, suicidality, or psychosis. Roughly one quarter of breast cancer patients will require psychiatric intervention for depression or anxiety during the course of their illness. Few studies have conclusively identified pharmacological treatments for psychiatric disorders in cancer patients, and principles of general psychiatry largely guide the standard of care in this population. Comprehensive treatment of depression and anxiety disorders in breast cancer patients includes treatment of exacerbating medical factors, talk therapy, and provision of psychotropic medication.

■ KEY POINTS

- While some sadness and anxiety is normal, mood disturbances in breast cancer patients are a cause for concern when they are severe, persistent, or accompanied by other psychological and somatic symptoms, such as insomnia or thoughts of death and dying. Symptoms such as these are worthy of further workup and, perhaps, consultation with a trained mental health professional.
- In addition to psychosocial stressors, medical factors, such as menopausal estrogen decline and pain,

can trigger or exacerbate symptoms such as fatigue, insomnia, and irritability in breast cancer patients.
- For the most part, antidepressants, anxiolytics, and hypnotics do not pose significant risk for drug-drug interactions with breast cancer medications; that said, fluoxetine, paroxetine, and, to a lesser extent, other antidepressants are metabolized along a shared cytochrome P450 pathway with tamoxifen and may decrease tamoxifen's efficacy by impeding its conversion to active metabolites.

■ REFERENCES

1. Fann JR, Thomas-Rich AM, Katon WJ, et al. Major depression after breast cancer: a review of epidemiology and treatment. *Gen Hosp Psychiatry*. 2007;30:112–126.
2. Lueboonthavatchai, P. Prevalence and psychosocial factors of anxiety and depression in breast cancer patients. *J Med Assoc Thai*. 2007;90(10):2164–2174.
3. Mehnert A, Koch U. Psychological comorbidity and health-related quality of life and its association with awareness, utilization, and need for psychosocial support in a cancer register-based sample of long-term breast cancer survivors. *J Psychosom Res*. 2008;64(4):383–391.
4. Massie MJ, Greenberg DB. Oncology. In: Levenson JL, ed. *Textbook of Psychosomatic Medicine*. Washington, DC: American Psychiatric Publishing; 2005:518.
5. Massie MJ, Popkin M. Depressive disorders. In: Holland JC, ed. *Psycho-Oncology*. New York, NY: Oxford University Press; 1998: 518–40.
6. Newport DJ, Nemeroff CB: Assessment and treatment of depression in the cancer patient. *J Psychosom Res*. 1998;45:215–237.
7. Bjorkenstam C, Edberg A, Ayoubi S, et al. Are cancer patients at higher suicide risk than the general population? *Scan J Public Health*. 2005;33:208–214.
8. Levi F, Buillard JL, La Vecchia C. Suicide risk among incident cases of cancer in the Swiss Canton of Vaud. *Oncology*. 1991;48: 44–47.
9. Louhivouri KA, Hakama M. Risk of suicide among cancer patients. *Am J Epidemiol*. 1979;109:59–65.
10. Daniels J, Kissane DW. Psychosocial interventions for cancer patients. *Curr Opin Oncol*. 2008;20(4);367–371.
11. Tatrow K, Montgomery GH. Cognitive behavioral therapy techniques for distress and pain in breast cancer patients: a meta-analysis. *J Behav Med*. 2006;29(1):17–27.
12. Classen C, Butler LD, Koopman C, et al. Supportive-expressive group therapy and distress in patients with metastatic breast cancer: a randomized clinical intervention trial. *Arch Gen Psychiatry*. 2001;58(5):494–501.
13. Classen C, Kraemer HC, Blasey C, et al. Supportive-expressive group therapy for primary breast cancer patients: a randomized prospective multicenter trial. *Psychooncology*. 2008;(17)5: 438–437.
14. Musselman DL, Somerset WI, Guo Y, et al. A double-blind, multicenter, parallel-group study of paroxetine, desipramine, or placebo in breast cancer patients (stage I, II, III, and IV) with major depression. *J Clin Psychiatry*. 2006;67(2):288–296.

14 Multidisciplinary Considerations: Racial Disparities in Breast Cancer

BEVERLY MOY

It is well established that despite lower incidence of breast cancer, black women are more likely than white women to die of the disease (1,2). Compared with white women, minority women have been found to have lower levels of mammography screening, to present at more advanced stages of breast cancer, and to have higher rates of breast cancer deaths (3–10).

This racial disparity in breast cancer survival is due to many contributing factors. Among the most significant factors are that ethnic minority populations have reduced access to cancer care, tend to have suboptimal treatment, and are more likely to have other comorbidities (11).

Breast cancer in black women is also more likely to have unfavorable biological characteristics, including higher proportions of estrogen receptor–negative tumors, high-grade tumors, and overexpression of cyclin E, p16, and p53 (12,13). Even after controlling for these biological factors, significant differences in survival remain between black and white breast cancer patients. For example, in five consecutive adjuvant breast cancer trials coordinated by the Southwest Oncology Group (SWOG), adjusted for age, receptor status, number of positive lymph nodes, and tumor size, black patients have significantly worse disease-free, overall, and cause-specific survival (14). Similarly, an analysis of breast cancer patients in the Surveillance, Epidemiology and End Results (SEER) database reveals that even after controlling for age, stage, histology, hormone receptor status, and residence area, black women have significantly worse survival than white women (15). It is also important to note that ethnic minority women are also underrepresented in cancer clinical trials (16).

This chapter will explore the racial disparities with regard to the multidisciplinary treatment of breast cancer.

■ RACIAL DISPARITIES IN BREAST CANCER SURGERY

Use of Sentinel Lymph Node Biopsy

Ascertaining the extent of lymph node involvement and accurately staging breast cancer are crucial components of breast cancer treatment. Axillary staging has traditionally been determined by surgical axillary lymph node dissection (ALND). While ALND allows for comprehensive evaluation of the extent of cancer spread, it may also lead to substantial morbidity, including lymphedema and functional deficits in the upper extremity (17–19). In the late 1990s, sentinel lymph node biopsy (SLNB) was established as a less invasive and effective alternative to ALND. Rates of regional recurrence are low among patients with negative SLNB results, sparing these patients from the morbidity of ALND (17,20). Therefore, National Comprehensive Cancer Network and American Society of Clinical Oncology guidelines recommend SLNB in lieu of upfront ALND for women with early-stage invasive breast cancer (21,22).

Despite these recommendations, SLNB is used less frequently in racial minority groups, those who have no health insurance, and lower socioeconomic groups (23,24). One study found that while the overall use of SLNB from 1998 to 2005 increased from 27% to 66%, black patients were 24% less likely than whites to have SLNB. In addition, patients without health insurance were 23% less likely to undergo SLNB. These disparities relating to receipt of SLNB are particularly important in light of the clinical advantages associated with this technique.

Breast-conserving Surgery Versus Mastectomy

For women diagnosed with early-stage breast cancer, breast-conserving surgery (BCS) plus radiation therapy has equivalent survival to mastectomy as initial treatment and can provide women with improved body image and emotional well-being (25,26). In 1990, the National

Institutes of Health released a consensus statement recommending use of BCS with adjuvant radiation instead of mastectomy for the treatment of early-stage breast cancer, whenever possible (27).

Despite these guidelines, disparities in the use of BCS exist by race/ethnicity, geographic region, and provider characteristics (28,29). Specifically, studies have found that Asian women are less likely to receive BCS than white women (30,31). Only 43% of foreign-born Asian women underwent BCS, compared with 56% of United States–born Asian women and white women. In addition, older women and women of lower socioeconomic status were less likely to receive BCS. Although the use of BCS does not influence mortality, its benefits in improving emotional well-being and quality of life warrants its use in all populations.

Use of Breast Reconstruction

If a patient and her physician decide that she should undergo a mastectomy, the option of breast reconstruction is often presented. The potential benefits of immediate reconstruction at the time of mastectomy include improved psychological well-being and improved cosmetic results. It has been found that patients who undergo mastectomy for breast cancer experience more postoperative psychosocial distress than patients who undergo other surgical procedures (32). Immediate breast reconstruction poses a minimal risk of delaying treatment and does not interfere with follow-up for recurrent cancer (33,34). In a randomized clinical trial, patients who underwent immediate reconstruction experienced higher physical self-esteem than patients who were offered delayed reconstruction 12 months after mastectomy (35).

Yet a racial disparity exists regarding breast reconstruction after mastectomy. A single institution study of 1,004 mastectomies showed that African American and Asian women underwent immediate breast reconstruction after mastectomy at significantly lower rates compared with white, Hispanic, and Asian women (36). Black women were less likely to be offered a referral for reconstruction, to accept a referral to plastic surgery when offered, and to elect a reconstruction when offered. The rate of delayed breast reconstruction was lower in African American and Asian women than in their white counterparts and did not affect the overall gap in reconstruction between those two groups and white women (36).

A more recent study of SEER data revealed that receipt of breast reconstruction varied significantly by patient race/ethnicity (37). These data demonstrated that 35.9% of whites, 28.4% of blacks, 35.7% of English-speaking Latinas, and only 13.2% of Spanish-speaking Latinas (P <0.001) received breast reconstruction after mastectomy (37). Compared with the other racial/ethnic groups, Spanish-speaking Latinas were least likely to be satisfied with their surgical decision and were most likely to face significant barriers to reconstruction, including lack of referral to a plastic surgeon.

■ RACIAL DISPARITIES IN RADIATION THERAPY

Radiation therapy is an integral part of treatment of early-stage breast cancer. As stated previously, BCS plus radiation therapy has equivalent survival to mastectomy in early-stage breast cancer since radiation significantly reduces the risk of recurrent disease. A clinical trial randomizing women with ductal carcinoma in situ to lumpectomy alone or lumpectomy plus radiation revealed that five-year event-free survival was significantly better in the women who received breast irradiation (38). Five-year event-free survival was 84% in women who received breast irradiation, compared with 73.8% for the women treated by lumpectomy alone. The improvement was due to a reduction in the occurrence of second ipsilateral breast cancers.

Similarly, a landmark clinical trial randomizing women with invasive breast cancer to BCS alone or BCS with radiation or mastectomy revealed that radiation significantly improves recurrence rates (39). Of the women treated with breast radiation after lumpectomy, 90% remained free of ipsilateral breast tumor, compared with 61% of those not treated with irradiation after lumpectomy.

Despite definitive data establishing radiation as a key component of the treatment of early-stage breast cancer, ethnic minority women are less likely to receive appropriate radiation therapy. A study of the SEER database from 1992 to 2002 revealed that the percentage of women who received BCS without radiotherapy increased from 10.8% to 19.8% for whites and from 13.6% to 27.7% for blacks (40). The disparity between blacks and whites increased during this period. Black women were 24% less likely than whites to receive the recommended radiation therapy, regardless of their year of diagnosis, geographic area, or patient or tumor characteristics (40).

These results were confirmed in an examination of the SEER database from 1988 to 2004, which revealed that as BCS has increasingly replaced mastectomy, fewer women received definitive breast radiotherapy after BCS (41). Significant persistent disparities remained evident for black and Latina women, with blacks being 23% less likely and Latinas 14% less likely to receive radiation (41).

■ RACIAL DISPARITIES IN MEDICAL ONCOLOGY

Chemotherapy

Large prospective randomized controlled trials demonstrate that adjuvant systemic chemotherapy for women with higher-risk early-stage breast cancer improves disease-free and overall survival (42). A potential contributor for racial disparities in breast cancer is the underutilization of chemotherapy (28,43,44). There are conflicting data about whether chemotherapy is as beneficial in ethnic minorities as it is in whites. Data from the Cancer and Leukemia Group B Trial showed that black women, white women, and women of other races treated with adjuvant chemotherapy for stage 2 breast cancer had similar benefits (45). Similarly, data from the National Surgical Adjuvant Breast and Bowel Project (NSABP) and the Piedmont Oncology Association showed that black and white women with breast cancer received similar benefits from chemotherapy (46,47).

In contrast, a study of 6,676 women enrolled in SWOG breast cancer adjuvant therapy trials between 1975 and 1995 revealed that black women had approximately 40% worse survival than women of other races, even after adjusting for differences in socioeconomic factors, baseline disease, and treatment variables (14). The investigators found similar racial disparities in ovarian and prostate cancer in the SWOG database.

Despite these conflicting results, the literature overwhelmingly supports the use of adjuvant chemotherapy in selected patients with early-stage breast cancer. Ethnic minority groups are less likely to receive chemotherapy than white women diagnosed with breast cancer. For example, a study of six New York City hospitals found that among 126 women with greater than stage 1A hormone receptor–negative tumors, black women were less likely than whites to receive chemotherapy (67% versus 78%; $P <0.01$) (48). Part of the underuse of chemotherapy in ethnic minority women may be explained by the facts that minority women have more comorbidities and are less likely to have insurance. However, after controlling for these factors, blacks and Latinas were more than twice as likely not to receive adjuvant systemic therapies.

Black women are also more likely to have suboptimal duration and number of chemotherapy treatment cycles. A study of the Henry Ford Health System tumor registry revealed that black women received less than 75% of the expected number of cycles of chemotherapy, and this was associated with poorer survival (49). Premature termination of chemotherapy was associated with both black race and poorer survival (49). Similarly, SEER data demonstrated that black women experience longer chemotherapy treatment delays (50). Blacks also receive lower than optimal doses of chemotherapy compared with whites, regardless of their weight, and all black women are more likely to have first-cycle dose reductions than whites (43).

The suboptimal delivery of or failure to deliver chemotherapy to ethnic minority women may contribute to documented disparities in breast cancer survival. What is somewhat reassuring is that a recent study of Los Angeles SEER data reports that in contrast to practice-based studies of chemotherapy use in cohorts treated in previous periods, there was no evidence of racial/ethnic or social disparities in the use of chemotherapy in this diverse population-based sample of recently treated women (51).

Endocrine Therapy

Large prospective randomized controlled trials demonstrate that adjuvant systemic endocrine therapy in women with hormone receptor–positive early-stage breast cancer significantly improves disease-free and overall survival (52). While black women have proportionately more hormone receptor–negative tumors than whites, the majority of breast cancers are still hormone receptor–positive in black women. Clinical trials of endocrine agents have not adequately included black women, and thus their efficacy and toxicity have yet to be fully defined in this ethnic population (53). Some studies suggest that endocrine therapies are as efficacious in ethnic minorities as they are in whites. NSABP trials show that African American and white women taking tamoxifen have the same risks of new contralateral breast cancers and similar risks of thromboembolic events (54). Specifically, the NSABP B-14 trial showed that tamoxifen improved event-free and overall survival equally in blacks and whites (54).

However, other studies question the benefit of endocrine therapy in ethnic minorities. The MA17 clinical trial showed that letrozole, an aromatase inhibitor (AI), improved disease-free survival in whites but possibly not in ethnic minorities (55). Minority women also had fewer side effects from AIs than whites, suggesting a differential treatment effect (55). Similarly, a preliminary analysis of the MA27 clinical trial (nonsteroidal AI anastrozole vs steroidal AI) in early-stage breast cancer patients showed better tolerability and fewer AI-induced hot flashes in minority women (56).

Despite the fully defined role of endocrine therapy in ethnic minorities, the overwhelming body of evidence supports the widespread use of endocrine therapy in hormone receptor–positive breast cancer among the population as a whole. However, racial disparities exist regarding the receipt of endocrine therapy.

A study of six New York City hospitals found that among 421 women with greater than stage 1A hormone receptor–positive tumors, black and Latina women were less likely to receive endocrine therapy (71% and 75%, respectively, versus 80%; $P <0.05$) (48).

Similarly, SEER data demonstrated that black women eligible for endocrine therapy were less likely to receive it than whites (50). Since endocrine therapy is a crucial component of the optimal treatment for breast cancer, this disparity could contribute to worsened clinical outcomes in these vulnerable populations.

■ RACIAL DISPARITIES IN CLINICAL TRIAL PARTICIPATION

Ethnic minorities are significantly underrepresented in breast cancer clinical trials (16,57,58), and their representation has been declining in recent years (59). Insufficient minority enrollment into prevention, early detection, and treatment trials leads to difficulty in addressing the disparity in mortality rates between minority and white cancer patients (59,60). Without adequate minority enrollment into clinical trials, it is not possible to distinguish the impact of socioeconomic status from the impact of race on responses to treatment and overall outcomes or to examine minority group differences (59,61). Physicians are therefore forced to extrapolate overall results of clinical trials to minority populations, which may not be accurate.

The first breast cancer prevention trials, NSABP P1, enrolled 12,800 women, of whom only 1.7% were African American (62). The NSABP follow-up prevention trial Study of Tamoxifen and Raloxifene (STAR) enrolled 19,470 women, of whom only 2.5% were African American (63). The pivotal joint analysis of NSABP B31 and NCCTG N9831, which led to the approval of adjuvant trastuzumab, enrolled a total of 3,350 patients, of whom only about 7% were African American (64). The results of these clinical trials have led to widespread global use of these drugs for the prevention and treatment of breast cancer. However, any definitive conclusions about their benefits in ethnic minority populations cannot be made due to poor minority participation in these clinical trials.

Increasing minority participation in cancer clinical trials requires a multipronged approach targeted at making changes to the doctor/patient relationship, performing systemwide changes within the oncologist's practice, and improving outreach and relationships within the community (16). These efforts would make great strides in improving care for minority cancer patients.

■ CONCLUSION

This chapter has reviewed the multidisciplinary considerations with regards to racial disparities in breast cancer treatment and outcome. The main purpose of this chapter was to increase awareness of these disparities among oncology providers in order to provide the highest level of care to all breast cancer patients.

The major contributor to racial disparities in breast cancer outcomes is decreased access to care among ethnic minority populations. However, ethnic minority patients who have access to medical care still have significantly suboptimal surgical, radiation, and medical treatment of breast cancer. The oncology community needs to develop more effective strategies for minority populations. Building community trust, identifying community leaders and networks, and ensuring more participation in clinical trials and research are examples of such strategies. The multidisciplinary team approach to the care of breast cancer patients, regardless of race or socioeconomic status, can improve overall care. Combining these strategies in the multidisciplinary care of breast cancer patients will be helpful in eliminating racial disparities in breast cancer care.

■ SUMMARY

- The major contributor to racial disparities in breast cancer outcomes is decreased access to care among ethnic minority populations.
- Despite a lower incidence of breast cancer, black women with breast cancer are more likely than whites to die of their disease.
- Ethnic minority breast cancer patients have been shown to have suboptimal surgical, radiation, and medical treatment of their disease.

■ REFERENCES

1. Surveillance Epidemiology, and End Results: SEER*Stat Database: Incidence: SEER 17 Regs Public-Use, Nov 2005 Sub (1973–2003 varying). Bethesda, MD: National Cancer Institute, Surveillance Research Program, Cancer Statistics Branch; 2006.
2. Ries LA, Harkins D, Krapcho M. SEER Cancer Statistics Review, 1975–2003. http://seer.cancer.gov/csr/1975_2003.
3. Elledge RM, Clark GM, Chamness GC, Osborne CK. Tumor biologic factors and breast cancer prognosis among white, Hispanic, and black women in the United States. [see comments]. *J Natl Cancer Inst.* 1994;86(9):705–712.
4. Elmore JG, Nakano CY, Linden HM, Reisch LM, Ayanian JZ, Larson EB. Racial inequities in the timing of breast cancer detection, diagnosis, and initiation of treatment. *Med Care.* 2005;43(2): 141–148.
5. Franzini L, Williams AF, Franklin J, Singletary SE, Theriault RL. Effects of race and socioeconomic status on survival of 1,332 black, Hispanic, and white women with breast cancer. *Ann Surg Oncol.* 1997;4(2):111–118.
6. Howard DL, Penchansky R, Brown MB. Disaggregating the effects of race on breast cancer survival. *Fam Med.* 1998;30(3): 228–235.
7. Joslyn SA, West MM. Racial differences in breast carcinoma survival. *Cancer.* 2000;88(1):114–123.
8. Lyman GH, Kuderer NM, Lyman SL, Cox CE, Reintgen D, Baekey P. Importance of race on breast cancer survival. *Ann Surg Oncol.* 1997;4(1):80–87.
9. Walker B, Figgs LW, Zahm SH. Differences in cancer incidence, mortality, and survival between African Americans and whites. *Environ Health Perspect.* 1995;103(Suppl 8):275–281.
10. Yood MU, Johnson CC, Blount A, et al. Race and differences in breast cancer survival in a managed care population. [comment]. *J Natl Cancer Inst.* 1999;91(17):1487–1491.

11. Bach PB, Schrag D, Brawley OW, Galaznik A, Yakren S, Begg CB. Survival of blacks and whites after a cancer diagnosis. [see comment]. *JAMA*. 2002;287(16):2106–2113.

12. Chlebowski RT, Chen Z, Anderson GL, et al. Ethnicity and breast cancer: factors influencing differences in incidence and outcome. [see comment]. *J Natl Cancer Inst*. 2005;97(6):439–448.

13. Porter PL, Lund MJ, Lin MG, et al. Racial differences in the expression of cell cycle-regulatory proteins in breast carcinoma. *Cancer*. 2004;100(12):2533–2542.

14. Albain KS, Unger JM, Hutchins LF. Outcome of African Americans on Southwest Oncology Group (SWOG) breast cancer adjuvant therapy trials. *Breast Cancer Res Treat*. 2003;82 (Suppl 1):S2.

15. Grann VR, Troxel AB, Zojwalla NJ, Jacobson JS, Hershman D, Neugut AI. Hormone receptor status and survival in a population-based cohort of patients with breast carcinoma. *Cancer*. 2005;103(11):2241–2251.

16. Park ER, Weiss ES, Moy B. Recruiting and enrolling minority patients to cancer clinical trials. *Community Oncology*. 2007; 4(4):254–257.

17. Blanchard DK, Donohue JH, Reynolds C, Grant CS. Relapse and morbidity in patients undergoing sentinel lymph node biopsy alone or with axillary dissection for breast cancer. *Arch Surg*. 2003;138(5):482–487; discussion 487–488.

18. Rietman JS, Dijkstra PU, Geertzen JH, et al. Treatment-related upper limb morbidity 1 year after sentinel lymph node biopsy or axillary lymph node dissection for stage I or II breast cancer. *Ann Surg Oncol*. 2004;11(11):1018–1024.

19. Schulze T, Mucke J, Markwardt J, Schlag PM, Bembenek A. Long-term morbidity of patients with early breast cancer after sentinel lymph node biopsy compared to axillary lymph node dissection. *J Surg Oncol*. 2006;93(2):109–119.

20. Badgwell BD, Povoski SP, Abdessalam SF, et al. Patterns of recurrence after sentinel lymph node biopsy for breast cancer. *Ann Surg Oncol*. 2003;10(4):376–380.

21. Lyman GH, Giuliano AE, Somerfield MR, et al. American Society of Clinical Oncology guideline recommendations for sentinel lymph node biopsy in early-stage breast cancer. [see comment]. *J Clin Oncol*. 2005;23(30):7703–7720.

22. McNeil C. Sentinel node biopsy: studies should bring needed data. *J Natl Cancer Inst*. 1998;90(10):728–730.

23. Chen AY, Halpern MT, Schrag NM, Stewart A, Leitch M, Ward E. Disparities and trends in sentinel lymph node biopsy among early-stage breast cancer patients (1998–2005). *J Natl Cancer Inst*. 2008;100(7):462–474.

24. Maggard MA, Lane KE, O'Connell JB, Nanyakkara DD, Ko CY. Beyond the clinical trials: how often is sentinel lymph node dissection performed for breast cancer? *Ann Surg Oncol*. 2005;12(1):41–47.

25. Fisher B, Anderson S, Redmond CK, Wolmark N, Wickerham DL, Cronin WM. Reanalysis and results after 12 years of follow-up in a randomized clinical trial comparing total mastectomy with lumpectomy with or without irradiation in the treatment of breast cancer. [see comment]. *New Engl J Med*. 1995; 333(22):1456–1461.

26. Kiebert GM, de Haes JC, van de Velde CJ. The impact of breast-conserving treatment and mastectomy on the quality of life of early-stage breast cancer patients: a review. *J Clin Oncol*. 1991;9(6):1059–1070.

27. Treatment of early-stage breast cancer. NIH Consensus Statement.Online 1990 June 18–21 (cited June 25, 2008):8(6):1–19. http://consensus.nih.gov/1990/1990EarlyStageBreastCancer081html.htm.

28. Joslyn SA. Racial differences in treatment and survival from early-stage breast carcinoma. *Cancer*. 2002;95(8):1759–1766.

29. Nattinger AB, Gottlieb MS, Veum J, Yahnke D, Goodwin JS. Geographic variation in the use of breast-conserving treatment for breast cancer. [see comment]. *New Engl J Med*. 1992;326(17):1102–1107.

30. Goel MS, Burns RB, Phillips RS, Davis RB, Ngo-Metzger Q, McCarthy EP. Trends in breast conserving surgery among Asian Americans and Pacific Islanders, 1992–2000. *J Gen Intern Med*. 2005;20(7):604–611.

31. Morris CR, Cohen R, Schlag R, Wright WE. Increasing trends in the use of breast-conserving surgery in California. *Am J Public Health*. 2000;90(2):281–284.

32. Psychological aspects of Breast Cancer Study Group. Psychological response to mastectomy. A prospective comparison study. *Cancer*. 1987;59(1):189–196.

33. Murphy RX Jr,. Wahhab S, Rovito PF, et al. Impact of immediate reconstruction on the local recurrence of breast cancer after mastectomy. *Ann Plast Surg*. 2003;50(4):333–338.

34. Osteen RT. Reconstruction after mastectomy. *Cancer*. 1995;76(10 Suppl):2070–2074.

35. Dean C, Chetty U, Forrest AP. Effects of immediate breast reconstruction on psychosocial morbidity after mastectomy. *Lancet*. 1983;1(8322):459–462.

36. Tseng JF, Kronowitz SJ, Sun CC, et al. The effect of ethnicity on immediate reconstruction rates after mastectomy for breast cancer. *Cancer*. 2004;101(7):1514–1523.

37. Alderman AK, Hawley ST, Hamilton AS, Katz SJ. Racial/ethnic disparities in breast reconstruction after mastectomy. Abstract presented at the American Society of Clinical Oncology annual meeting, Chicago, Illinois, 2008. Abstract 6510.

38. Fisher B, Costantino J, Redmond C, et al. Lumpectomy compared with lumpectomy and radiation therapy for the treatment of intraductal breast cancer. [see comment]. *New Engl J Med*. 1993; 328(22):1581–1586.

39. Fisher B, Redmond C, Poisson R, et al. Eight-year results of a randomized clinical trial comparing total mastectomy and lumpectomy with or without irradiation in the treatment of breast cancer. [see comment]. *New Engl J Med*. 1989;320(13):822–828. [erratum appears in *New Engl J Med*. 1994;330(20):1467].

40. Du X, Gor B. Racial disparities and trends in radiation therapy after breast-conserving surgery for early-stage breast cancer in women, 1992 to 2002. *Ethn Dis*. 2007;17(1):122–128.

41. Freedman RA, He Y, Winer EP, Keating NL. Racial disparity trends in definitive primary therapy of early stage breast cancer. Abstract presented at the American Society of Clinical Oncology annual meeting, Chicago, Illinois, 2008. Abstract 535.

42. Early Breast Cancer Trialists' Collaborative Group. Polychemotherapy for early breast cancer: an overview of the randomised trials. *Lancet*. 1998;352(9132):930–942.

43. Griggs JJ, Sorbero ME, Stark AT, Heininger SE, Dick AW. Racial disparity in the dose and dose intensity of breast cancer adjuvant chemotherapy. *Breast Cancer Res Treat*. 2003;81(1):21–31.

44. Newman LA, Theriault R, Clendinnin N, Jones D, Pierce L. Treatment choices and response rates in African-American women with breast carcinoma. *Cancer*. 2003;97(1 Suppl):246–252.

45. Roach M 3rd, Cirrincione C, Budman D, et al. Race and survival from breast cancer: based on Cancer and Leukemia Group B trial 8541. [see comment]. *Cancer J Sci Am*. 1997;3(2):107–112.

46. Dignam JJ, Redmond CK, Fisher B, Costantino JP, Edwards BK. Prognosis among African-American women and white women with lymph node negative breast carcinoma: findings from two randomized clinical trials of the National Surgical Adjuvant Breast and Bowel Project (NSABP). *Cancer*. 1997;80(1):80–90.

47. Kimmick G, Muss HB, Case LD, Stanley V. A comparison of treatment outcomes for black patients and white patients with metastatic breast cancer. The Piedmont Oncology Association experience. *Cancer*. 1991;67(11):2850–2854.

48. Bickell NA, Wang JJ, Oluwole S, et al. Missed opportunities: racial disparities in adjuvant breast cancer treatment. *J Clin Oncol*. 2006;24(9):1357–1362.

49. Hershman D, McBride R, Jacobson JS, et al. Racial disparities in treatment and survival among women with early-stage breast cancer. *J Clin Oncol*. 2005;23(27):6639–6646.

50. Lund MJ, Brawley OP, Ward KC, Young JL, Gabram SS, Eley JW. Parity and disparity in first course treatment of invasive breast cancer. *Breast Cancer Res Treat.* 2008;109(3):545–557.

51. Griggs JJ, Abrahamse PH, Hamilton AS, et al. Adjuvant chemotherapy use in a diverse population-based sample of women with breast cancer. Abstract presented at the American Society of Clinical Oncology annual meeting, Chicago, Illinois, 2008. Abstract 6539.

52. Early Breast Cancer Trialists' Collaborative Group. Tamoxifen for early breast cancer: an overview of the randomised trials. *Lancet.* 1998;351(9114):1451–1467.

53. Moy B, Goss PE. Identifying the role of hormonal therapy in African Women. Capetown, South Africa: African Organisation for Research and Training in Cancer (AORTIC); 2007.

54. McCaskill-Stevens W, Wilson J, Bryant J, et al. Contralateral breast cancer and thromboembolic events in African American women treated with tamoxifen. *J Natl Cancer Inst.* 2004;96(23):1762–1769. [erratum appears in *J Natl Cancer Inst.* 2005;97(1):71].

55. Moy B, Tu D, Pater JL, et al. Clinical outcomes of ethnic minority women in MA 17: a trial of letrozole after 5 years of tamoxifen in postmenopausal women with early stage breast cancer. *Ann Oncol.* 2006;17(11):1637–1643.

56. Moy B, Elliot CR, J.W. C, Pater JL, Ding Z, Goss PE. NCIC CTG MA 27: Menopausal symptoms of ethnic minority women. Abstract presented at the San Antonio Breast Cancer Symposium, San Antonio, Texas, 2006. p. S144. Abstract 3059.

57. Giuliano AR, Mokuau N, Hughes C, et al. Participation of minorities in cancer research: the influence of structural, cultural, and linguistic factors. *Ann Epidemiol.* 2000;10(8 Suppl):S22–S34.

58. Paskett ED, Katz ML, DeGraffinreid CR, Tatum CM. Participation in cancer trials: recruitment of underserved populations. *Clin Adv Hematol Oncol.* 2003;1(10):607–613.

59. Christian MC, Trimble EL. Increasing participation of physicians and patients from underrepresented racial and ethnic groups in National Cancer Institute-sponsored clinical trials. *Cancer Epidemiol Biomarkers Prev.* 2003;12(3):277s–283s.

60. Brawley OW, Tejada H. Minority inclusion in clinical trials issues and potential strategies. *J Natl Cancer Inst Monogr.* 1995:55–57.

61. Sateren WB, Trimble EL, Abrams J, et al. How sociodemographics, presence of oncology specialists, and hospital cancer programs affect accrual to cancer treatment trials. *J Clin Oncol.* 2002;20(8):2109–2117.

62. Fisher B, Costantino JP, Wickerham DL, et al. Tamoxifen for prevention of breast cancer: report of the National Surgical Adjuvant Breast and Bowel Project P-1 Study. [see comment]. *J Natl Cancer Inst.* 1998;90(18):1371–1388.

63. Vogel VG, Costantino JP, Wickerham DL, et al. Effects of tamoxifen vs raloxifene on the risk of developing invasive breast cancer and other disease outcomes: the NSABP Study of Tamoxifen and Raloxifene (STAR) P-2 trial. [see comment]. *JAMA.* 2006;295(23):2727–2741. [erratum appears in *JAMA.* 2006;296(24):2926].

64. Romond EH, Perez EA, Bryant J, et al. Trastuzumab plus adjuvant chemotherapy for operable HER2-positive breast cancer. [see comment]. *New Engl J Med.* 2005;353(16):1673–1684.

15 Multidisciplinary Breast Cancer Care in the Community

KAREN KRAG

ROBIN SCHOENTHALER

JEANNE YU

Almost one and a half million people are diagnosed with cancer every year in the United States, 85% of them at hospitals in their communities. The other 15% are diagnosed at National Cancer Institute (NCI)–designated cancer centers, 63 academic institutions located mainly in urban areas (1). Even after diagnosis, most patients continue treatment at community-based institutions for personal, logistic, or economic reasons. A retrospective analysis of operative cases of invasive ductal carcinoma from 1994 to 2000 from the Florida Cancer Data System found that 89% of patients were treated at community hospitals, whereas 11% were treated at one of the state's eight teaching hospitals. Patients treated at community hospitals were generally older (median age 67 years versus 59 years at teaching hospitals) and more likely to have low-grade tumors and regionalized disease than those treated at teaching institutions (2). Data from our own practices in the Boston area confirm these findings: In five local community hospitals, 26% to 36% of breast cancer patients are over 70 years old, and 9% to 13% are over 80. This contrasts with data from two of our regional academic centers, where only 13% to 16% of breast cancer patients are over 70, and only 4% are over 80.

Patients treated in the community are therefore slightly different from those treated in academic centers, but is the care any different? From a surgical standpoint, it appears to be. In the United States, surgical treatment of breast cancer is predominantly performed by general surgeons (3), with breast diseases comprising approximately 20% of general surgeons' practice volume. However, data collected by the American Board of Surgery for surgeons applying for recertification show that 50% of general surgeons do fewer than two lumpectomy and axillary dissections and fewer than two modified radical mastectomies in any given year (4). In an analysis looking at Surveillance, Epidemiology and End Results (SEER) program data, women who had surgery in hospitals that performed fewer than 20 breast cancer surgeries (all surgeons combined) per year had a slightly higher all-cause mortality and breast cancer mortality than women who had surgery in hospitals with higher volumes [all-cause mortality relative risk (RR) 0.83 and breast cancer mortality RR 0.80 in medium- and high-volume hospitals compared with low-volume hospitals] (5). However, breast surgery perioperative mortality is extremely low in all settings, and some of the differences in long-term mortality may be due to differences in patient factors or, more likely, to differences in multidisciplinary care. If individual surgeons rather than hospitals are assessed, there is again an improvement in mortality. Women whose surgery was performed by surgical oncologists had a 5-year overall survival of 86%, whereas those whose surgery was performed by general surgeons had a 5-year survival of 79%. When data were controlled for age, stage, race, and hospital tumor volume, patients of a surgical oncologist had an RR of death of 0.77 compared with patients of a general surgeon (6).

In addition to affecting overall survival, the breast cancer operation itself can have a significant impact on short-term outcomes. Zork and colleagues examined the effect of dedicated breast cancer surgeons on practice patterns by performing a retrospective review of patients who underwent their primary surgical breast cancer treatment at a single county hospital breast clinic between 1997 and 2006. Patients treated by breast surgeons were significantly more likely to undergo breast conservation and to have negative margins and lower rates of re-excision despite smaller average volumes of excision; and they were more likely to undergo a less morbid sentinel node procedure (SLNB) rather than axillary lymph node dissection (ALND) (7). In another study, Chen and colleagues examined the National Cancer Database to compare the use of sentinel lymph node biopsy and ALND from 1998 through 2005 at facilities accredited by the American College of Surgeons Commission on Cancer. The participating treatment facilities were classified into community cancer programs, comprehensive community cancer programs (defined as those that treat more than 750 cancer patients per year and conduct weekly cancer conferences), and teaching or research facilities (facilities with residency programs and ongoing cancer research). The authors found that patients who received treatment in facilities other than a teaching or research hospital were 15% less likely to undergo SLNB (8).

In radiation oncology, there may be fewer differences between techniques utilized in academic and community practices. By the end of 2007, 97% of all US sites had computed tomography based treatment planning systems, a technological advance virtually unknown only a decade before. Intensity modulated radiation therapy (IMRT) was available at a single institution in 1999 but by 2007 had been adopted by 87% of all radiation oncology sites in the United States. The number of centers using image-guided radiation therapy (IGRT) treatment capabilities is a particularly telling example of rapid adoption of new technology in radiation oncology. While only 15% of centers had any IGRT capabilities in 2004 (either dedicated IGRT devices or portal vision), and only one third reported its availability in 2006, by 2007, more than 50% of all US radiation oncology centers were using this technology.

The explosive growth of partial breast irradiation is another example of rapid acquisition of technology in the community setting. As an example, the MammoSite Radiation Therapy System balloon-brachytherapy system received Food and Drug Administration approval as a boost technique in breast cancer radiotherapy management in 2002 based on safety data in 43 women. By 2006, 5,000 women had received definitive partial breast cancer radiotherapy via MammoSite. By 2008, 32,000 women in both academic and community settings had been treated using the MammoSite system (www.cytyc.com).

Many medical oncology practice patterns vary little between community and academic settings. Once patients meet their oncologist, recommendations in both settings adhere fairly well to clinical guidelines. Mariotto and colleagues coordinated SEER data with population-based patterns of care data and found that clinical trial information about adjuvant treatment is disseminated rapidly to the community (9). Harlan and colleagues also reported that community physicians' treatment patterns actually at times precede guidelines recommendations, since the studies that support the guidelines are reported and published prior to the guidelines (10). Data from the Network for Oncology Communication and Research (NOCR) also suggest that in an adjuvant setting, patients are treated similarly in the community and in academic institutions, with comparable drug regimens chosen. In both settings, there is a significant minority who choose unusual treatment plans (NOCR 2007/2008 data, personal communication).

■ MULTIDISCIPLINARY CLINICS

Multidisciplinary clinics are now standard at most academic centers, where the majority of breast cancer patients receive care in a coordinated, streamlined interdisciplinary fashion by subspecialty oncologists. Can this model be followed in the community, where subspecialists are not as common, physicians often practice at different sites, and there are different economic incentives? And are there truly benefits to this approach that outweigh the difficulties in setting up these clinics?

Role of Multidisciplinary Clinics in Coordinating Care

Historically, breast cancer has been a surgical disease. Radical mastectomy, oophorectomy, adrenalectomy, and hypophysectomy were the treatments available to women 50 years ago. In the 1970s, radiation oncologists became increasingly involved, as the results of trials of breast conservation became solidly established. At that time, medical oncologists had little role in the adjuvant setting, as few women received either chemotherapy or tamoxifen. However, NCI and American Society of Clinical Oncology (ASCO) guidelines in the 1990s extended recommendations for adjuvant therapy, and breast cancer has become a disease that must be treated in a multidisciplinary fashion. These guidelines were quickly accepted both in the community and in academic centers. Now only a minority of patients are treated with surgery alone. In our own regional experience in two Boston academic centers, only 17% to 20% of patients were treated with surgery alone, whereas this number ranged from 13% to 29% among surveyed local community centers. Interestingly, the highest percentage of patients treated with surgery alone was seen in a hospital without multidisciplinary breast clinics, and the lowest percentage in one with a very active multidisciplinary clinic (personal communication).

Community breast cancer care is often given in a linear fashion. Radiologists see and diagnose the patients, surgeons proceed with local excision, radiation oncologists complete the local treatment, and then medical oncologists determine further adjuvant therapies. Care is not always in one location, as practice settings for private radiologists, private surgeons, and unaffiliated medical oncologists may be quite scattered. This is not ideal for several reasons.

The linear approach has inherent delays, as women wait for the results and recommendations from one discipline prior to even making the appointment—and waiting—for the next discipline. In one study of a multidisciplinary clinic in Delaware, patients reduced time from diagnosis to final treatment recommendations by 3 weeks (11). More important, the ordering of treatments is not as straightforward as it once was, with chemotherapy and hormonal therapies sometimes used before surgery, and hormonal therapies sometimes substituting for radiation.

Referral to multidisciplinary clinics can occur at any point, and does so both in the community and in academic centers. In some settings, the surgeon is comfortable explaining the diagnosis and treatment options, then proceeding with staging followed by local surgery and nodal sampling, and only then referring the patient to a multidisciplinary clinic for further recommendations. In that case, the medical oncologist already has full staging information and can make treatment decisions. Some surgeons prefer multidisciplinary clinic referral prior to definitive surgery. In that case, the medical oncologist's role is a little more difficult, as prior to definitive surgery there are many questions that must be resolved before final treatment recommendations can be made: Will the nodes be positive or negative? Is there metastatic disease? Will there be clear margins?

Some centers are using a breast navigator, often a nurse practitioner, who guides patients with abnormal mammograms through the diagnostic process. This clinician can be invaluable in understanding how the system works, how the disease progresses, and how an individual patient needs each of the various healthcare providers. The navigator can make a referral for other needed care at a time appropriate for the individual patient.

In academic centers, earlier multidisciplinary consultation is often preferred, as neoadjuvant therapy is used more frequently. Wider use of neoadjuvant therapy in tertiary centers is not solely to downstage advanced disease, as locally advanced cancer is uncommon in both settings. Data from our local practices shows 4.2% to 10.8% of women presenting with stage III disease, whereas in the two academic centers, 6.8% or 12% have stage III cancer (personal communication). But when presented with locally advanced disease, academic practices refer more commonly to medical oncology. Data from the NOCR show that women with T2 lesions who would benefit from downstaging are referred to medical oncology 25% more frequently in an academic setting (NOCR analytic data 2006, personal communication). Once patients have been referred, equal numbers of medical oncologists in the NOCR data set recommend neoadjuvant therapy, and equal numbers involve a radiation oncologist at that time (30% in the academic setting, 33% in the community), suggesting that these women are then seen in a multidisciplinary setting.

Early systemic treatment is also a valuable approach to evaluate new drugs, as active agents can be identified without the extended follow-up required in adjuvant trials in a disease that has a long natural history. Complex neoadjuvant trials are more suited to an academic practice, as they often involve multiple extra biopsies, specimen banking, and coordination with multiple disciplines, but as community trial activity increases, we may see more neoadjuvant trial activity outside of an academic setting.

One situation seen frequently in the community is that of a frail elderly woman who is not a candidate for standard surgical approaches. Such women benefit greatly from a discussion that includes how best to palliate—whether it be through surgery (even without clear margins), hormonal therapy alone, chemotherapy in selected patients, or even a decision to observe without treatment. There is increasing recognition that breast cancer is a heterogeneous disease, and while chemotherapy may not improve the prognosis of an elderly woman with an unresectable estrogen receptor–positive tumor, it may be critically important for an elderly woman with estrogen receptor–negative disease.

There are multiple benefits to the patient when care is coordinated effectively. In a multidisciplinary setting, visits to different providers occur on the same day, shortening the anxiety-provoking time while awaiting a treatment plan. Women who decide to be treated in the community may be more motivated to minimize the time spent getting care since they have chosen to avoid travel to an academic center, so a multidisciplinary approach may be especially appealing.

In addition to more effective use of the patient's time, women may feel very well cared for with a team approach. This is best described in a wonderful article by Frances Bolye and colleagues: "Multidisciplinary care in cancer: the fellowship of the ring" (12). Boyle compares the patient tackling the cancer alone to Tolkien's Gollum, and the patient cared for by many to Frodo, who is supported by the Fellowship—all the different disciplines present in a multidisciplinary clinic.

Role of Multidisciplinary Clinics in Promoting Quality

One of the major initiatives for promoting quality in cancer care is the development of guidelines. These are widely available from many sources, not all of which agree as to optimal care. The St. Gallen guidelines are different from the National Cancer Center Network (NCCN) guidelines, which are in turn different from the ASCO guidelines, but all provide a structure within which lies appropriate care. It is quite useful if a community practice can use these available resources to develop its own guidelines. While treatment recommendations by each community physician do not need to be identical (they are not identical in academic centers), and indeed can and should evolve over time, it is very useful if all agree on a treatment plan, and if visits to Dr. X do not lead to radically different recommendations from visits to Dr. Y. Using these guidelines, recommendations will not vary too widely week to week, and this is very helpful not just to patients but to nurses, referring doctors, primary care physicians, and all in the community.

While it may not be feasible to demand breast oncology subspecialization by physicians participating in multidisciplinary clinics, those participating in multidisciplinary clinics should be held to high professional standards and should be able to demonstrate experience and knowledge in the field of breast cancer.

Community oncology practices are rarely large enough to have multiple subspecialized breast oncologists. Therefore, face-to-face staffing of a multidisciplinary clinic is often by a single breast oncologist or multiple general oncologists. The oncologist who staffs the breast clinic should have have both interest and expertise in breast cancer care. Performance criteria could include attendance at breast oncology seminars or conferences on a national, regional, or local scale, documentation of continuing medical education credits in breast oncology–related topics, attendance at a prescribed percentage of breast tumor conferences, participation in professional cancer organizations or committees, and focused interest in a breast subspecialty.

Another option is to have the clinic staffed by general oncologists but to have a breast oncology subspecialist present at the discussion and data review. This is not only beneficial for the patients, who benefit from the added expertise available at the time that data are reviewed and clinical recommendations are generated, but it is also a learning opportunity for all those present. Tertiary care centers are now increasingly aligning with community practices regularly providing a subspecialty physician to provide additional expertise at working conferences.

Academic and community center collaboration can also be achieved through telemedicine. One such model is a statewide community cancer videoconferencing program in Delaware. Early reports have shown an increase in clinical trial accrual and a high level of adherence to ASCO and NCCN treatment guidelines following the use of a weekly prospective clinical videoconferencing program (13). This approach has also been used in a community hospital in the Boston area and has led to greater retention of breast cancer cases within community care settings (personal communication).

Thorough pathology and radiology review, often including a second opinion review of slides and images, is necessary for care of women with breast cancer. This review can be done at the conference by onsite physicians or through telemedicine. Studies have looked at changes in recommendations after review of radiology and pathology specimens. One study demonstrated a change in surgical recommendation from review of imaging studies in 10.7% of patients usuallya second cancer detected precluding breast conservation. In addition, they also showed nd a change in surgical recommendation after pathology review in 8.7% of patients, most commonly the need for a re-excision (14). While this study evaluated women who had an initial diagnosis in the community and had their data reviewed at an academic center, our experience in a community practice clearly demonstrates that recommendations can change when all disciplines review the mammograms and pathology together.

Multidisciplinary clinics provide the opportunity for physicians in different oncology disciplines to learn about the important contributions of each specialty to breast cancer care. Through discussions with surgeons, colleagues learn about complications from different surgical approaches, about cosmetic outcomes with different techniques, and about long-term issues in surgical management. From the radiation oncologists, colleagues learn about treatment planning and skin toxicities and are kept up to date about technologic advances. From the medical oncologists, colleagues learn about weighing the risks and benefits of new systemic therapies. Radiologists and pathologists are also key, as they help colleagues quantitate information, teach about the advantages and disadvantages of new technologies, and help analyze data within a clinical scenario. The interplay between disciplines at the conference may lead to practice changes. For example, discussions about margins lead the surgeon to more precise operative reports and specimen orientation, while the pathologist may understand more fully the need for specific details in a pathology report in guiding subsequent treatment decisions. This in turn helps the radiation oncologist tailor the radiation field, plan the boost, and determine whether nodal groups should be treated.

These discussions also provide an impetus for all practitioners to keep up with new data. When colleagues return from national oncology conferences, results of recent studies are discussed and new policies are developed. We all learn by teaching, and this provides an opportunity for us to teach our colleagues—to define for others exactly how we approach different situations. And when others question our decisions, we are able to learn from each other and ultimately provide the patient with the best treatment options.

Some multidisciplinary clinics can include participation of many other disciplines. These could include social workers, geriatricians, plastic surgeons, dieticians, internists, psychiatrists, palliative care specialists, clinical trials specialists, and other individuals whose expertise might favorably impact care for these women. One new focus of oncologic care is survivorship, with ASCO planning to mandate breast survivorship care. Some multidisciplinary clinics begin their survivorship programs at the first multidisciplinary visit, so that patients immediately know that after chemotherapy, surgery, and radiation, survivorship issues will be addressed. Many centers are developing survivorship clinics that include nurse practitioners and physician assistants in central roles, working collaboratively with other oncology specialists.

Clinical trials are now widely supported by community oncologists. Certainly there is a wider variety of trials in most academic centers than in most community settings, but with the development of national cooperative trials, the Community Clinical Oncology Program (CCOP), and the NCI-sponsored Clinical Trials Support Unit (CTSU), it is now relatively easy for the community oncologist to enroll patients in treatment trials. A multidisciplinary approach can facilitate this. If physicians and the breast navigator are familiar with available trials and talk about trial eligibility in conferences, trial participation can be increased and providers educated.

Setting up a clinical trials program in the community does require additional financial support. This can initially come from the affiliated hospital(s) or from philanthropic donations. Establishment of a dedicated, enthusiastic research team can then grow a self-supporting program with trials funded through national cooperative groups and industry.

Economics of Community Multidisciplinary Clinics

Setting up a multidisciplinary clinic is costly. While reimbursement is possible for individual physicians' services and facility fees, there is substantial non-reimbursible activity involved in multidisciplinary care. Nevertheless, multidisciplinary clinics may provide definite financial benefits to their institution, including higher rates of retention of patients in the community facility for their care. One of our local hospitals noted significantly increased retention of patients for chemotherapy and follow-up care after the institution of a breast multidisciplinary clinic, suggesting that patients prefer this approach. Adherence to care guidelines may also be increased. Our own data from five community hospitals found that 7.4% to 8.9% of women received chemotherapy in hospitals with no multidisciplinary care, as compared with 16% to 27% of those in facilities with multidisciplinary clinics.

■ CONCLUSIONS

- Multidisciplinary care of breast cancer patients can occur in the community as well as in academic centers.
- Challenges of multidisciplinary care in the community setting include staffing the clinic with caregivers who have expertise in breast cancer care and meeting the upfront costs of establishing a multidisciplinary center.
- Benefits of multidisciplinary care in the community setting include a more streamlined patient experience, increased physician collaboration and knowledge, and likely both increased trial participation and patient retention.
- Multidisciplinary practice in a community setting enables breast care that is more timely and more evidence based.

■ REFERENCES

1. Petrelli NJ, Grusenmeyer PA. Establishing the multidisciplinary care of patients with cancer in the state of Delaware. *Cancer.* 2004;101(2):220–225.
2. Gutierrez JC, Hurley JD, Housri N, et al. Are many community hospitals undertreating breast cancer? Lessons from 24,834 patients. *Ann Surg.* 2008;248(2):154–162.
3. Hillner BE, Smith TJ, Desch CE. Hospital and physician volume or specialization and outcomes in cancer treatment: importance in quality of cancer care. *J Clin Oncol.* 2000;18(11):2327–2340.
4. Pass HA, Klimberg SV, Copeland EM 3rd. Are "breast-focused" surgeons more competent? *Ann Surg Oncol.* 2008;15(4):953–955.
5. Gilligan MA, Neuner J, Zhang X, et al. Relationship between number of breast cancer operations performed and 5-year survival after treatment for early-stage breast cancer. *Am J Public Health.* 2007;97(3):539–544.
6. Skinner KA, Helsper JT, Deapen D, et al. Breast cancer: do specialists make a difference? *Ann Surg Oncol.* 2003;10(6):606–615.
7. Zork NM, Komenaka IK, Pennington RE Jr., et al. The effect of dedicated breast surgeons on the short-term outcomes in breast cancer. *Ann Surg.* 2008;248(2):280–285.
8. Chen AY, Halpern MT, Schrag NM, et al. Disparities and trends in sentinel lymph node biopsy among early-stage breast cancer patients (1998–2005). *J Natl Cancer Inst.* 2008;100(7):462–474.
9. Mariotto A, Feuer EJ, Harlan LC, Wun L-M, Johnson KA, Abrams J. Trends in use of adjuvant multi-agent chemotherapy and tamoxifen for breast cancer in the United States: 1975–1999. *J Natl Cancer Inst.* 2002;94(21):1626–1634.
10. Harlan LC, Abrams J, Warren JL, Clegg L, Stevens J, Ballard-Barbash R. Adjuvant therapy for breast cancer: practice patterns of community physicians. *J Clin Oncol.* 2002;20(7):1809–1817.
11. Petrelli NJ, Grubbs S, Price K, et al. A multidisciplinary team approach to cancer care in a community based teaching hospital: 6102 [Abstract]. *J Clin Oncol.* 2004;22(Suppl 14):544s.
12. Boyle FM, Robinson E, Dunn SM, Heinrich PC. Multidisciplinary care in cancer: the fellowship of the ring. *J Clin Oncol.* 2005; 23:916–920.
13. Dickson-Witmer D, Petrelli NJ, Witmer DR, et al. A statewide community cancer center videoconferencing program. *Ann Surg Oncol.* 2008;15:3058–3064.
14. Newman EA, Guest AB, Helvie MA, et al. Changes in surgical management resulting from case review at a breast cancer multidisciplinary tumor board. *Cancer.* 2006;107(10):2346–2351.

16 Future Directions in the Treatment of Breast Cancer

Surgical Innovations in Breast Cancer

AMANDA WHEELER

BARBARA L. SMITH

The surgical management of breast cancer has changed dramatically over the past two decades. Needle biopsy techniques have replaced open surgical biopsy for diagnosis of most breast cancers, breast-conserving surgery is a viable alternative to mastectomy for many patients, and sentinel node biopsy rather than axillary dissection is the standard of care for patients with clinically negative axillary nodes.

Progress continues toward more precise and less invasive treatment for breast cancer. Future innovations in breast surgery will reduce re-excision rates through improved preoperative imaging and improved methods for assessment of lumpectomy margins. Technical innovations will continue to improve cosmetic results of lumpectomy and mastectomy procedures. Nonsurgical methods for axillary staging and for ablation of breast tumors may be incorporated into standard practice. Advanced breast imaging technologies are likely to enhance diagnosis and management. With these changes, the surgeon's role in guiding a patient from initial diagnosis through complex multidisciplinary care will continue to evolve. This chapter will review progress to date in these areas and highlight ongoing areas of investigation.

■ IMPROVED MARGIN ASSESSMENT

It is essential to obtain tumor-free margins on all aspects of a lumpectomy specimen, as even microscopic involvement of margins by tumor increases rates of local recurrence. If clear margins are not obtained on the initial lumpectomy, re-excision of any positive margins is required.

A number of factors are associated with higher rates of margin involvement and need for re-excision after a lumpectomy attempt. Positive margins are more common for tumors with extensive ductal carcinoma in situ (DCIS) (1) and for invasive lobular cancers where the borders of the tumor are not easily palpable and may not be visualized on preoperative imaging studies. Reported rates of re-excision for positive margins vary widely for DCIS, and may be as high as 48% to 59% (2).

Re-excision rates are lower for patients diagnosed by core than by surgical biopsy. Lind and colleagues (3) found positive margins in only 6% of patients diagnosed by core needle biopsy, compared with 55% of those initially diagnosed by surgical biopsy. Smitt and colleagues (4) reported a 34% re-excision rate for patients diagnosed by core needle biopsy, compared with 61% for those diagnosed by surgical biopsy (P <0.0001). Use of multiple localizing wires for large or irregularly shaped mammographic lesions has also been shown to reduce re-excision rates (5).

Intraoperative Margin Assessment

There is great interest in development of technologies to allow real-time identification of tumor at the margins of a lumpectomy specimen or in cavity walls in the breast to allow excision of positive margins during the initial lumpectomy procedure. In practice, rapid and accurate intraoperative assessment of lumpectomy margins remains difficult. Frozen section assessment of margins may reduce re-excision rates (2) but is limited by histological changes associated with tissue freezing and is too time-consuming for application in most practice settings. Touch prep cytology for margin assessment has been proposed as a rapid and accurate method for intraoperative margin assessment (6), but the required cytology expertise is not widely available.

A number of devices are under development to exploit differences in tumor and normal tissue properties to provide accurate intraoperative margin assessment and reduce re-excision rates. Ramen spectroscopy, optical coherence tomography (OCT), and radiofrequency (RF) spectroscopy have been used in pilot studies for margin assessment of breast specimens.

Raman spectroscopy is an optical modality that provides quantitative chemical information about a tissue sample. In Raman spectroscopy a molecule simultaneously absorbs an incident photon and emits a Raman photon, accompanied by a transition from one energy level to another. Because the energy levels are unique for each molecule, Raman spectra are chemical-specific. Raman spectroscopy is particularly amenable to in vivo measurements, as the excitation wavelengths used cause no tissue damage and have a relatively large penetration depth (7). Haka and colleagues (8) used Ramen spectral-based tissue characterization to assess 31 cavity margins in nine patients undergoing lumpectomy. Data acquisition for assessment of each margin took only one second and showed 100% sensitivity and 100% specificity for distinguishing benign from malignant tissue.

OCT uses low-coherence interferometry to produce a high-resolution two-dimensional image of optical scattering from internal tissue microstructures (9). OCT is analogous to ultrasound but measures reflections of near-infrared light rather than sound. While depth of imaging is limited to only a few millimeters in breast tissue, imaging resolution is in the microns range. Real-time image acquisition is possible using an optical beam from a surgical microscope, a handheld probe in the open surgical field, or with needle biopsy probes (10). Hsiung and colleagues (11) performed OCT imaging in 119 freshly excised specimens from 35 women. Microstructure of normal breast parenchyma, DCIS, and infiltrating cancer correlated with corresponding histopathological findings. Breast structures as small as 25 μm in diameter could be visualized.

Use of RF spectroscopy to assess margins on the basis of different electromagnetic responses of malignant and normal breast cells is also under investigation (12).

■ NONSURGICAL TUMOR ABLATION TECHNIQUES

The success of in situ ablation of hepatic tumor deposits via minimally invasive techniques such as cryoablation, high-intensity focused ultrasound, laser ablation, and RF ablation has led to consideration of these techniques for nonsurgical ablation of breast tumors (13–16). Cryoablation results in tumor killing by freezing a sphere of tissue with resulting cell lysis, while other techniques produce localized tissue heating that results in cell death.

Technical factors have limited the utility of ultrasound and microwave ablation approaches in the breast. Focused ultrasound requires sequential targeting and heating of individual small areas within a mass, of approximately 1 × 9 mm in size, for 10 seconds each (17). Although focused ultrasound has the advantage of producing no skin incision, killing has been shown to be patchy and incomplete (17,18), significantly limiting its application for treating malignancies. Use of focused microwave array ablation also showed only incomplete tumor killing, with additional difficulties caused by the heat generated in surrounding tissue (19).

RF ablation, cryoablation, and laser ablation are the most promising approaches for breast tumor ablation as they produce a circumferentially expanding kill zone around a probe placed within a mass under image guidance. Nearly all the information currently available that addresses the efficacy of these techniques comes from studies where percutaneous ablation is performed followed by surgical excision and histological assessment of tumor viability.

RF Ablation

For RF ablation of breast masses (20), an RF probe is placed into the tumor under ultrasound guidance, killing tumor cells through frictional heating caused when ions in the tissue attempt to follow the changing directions of a high-frequency alternating current. Real-time ultrasound monitoring is used to monitor the diameter of the treated area. Target tissue is heated to temperatures ranging from 50°C to 95°C for 10 to 15 minutes, which may require general anesthesia and limits use to tumors more than 1 cm from skin and chest wall to avoid thermal injury to skin and muscle. More recently, Burak and colleagues showed that RF ablation of small breast malignancies was feasible under local anesthesia (21).

Experience to date with RF ablation has demonstrated fairly high rates of tumor cell death, but with occasional residual viable-appearing tumor cells. Jeffrey and colleagues (22) first demonstrated the feasibility of RF ablation in locally advanced invasive breast cancers, with complete cell death within an ablation zone of 0.8 to 1.8 cm documented on excision performed immediately following ablation.

Izzo and colleagues reported complete necrosis in 25 of 26 tumors (96%) smaller than 3 cm with RF (23). One patient developed a full-thickness burn of the skin overlying the tumor following RF ablation.

Fornage and colleagues (24) reported RF ablation of 21 breast cancers (tumor size 2.0 cm or smaller) immediately before surgical excision. Tumor kill was assessed using a nicotinamide adenine dinucleotide (NADH) diaphorase stain to confirm thermal cell injury and lack of viability as this proved more reliable for assessing RF kill than hematoxylin and eosin staining. Complete ablation of the target lesion as assessed by ultrasound was achieved in all cases, but one patient had residual viable invasive carcinoma outside the ablated area on histopathological examination. There were no procedure-related complications observed.

Noguchi and colleagues performed RF ablation for 10 breast tumors (mean 1.1 cm, range 0.5 to 2.0 cm), with no viable tumor cells seen in excised specimens with NADH-diaphorase staining (25,26). Imoto and colleagues (27) evaluated RF ablation in 30 patients with clinical T1N0 breast cancer. Adverse events were observed in nine patients, including skin and muscle burns. Tumor killing was complete in 24 of 26 cases (92%), as assessed by NADH-diaphorase staining.

Residual viable tumor cells were seen in 3 of 10 locally recurrent tumors treated with RF ablation followed by mastectomy (28), with the authors concluding that RF ablation was not sufficiently effective for this use.

Cryoablation and Laser Ablation

Roubidoux and colleagues (29) performed outpatient cryoablation of nine breast tumors with a mean size of 1.2 cm using a 2.7 mm cryoprobe with a tabletop argon gas–based cryoablation system and a double freeze-thaw protocol. Tumor sites were excised at lumpectomy 2 to 3 weeks after cryoablation. Specimens were found to contain fat necrosis at excision, and two of nine excised tumors (22%) contained residual viable tumor cells.

Cryoablation has also been used to ablate benign lesions where there is a desire to eliminate a palpable lesion but no concern about leaving residual viable cells. Cryoablation was performed for 78 fibroadenomas and other benign breast lesions using a double freeze-thaw cycle lasting 6 to 30 minutes (30). At 1 year, tumor volume resorption was 88.3% overall on ultrasound, with minimal residual density and no calcifications on mammography. Cosmesis was excellent, with no visual or palpable tissue defect after treatment. The overall utility of such ablation techniques for benign breast lesions remains under investigation.

Dowlatshahi and colleagues (31) performed laser ablation for 54 tumors with a mean size of 12 mm using an 805 nm laser beam via a fiber in a 16-gauge needle, with complete killing in 93% of tumors in one 14-patient cohort and complete killing in 100% of tumors in another 14-patient cohort. Tumor killing by ablation with an 805 nm diode laser was also inconsistent in a series of 44 breast tumors reported by Harries and colleagues. (32)

Follow-up of Ablation Procedures: Local Control, Cosmesis, and Imaging Findings

Few data exist on long-term local control rates or cosmetic results for tumors ablated percutaneously and left in place. Fat necrosis with oil cyst formation at the treated site seems common after percutaneous ablation. Marcy and colleagues (33) performed RF ablation without subsequent surgical resection in five elderly women with T1 to T2 tumors. A firm 4 × 5 cm mass was present in all patients within the first 3 months, with fat necrosis and an oil cyst seen in the area on imaging. One of five patients developed a local recurrence within four months after RF ablation, and another patient developed an abscess in the treatment site at nine months that required aspiration and excision. Akimov and colleagues (34) performed laser ablation in 35 breast cancers using a neodymium-doped yttrium-aluminium-garnet (Nd:YAG) (1,064 nm) pulse-wave laser. Among seven patients treated without surgery, local tumor control was achieved in five.

Development of a 2 to 3 cm oil cyst with fibrosis was seen on needle core biopsies in two patients treated with laser ablation without surgical excision (31). Skin puckering was seen immediately after RF ablation in 2 of 15 patients, requiring excision of affected skin (35).

Noguchi and colleagues (36) summarized significant problems to be resolved before widespread application of RF ablation, including current inability to precisely determine tumor size (and ablation target) on pretreatment imaging, inability to assess completeness of tumor cell killing without surgery, inability to assess margins, uncertainty as to whether ablation procedure scarring will hamper detection of local recurrence, and uncertainty as to long-term cosmetic outcome. These concerns apply to all forms of nonsurgical tumor ablation.

■ IMPACT OF ADVANCED IMAGING APPROACHES IN GUIDING SURGERY

It is hoped that new imaging approaches will enable earlier detection of breast tumors and provide increased sensitivity and specificity for screening. In addition, it is hoped that future imaging technologies will provide a more accurate definition of tumor geometry to permit more precise lumpectomies with fewer positive margins, and potentially provide specific enough information to accurately guide nonsurgical ablation techniques. These approaches may also be useful for early and ongoing assessment of tumor response to neoadjuvant systemic therapy.

Breast Tomosynthesis

Breast tomosynthesis, an approach derived from digital mammography technology, is currently in development. In breast tomosynthesis, low–radiation dose digital mammogram images are acquired as the x-ray source is moved in an arc above the stationary breast and digital detector (37). Images of individual "slices" of breast volume are produced, resulting in a three-dimensional digital image and reducing the problem of interpreting mammographic features produced by tissue overlap.

Functional Imaging

Mammography and ultrasound are anatomical imaging modalities that create images on the basis of differences in the physical structure of tumors (x-ray density and reflection of ultrasound waves) relative to normal tissue. Functional imaging exploits unique aspects of tumor physiology that distinguish tumor cells from adjacent normal tissues. For example, magnetic resonance imaging (MRI) takes advantage of differences in tumor vasculature that result in increased gadolinium enhancement relative to normal breast tissue, and positron emission tomography (PET) scans take advantage of the increased metabolic activity of tumors relative to normal tissue and identifies tumors as areas of labeled FD-glucose uptake.

Several functional imaging technologies currently being applied to breast cancer imaging are likely to have an impact on future surgical management of breast cancer.

Magnetic Resonance Imaging

Breast MRI already has an increasing role in assessing extent of disease and may identify unsuspected ipsilateral or contralateral lesions in as many as 3% to 5% of newly diagnosed breast cancer patients overall (38,39) and in as many as 12% of women aged 40 or younger at diagnosis (40). Breast MRI is also being studied for its ability to assess tumor response in patients being considered for breast conservation after neoadjuvant systemic therapy. However, MRI may either underestimate or overestimate the extent of DCIS present (41), requiring caution in using MRI findings to determine extent of surgery.

Breast-specific Gamma Imaging

During use of ^{99m}Tc-sestimibi for assessment of myocardial perfusion, it was noted that certain tumors, including breast cancers, showed high levels of uptake relative to normal tissue (42). ^{99m}Tc-sestimibi is a lipophilic cationic complex whose uptake has been related to regional blood flow, plasma and mitochondrial membrane potential, angiogenesis, and apoptosis. It accumulates in the mitochondria of tumor cells at rates fourfold to ninefold greater than in benign cells.

Use of ^{99m}Tc-sestimibi in breast imaging, termed scintimammography, is reported to be more specific for diagnosis of malignancy than mammography and has the advantage of being equally accurate in dense and fatty breasts. However, its application has been limited by decreased sensitivity for identifying small breast lesions. In a meta-analysis of 5,340 patients assessed for breast cancer with scintimammography, overall results showed sensitivity of 85.2% and specificity of 86.6% in tumor diagnosis. For patients with a palpable mass, the sensitivity and specificity were 87.8% and 87.5%, respectively, but for patients without a palpable mass the sensitivity was only 66.8%, with 86.9% specificity (43).

A high-resolution, small-field-of-view gamma camera, optimized to perform metabolic analyses of breast parenchyma, has been developed to increase sensitivity of ^{99m}Tc-sestimibi imaging in breast applications. This breast-specific gamma imaging (BSGI) can permit identification of subcentimeter malignancies. In a recent study of 167 breast lesions in 146 patients, BSGI had high sensitivity (96.4%) and moderate specificity (59.5%) in detecting breast cancers, and it identified additional foci of malignancy not seen on mammography or ultrasound in 7% of patients (44). This imaging modality was able to detect both invasive cancer and DCIS foci measuring only 1 mm.

BSGI may be particularly useful for identification of invasive lobular carcinoma. In 26 women with 28 biopsy-proven invasive lobular cancers, BSGI showed the highest sensitivity for the detection of invasive lobular carcinoma, with a sensitivity of 93%, while mammography, ultrasound, and MRI showed sensitivities of 79%, 68%, and 83%, respectively (45).

[99m]Tc-sestimibi imaging is also being explored to assess tumor response to neoadjuvant chemotherapy. The ^{99m}Tc-sestimibi tracer is a transport substrate for the P-glycoprotein, which is commonly associated with the development of the multidrug-resistance phenotype. As a result, ^{99m}Tc-sestimibi uptake correlates with P-glycoprotein expression. Tumor retention of ^{99m}Tc-sestamibi has been associated with good tumor response, while rapid clearance was associated with decreased response (46–48).

Wider implementation of BSGI is unlikely unless technical improvements enhance its ability to detect small breast cancers. However, the increased sensitivity and specificity of BSGI over mammography, and the reduced cost of BSGI relative to MRI, may provide a role for BSGI in diagnostic breast imaging.

■ IMPROVING AXILLARY STAGING

Although the use of sentinel lymph node mapping has greatly reduced the morbidity of surgical staging of the axilla, interest remains in exploring options to reduce further or eliminate surgery for axillary staging. Clinical trials addressing use of axillary radiation rather than completion dissection for patients with positive sentinel nodes (49,50) or systemic therapy and standard tangent radiation without completion axillary dissection (51) have been conducted, and the results are pending. Advanced imaging technologies are also being assessed for their capacity to accurately stage the axilla without surgery in breast cancer patients.

Ultrasound Staging of the Axilla

A number of ultrasound features of axillary nodes have been suggested to predict the presence of breast cancer metastases, including asymmetric cortical thickening or lobulations, loss or compression of the hyperechoic medullary region, absence of fatty hilum, abnormal lymph node shape, hypoechoic cortex, admixture of normal-appearing and abnormal-appearing nodes, and increased peripheral blood flow (52).

These ultrasound features are fairly nonspecific. Bedrosian and colleagues reported use of axillary ultrasound in 208 breast cancer patients with clinically negative axillae (53). Final pathological examinations revealed positive nodes in 39 of 180 (22%) with negative ultrasonographic findings and 14 of 28 (50%) with indeterminate or suspicious ultrasonographic findings.

It has been suggested that axillary ultrasound is most useful for guiding fine-needle biopsy of potentially suspicious axillary nodes, allowing those with positive fine-needle biopsies to proceed directly to axillary dissection without an unnecessary sentinel node biopsy (54,55). Sentinel node biopsy is still required for patients with benign-appearing axillary nodes or those whose fine-needle biopsies are negative or nondiagnostic.

MRI Staging of the Axilla

Kvistad and colleagues (56) performed MRI prior to axillary dissection in 65 patients with breast cancer. When using a signal intensity increase in the lymph nodes of more than 100% during the first postcontrast image as a threshold for malignancy, 57 of 65 patients were correctly classified (sensitivity 83%, specificity 90%, accuracy 88%). These results were not improved when lymph node size and morphology were used as additional criteria.

Use of additional MRI contrast agents to improve detection of lymph node metastases is under investigation. Iron-based contrast agents, including ultrasmall superparamagnetic iron oxide (USPIO)–enhanced MRI (57,58), may allow detection of smaller nodal deposits for breast cancers and other tumors.

Fluorodeoxyglucose–Positron Emission Tomography Staging of the Axilla

The role of fluorodeoxyglucose (FDG)–PET imaging in breast cancer staging is evolving (59). FDG-PET imaging has been reported to have a higher sensitivity and specificity than computed tomography (CT), MRI, or ultrasound (US) for predicting axillary nodal status (60–62).

Veronisi and colleagues (63) reported results of 236 patients with breast cancer and a clinically negative axilla who underwent FDG-PET imaging before sentinel node biopsy. Patients underwent axillary lymph node dissection for a positive FDG-PET scan or a positive sentinel node. Sensitivity of FDG-PET for detection of axillary node metastases was low (37%), but specificity and positive predictive values were felt to be acceptable (96% and 88%, respectively). The authors concluded that high PET specificity allows patients with a PET-positive axilla to proceed directly to axillary dissection. In contrast, poor FDG-PET sensitivity for detection of axillary metastases requires sentinel node biopsy where PET is negative in the axilla.

Kim and colleagues performed FDG-PET/CT imaging in 137 patients with biopsy-proven breast cancers, with 27 patients (19.7%) predicted to have axillary metastases. The overall sensitivity, specificity, positive predictive value, and overall accuracy of FDG-PET/CT in predicting axillary metastasis were 77.1%, 100%, 100%, and 94.2%, respectively (64). There were eight false-negative scans and no false-positive scans.

Imaging for Axillary Staging: Conclusions

A number of imaging techniques, such as FDG-PET/CT, have a high positive predictive value in identifying patients with positive axillary nodes who might go directly to axillary dissection without sentinel node biopsy. It is as yet unclear whether the use of such imaging approaches for axillary staging will prove cost-effective when compared with sentinel node biopsy at the time of definitive surgical excision of the primary tumor.

Unfortunately, all axillary imaging approaches applied to date have significant false negative rates, generally in the 20% to 30% range, for predicting axillary involvement. As a result, no current axillary imaging technique is likely to be considered accurate enough to deem a patient node-negative for systemic and local therapy decision-making purposes.

■ IMPROVING COSMETIC OUTCOME

Oncoplastic Approaches for Breast-conserving Surgery

While the primary goal of breast-conserving surgery is effective local control, achievement of a pleasing cosmetic result is an important secondary goal. Many breast surgeons now incorporate a variety of plastic surgery techniques into breast cancer resections, in an approach being termed "oncoplastic" surgery (65). Local advancement flaps, concurrent mastopexy or reduction mammoplasty, creative incision placement, and other procedures may be incorporated into excision of the breast tumor and closure of the resulting defect. These oncoplastic techniques allow extensive resections that may extend eligibility for breast conservation and improve overall cosmetic outcome.

Although cosmetic outcome is difficult to quantify, use of oncoplastic techniques resulted in larger lumpectomy volumes (66,67) and achieved wider clear margins (66) than standard lumpectomy techniques. Local recurrence rates and overall survival do not seem to be negatively affected by use of oncoplastic techniques. Clough and colleagues (68) reported 3.8-year follow-up results of oncoplastic breast-conserving surgery in 101 patients at the Institut Curie with a median tumor size of 32 mm and mean lumpectomy weight of 222 g. All received preoperative or postoperative radiotherapy. The actuarial 5-year local recurrence rate was 9.4%, the overall survival rate was 95.7%, and the metastasis-free survival rate was 82.8%—all felt to be comparable to results in similar patients undergoing standard breast-conserving surgery. Cosmesis was favorable in 82% of cases, despite the fairly large median tumor size.

Immediate repair of lumpectomy defects using local advancement flaps resulted in a lower risk of complications and better aesthetic outcome than immediate repair of partial mastectomy defects with a latissimus dorsi flap (69). Complication rates were higher when repair of the lumpectomy defect was delayed until after completion of radiation.

Nipple-sparing Mastectomy

The efficacy of skin-sparing mastectomy in achieving local control has led to consideration of nipple-sparing mastectomy for selected patients with early-stage breast cancer (70). In nipple-sparing mastectomy all skin, including the nipple and areola, is left in place, with the mastectomy performed through an incision that is closed primarily. For many patients, the cosmetic result possible with this approach is superior to that achieved with skin-sparing mastectomy and nipple reconstruction. Increased use of nipple-sparing mastectomy is likely if early results that suggest excellent local control are confirmed and if ongoing efforts to identify eligible patients preoperatively prove successful.

Early follow-up of nipple-sparing mastectomy in selected patients has shown low rates of nipple recurrence and acceptable rates of nipple necrosis (71–74). Brachtel and colleagues (75) reported a 22% rate of nipple involvement in a recent series of 316 consecutive mastectomy specimens. Rusby and colleagues have created a calculator to predict risk of nipple involvement for breast cancer patients being considered for nipple-sparing mastectomy (76). The potential benefits of intraoperative radiation to improve local control with nipple-sparing mastectomy are being explored (73).

■ THE EVOLVING ROLE OF THE SURGEON IN MULTIDISCIPLINARY CARE

For many patients with a new diagnosis of breast cancer, the surgeon is the specialist who will serve as their guide through the initial staging and treatment of their breast cancer. In addition, although an increasing percentage of patients will have an image-guided needle biopsy for diagnosis, there are still a significant number of patients for whom a surgical biopsy is required for diagnosis. The surgeon is often the specialist who communicates the results of definitive surgery and its prognostic implications. In many practice settings the surgeon is also responsible for referring patients to medical and radiation oncologists for adjuvant therapy, and for initiating any other consultations required.

The current importance of this role is demonstrated by studies that report that patients treated by surgeons and hospitals with a high breast case volume have improved survival relative to patients treated by low-volume surgeons and hospitals.

Analysis of the New York State hospital discharge database found that breast cancer patients from very-low-volume hospitals had a 60% greater risk of all-cause mortality at 5 years than patients from high-volume hospitals (77). Review of 29,666 breast cancer patients in the Cancer Surveillance Program database for Los Angeles County found that type of surgeon was an independent predictor of survival, as were both hospital and surgeon case volume. Treatment by a surgical oncologist resulted in a 33% reduction in the risk of death at 5 years (78). Using the Surveillance, Epidemiology, and End Results (SEER) tumor registry data and Medicare claims data for 11,225 Medicare patients who had undergone surgery for early-stage breast cancer from 1994 to 1996, Gilligan and colleagues found that treatment in a high-volume hospital was associated with hazard ratios of 0.83 (95% confidence interval 0.75 to 0.92) for all-cause mortality and 0.80 (95% confidence interval 0.66 to 0.97) for breast cancer–specific mortality when compared with treatment at a low-volume hospital (79). Others have suggested that other patient factors, rather than surgeon or hospital volume contribute to these results (80).

In the future, it is likely that the surgeon's role as guide and gatekeeper will have increasing importance as more and increasingly complex breast cancer treatment options become available. It will be essential for a surgeon to maintain up-to-date knowledge of diagnosis and treatment options to assure patients timely and maximally effective treatment. For example, modern breast surgical expertise now includes

- Awareness of evolving indications for neoadjuvant therapy rather than primary surgery with appropriate referral of patients for medical oncology consultation prior to surgery
- Careful assessment of treatment options for elderly breast cancer patients. Many elderly patients with estrogen receptor–positive tumors may be effectively treated with excision of their primary tumor followed by endocrine therapy, without axillary surgery or radiation, and the frail elderly may be treated by endocrine therapy without surgery or radiation. Appropriate assessment of each elderly patient's tumor and general medical health is essential in

selecting treatment that will be effective and result in minimal morbidity

- Awareness of appropriate immediate or delayed reconstruction candidates, with prompt referral of reconstruction candidates for plastic surgery consultation
- Early referral of high-risk patients for genetic counseling, making genetic test results available prior to any surgical procedure. A patient found to be a mutation carrier may be better served by bilateral mastectomies rather than a lumpectomy, and reconstruction options may be limited by a poorly placed biopsy or lumpectomy incision
- Awareness of options for fertility preservation and timely referral to reproductive medicine specialists for patients who wish to consider embryo banking. There is only a very narrow window of opportunity for embryo banking if it is to be performed without causing a delay in initiation of chemotherapy. If referral is not made promptly at diagnosis, and often prior to any surgical procedures, the opportunity for fertility preservation may be lost

The surgeon will play a critical role in ongoing efforts to provide care that is cost-effective as well as high quality. The surgeon will continue to make decisions about use of expensive diagnostic modalities such as breast MRI and will drive adherence to guidelines for MRI utilization (81). Initiatives to create effective guidelines and standards are under way (82,83), including the American Society of Breast Surgeons Mastery of Breast Surgery Pilot Program (84), which allows individual surgeons to report and track their performance on a number of quality measures.

■ REFERENCES

1. Dzierzanowski M, Melville KA, Barnes PJ, et al. Ductal carcinoma in situ in core biopsies containing invasive breast cancer: correlation with extensive intraductal component and lumpectomy margins. *J Surg Oncol.* 2005;90:71–76.
2. Chagpar A, Yen T, Sahin A, et al. Intraoperative margin assessment reduces reexcision rates in patients with ductal carcinoma in situ treated with breast-conserving surgery. *Am J Surg.* 2003;186:371–377.
3. Lind DS, Minter R, Steinbach B, et al. Stereotactic core biopsy reduces the reexcision rate and the cost of mammographically detected cancer. *J Surg Res.* 1998;78:23–26.
4. Smitt MC, Horst K. Association of clinical and pathologic variables with lumpectomy surgical margin status after preoperative diagnosis or excisional biopsy of invasive breast cancer. *Ann Surg Oncol.* 2007;14:1040–1044.
5. Kirstein L, Rafferty E, Moore R, et al. Outcome of multiple wire localization for larger breast cancers: when can mastectomy be avoided? *J Am Coll Surg.* 2008;207:342–346.
6. Klimberg VS, Westbrook KC, Korourian S. Use of touch preps for diagnosis and evaluation of surgical margins in breast cancer. *Ann Surg Onc.* 1998;5:220–226.
7. Haka AS, Shafer-Peltier KE, Fitzmaurice M, et al. Diagnosing breast cancer using Raman spectroscopy. *Proc Natl Acad Sci USA.* 2005;102:12371–12376.
8. Haka AS, Zoya Volynskaya Z, Gardecki JA, et al. In vivo margin assessment during partial mastectomy breast surgery using Raman spectroscopy. *Cancer Res.* 2006;66:3317–3322.
9. Huang D, Swanson EA, Lin CP, et al. Optical coherence tomography. *Science.* 1991;254:1178–1181.
10. Boppart SA, Luo W, Marks DL, Singletary KW. Optical coherence tomography: feasibility for basic research and image-guided surgery of breast cancer. *Breast Cancer Res Treat.* 2004;84:85–97.
11. Hsiung P-L, Phatak DR, Chen Y, et al. Benign and malignant lesions in the human breast depicted with ultrahigh resolution and three-dimensional optical coherence tomography. *Radiology.* 2007;244:865–874.
12. Karni T, Pappo I, Sandbank J, et al. A device for real-time, intraoperative margin assessment in breast-conservation surgery. *Am J Surg.* 2007;194:467–473.
13. Vlastos G, Verkooijen HM. Minimally invasive approaches for diagnosis and treatment of early-stage breast cancer. *Oncologist.* 2007;12:1–10.
14. Bland K, Gass J, Klimberg V. Radiofrequency, cryoablation, and other modalities for breast cancer ablation. *Surg Clinics N Amer.* 2007;87:539–550.
15. Simmons RM. Ablative techniques in the treatment of benign and malignant breast disease. *J Am Coll Surg.* 2003;197:334–338.
16. Singletary SE, Fornage BD, Sneige N, et al. Radiofrequency ablation of early-stage invasive breast tumors: an overview. *Cancer J.* 2002;8(2):177–180.
17. Huber PE, Jenne JW, Rastert R, et al. A new noninvasive approach in breast cancer therapy using magnetic resonance imaging-guided focused ultrasound surgery. *Cancer Res.* 2001;61:8441–8447.
18. Hynynen K, Pomeroy O, Smith DN, et al. MR imaging-guided focused ultrasound surgery of fibroadenomas in the breast: a feasibility study. *Radiology.* 2001;219:176–185.
19. Gardner RA, Vargas HI, Block JB, et al. Focused microwave phased array thermotherapy for primary breast cancer. *Ann Surg Oncol.* 2002;9:326–332.
20. Singletary, SE. Feasibility of radiofrequency ablation for primary breast cancer. *Breast Cancer.* 2003;10:4–9.
21. Burak WE Jr, Agnese DM, Povoski SP, et al. Radiofrequency ablation of invasive breast carcinoma followed by delayed surgical excision. *Cancer.* 2003;98:1369–1376.
22. Jeffrey SS, Birdwell PL, Ikeda DM, et al. Radiofrequency ablation of breast cancer: first report of an emerging technology. *Arch Surg.* 1999;134:1064–1068.
23. Izzo F, Thomas R, Delrio P, et al. RFA in patients with primary breast carcinoma: a pilot study in 26 patients. *Cancer.* 2001;92:2036–2044.
24. Fornage BD, Sneige N, Ross MI, et al. Small (<2-cm) breast cancer treated with US-guided radiofrequency ablation: feasibility study. *Radiology.* 2004;231:215–224.
25. Noguchi M, Earashi M, Fujii H, Yokoyama K, Harada K, Tsuneyama K. Radiofrequency ablation of small breast cancer followed by surgical resection. *J Surg Oncol.* 2006;93:120–128.
26. Earashi M, Noguchi M, Motoyoshi A, Fujii H. Radiofrequency ablation therapy for small breast cancer followed by immediate surgical resection or delayed Mammotome excision. *Breast Cancer.* 2007;14:39–47.
27. Imoto S, Wada N, Sakemura N, Hasebe T, Murata Y. Feasibility study on radiofrequency ablation followed by partial mastectomy for stage I breast cancer patients. *Breast.* 2009;18:130–134.
28. Garbay J-R, Mathieu M-C, Lamuraglia M, et al. Radiofrequency thermal ablation of breast cancer local recurrence: a phase II clinical trial. *Ann Surg Oncol.* 2008;15:3222–3226.
29. Roubidoux MA, Sabel MS, Bailey JE, et al. Small (<2.0-cm) breast cancers: mammographic and US findings at US-guided cryoablation—initial experience. *Radiology.* 2004;233:857–867.
30. Kaufman C, Bachman B, Littrup P, et al Cryoablation treatment of benign breast lesions with 12-month follow-up. *Am J Surg.* 2004;188:340–348.

31. Dowlatshahi K, Francescatti DS, Bloom KJ. Laser therapy for small breast cancers. *Am J Surg.* 2002;184(4):359–363.

32. Harries SA, Amin Z, Smith MEF, et al. Interstitial laser photocoagulation as a treatment for breast cancer. *Br J Surg.* 2005; 81:1617–1619.

33. Marcy P-Y, Magné N, Castadot P, Bailet C, Namer, M. Ultrasound-guided percutaneous radiofrequency ablation in elderly breast cancer patients: preliminary institutional experience. *Br J Radiol.* 2007;80:267–273.

34. Akimov AB, Seregin VE, Rusanov KV, et al. Nd:YAG interstitial laser thermotherapy in the treatment of breast cancer. *Lasers Surg Med.* 1998;22:257–267.

35. Khatri VP, McGahan JP, Ramsamooj R, et al. A phase II trial of image-guided radiofrequency ablation of small invasive breast carcinomas: use of saline-cooled tip electrode. *Ann Surg Oncol.* 2007;14:1644–1652.

36. Noguchi M. Is radiofrequency ablation treatment for small breast cancer ready for "prime time"? *Breast Cancer Res Treat.* 2007; 106:307–314.

37. Niklason LT, Christian BT, Niklason LE, et al. Digital tomosynthesis in breast imaging. *Radiology.* 1997;205:399–406.

38. Lehman CD, Gatsonis C, Kuhl CK, et al. MRI evaluation of the contralateral breast in women with recently diagnosed breast cancer. *New Engl J Med.* 2007;356:1295–1303.

39. Liberman L, Morris EA, Kim CM, et al. MR imaging findings in the contralateral breast of women with recently diagnosed breast cancer. *AJR Am J Roentgenol.* 2003;180:333–341.

40. Samphao S, Wheeler AJ, Rafferty E, et al. Diagnosis of breast cancer in women age 40 and younger: delays in diagnosis result from underutilization of genetic testing and breast imaging. *Am J Surg.* In press.

41. Schouten van der Velden AP, Boetes C, Bult P, Wobbes T. The value of magnetic resonance imaging in diagnosis and size assessment of in situ and small invasive breast carcinoma. *Am J Surg.* 2006;192:172–178.

42. Stuntz ME, Khalkhali I, Kakuda KT, et al. Scintimammography. *Semin Breast Dis.* 1999;2:97–106.

43. Liberman M, Sampalis F, Mulder DS, Sampalis JS. Breast cancer diagnosis by scintimammography: a meta-analysis and review of the literature. *Breast Cancer Res Treat.* 2003;80:115–126.

44. Brem RF, Floerke AC, Rapelyea JA, et al. Breast-specific gamma imaging as an adjunct imaging modality for the diagnosis of breast cancer. *Radiology.* 2008;247:651–657.

45. Brem RF, Ioffe M, Rapelyea JA, et al. Invasive lobular carcinoma: detection with mammography, sonography, MRI, and breast-specific gamma imaging. *AJR Am J Roentgenol.* 2009;192: 379–383.

46. Ciarmiello A, Vecchio SD, Silvestro P, et al. Tumor clearance of technetium 99m-sestamibi as a predictor of response to neoadjuvant chemotherapy for locally advanced breast cancer. *J Clin Oncol.* 1998;16:1677–1683.

47. Salvatore M, Del Vecchio S. Dynamic imaging: scintimammography. *Eur J Radiol.* 1998;27(Suppl 2):S259–S264.

48. Sciuto R, Pasqualoni R, Bergomi S, et al. Prognostic value of ^{99m}Tc-sestamibi washout in predicting response of locally advanced breast cancer to neoadjuvant chemotherapy. *J Nucl Med.* 2002;43:745–751.

49. Gadd M, Harris J, Taghian A, et al. Prospective study of axillary radiation without axillary dissection for breast cancer patients with a positive sentinel node. Oral presentation, San Antonio Breast Cancer Symposium 2005.

50. Rutgers E, Meijnen P, Bonnefoi H. Clinical trials update of the European Organization for Research and Treatment of Cancer Breast Cancer Group. *Breast Cancer Res.* 2004;6:165–169.

51. Lucy A, Mackie-McCall L, Beitsch PD, et al. Surgical complications associated with sentinel lymph node dissection (SLND) plus axillary lymph node dissection compared with SLND alone in the American College of Surgeons Oncology Group Trial Z0011. *J Clin Oncol.* 2007;25:3657–3663.

52. Moore A, Hester M, Nam M-W, et al. Distinct lymph nodal sonographic characteristics in breast cancer patients at high risk for axillary metastases correlate with the final axillary stage. *Br J Radiol.* 2008;81:630–636.

53. Bedrosian I, Bedi D, Kuerer HM, et al. Impact of clinicopathological factors on sensitivity of axillary ultrasonography in the detection of axillary nodal metastases in patients with breast cancer. *Ann Surg Oncol.* 2003;10:1025–1030.

54. Hinson JL, McGrath P, Moore A, et al. The critical role of axillary ultrasound and aspiration biopsy in the management of breast cancer patients with clinically negative axilla. *Ann Surg Oncol.* 2008;15:250–255.

55. Jain A, Haisfield-Wolfe ME, Lange J, et al. The role of ultrasound-guided fine-needle aspiration of axillary nodes in the staging of breast cancer. *Ann Surg Oncol.* 2008;15: 462–471.

56. Kvistad KA, Rydland J, Smethurst H-B, et al. Axillary lymph node metastases in breast cancer: preoperative detection with dynamic contrast-enhanced MRI. *Eur Radiol.* 2000;10:1464–1471.

57. Harisinghani MG, Dixon WT, Saksena MA, et al. MR lymphangiography: imaging strategies to optimize the imaging of lymph nodes with ferumoxtran-10. *Radiographics.* 2004;24:867–878.

58. Memarsadeghi M, Riedl CC, Kaneider A, et al. Axillary lymph node metastases in patients with breast carcinomas: assessment with nonenhanced versus USPIO-enhanced MR imaging. *Radiology.* 2006;241:367–377.

59. Hodgson NC, Gulenchyn KY. Is there a role for positron emission tomography in breast cancer staging? *J Clin Oncol.* 2008;26: 712–720.

60. Kao CH, Hsieh JF, Tsai SC, et al. Comparison and discrepancy of ^{18}F-2-deoxyglucose positron emission tomography and Tc-99m MDP bone scan to detect bone metastasis. *Anticancer Res.* 2000; 20:2189–2192.

61. Kostakoglu L, Goldsmith SJ. ^{18}F-FDG PET evaluation of the response to therapy for lymphoma and for breast, lung, and colorectal carcinoma. *J Nucl Med.* 2003;44:224–239.

62. Eubank WB, Mankoff DA, Vesselle HJ, et al. Detection of locoregional and distant recurrences in breast cancer patients by using FDG PET. *Radiographics.* 2003;22:5–17.

63. Veronesi U, De Cicco C, Galimberti VE, et al. A comparative study on the value of FDG-PET and sentinel node biopsy to identify occult axillary metastases. *Ann Oncol.* 2007;18:473–478.

64. Kim J, Lee J, Chang E, et al. Selective sentinel node plus additional non-sentinel node biopsy based on an FDG-PET/CT scan in early breast cancer patients: single institutional experience. *World J Surg.* 2009;33:943–949.

65. Masetti R, Di Leone A, Franceschini G, et al. Oncoplastic techniques in the conservative surgical treatment of breast cancer: an overview. *Breast J.* 2006;12(Suppl 2):S174–S180.

66. Giacalone P-L, Roger P, Dubon O, et al. Comparative study of the accuracy of breast resection in oncoplastic surgery and quadrantectomy in breast cancer. *Ann Surg Oncol.* 2007;14:605–614.

67. Kaur N, Petit J-Y, Rietjens M, et al. Comparative study of surgical margins in oncoplastic surgery and quadrantectomy in breast cancer. *Ann Surg Oncol.* 2005;12:539–545.

68. Clough KB, Lewis JS, Couturaud B, et al. Oncoplastic techniques allow extensive resections for breast-conserving therapy of breast carcinomas. *Ann Surg.* 2003;237:26–34.

69. Kronowitz SJ, Feledy JA, Hunt KK, et al. Determining the optimal approach to breast reconstruction after partial mastectomy. *Plastic Reconst Surg.* 2006;117:1–11.

70. Chung A, Sacchini V. Nipple-sparing mastectomy: where are we now? *Surg Oncol.* 2008;17:261–266.

71. Stolier AJ, Sullivan SK, Dellacroce FJ. Technical considerations in nipple-sparing mastectomy: 82 consecutive cases without necrosis. *Ann Surg Oncol.* 2008;15:1341–1347.

72. Caruso F, Ferrara M, Castiglione G, et al. Nipple sparing subcutaneous mastectomy: sixty-six months follow-up. *Eur J Surg Oncol.* 2006;32(9):937–940.

73. Petit JY, Veronesi U, Orecchia R, et al. Nipple-sparing mastectomy in association with intra operative radiotherapy (ELIOT): a new type of mastectomy for breast cancer treatment. *Breast Cancer Res Treat.* 2006;96:47–51.

74. Sacchini V, Pinotti JA, Barros AC, et al. Nipple-sparing mastectomy for breast cancer and risk reduction: oncologic or technical problem? *J Am Coll Surg.* 2006;203:704–714.

75. Brachtel EF, Rusby JE, Michaelson JS, Smith BL, Koerner FC. Histologic patterns of occult nipple involvement in breast cancer: a prospective study of 316 mastectomies. *J Clin Oncol.* 2009; 27:4948–54.

76. Rusby JE, Brachtel EF, Michaelson JS, Koerner FC, Smith BL. Predictors of occult nipple involvement to aid selection of patients for nipple-sparing mastectomy. *Br J Surg.* 2008;95:1356–1361.

77. Roohan PJ, Bickell NA, Baptiste MS, et al. Hospital volume differences and five-year survival from breast cancer. *Am J Public Health.* 1998;88:454–457.

78. Skinner KA, Helsper JT, Deapen D, Ye W, Sposto R. Breast cancer: do specialists make a difference? *Ann Surg Oncol.* 2003;10: 606–615.

79. Gilligan MA, Neuner, J, Zhang X, et al. Relationship between number of breast cancer operations performed and 5-year survival after treatment for early-stage breast cancer. *Am J Public Health.* 2007;97:539–544.

80. Nattinger AB, Laud PW, Sparapani RA, et al. Exploring the surgeon volume outcome relationship among women with breast cancer. *Arch Intern Med.* 2007;167:1958–1963.

81. Saslow D, Boetes C, Burke W, et al. American Cancer Society guidelines for breast screening with MRI as an adjunct to mammography. *CA Cancer J Clin.* 2007;57:75–89.

82. Hassett MJ, Hughes ME, Niland JC, et al. Selecting high priority quality measures for breast cancer quality improvement. *Med Care.* 2008;46:762–770.

83. Desch CE, McNiff KK, Schneider EC, et al. American Society of Clinical Oncology/National Comprehensive Cancer Network quality measures. *J Clin Oncol.* 2008;26:3631–3637.

84. American Society of Breast Surgeons. Mastery of breast surgery pilot program. Available at www.breastsurgeons.org/mastery/mastery_faq.php.

Evolving Innovations for Breast Radiotherapy

SHANNON M. MACDONALD

ALPHONSE G. TAGHIAN

Almost immediately following the discovery of x-rays and their diagnostic capabilities by Wilhelm Roentgen in 1895, it became apparent in scientific and academic communities that radiation had potential for therapeutic applications as well. In the early 1900s, reports of the use of radiation for palliation of recurrent breast cancer surfaced (1,2). In 1904, Antoine Béclère published results documenting therapeutic benefits with the use of radium for two patients with recurrent breast cancer treated at Pierre Curie's laboratory (2). He documented acute skin toxicities and regression of tumor following administration of radium. There was no method of measuring dose at this time and no knowledge of the benefits of fractionated radiation therapy. Nor were there multiple modalities of radiation from which to choose. Suffice to say, we have come a very long way since the initial utilization of radiation therapy for breast cancer depicted in the painting by Chicotot reproduced in Figure 16.1. Since the beginning of the twentieth century, radiation therapy has been established as an important component of curative treatment for early-stage and locally advanced breast cancer. For early-stage breast cancer, radiation allows for breast conservation with equivalent survival and comparable local control to mastectomy (3,4). In more advanced cases of breast cancer, postmastectomy or comprehensive radiation provides a substantial decrease in locoregional recurrence, and improved disease-free and overall survival has been demonstrated in several studies (5–7). Increased understandings of breast disease and technological advances in the past century have led to dramatic progress in the management and outcomes of patients receiving radiation. It is exciting to imagine what the next century will hold.

■ TARGET DEFINITION/USING ADVANCES IN RADIOLOGY

In the past three decades advances in diagnostic radiology and computer technology have enabled marked advances in radiation delivery. Before the advent of computed tomography (CT), radiation planning was performed with x-rays or plain films (two-dimensional treatment planning). Measurements were obtained in one axial plane in

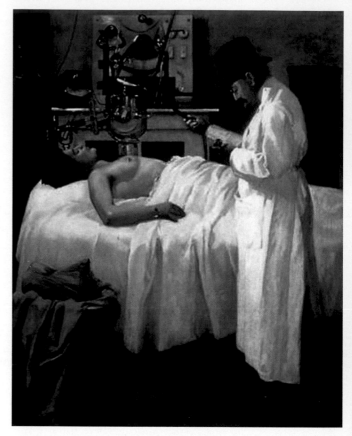

FIGURE 16.1 A painting by Chicotot that hangs in the Museum de la Assistance Publique Chicotot depicting the application of radium for carcinoma of the breast and representing one of the first therapeutic applications of radiation. (Reproduced with permission.)

the center of the breast, and these measurements were used to determine dose for the whole breast, but changes in contour of the breast superior and inferior to this plane could not be accounted for. Three-dimensional treatment planning (3D-CRT) enables visualization at all planes through the breast tissue, providing the ability to better compensate for changes in tissue throughout the entire breast and deliver a homogeneous dose distribution. This results in improved target volume coverage with fewer unwanted regions above and below the prescribed dose. CT planning also allows for better visualization of the tumor bed to ensure optimal coverage of this volume during whole breast irradiation and to allow for accurate delineation for targeting the tumor bed alone for either boost or partial breast irradiation (PBI). Cardiac and pulmonary tissues can be better visualized, and we can now determine the amount of these critical structures receiving a certain dose of radiation. In addition, with improved visualization, we

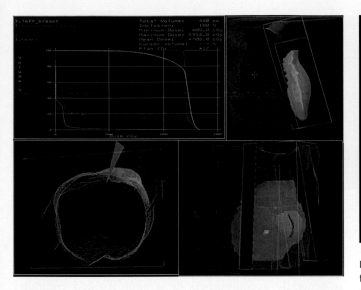

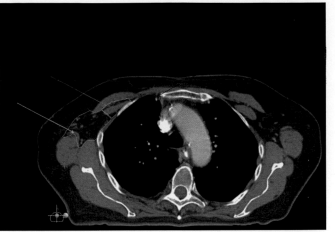

FIGURE 16.2 Three-dimensional treatment planning (3D-CRT) with visualization at all planes through the breast tissue, tumor bed, and cardiac and pulmonary tissues. Dose-volume histograms allow the determination of the volume of these critical structures receiving a certain dose of radiation.

FIGURE 16.3 Lymph node contours used for three-dimensional treatment planning. The figure depicts an axial computed tomography slice with level I, II, and III axilla contoured. Nodal contours may ensure adequate dose coverage of target areas.

can better determine the optimum treatment parameters to minimize dose to these critical structures. Although it remains current practice to minimize dose to these structures, at present, no clear dosimetric constraints for these tissues exist for the treatment of breast cancer (i.e., V10, V20, and V30 for cardiac and pulmonary tissues). Many breast radiation oncologists are actively accumulating these data, and more definitive volumetric constraints for standard and hypofractionated treatments should become available in coming years. Figure 16.2 illustrates three-dimensional treatment planning (3D-CRT) and a dose-volume histogram.

While 3D-CRT planning has led to improved dose homogeneity in breast tissue and better visualization of normal tissues, its full potential for truly conformal treatment is not yet used routinely. Targets such as the supraclavicular fossa, axilla nodal regions (levels I, II, and III), and the internal mammary lymph nodes are not routinely contoured and employed for treatment planning. Supraclavicular and axillary fields are still largely based on bony landmarks, and dose is prescribed to traditional prescription points. While three-dimensional plans can be performed without contouring structures, more advanced radiation modalities such as intensity-modulated radiation therapy (IMRT) and proton radiation require that all targets be clearly defined. The lack of routine contouring of these structures is likely, at least in part, due to the complexity of contouring these regions and the lack of available guidelines for defining these regions. The Radiation Therapy Oncology Group (RTOG) has recognized the need for guidelines for the contouring of target and avoidance volumes to allow the full potential of 3D-CRT to be

utilized. A committee of breast radiation oncologists in consultation with surgeons and radiologists formed written consensus guidelines for defining these structures. This exercise underscored the importance of consensus guidelines as it demonstrated substantial variability even among experienced breast radiation oncologists (8). The RTOG has formed a consensus CT breast atlas that is available on the RTOG website (9). Figure 16.3 demonstrates contoured lymphatic volumes according to these guidelines. Utilized by some radiation oncologists today, this practice will, we believe, become routine with the help of standard guidelines.

Further advances in radiology may also be of benefit for radiation planning for treatment to the regional lymphatics. This will be imperative if ongoing studies support axillary radiation in place of surgery for patients with microscopic involvement of axillary lymph nodes. While the removal of axillary contents provides both diagnostic and therapeutic benefit, it is considered the primary cause of surgical morbidity. Sentinel lymph node biopsy has been proven to decrease morbidity for many patients, but axillary node dissection following a positive sentinel lymph node biopsy is currently considered the standard of care. There is much interest in substituting radiation therapy for axillary dissection following a positive sentinel lymph node biopsy. Excellent outcomes for radiation treatment in place of full axillary lymph node dissection have been reported (10). The European Organisation for Research and Treatment of Cancer (EORTC) AMAROS (after mapping of the axilla radiotherapy or surgery) phase III randomized trial is currently examining this question of whether radiation therapy can be substituted for full axillary node dissection (11). If radiation is being considered as an alternative to surgical dissection, it is of paramount

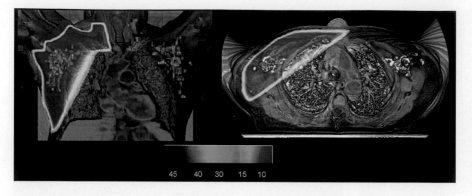

FIGURE 16.4 Advances in delineation of lymph nodes using lymphotrophic nanoparticle-enhanced magnetic resonance imaging (LN-MRI). Radiation doses seen on the patient's right overlaying lymph nodes mapped by LN-MRI (gray). On the patient's left side, LN-MRI lymph nodes without radiation dose wash. (Reproduced with permission from Ref. 90.)

importance that these areas be defined accurately. In addition, if the purpose of radiation therapy is to decrease the toxicities of axillary dissection, better definition of the lymph node locations may provide an improved toxicity profile for radiation therapy by allowing more conformal treatment to lymph nodes at risk. Lymphotrophic nanoparticles have been demonstrated to allow for the identification of lymph node metastasis of breast cancer with very high accuracy (12,13). Ferumoxtran-10 (Combidex; Advanced Magnetics, Cambridge, Mass.) is an iron-containing nanoparticle administered in solution intravenously. These particles circulate systemically and travel to the interstitium, where they are internalized by macrophages. They accumulate in normal lymph nodes and cause changes in magnetic resonance imaging (MRI) signal. This information can assist in delineation of the location of both the normal lymphatics and lymph nodes harboring metastatic disease. Lymphotrophic nanoparticle-enhanced MRI (LN-MRI) has the sensitivity to detect disease as minute as 1 to 2 mm, surpassing positron emission tomography in the ability to detect small amounts of disease in the lymphatics. LN-MRI has been evaluated to determine adequacy of radiation fields and defined nodal volumes (Figure 16.4) (90). In the future, this or other advanced imaging modalities may play a role in defining targets for individual patients undergoing radiation therapy and ensuring that involved lymphatics receive adequate dose.

■ INTENSITY-MODULATED RADIATION THERAPY

IMRT is the most sophisticated form of three-dimensional photon radiation currently available. IMRT achieves excellent conformity to target volumes while decreasing high dose to specified avoidance structures by delivering radiation with multiple treatment beams that vary in intensity to produce a nonuniform fluency in order to optimize specified constraints determined by the treating physician.

This is in contrast to 3D-CRT, which determines the final plan by manual iteration (i.e., human adjustments). IMRT is generally accomplished by a sophisticated computer planning system that performs hundreds of iterations and determines the best fit for defined constraints (14). As mentioned previously, in order to utilize computer-based or inverse planning, all targets and avoidance structures must be contoured. IMRT has been shown to improve homogeneity for whole breast irradiation and to decrease acute side effects of moist desquamation and skin toxicity in a phase III randomized trial (15,16). IMRT has not yet been universally accepted as the standard of care for whole breast irradiation. This is in large part due to a substantial increase in the cost of treatment with IMRT (17). In time, further benefits may justify increased costs to all parties involved in determining reimbursement, or more appropriate compensation may be agreed on for this less complex IMRT treatment of the breast.

Despite the extensive use of IMRT for breast cancer, its use in clinical trials has been limited mainly to the breast or tumor bed (15,18,19). Treatment of locally advanced cancer requires coverage of the breast or chest wall, or both, and regional lymphatics, including the supraclavicular lymph nodes, axilla (apex or full axilla), and possibly the internal mammary nodes. Multiple 3D-CRT photon techniques exist, but all have some limitations. It may be difficult or impossible to provide homogeneous coverage of the target volume while producing acceptable doses to the heart and lung. The clinical experience with IMRT in this setting is extremely limited, but dosimetric comparisons exist (20–23). One of the major disadvantages of IMRT is the potential increase in integral-dose or low-dose radiation to a larger amount of normal tissue. It is almost certain that the role of IMRT for treatment of the regional lymphatics will be further explored and will play a role in the treatment of locally advanced breast cancer in the coming years. It remains to be seen whether decreased morbidity can be achieved with IMRT to regional lymphatics and whether increased integral dose delivered as a result of IMRT technique will be of consequence.

■ THE USE OF PROTONS BEAMS IN THE TREATMENT OF BREAST CANCER

Proton radiation therapy is a form of particle radiation therapy currently available at only a handful of radiation treatment centers. Mainly due to restricted availability and increased costs, the clinical use of protons has been limited, for the most part, to tumors requiring high doses or in close proximity to critical structures, and children (24–29). Over the past several years, the substantial benefit of this radiation modality has been recognized. Despite substantial capital and operational costs, several proton facilities in both the private and academic sectors are in the planning or construction phases. Given the increased availability and substantial costs of proton therapy, it is important to explore in academic centers the potential benefit for additional malignancies such as breast cancer.

Protons are charged particles that enter tissue and deliver a small and constant dose until near the end of the proton range, where the majority of dose is delivered (30). Beyond this distal portion of the proton beam no dose is delivered. This enables complete sparing of uninvolved tissues and organs distal to the target volume. This is in contrast to photons that must deliver dose both proximal and distal to the region targeted. Proton radiation is prescribed in Gray RBE as opposed to Gray, which is used for prescribing photon radiation. This takes into account the slightly higher relative biological effectiveness (RBE) of protons. Thus, for a given prescribed dose, the biological effect in tissues is the same for protons and photons, and benefits are due to physical properties of the proton beam (31–33).

At his time, the predominant mode of proton delivery is through passive beam scattering methods or three-dimensional conformal proton therapy. Scattering foils, range compensators, and apertures are designed to deliver a homogeneous dose distribution to the target, with optimal dose conformity at the distal target region for each field (30). There is some degree of intensity modulation in these proton plans, but increased modulation is possible through scanning techniques. Plans that use scanning techniques are referred to as intensity-modulated proton therapy (IMPT) plans (34,35). Similar to IMRT, IMPT refers to plans that deliver a homogeneous dose to the target, with the superimposition of individually inhomogeneous fields (36). Although this increases the complexity of the plan, it allows for increased dose-shaping capabilities with optimal conformity not only at the distal region of the target but also to the proximal target edge. IMPT may also facilitate the treatment of fields large enough for comprehensive breast or chest wall treatment.

As mentioned in the previous section on IMRT, homogeneous coverage of targets and optimal sparing of cardiac and pulmonary structures can be a challenge, especially for the treatment of locally advanced breast cancer. Clinical data are not currently available for treatment of comprehensive breast or for regional lymphatic irradiation, but studies evaluating the dosimetry for such case studies have been reported (37,38). Lomax and colleagues reported results of comparative treatment planning using standard photons, IMRT, and IMPT for radiation of the breast and regional nodes for a patient with left-sided breast cancer (37). The IMPT plan provided improved target coverage and dose homogeneity, decreased dose to cardiac and pulmonary structures, and the lowest integral dose to surrounding tissues. Johansson and colleagues also examined the potential benefit of protons for left-sided locally advanced breast cancer (38). This study evaluated two conventional plans (tangents and mixed photon/electron technique), IMRT, and three-dimensional conformal proton treatment plans for 11 patients. The authors used normal tissue complication probabilities (NTCPs) for evaluation of plans (39). Mean calculated NTCP values for cardiac mortality and pneumonitis were substantially lower for the proton plan than for all other plans. Although IMRT reduced the NTCP for the heart, it did not decrease NTCP for radiation pneumonitis in this study. Both conventional and IMRT plans showed increased integral dose compared with the proton plan. In summary, the authors concluded that proton therapy has the potential to offer a major advantage in decreasing the risk of normal tissue complications in the treatment of left-sided node-positive breast cancer. At the Massachusetts General Hospital, we have also analyzed plans for both three-dimensional conformal protons and IMPT for the treatment of patients requiring postmastectomy radiation therapy (PMRT) for left-sided breast cancer. We compared these treatment plans with partially wide tangent fields (PWTFs) and mixed photon/electron technique. Three-dimensional proton plans were superior to PWTF and photon/electron technique. Figure 16.5

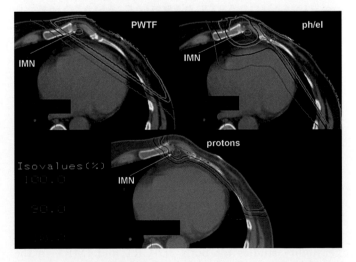

FIGURE 16.5 Axial images at the level of the heart comparing a partially wide tangent technique (PWTF), mixed photon/electron technique, and three-dimensional conformal protons. Protons allow for maximal sparing of the heart and lung with minimal hotspots.

depicts the advantages of three-dimensional proton plans over both of these techniques. IMPT was superior to all other treatment plans for target coverage and sparing of critical structures. Although no clinical experience for this treatment has been reported to date, phase I/II clinical trials to evaluate toxicity and clinical outcomes for patients treated with proton radiation (3D-CRT or IMPT) and for patients requiring left PMRT are likely in the near future. As the number of proton facilities increase, it is likely that additional centers will explore the use of protons for locally advance breast cancer.

Despite lack of clinical data for advanced breast cancer, feasibility studies using protons for PBI have been published. The Massachusetts General Hospital and Loma Linda have both published favorable early outcomes for patients treated with three-dimensional conformal proton PBI. Both institutions concluded that proton PBI provided an external beam technique with the advantages of such (decreased invasiveness, ability to evaluate pathology prior to treatment, decreased technical limitations, and less specialized training). However, proton radiation was superior to photon radiation in its ability to spare uninvolved breast tissue, perceived to be one of the major disadvantages of photon external beam treatment (40–42). Moderate improvements in dose to lung and heart were seen, but this is of unknown clinical significance given the minimal cardiac and pulmonary doses with photon PBI. Proton PBI was found to be best delivered by multiple fields due to increased skin toxicity. However, IMPT, which allows decreased proximal or skin dose, may allow for proton PBI treatments from a single entry point for select patients.

■ ADDITIONAL CARDIAC SPARING TECHNIQUES FOR PATIENTS WITH UNFAVORABLE CARDIAC ANATOMY

A major goal of technological advances such as IMRT and proton therapy is to spare critical structures. However, these modalities are typically costly, and treatment planning to avoid cardiac and pulmonary structures can be time-consuming. Positioning techniques that move cardiac and pulmonary tissues away from the breast tissue or chest wall have been explored and, when feasible and successful, allow a relatively simple and cost-effective method of decreasing radiation dose to critical structures without compromising target coverage. Prone positioning has been examined as one technique capable of providing improved separation between the heart and breast tissue for many patients while decreasing the effects of respiratory motion. Feasibility studies for both 3D-CRT and IMRT in the prone position have been published (18,43–46). There are several commercially available prone breast boards. Patient comfort and reproducibility must be given a great deal of consideration when using this technique. New developments in prone breast radiation are focused on superior patient comfort, along with improved immobilization. Another relatively straightforward maneuver to decrease the volume of heart in the radiation field for left-sided breast cancer is to have patients hold their breath at deep inspiration (47,48). Despite the findings that breath-holding techniques are poorly tolerated during radiation for lung cancer, because most patients with breast cancer do not have pulmonary compromise and radiation delivery for breast cancer is relatively short, breath holding is, overall, well tolerated. Several reports demonstrating feasibility and reduced radiation doses to the heart with deep inspiration have been published (47,49–56). Modalities to ensure reproducibility are available, and more are in development.

■ THE USE OF HYPOFRACTIONATION IN WHOLE BREAST RADIATION

Although the benefit of fractionated radiation has been clear since the early 1900s, the number of fractions necessary to avoid increased complications while providing adequate tumor control is not clear. Fractionated whole breast irradiation followed lumpectomy delivered in approximately 25 to 28 fractions generally, with an additional 5 to 8 fractions of treatment to the primary tumor site, has proven a successful and well-tolerated regimen and has remained the accepted standard for decades (57–59). One negative aspect is that the time required for a course of whole breast irradiation ranges from six to seven weeks. It has been suggested that many patients choose mastectomy over breast conservation due to an inability to travel to a radiation center for several weeks of treatment, and decreased rates of adjuvant radiation have been reported for the elderly and those with multiple comorbidities (60–62). In addition, in vitro studies for breast adenocarcinoma suggest that an α/β value of 4 Gy may be more appropriate than the more common tumor value of 10 Gy (63–65). This suggests that biologically hypofractionation may allow for equivalent, or even superior, tumor control. Several phase I/II studies show feasibility with excellent local control and little toxicity for whole breast hypofractionated treatments (44,46,66). In addition, multiple randomized trials from the United Kingdom and Canada supporting hypofractionated whole breast irradiation have recently been published (67–71). These trials compared standard fractionation (50 Gy in 25 fractions) with delivery of radiation therapy in 13 to 16 fractions and demonstrated equivalent local recurrence, cosmesis, and toxicities. We should note that the Canadian study included only patients with negative lymph nodes, only 11% received adjuvant chemotherapy, patients with separation larger than 25 cm were excluded, and boost was not utilized in this study. The 12-year follow-up data have been presented (T. Whelan, personal communication) and show that both arms are equivalent on cosmetic results, local control, disease-free survival, and overall survival. The British studies included patients with negative lymph nodes and have only five years of follow-up. The results are encouraging (70–71). Further research is still needed to determine whether a boost to the tumor bed can be safely incorporated into a hypofractionated regimen following radiation or concurrently with whole breast irradiation, but the low rate of acute toxicity and favorable early outcomes reported in phase I/II studies are encouraging (44,46). The RTOG plans for a randomized trial to compare standard fractionation and hypofractionated whole breast radiation with a concurrent boost to the tumor bed (F. Vicini, personal communication). Additional studies are ongoing to determine whether radiation can be hypofractionated further to allow for a still shorter course of treatment. Although at this time "standard" whole breast irradiation, at least in the United States, is considered delivery of radiation at 1.8 to 2.0 Gy per fraction, sufficient data exist to support hypofractionation, and this standard is likely to change for many patients over the coming years.

ACCELERATED PARTIAL BREAST IRRADIATION FOR SELECTED PATIENTS WITH EARLY BREAST CANCER

Perhaps the most extreme example of hypofractionation for breast cancer is accelerated partial breast irradiation (APBI). For APBI, the breast volume targeted for treatment includes the surgical cavity and 1.5 to 2 cm margins; the dose per fraction can then increase from 1.8 to 2 Gy to 3.4 to 5 Gy, the total dose can be reduced from 60 Gy to 30 to 40 Gy, and the overall treatment time can be reduced from six to seven weeks to one to two weeks. Highly conformal techniques should be used to avoid toxicity.

The hypothesis that APBI may offer control equivalent to whole breast irradiation comes from the observation that the vast majority of in-breast recurrences occur either within or in close proximity to the tumor bed (72). Several randomized trials comparing local excision alone with excision followed by radiation report that most recurrences in nonirradiated patients occur in the region of the resection cavity (58,73–76). Some studies have demonstrated that the risk of recurrence outside the region of the tumor bed is similar to the risk of developing a contralateral breast cancer (58,72,77–79). These observations suggest that the benefit of whole breast irradiation is derived mainly from the delivery of radiation to the breast tissue in the region of the tumor bed. Decreasing the volume of the breast and other healthy tissues in the radiation field may make radiation in a single fraction or over one week feasible, making radiation treatment more accessible and less tedious for many patients (61,62,80–84).

Several approaches exist for the administration of APBI. These delivery systems include interstitial brachytherapy, the MammoSite balloon catheter system, external beam radiation, and intraoperative radiation. Each of these methods has certain advantages and disadvantages. Physician and patient preference play a major role in determining the modality of choice in each case or setting; as data and experience increase, tumor characteristics play an increasing role. The current National Surgical Adjuvant Breast and Bowel Project (NSABP)/RTOG trial has shown external beam techniques to be chosen most often (F. Vicini, personal communication). Figure 16.6 depicts an example of an external beam APBI plan.

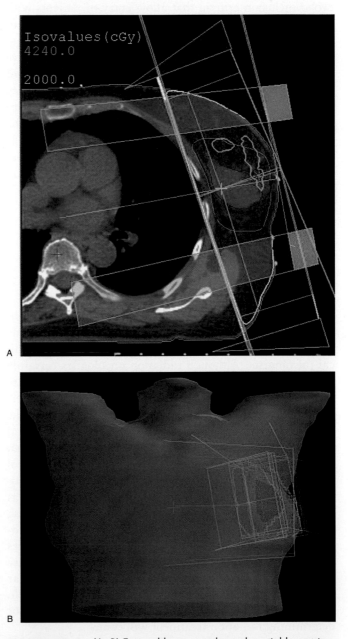

FIGURE 16.6 (A, B) External beam accelerated partial breast irradiation using a mixed photon/electron technique prescribing a dose of 40 Gy to the lumpectomy cavity plus a margin.

At this time, APBI is considered an experimental therapy and should be administered only on a clinical trial. It is clear that APBI is more convenient for patients, to such an extent that it is predicted more patients will choose breast conservation if APBI is an option. In addition, it is more desirable to avoid normal tissues, including heart, lung, ribs, and uninvolved breast tissue. However, it is not anticipated that APBI will improve upon the exceptional rates of local control provided by whole breast irradiation (85). If outcomes can be maintained while patients are treated more efficiently, APBI will likely become the standard of care for select patients in the future. At this time, the NSABP B-39/RTOG 0413 phase III randomized, controlled trial continues to accrue patients. This study has broad inclusion criteria that allow entry of patients with stage 0 to 2 breast cancer, with tumors measuring up to 3 cm, and with 0 to 3 positive lymph nodes. While accrual has been completed for older patients with node-negative disease, the trial continues to accrue patients younger than 50 years of age and those with less favorable primary tumor characteristics or node-positive disease. In years to come, this trial should provide an answer regarding the potential to replace whole breast irradiation with APBI for at least a subset of patients. However, long follow-up is required, and definitive results of this trial are years away.

■ THE USE OF MOLECULAR PROFILES AND TUMOR RECEPTORS FOR RADIATION PLANNING

Over the past decade, the predictive and prognostic implications of molecular profiles in breast cancer have become increasingly valued in clinical decision making for medical oncologists. Although radiation oncologists certainly consider receptor status and genomic profiles, they are rarely utilized to guide recommendations for local therapy. Retrospective analyses are beginning to surface in the literature, some showing profiles to be predictive of local outcomes and others showing no association between receptor status (estrogen, progesterone, and HER2/neu) and local recurrence (86–89). The utility of receptor profiles and commercially available multigene assays such as Onco*type* DX and MammoPrint for decisions regarding radiation management is currently unclear. Modern prospective trials are needed, and the use of these profiles for radiation recommendations and the appropriate use of these tests may take years to be recognized. Molecular profiles do, however, represent an area of active research, and in all likelihood the use of molecular profiles for determining radiation treatment will come.

■ THE VALUE OF THE MULTIDISCIPLINARY APPROACH

Breast cancer is a disease that routinely involves therapy from multiple disciplines and also one in which a patient's choice regarding one form of management may affect other therapies. Surgical management often alters the need for irradiation. Radiation therapy may alter breast reconstruction recommendations and options. Chemotherapy may alter the type of surgery feasible or the timing of surgery or radiation. There is often more than one option for a patient with newly diagnosed breast cancer. Treatment decisions can be difficult, and it is valuable for the patient to discuss therapy with potentially involved disciplines at diagnosis. It is also important for there to be good communication between physicians regarding an individual's management. The optimal management for patients with breast cancer and their education and confidence in the choices they make is made possible through a multidisciplinary approach. Multidisciplinary clinics and conferences are available at many hospitals and institutions. In our opinion, the multidisciplinary approach provides a means to determine a cohesive and clear set of recommendations and treatment options for the patient and facilitates optimal care for each individual with breast cancer.

■ CONCLUSIONS

While it is clear that we have made tremendous progress over the past century, further improvements, both anticipated and beyond our imagination, are sure to occur over the next century. Technical innovations in radiology and radiation oncology will allow for better avoidance of normal healthy tissues while ensuring adequate delivery of radiation to all areas of disease. More convenient treatment schedules are already surfacing in practice, and shorter radiation courses may become the standard of care over the next few years. Molecular profiles that currently dictate chemotherapeutic regimens and indicate which patients may have more biologically aggressive disease are likely to play a larger role in determining which patients may benefit from radiation therapy and for which patients radiation can be omitted. Continued improvements in systemic therapy may allow us to avoid radiation therapy in some patients, while adding to the benefit for others in whom local control becomes of increased importance due to eradication of systemic metastatic disease. It is certain that these developments, along with advances in the cancer disciplines of surgery and medicine, will allow for increased survival as well as an improvement in the quality of life for our patients.

■ KEY POINTS

- Advances in the field of radiology have been adapted to provide improved treatment planning.
- Hypofractionated regimens may increase convenience of radiation for selected patients in the future.
- Technical innovations may allow for better sparing of cardiac and pulmonary tissues.
- Molecular advances widely used to determine systemic treatment may affect radiation recommendations in the future.

■ REFERENCES

1. Keynes G. The place of radium in the treatment of cancer of the breast. *Ann Surg.* 1937;106:619–630.
2. Béclère A. Une note sur la radiotherapie des neoplasms du sein. *Bull et Mem Doc Nat de Chir.* 1904;30:996–1003.
3. Fisher B, Jeong JH, Anderson S, Bryant J, Fisher ER, Wolmark N. Twenty-five-year follow-up of a randomized trial comparing radical mastectomy, total mastectomy, and total mastectomy followed by irradiation. *New Engl J Med.* 2002;347:567–575.
4. Veronesi U, Cascinelli N, Mariani L, et al. Twenty-year follow-up of a randomized study comparing breast-conserving surgery with radical mastectomy for early breast cancer. *New Engl J Med.* 2002; 347:1227–1232.
5. Overgaard M, Hansen PS, Overgaard J, et al. Postoperative radiotherapy in high-risk premenopausal women with breast cancer who receive adjuvant chemotherapy. Danish Breast Cancer Cooperative Group 82b trial. *New Engl J Med.* 1997;337:949–955.
6. Overgaard M, Jensen MB, Overgaard J, et al. Postoperative radiotherapy in high-risk postmenopausal breast-cancer patients given adjuvant tamoxifen: Danish Breast Cancer Cooperative Group DBCG 82c randomised trial. *Lancet.* 1999;353:1641–1648.
7. Ragaz J, Olivotto IA, Spinelli JJ, et al. Locoregional radiation therapy in patients with high-risk breast cancer receiving adjuvant chemotherapy: 20-year results of the British Columbia randomized trial. *J Natl Cancer Inst.* 2005;97:116–126.
8. Li XA, Tai A, Arthur DW, et al. Variability of target and normal structure delineation for breast cancer radiotherapy: an RTOG multi-institutional and multiobserver study. *Int J Radiat Oncol Biol Phys.* 2009;73:944–951.
9. White J, Buchholz T, MacDonald S, et al. Breast cancer atlas for radiation planning; consensus definitions; Radiation Therapy Oncology Group (RTOG). Available at www.rtog.org/pdf_file2. html?pdf_document=BreastCancerAtlas.pdf.
10. Galper S, Recht A, Silver B, et al. Is radiation alone adequate treatment to the axilla for patients with limited axillary surgery? Implications for treatment after a positive sentinel node biopsy. *Int J Radiat Oncol Biol Phys.* 2000;48:125–132.
11. Hurkmans CW, Borger JH, Rutgers EJ, van Tienhoven G. Quality assurance of axillary radiotherapy in the EORTC AMAROS trial 10981/22023: the dummy run. *Radiother Oncol.* 2003; 68:233–240.
12. Harada T, Tanigawa N, Matsuki M, Nohara T, Narabayashi I. Evaluation of lymph node metastases of breast cancer using ultrasmall superparamagnetic iron oxide-enhanced magnetic resonance imaging. *Eur J Radiol.* 2007.
13. Memarsadeghi M, Riedl CC, Kaneider A, et al. Axillary lymph node metastases in patients with breast carcinomas: assessment with nonenhanced versus USPIO-enhanced MR imaging. *Radiology.* 2006;241:367–377.
14. Kahan FM. *The Physics of Radiation Therapy.* 3rd ed. Philadelphia: Lippincott Williams & Wilkins; 2003.
15. Pignol JP, Olivotto I, Rakovitch E, et al. A multicenter randomized trial of breast intensity-modulated radiation therapy to reduce acute radiation dermatitis. *J Clin Oncol.* 2008;26:2085–2092.
16. Donovan E, Bleakley N, Denholm E, et al. Randomised trial of standard 2D radiotherapy (RT) versus intensity modulated radiotherapy (IMRT) in patients prescribed breast radiotherapy. *Radiother Oncol.* 2007;82:254–264.
17. Haffty BG, Buchholz TA, McCormick B. Should intensity-modulated radiation therapy be the standard of care in the conservatively managed breast cancer patient? *J Clin Oncol.* 2008; 26:2072–2074.
18. Croog VJ, Wu AJ, McCormick B, Beal KP. Accelerated whole breast irradiation with intensity-modulated radiotherapy to the prone breast. *Int J Radiat Oncol Biol Phys.* 2008.
19. Vicini FA, Sharpe M, Kestin L, et al. Optimizing breast cancer treatment efficacy with intensity-modulated radiotherapy. *Int J Radiat Oncol Biol Phys.* 2002;54:1336–1344.
20. Caudrelier JM, Morgan SC, Montgomery L, Lacelle M, Nyiri B, Macpherson M. Helical tomotherapy for locoregional irradiation including the internal mammary chain in left-sided breast cancer: dosimetric evaluation. *Radiother Oncol.* 2009;90:99–105.
21. Krueger EA, Fraass BA, McShan DL, Marsh R, Pierce LJ. Potential gains for irradiation of chest wall and regional nodes with intensity modulated radiotherapy. *Int J Radiat Oncol Biol Phys.* 2003;56:1023–1037.
22. Krueger EA, Fraass BA, Pierce LJ. Clinical aspects of intensity-modulated radiotherapy in the treatment of breast cancer. *Semin Radiat Oncol.* 2002;12:250–259.
23. Dogan N, Cuttino L, Lloyd R, Bump EA, Arthur DW. Optimized dose coverage of regional lymph nodes in breast cancer: the role of intensity-modulated radiotherapy. *Int J Radiat Oncol Biol Phys.* 2007;68:1238–1250.
24. MacDonald SM, Safai S, Trofimov A, et al. Proton radiotherapy for childhood ependymoma: initial clinical outcomes and dose comparisons. *Int J Radiat Oncol Biol Phys.* 2008;71:979–986.
25. Yock T, Schneider R, Friedmann A, Adams J, Fullerton B, Tarbell N. Proton radiotherapy for orbital rhabdomyosarcoma: clinical outcome and a dosimetric comparison with photons. *Int J Radiat Oncol Biol Phys.* 2005;63:1161–1168.
26. DeLaney TF, Trofimov AV, Engelsman M, Suit HD. Advanced-technology radiation therapy in the management of bone and soft tissue sarcomas. *Cancer Control.* 2005;12:27–35.
27. Gragoudas ES, Marie Lane A. Uveal melanoma: proton beam irradiation. *Ophthalmol Clin North Am.* 2005;18:111–118, ix.
28. Hug EB, Muenter MW, Archambeau JO, et al. Conformal proton radiation therapy for pediatric low-grade astrocytomas. *Strahlenther Onkol.* 2002;178:10–17.
29. Hug EB, Sweeney RA, Nurre PM, Holloway KC, Slater JD, Munzenrider JE. Proton radiotherapy in management of pediatric base of skull tumors. *Int J Radiat Oncol Biol Phys.* 2002;52: 1017–1024.
30. Bussiere MR, Adams JA. Treatment planning for conformal proton radiation therapy. *Technol Cancer Res Treat.* 2003;2:389–399.
31. Hall EJ. *Radiobiology for the Radiologist.* 5th ed. Philadelphia: Lippincott Williams & Wilkins; 2000.
32. Paganetti H, Niemierko A, Ancukiewicz M, et al. Relative biological effectiveness (RBE) values for proton beam therapy. *Int J Radiat Oncol Biol Phys.* 2002;53:407–421.
33. Mason KA, Gillin MT, Mohan R, Cox JD. Preclinical biologic assessment of proton beam relative biologic effectiveness at Proton Therapy Center Houston. *Int J Radiat Oncol Biol Phys.* 2007;68:968–970.

34. Oelfke U, Bortfeld T. Intensity modulated radiotherapy with charged particle beams: studies of inverse treatment planning for rotation therapy. *Med Phys.* 2000;27:1246–1257.

35. Oelfke U, Bortfeld T. Inverse planning for photon and proton beams. *Med Dosim.* 2001;26:113–124.

36. Lomax AJ, Boehringer T, Coray A, et al. Intensity modulated proton therapy: a clinical example. *Med Phys.* 2001;28:317–324.

37. Lomax AJ, Cella L, Weber D, Kurtz JM, Miralbell R. Potential role of intensity-modulated photons and protons in the treatment of the breast and regional nodes. *Int J Radiat Oncol Biol Phys.* 2003;55:785–792.

38. Johansson J, Isacsson U, Lindman H, Montelius A, Glimelius B. Node-positive left-sided breast cancer patients after breast-conserving surgery: potential outcomes of radiotherapy modalities and techniques. *Radiother Oncol.* 2002;65:89–98.

39. Kallman P, Agren A, Brahme A. Tumour and normal tissue responses to fractionated non-uniform dose delivery. *Int J Radiat Biol.* 1992;62:249–262.

40. Kozak KR, Doppke KP, Katz A, Taghian AG. Dosimetric comparison of two different three-dimensional conformal external beam accelerated partial breast irradiation techniques. *Int J Radiat Oncol Biol Phys.* 2006;65:340–346.

41. Formenti SC, Truong MT, Goldberg JD, et al. Prone accelerated partial breast irradiation after breast-conserving surgery: preliminary clinical results and dose-volume histogram analysis. *Int J Radiat Oncol Biol Phys.* 2004;60:493–504.

42. Vicini F, Winter K, Straube W, et al. A phase I/II trial to evaluate three-dimensional conformal radiation therapy confined to the region of the lumpectomy cavity for Stage I/II breast carcinoma: initial report of feasibility and reproducibility of Radiation Therapy Oncology Group (RTOG) study 0319. *Int J Radiat Oncol Biol Phys.* 2005;63:1531–1537.

43. DeWyngaert JK, Jozsef G, Mitchell J, Rosenstein B, Formenti SC. Accelerated intensity-modulated radiotherapy to breast in prone position: dosimetric results. *Int J Radiat Oncol Biol Phys.* 2007;68:1251–1259.

44. Formenti SC, Gidea-Addeo D, Goldberg JD, et al. Phase I-II trial of prone accelerated intensity modulated radiation therapy to the breast to optimally spare normal tissue. *J Clin Oncol.* 2007;25: 2236–2242.

45. Stegman LD, Beal KP, Hunt MA, Fornier MN, McCormick B. Long-term clinical outcomes of whole-breast irradiation delivered in the prone position. *Int J Radiat Oncol Biol Phys.* 2007;68: 73–81.

46. Freedman GM, Anderson PR, Goldstein LJ, et al. Four-week course of radiation for breast cancer using hypofractionated intensity modulated radiation therapy with an incorporated boost. *Int J Radiat Oncol Biol Phys.* 2007;68:347–353.

47. Jagsi R, Moran JM, Kessler ML, Marsh RB, Balter JM, Pierce LJ. Respiratory motion of the heart and positional reproducibility under active breathing control. *Int J Radiat Oncol Biol Phys.* 2007;68:253–258.

48. Moran JM, Balter JM, Ben-David MA, Marsh RB, Van Herk M, Pierce LJ. Short-term displacement and reproducibility of the breast and nodal targets under active breathing control. *Int J Radiat Oncol Biol Phys.* 2007;68:541–546.

49. Korreman SS, Pedersen AN, Aarup LR, Nottrup TJ, Specht L, Nystrom H. Reduction of cardiac and pulmonary complication probabilities after breathing adapted radiotherapy for breast cancer. *Int J Radiat Oncol Biol Phys.* 2006;65:1375–1380.

50. Korreman SS, Pedersen AN, Josipovic M, et al. Cardiac and pulmonary complication probabilities for breast cancer patients after routine end-inspiration gated radiotherapy. *Radiother Oncol.* 2006;80:257–262.

51. Korreman SS, Pedersen AN, Nottrup TJ, Specht L, Nystrom H. Breathing adapted radiotherapy for breast cancer: comparison of free breathing gating with the breath-hold technique. *Radiother Oncol.* 2005;76:311–318.

52. Chen MH, Cash EP, Danias PG, et al. Respiratory maneuvers decrease irradiated cardiac volume in patients with left-sided breast cancer. *J Cardiovasc Magn Reson.* 2002;4:265–271.

53. Lu HM, Cash E, Chen MH, et al. Reduction of cardiac volume in left-breast treatment fields by respiratory maneuvers: a CT study. *Int J Radiat Oncol Biol Phys.* 2000;47:895–904.

54. Remouchamps VM, Letts N, Vicini FA, et al. Initial clinical experience with moderate deep-inspiration breath hold using an active breathing control device in the treatment of patients with left-sided breast cancer using external beam radiation therapy. *Int J Radiat Oncol Biol Phys.* 2003;56:704–715.

55. Remouchamps VM, Vicini FA, Sharpe MB, Kestin LL, Martinez AA, Wong JW. Significant reductions in heart and lung doses using deep inspiration breath hold with active breathing control and intensity-modulated radiation therapy for patients treated with locoregional breast irradiation. *Int J Radiat Oncol Biol Phys.* 2003;55:392–406.

56. Sixel KE, Aznar MC, Ung YC. Deep inspiration breath hold to reduce irradiated heart volume in breast cancer patients. *Int J Radiat Oncol Biol Phys.* 2001;49:199–204.

57. Fisher B, Anderson S, Bryant J, et al. Twenty-year follow-up of a randomized trial comparing total mastectomy, lumpectomy, and lumpectomy plus irradiation for the treatment of invasive breast cancer. *New Engl J Med.* 2002;347:1233–1241.

58. Veronesi U, Cascinelli N, Mariani L, et al. Twenty-year follow-up of a randomized study comparing breast-conserving surgery with radical mastectomy for early breast cancer. *New Engl J Med.* 2002;347:1227–1232.

59. Arriagada R, Le MG, Rochard F, Contesso G. Conservative treatment versus mastectomy in early breast cancer: patterns of failure with 15 years of follow-up data. Institut Gustave-Roussy Breast Cancer Group. *J Clin Oncol.* 1996;14:1558–1564.

60. Schroen AT, Brenin DR, Kelly MD, Knaus WA, Slingluff CL Jr. Impact of patient distance to radiation therapy on mastectomy use in early-stage breast cancer patients. *J Clin Oncol.* 2005; 23:7074–7080.

61. Buchholz TA, Theriault RL, Niland JC, et al. The use of radiation as a component of breast conservation therapy in National Comprehensive Cancer Network Centers. *J Clin Oncol.* 2006;24: 361–369.

62. Truong PT, Wong E, Bernstein V, Berthelet E, Kader HA. Adjuvant radiation therapy after breast-conserving surgery in elderly women with early-stage breast cancer: controversy or consensus? *Clin Breast Cancer.* 2004;4:407–414.

63. Williams MV, Denekamp J, Fowler JF. A review of alpha/beta ratios for experimental tumors: implications for clinical studies of altered fractionation. *Int J Radiat Oncol Biol Phys.* 1985; 11:87–96.

64. Yamada Y, Ackerman I, Franssen E, MacKenzie RG, Thomas G. Does the dose fractionation schedule influence local control of adjuvant radiotherapy for early stage breast cancer? *Int J Radiat Oncol Biol Phys.* 1999;44:99–104.

65. Matthews JH, Meeker BE, Chapman JD. Response of human tumor cell lines in vitro to fractionated irradiation. *Int J Radiat Oncol Biol Phys.* 1989;16:133–138.

66. Livi L, Stefanacci M, Scocciant S, et al. Adjuvant hypofractionated radiation therapy for breast cancer after conserving surgery. *Clin Oncol (R Coll Radiol).* 2007;19:120–124.

67. Whelan T, MacKenzie R, Julian J, et al. Randomized trial of breast irradiation schedules after lumpectomy for women with lymph node-negative breast cancer. *J Natl Cancer Inst.* 2002; 94:1143–1150.

68. Bentzen SM, Agrawal RK, Aird EG, et al. The UK Standardisation of Breast Radiotherapy (START) Trial B of radiotherapy hypofractionation for treatment of early breast cancer: a randomised trial. *Lancet.* 2008;371:1098–1107.

69. Bentzen SM, Agrawal RK, Aird EG, et al. The UK Standardisation of Breast Radiotherapy (START) Trial A of radiotherapy

hypofractionation for treatment of early breast cancer: a randomised trial. *Lancet Oncol.* 2008;9:331–341.

70. Owen JR, Ashton A, Bliss JM, et al. Effect of radiotherapy fraction size on tumour control in patients with early-stage breast cancer after local tumour excision: long-term results of a randomised trial. *Lancet Oncol.* 2006;7:467–471.

71. Yarnold J, Ashton A, Bliss J, et al. Fractionation sensitivity and dose response of late adverse effects in the breast after radiotherapy for early breast cancer: long-term results of a randomised trial. *Radiother Oncol.* 2005;75:9–17.

72. Smith TE, Lee D, Turner BC, Carter D, Haffty BG. True recurrence vs. new primary ipsilateral breast tumor relapse: an analysis of clinical and pathologic differences and their implications in natural history, prognoses, and therapeutic management. *Int J Radiat Oncol Biol Phys.* 2000;48:1281–1289.

73. Fisher B, Anderson S, Bryant J, et al. Twenty-year follow-up of a randomized trial comparing total mastectomy, lumpectomy, and lumpectomy plus irradiation for the treatment of invasive breast cancer. *New Engl J Med.* 2002;347:1233–1241.

74. Clark RM, Whelan T, Levine M, et al. Randomized clinical trial of breast irradiation following lumpectomy and axillary dissection for node-negative breast cancer: an update. Ontario Clinical Oncology Group. *J Natl Cancer Inst.* 1996;88:1659–1664.

75. Holli K, Saaristo R, Isola J, Joensuu H, Hakama M. Lumpectomy with or without postoperative radiotherapy for breast cancer with favourable prognostic features: results of a randomized study. *Br J Cancer.* 2001;84:164–169.

76. Liljegren G, Holmberg L, Bergh J, et al. 10-year results after sector resection with or without postoperative radiotherapy for stage I breast cancer: a randomized trial. *J Clin Oncol.* 1999;17:2326–2333.

77. Fisher ER, Costantino J, Fisher B, et al. Pathologic findings from the National Surgical Adjuvant Breast Project (NSABP) Protocol B-17. Five-year observations concerning lobular carcinoma in situ. *Cancer.* 1996;78:1403–1416.

78. Arthur DW, Vicini FA. Accelerated partial breast irradiation as a part of breast conservation therapy. *J Clin Oncol.* 2005;23:1726–1735.

79. Fisher ER, Dignam J, Tan-Chiu E, et al. Pathologic findings from the National Surgical Adjuvant Breast Project (NSABP) eight-year update of protocol B-17: intraductal carcinoma. *Cancer.* 1999;86:429–438.

80. Schroen AT, Brenin DR, Kelly MD, Knaus WA, Slingluff CL, Jr. Impact of patient distance to radiation therapy on mastectomy use in early-stage breast cancer patients. *J Clin Oncol.* 2005;23:7074–7080.

81. Rutqvist LE, Lax I, Fornander T, Johansson H. Cardiovascular mortality in a randomized trial of adjuvant radiation therapy versus surgery alone in primary breast cancer. *Int J Radiat Oncol Biol Phys.* 1992;22:887–896.

82. Gagliardi G, Lax I, Ottolenghi A, Rutqvist LE. Long-term cardiac mortality after radiotherapy of breast cancer—application of the relative seriality model. *Br J Radiol.* 1996;69:839–846.

83. Rutqvist LE, Johansson H. Mortality by laterality of the primary tumour among 55,000 breast cancer patients from the Swedish Cancer Registry. *Br J Cancer.* 1990;61:866–868.

84. Hiatt JR, Evans SB, Price LL, Cardarelli GA, Dipetrillo TA, Wazer DE. Dose-modeling study to compare external beam techniques from protocol NSABP B-39/RTOG 0413 for patients with highly unfavorable cardiac anatomy. *Int J Radiat Oncol Biol Phys.* 2006;65:1368–1374.

85. Prosnitz LR, Marks LB. Partial breast irradiation: a cautionary note. *Int J Radiat Oncol Biol Phys.* 2006;65:319–321.

86. Nguyen PL, Taghian AG, Katz MS, et al. Breast cancer subtype approximated by estrogen receptor, progesterone receptor, and HER-2 is associated with local and distant recurrence after breast-conserving therapy. *J Clin Oncol.* 2008;26:2373–2378.

87. Haffty BG, Yang Q, Reiss M, et al. Locoregional relapse and distant metastasis in conservatively managed triple negative early-stage breast cancer. *J Clin Oncol.* 2006;24:5652–5657.

88. Cheng SH, Horng CF, West M, et al. Genomic prediction of locoregional recurrence after mastectomy in breast cancer. *J Clin Oncol.* 2006;24:4594–4602.

89. Kyndi M, Sorensen FB, Knudsen H, Overgaard M, Nielsen HM, Overgaard J. Estrogen receptor, progesterone receptor, HER-2, and response to postmastectomy radiotherapy in high-risk breast cancer: the Danish Breast Cancer Cooperative Group. *J Clin Oncol.* 2008;26:1419–1426.

90. Macdonald SM, Harisinghani MG, Katkar A, et al. Nanoparticle-enhanced MRI to evaluate radiation delivery to the regional lymphatics for patients with breast cancer. *Int J Radiat Oncol Biol Phys.* 2009; in press.

Hormonal Therapy in the Treatment of Breast Cancer

KATHRIN STRASSER-WEIPPL

PAUL E. GOSS

For many years, postmenopausal women with endocrine-responsive breast cancer have been treated with 5 years of adjuvant tamoxifen (1–4). On the basis that the majority of patients experiencing a relapse do so after 5 years, longer durations of endocrine therapy have been and are being evaluated. However, on the basis of currently available data, the use of tamoxifen beyond 5 years is of minimal, if any, additional benefit and substantially increases toxicity (5,6). Inhibiting estrogen synthesis with aromatase inhibitors (AIs) demonstrated superiority over 5 years of tamoxifen—in terms of reducing recurrence risk—in several clinical trial settings, including as an alternative to tamoxifen or in sequence with it (3,7–9). This chapter reviews the benefits of extended adjuvant AI therapy in reducing the risk of late recurrences of breast cancer in postmenopausal women and discusses recent analyses of late extended adjuvant AI therapy, in which treatment was started years after completing 5 years of tamoxifen. Current trials evaluating the optimal duration of AI therapy and a trial confirming the value of late extended therapy following at least 1 year off any prior adjuvant endocrine therapy are reviewed in this chapter.

■ LATE RECURRENCE RISK AND THE NEED FOR EXTENDED ADJUVANT THERAPY

The substantial risk of breast cancer recurrence up to 15 years following diagnosis and primary treatment is well established (2,10). Results from the Early Breast Cancer Trialists' Collaborative Group (EBCTCG) showed that more than half of breast cancer recurrences and two thirds of breast cancer deaths occur beyond the initial 5 years of tamoxifen (2). Notably, distant metastases are the most common type of late recurrence (11,12). Among 1,086 patients from the British Columbia Breast Cancer Outcomes database, 159 patients (15%) developed a breast cancer event between 5 and 10 years following initial presentation, 53% of whom had distant metastases (11).

On the basis of data from 10 adjuvant breast cancer trials conducted by the Eastern Cooperative Oncology Group in estrogen receptor–positive (ER+) breast cancer patients, the annual rate of recurrence in ER+ breast cancer

patients is substantial in the later years, at 4.3% per year between years 5 and 12 postoperatively, and after year 4 it is also higher than that of ER– breast cancer (10). Among ER+ patients not receiving adjuvant therapy, breast cancer demonstrates a continuous recurrence rate over 15 or more years (10,13). The ongoing EBCTCG meta-analysis reports that in ER+ patients, 5 years of tamoxifen reduces recurrence and contralateral breast cancer by approximately 41% and breast cancer mortality by 34% (2). The EBCTCG established that among patients completing a full 5-year course of adjuvant tamoxifen, the risk of breast cancer relapse continues during years 5 to 15 following surgery, without any indication of a decrease (2,14).

■ EXTENDED ADJUVANT THERAPY USING TAMOXIFEN

On the basis of the ongoing recurrence risk for patients with ER+ breast cancer, the use of tamoxifen beyond 5 years was tested in the National Surgical Adjuvant Breast and Bowel Project (NSABP) B-14 trial. This study showed that more than 5 years of tamoxifen is not associated with any further benefit and is associated with an increased risk of stroke, endometrial cancer, and pulmonary embolism (5). Similar results were seen in another study, which showed that the annual rate of relapse after 5 years of tamoxifen was similar in both the long- and short-term tamoxifen groups, suggesting that there is no benefit in receiving tamoxifen for more than 5 years (15). The first analysis of the Adjuvant Tamoxifen Longer Against Shorter (ATLAS) trial presented at the December 2007 San Antonio Breast Cancer Symposium shows a small improvement with ongoing tamoxifen, but no safety information was provided (6). Of note, a substantial increased cumulative toxicity, especially for serious life-threatening events (i.e., venous thromboembolism, endometrial cancer), has been reported in several trials that were investigating the use of tamoxifen for more than five years (5,16). The adjuvant Tamoxifen Treatment offer more (aTTom) trial will provide additional evidence as to the potential efficacy of longer durations of tamoxifen (17). Currently, its use beyond 5 years is not routinely recommended (5,18).

■ THE LANDMARK MA.17 TRIAL

The randomized, double-blind, placebo-controlled National Cancer Institute of Canada Clinical Trials Group (NCIC

CTG) trial (NCIC MA.17) was designed to test the effectiveness of 5 years of letrozole daily in postmenopausal women with primary breast cancer who had completed 4½ to 6 years of tamoxifen before randomization. A planned interim analysis was conducted when 171 recurrences (events) occurred (19). Analysis at 2.4 years (207 events) showed a highly significant improvement in the estimated 4-year disease-free survival (DFS) for letrozole-treated patients (93% with letrozole versus 87% for placebo). Extended adjuvant letrozole offered a 43% reduction in recurrence risk [75 with letrozole versus 132 with placebo; hazard ratio (HR) 0.57, 95% confidence interval (CI) 0.43 to 0.75, $P \leq 0.00008$] (19,20). Because of this strong treatment effect, early unblinding of the study was recommended by the data and safety monitoring committee (19). On the basis of these impressive initial results from the MA.17 trial, extended adjuvant letrozole represents a new paradigm for breast cancer treatment. With letrozole, postmenopausal, hormone receptor–positive women now have the opportunity to effectively reduce their risk of late recurrence without the risk of life-threatening side effects associated with tamoxifen (19). Updated trial findings at a median follow-up of 30 months revealed a continued significant reduction in recurrence risk of 42% ($P < 0.001$) with letrozole, a significant 40% improvement in distant DFS (DDFS) ($P = 0.002$), and a significant survival advantage in patients with node-positive disease (HR, 0.61, $P = 0.04$), supporting the initial decision to unblind the trial (Table 16.1) (21,22). A more recent analysis supported the conclusion of the safety monitoring committee to unmask MA.17 early. This analysis showed support for the initial decision to release the interim analysis results and to allow patients on placebo to cross over to letrozole; patients who went on letrozole after placebo had a significantly lower risk of recurrence than those who declined placebo (DFS: HR 0.37, $P < 0.0001$; DDFS: HR 0.38, $P = 0.004$; contralateral breast cancer: HR 0.18, $P < 0.0001$) (19,20,23).

The benefits of extended adjuvant therapy were further confirmed in two trials, one using anastrozole and the other using exemestane (24,25). In the NSABP B-33 trial, extended adjuvant exemestane compared with placebo was investigated in patients who were disease-free after 5 years of tamoxifen (24). This trial was unblinded after enrollment of about half (N = 1,598) of the planned 3,000 patients following the results of NCIC MA.17 in 2003. At the time of unblinding, the NSABP B-33 study found a significant improvement in relapse-free survival (RFS), which included local, regional, distant, and opposite breast recurrence, after 30 months (96% versus 94%, $P = 0.03$) and, although not reaching statistical significance, a trend toward improvement in DFS, which additionally included second primary nonbreast cancer and death (91% versus 89%, $P = 0.07$) or in DDFS (HR 0.69, $P = 0.13$) (24).

The Austrian Breast and Colorectal Cancer Study Group (ABCSG) compared anastrozole (n = 387) with placebo (n = 469) at 5 years of follow-up. While this small open-label trial (N = 856) displayed unbalanced treatment arms, significantly fewer patients in the anastrozole group experienced disease recurrence compared with the placebo group (30 versus 56 patients; HR 0.64, $P = 0.047$) (25). These trials, while not as robust as MA.17, lend further support to the use of AIs in the extended adjuvant setting, with letrozole remaining the only AI with this indication approved by regulatory authorities.

MA.17: Safety and Quality of Life

The AIs have a safety profile different from that of tamoxifen, in that they are not associated with increased risk of rare serious life-threatening adverse events such as thromboembolism or uterine cancer (1,3,5,8,9). MA.17 was the only large blinded trial of an AI in which not only self-reported side effects but also their impact on quality of life (QoL) was evaluated against a placebo (19,21,26). Important to the interpretation of toxicity and QoL data from MA.17 is that patients were selected on the basis of having been able to complete 5 years of prior tamoxifen.

■ **Table 16.1** MA.17 updated efficacy analysis				
	Intent-to-Treat (All Patients)		**Node-Positive**	
Outcome	Hazard Ratio[a]	P Value	Hazard Ratio[b]	P Value
Disease-free survival (DFS)	0.58	<0.001	0.61	95% confidence interval 0.39–0.98
Distant DFS	0.60	0.002	Not reported	0.001
Overall survival	0.82	0.3	0.61	0.04
Contralateral breast cancer	0.63	0.12	Not reported	Not reported

[a]Letrozole versus placebo.
[b]Placebo followed by letrozole versus no treatment.
Source: Data from Refs. 21 and 22.

Women most vulnerable to problems with endocrine therapy therefore may not be represented by the patients in this trial. With this proviso, letrozole was generally well tolerated, with overall toxicities as expected (21). The incidence of hot flashes (58% versus 54%), myalgia (15% versus 12%), arthralgia (25% versus 21%), and alopecia (5% versus 3%) was significantly higher in patients receiving letrozole. These adverse events were considered to be due to patients' depleted estrogen levels, and the majority of such side effects can be effectively managed (21). It is interesting to note that these side effects also were frequently experienced by patients receiving placebo, in whom the rate of arthralgia was also high.

The incidence of new-onset clinical osteoporosis was 8.1% in letrozole-treated patients, compared with 6.0% in placebo-treated patients. While there was a trend toward a numerical increase in clinical fractures in patients taking letrozole (5.3%) compared with placebo (4.6%), this difference was not statistically significant (Table 16.2) (21). In those patients experiencing a fracture, median time from randomization to a fracture event was 1.06 years, compared with 0.86 years for placebo-treated patients. The median time to any fracture occurrence for those receiving letrozole was 0.70 years, compared with 0.52 years for those receiving placebo (21).

To further define the effects of letrozole on skeletal health, a subset of 226 patients enrolled in MA.17 were followed for bone mineral density (BMD) and bone turnover markers (27). Although at 12 months there was no statistically significant difference between the two groups of patients, among those patients remaining in the cohort at 24 months, there was a significantly greater decrease in total hip BMD among women taking letrozole (-3.60 versus -0.71, $P = 0.044$) (27). Evaluation of the bone resorption marker urine N-telopeptide correlated with the BMD findings. Patients treated with letrozole had an increase in N-telopeptide at 6 months ($P = 0.054$), 12 months ($P < 0.001$), and 24 months ($P = 0.016$) (27). However, more patients receiving placebo (10.6%), compared with letrozole (4.1%), were using bisphosphonates, which could have had a positive impact on their BMD. Another observation was that BMD scores were more likely to show a significant drop in women who were osteopenic at the initiation of letrozole than in those with BMD within the normal range (27).

The incidence of cardiovascular (CV) disease in patients enrolled in MA.17 was similar among patients in the two groups (5.8% letrozole versus 5.6% placebo), as was the incidence of hypercholesterolemia (16% in both arms) (see Table 16.2) (21). In the MA.17 lipid substudy, total cholesterol, high-density lipoprotein (HDL) cholesterol, low-density lipoprotein (LDL) cholesterol, lipoprotein (a), and triglycerides were measured at baseline ($N = 347$), at 6 and 12 months, and yearly thereafter up to 36 months (28). The only differences among the two cohorts were marginally significant differences in the percentage changes in HDL cholesterol at 6 months (decreased HDL with letrozole vs increased HDL with placebo; $P = 0.049$), in LDL cholesterol at 12 months (increased LDL with both letrozole and placebo; $P = 0.033$), and in triglycerides at 24 months (increased triglycerides with letrozole versus decreased triglycerides with placebo; $P = 0.036$), but not at any other time points (28). These findings confirm that AI therapy with letrozole does not increase the risk of hypercholesterolemia, supporting previous findings that while AIs lack the potential cardioprotective effects of tamoxifen, they do not increase the overall risk of CV events (29).

In this aging population treated with endocrine therapy, an increasing CV risk competes with recurrence as a cause of mortality, making women with CV disease more likely to die from non-breast-cancer-related causes (3,8,9,30). In fact, long-term follow-up of all survivors in the MA.17 trial demonstrated that non–breast cancer occurrences accounted for 72% of deaths among patients 70 years or older and 48% of deaths among those younger than 70 years (31).

MA.17: QoL Analyses

While it is clear that adjuvant AI therapy results in substantial improvements in DFS and overall survival (OS), the QoL associated with AI treatment is an important consideration for clinical decision making. To address this issue, the MA.17 trial evaluated a group of healthy women free of recurrent cancer. Data were collected using two surveys: a general QoL instrument, the Short Form 36-item Health Survey (SF-36), and a symptom-specific instrument, the Menopause Specific Quality of Life Questionnaire (MENQOL). The SF-36 evaluates 36 items, including general physical function, pain, general health, vitality, social functioning, and mental health. From this information,

■ Table 16.2 MA.17 updated safety analysis

Side Effect	Letrozole (%)	Placebo (%)	P Value
Clinical bone fractures	5.3	4.6	0.25
New osteoporosis	8.1	6.0	0.003
Hypercholesterolemia	16	16	0.79
Cardiovascular disease	5.8	5.6	0.76
Hot flashes	58	54	0.003
Myalgia	15	12	0.004
Arthralgia	25	21	<0.001
Alopecia	5	3	0.01

Source: Data from Ref. 21.

individual and global summary scores of physical and mental status are derived. The MENQOL assesses symptoms specifically related to menopause and estrogen depletion that might be affected by AIs (26,32,33).

In the MA.17 QoL substudy, mental and physical summary scores on the SF-36 were similar between patients taking placebo and patients taking letrozole, although some small differences were noted in the bodily pain domain (26). On the MENQOL questionnaire, only the vasomotor domain showed a significant difference between groups, with 22% of the placebo group and 29% of the letrozole group reporting worsening in QoL related to vasomotor symptoms (P <0.001) (26). These symptoms improved over time for both patient groups. Together, the results demonstrated that compared with placebo, letrozole did not have a detrimental effect on overall QoL after 36 months of treatment (26).

Bothersome symptoms were noted by a minority of patients in both the placebo and letrozole groups, and of these only hot flashes (17% placebo versus 22% letrozole; P = 0.0002) and sweating (14% placebo versus 18% letrozole; P = 0.003) were significantly different between groups. The incidences of night sweats, vaginal dryness, aching in muscles and joints, difficulty sleeping, change in sexual desire, avoidance of intimacy, poor memory, feeling depressed, or weight gain did not differ significantly between treatment arms.

Additional MA.17 Analyses

Several additional analyses of women enrolled in MA.17 have been conducted. A cohort analysis of all events up to the date of study unblinding by length of time on therapy showed that the hazard ratios significantly decreased, from 0.59 at 6 months to 0.19 at 48 months (P <0.0001), corresponding to a 41% to 81% reduction in recurrence risk over time. These significantly decreasing hazard ratios achieved with letrozole for up to 48 months for the primary study endpoint of DFS suggest a greater benefit with letrozole the longer patients remain on therapy. In this analysis, DDFS showed a similar pattern of increasing superiority for letrozole over time, with the test for trend being highly significant (P <0.0013) (34).

A retrospective analysis of the effect of hormone receptor status on clinical outcome with extended adjuvant letrozole was also performed. Letrozole demonstrated the greatest efficacy in women with ER+/progesterone receptor–positive (PR+) tumors (n = 3,809), the most hormone-dependent subset. A significant survival benefit was also seen in this large ER+/PR+ patient population. Women in this group showed a 51% reduction in DFS compared with placebo. Those with ER–/PR+ tumors (n = 200), although a very small subset, also appeared to benefit, with a 44% reduction in events compared with placebo. By comparison, women with ER+/PR– tumors

(n = 636) did not appear to experience a DFS benefit with letrozole. However, the following caveats should be considered: The 95% CI in the ER+/PR– subgroup for DFS was very wide (0.63 to 2.34), and the receptor levels were measured locally (35). While the best outcomes were seen in the ER+/PR+ patients, because receptor levels were measured locally rather than centrally, and in light of the small number of patients in the other subgroups, the data require confirmation before PR is incorporated into treatment decisions (35).

The benefits of letrozole in postmenopausal women with early-stage breast cancer were independent of age. Benefits in DFS and DDFS were observed with letrozole in all age groups. In particular, among patients 70 years of age or older and in good health, the benefits of letrozole were similar to those seen in younger patients, without any increase in toxicity or decrease in QoL compared with placebo (36).

A separate intent-to-treat (ITT) analysis, which assessed all outcomes (DFS, DDFS, OS, and contralateral breast cancer), was also performed. It did not take into account whether patients in the placebo group switched to letrozole at the unblinding of the data. This ITT analysis, which included all events before and after the unblinding, based on the original randomization to letrozole or placebo, showed a significant benefit for women originally randomized to letrozole compared with those who initially received placebo at a median follow-up of 54 months (37). Furthermore, those women originally randomized to letrozole within 3 months of completing tamoxifen did better than placebo patients, even though 73% of placebo patients crossed to letrozole after unblinding. This benefit was noted for DFS (P = 0.0002), DDFS (P = 0.041), and contralateral breast cancer (P = 0.037) (37).

An additional post-unblinding analysis also showed the benefit of late extended adjuvant letrozole. When MA.17 was unblinded in 2003, most patients who were receiving letrozole chose to continue their 5 years of planned therapy. Those who had been receiving placebo were given the chance to switch to letrozole; about two thirds of placebo-treated patients (n = 1,579) crossed over to letrozole, but 804 patients decided to be followed annually and not receive treatment (23,38,39). This analysis was done after a median follow-up of 63.6 months in all patients who had a recurrence, or died, before unblinding or discontinued treatment because of any toxicity. The two groups studied also had different baseline characteristics, with the women electing to switch to letrozole at increased risk for disease recurrence (i.e., younger age, node-positive disease, prior chemotherapy). The multivariate analysis was adjusted for all known risk factor imbalances. Efficacy results from the post-unblinding analysis showed that patients who received late extended adjuvant letrozole experienced a significant reduction in DFS (HR 0.37, P <0.0001), DDFS (HR 0.38, P = 0.004), and risk of contralateral breast cancer

(HR 0.18, P = 0.004), and an improvement in OS (HR 0.30, P <0.0001), despite a gap between the completion of tamoxifen and the initiation of letrozole. Safety analysis post-unblinding was comparable to that seen in the main trial. In patients who received late extended adjuvant letrozole, there was an increased incidence of osteoporosis (self-reported) (5.3% versus 1.6%) and fractures (5.2% versus 3.1%) but no increase in the incidence of CV events (4.2% versus 3.1%) (23).

■ ONGOING TRIALS OF EXTENDED ADJUVANT AI THERAPY

To determine whether adjuvant AI therapy for more than 5 years is better than therapy for 5 years, a randomized, placebo-controlled trial (MA.17R) is being conducted. This trial randomizes women completing 5 years of any AI, after any duration of prior tamoxifen or no prior tamoxifen, to either 5 more years of letrozole or placebo (Figure 16.7). This trial includes women who completed 5 years of letrozole after 5 years of tamoxifen in the original MA.17 trial (29,40,41). Disease stratification includes receptor status (positive versus unknown), lymph node status (negative, positive, unknown), prior adjuvant chemotherapy (yes or no), interval between last dose of AI and randomization (less than 6 months, 6 months, 2 years), and duration of tamoxifen use (0 years, less than 2 years, 2 to 4½ years, more than 4½ years) (41). Companion translational studies in this trial will examine whether common genetic single nucleotide polymorphisms, for genes encoding proteins involved in the pharmacokinetic or pharmacodynamic pathways for letrozole, contribute to a variation in toxicity and efficacy of letrozole in individual patients (41). This trial completed accrual in May 2009.

In addition to the extension of MA.17, several other trials are under way to determine the optimal duration of AI therapy. The NSABP B-42 trial will examine specifically whether 10 years of endocrine therapy is superior to 5 years. Women who have completed 5 years of endocrine treatment with any AI or 2 to 3 years of tamoxifen followed by 2 to 3 years of AI will be randomized to

receive letrozole for an additional 5 years or placebo (42). In a similar trial using anastrozole [ABCSG-16 Secondary Adjuvant Long-term Study in Arimidex (SALSA)], more than 1,700 postmenopausal patients (of a total 3,500) who were free of breast cancer recurrence after approximately 5 years of any endocrine therapy have already been enrolled. Patients are randomized to receive either 2 or 5 years of extended adjuvant anastrozole. The primary outcome measure is DFS, and assessments of OS and fracture rates are planned (43,44).

Two additional trials will evaluate letrozole use in patients treated with 2 to 3 years of tamoxifen following primary resection. In the LEAD (LEtrozole Adjuvant therapy Duration) study, patients will be randomized to receive shorter-term letrozole for 2 to 3 years or letrozole for 5 years (45). In a similar population, the Dutch DATA trial (Different Durations of Adjuvant Anastrozole Therapy after 2 to 3 years of Tamoxifen) will analyze differences between 3 and 6 years of anastrozole in postmenopausal women with hormone-sensitive breast cancer (46). A primary endpoint of DFS has been established for both trials (46).

In Figure 16.8, the designs of ongoing trials evaluating the duration of adjuvant AI therapy are shown.

■ CONCLUSIONS

In women with early-stage hormone receptor–positive breast cancer, the risk of disease recurrence is highest after 5 years, with the most common and serious late relapse event being distant metastases. This risk is seen both in patients treated with tamoxifen and in untreated patients. The MA.17 trial has demonstrated that extended adjuvant letrozole allows patients to further reduce their risk of relapse following 5 years of tamoxifen. Extended adjuvant letrozole significantly reduced the risk of recurrence by 42% and distant metastases by 40%. These results from the MA.17 trial have led to letrozole becoming the only approved extended adjuvant therapy.

All current guidelines support the use of letrozole as an extended adjuvant therapy (47,48), and results from the MA.17 cohort analysis show that the longer the use of letrozole, the greater the benefit (at least out to 4 years) (34). When considering extended adjuvant hormonal therapy after the completion of 5 years of tamoxifen, clinicians and patients should consider the residual risk of recurrence and individual patient preferences (47). The MA.17 results clearly show that the benefit of extended adjuvant letrozole is seen irrespective of nodal status and that the option of extended adjuvant therapy should be discussed with all patients completing tamoxifen. The worth of extending tamoxifen treatment past 5 years will be clarified by longer follow-up of both ATLAS and aTTom trials.

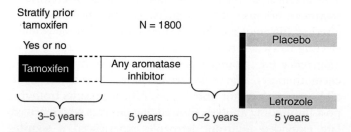

FIGURE 16.7 MA.17R re-randomization recruitment criteria and protocol.

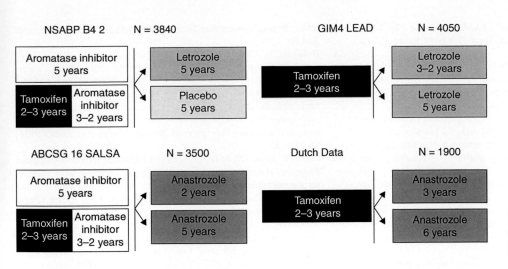

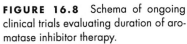

FIGURE 16.8 Schema of ongoing clinical trials evaluating duration of aromatase inhibitor therapy.

MA.17 post-unblinding results show that women with hormone-dependent breast cancer who were prescribed letrozole following a prolonged delay after completing tamoxifen also experienced a significant improvement in outcomes. Women who have not been given letrozole immediately after completing tamoxifen should be considered candidates for late extended adjuvant therapy. Of note, AIs and tamoxifen are now appropriate choices for initial adjuvant therapy for postmenopausal women with hormone-sensitive breast cancer (48). For those patients who have received initial adjuvant tamoxifen, extended adjuvant and late extended adjuvant letrozole therapy offers an opportunity for further protection against late relapses. The results of the MA.17R re-randomization trial and other trials, including NSABP B-42, will build on current information and help determine the optimal duration of AI therapy for women with hormone receptor–positive breast cancer.

■ SUMMARY

- ER+ early breast cancer is a chronic relapsing disease.
- Extended adjuvant endocrine therapy of 10 years versus 5 years reduces the risk of recurrences significantly.
- Confirmatory trials of more than 5 years of adjuvant endocrine therapy are under way, as are studies to identify those at risk of late recurrences and those most likely to experience toxicities.

■ REFERENCES

1. Duffy S, Jackson TL, Lansdown M, et al. The ATAC ('Arimidex', Tamoxifen, Alone or in Combination) adjuvant breast cancer trial: first results of the endometrial sub-protocol following 2 years of treatment. *Hum Reprod.* 2006;21:545–553.
2. Early Breast Cancer Trialists' Collaborative Group (EBCTCG). Effects of chemotherapy and hormonal therapy for early breast cancer on recurrence and 15-year survival: an overview of the randomised trials. *Lancet.* 2005;365:1687–1717.
3. Howell A, Cuzick J, Baum M, et al.; ATAC Trialists' Group. Results of the ATAC (Arimidex, Tamoxifen, Alone or in Combination) trial after completion of 5 years' adjuvant treatment for breast cancer. *Lancet.* 2005;365:60–62.
4. Adjuvant Therapy for Breast Cancer. NIH Consensus Statement. 2000;17:1–35.
5. Fisher B, Dignam J, Bryant J, et al. Five versus more than five years of tamoxifen for lymph node-negative breast cancer: updated findings from the National Surgical Adjuvant Breast and Bowel Project B-14 randomized trial. *J Natl Cancer Inst.* 2001;93:684–690.
6. Peto R, Davies C. ATLAS (Adjuvant Tamoxifen, Longer Against Shorter): international randomized trial of 10 versus 5 years of adjuvant tamoxifen among 11500 women—preliminary results. *Breast Cancer Res Treat.* 2007;106(suppl 1) (Abstract 48).
7. Mouridsen H, Gershanovich M, Sun Y, et al. Phase III study of letrozole versus tamoxifen as first-line therapy of advanced breast cancer in postmenopausal women: analysis of survival and update of efficacy from the International Letrozole Breast Cancer Group. *J Clin Oncol.* 2003;21:2101–2109.
8. Thurlimann B, Keshaviah A, Coates AS, et al.; Breast International Group (BIG) 1–98 Collaborative Group. A comparison of letrozole and tamoxifen in postmenopausal women with early breast cancer. *New Engl J Med.* 2005;353:2747–2757.
9. Coombes RC, Kilburn LS, Snowdon CF, et al. Exemestane study. Survival and safety of exemestane versus tamoxifen after 2–3 years' tamoxifen treatment (Intergroup Exemestane Study): a randomised controlled trial. *Lancet.* 2007;369:559–570.
10. Saphner T, Tormey DC, Gray R. Annual hazard rates of recurrence for breast cancer after primary therapy. *J Clin Oncol.* 1996; 14:2738–2746.
11. Kennecke HF, Olivotto IA, Speers C, et al. Late risk of relapse and mortality among postmenopausal women with estrogen responsive early breast cancer after 5 years of tamoxifen. *Ann Oncol.* 2007;18:45–51.
12. Lamerato L, Havstad S, Ganhdi S, et al. Breast cancer recurrence and related mortality in US pts with early breast cancer. *J Clin Oncol.* 2005;23(16 suppl):62s (Abstract 738).
13. Chia SK, Speers CH, Bryce CJ, et al. Ten-year outcomes in a population-based cohort of node-negative, lymphatic, and vascular invasion-negative early breast cancers without adjuvant systemic therapies. *J Clin Oncol.* 2004;22:1630–1637.
14. Freedman GM, Anderson P, Li T, et al. Identifying breast cancer patients most likely to benefit from aromatase inhibitor therapy after adjuvant radiation and tamoxifen. *Cancer.* 2006;107:2552–2558.
15. Delozier T, Spielmann M, Janvier M, et al. Optimal duration of adjuvant tamoxifen (TAM) in early breast cancer (EBC): ten

year results of a randomized trial (TAM-01) of the FNCLCC Breast Group. *Breast Cancer Res Treat.* 2005;94(Suppl 1):S10 (Abstract 14).

16. McDonald CC, Alexander FE, Whyte BW, et al. Cardiac and vascular morbidity in women receiving adjuvant tamoxifen for breast cancer in a randomised trial. The Scottish Cancer Trials Breast Group. *Br Med J.* 1995;311:977–980.

17. Gray RG, Rea DW, Handley K, et al. aTTom (adjuvant Tamoxifen—To offer more?): randomized trial of 10 versus 5 years of adjuvant tamoxifen among 6,934 women with estrogen receptor-positive (ER+) or ER untested breast cancer—preliminary results. *J Clin Oncol.* 2008;26(15 suppl):513.

18. Bryant J, Fisher B, Dignam J. Duration of adjuvant tamoxifen therapy. *J Natl Cancer Inst Monogr.* 2001;30:56–61.

19. Goss PE, Ingle JN, Martino S, et al. A randomized trial of letrozole in postmenopausal women after five years of tamoxifen therapy for early-stage breast cancer. *New Engl J Med.* 2003;349:1793–1802.

20. Pater J, Tu D, Shepherd L, et al. Decision making in adjuvant trials in breast cancer: the NCIC CTG MA.17 trial as an example. *Breast Cancer Res Treat.* 2008;108:265–269.

21. Goss PE, Ingle JN, Martino S, et al. Randomized trial of letrozole following tamoxifen as extended adjuvant therapy in receptor-positive breast cancer: updated findings from NCIC CTG MA.17. *J Natl Cancer Inst.* 2005;97:1262–1271.

22. Kaufmann M, Rody A. Long-term risk of breast cancer recurrence: the need for extended adjuvant therapy. *J Cancer Res Clin Oncol.* 2005;131:487–494.

23. Goss PR, Ingle JN, Palmer MJ, et al. Updated analysis of NCIC CTG MA.17 (letrozole vs placebo to letrozole vs placebo) post unblinding. *J Clin Oncol.* 2008;26:1948–1955.

24. Mamounas E, Jeong JH, Wickerham DL, et al. Benefit from exemestane (EXE) as extended adjuvant therapy after 5 years of tamoxifen (TAM): intent-to-treat analysis of NSABP B-33. *J Clin Oncol.* 2008;26:1965–1971.

25. Jakesz R, Samonigg H, Greil R, et al. on behalf of the ABCSG. Extended adjuvant treatment with anastrozole: results from the Austrian Breast and Colorectal Cancer Study Group trial 6a (ABCSG-6a). *J Clin Oncol.* 2005;23(16 suppl):10s (Abstract 526).

26. Whelan TJ, Goss PE, Ingle JN, et al. Assessment of quality of life in MA.17: a randomized, placebo-controlled trial of letrozole after 5 years of tamoxifen in postmenopausal women. *J Clin Oncol.* 2005;23:6931–6940.

27. Perez EA, Josse RG, Pritchard KI, et al. Effect of letrozole versus placebo on bone mineral density in women with primary breast cancer completing 5 or more years of adjuvant tamoxifen: a companion study to NCIC CTG MA.17. *J Clin Oncol.* 2006;24:3629–3635.

28. Wasan KM, Goss PE, Pritchard PH, et al. The influence of letrozole on serum lipid concentrations in postmenopausal women with primary breast cancer who have completed 5 years of adjuvant tamoxifen (NCIC CTG MA.17L). *Ann Oncol.* 2005;16:707–715.

29. Goss P. Update on the MA.17 extended adjuvant trial. *Best Pract Res Clin Endocrinol Metab.* 2006;20(Suppl 1):S5–S13.

30. Monnier A, Sakek N, Aladen S. Comparing AI cardiovascular safety data: trial comparators and outcomes. *Ann Oncol.* 2006;17(Suppl 9):ix100 (Abstract 266).

31. Chapman J, Meng D, Shepherd L, et al. Competing causes of death in NCIC CTG MA.17, a placebo-controlled trial of letrozole as extended adjuvant therapy for breast cancer patients. *J Clin Oncol.* 2007;25(18 suppl):12s (Abstract 540).

32. Abetz L, Barghout V, Thomas S, et al. Letrozole did not worsen quality of life relative to placebo in post-menopausal women with early breast cancer: results from the US subjects of the MA-17

study. *Breast Cancer Res Treat.* 2005;94(Suppl 1):S100 (Abstract 2047).

33. Barghout V, Abetz L, Thomas S, et al. Impact of letrozole on quality of life in post-menopausal women with early breast cancer: does age matter? *Breast Cancer Res Treat.* 2005;94(Suppl 1):S97 (Abstract 2040).

34. Ingle JN, Tu D, Pater JL, et al. Duration of letrozole treatment and outcomes in the placebo-controlled NCIC CTG MA.17 extended adjuvant therapy trial. *Breast Cancer Res Treat.* 2006;99:295–300.

35. Goss PE, Ingle JN, Martino S, et al. Efficacy of letrozole extended adjuvant therapy according to estrogen receptor and progesterone receptor status of the primary tumor: National Cancer Institute of Canada Clinical Trials Group MA.17. *J Clin Oncol* 2007;25:2006–2011.

36. Muss HB, Tu D, Ingle JN, et al. Efficacy, toxicity and quality of life in older women with early stage breast cancer treated with letrozole or placebo after five years of tamoxifen: NCIC CTG Intergroup trial MA.17. *J Clin Oncol.* 2008;26:1956–1964.

37. Ingle JN, Tu D, Pater JL, et al. Intent-to-treat analysis of the placebo-controlled trial of letrozole for extended adjuvant therapy in early breast cancer: NCIC CTG MA. *Ann Oncol.* 2008;19:877–882.

38. Goss PR, Ingle JN, Palmer MJ, et al. Updated analysis of NCIC CTG MA.17 (letrozole vs placebo to letrozole vs placebo) post unblinding. *Breast Cancer Res Treat.* 2005;94(Suppl 1):S10–S11 (Abstract 16).

39. Robert NJ, Goss PE, Ingle JN, et al. Updated analysis of NCIC CTG MA.17 (letrozole vs. placebo to letrozole vs placebo) post unblinding. *J Clin Oncol.* 2006;24(18 suppl):15s (Abstract 550).

40. Pritchard KI, Goss PE, Shepherd L. The extended adjuvant NCIC CTG MA.17 trials: initial and re-randomization studies. *Breast.* 2006;15(1 suppl):14–20.

41. NCT00003140 NCI. National Cancer Institute. Letrozole after tamoxifen in treating women with breast cancer. Available at http://www.clinicaltrials.gov.

42. Mamounas EP, Lembersky B, Jeong JH, et al. NSABP B-42: a clinical trial to determine the efficacy of five years of letrozole compared with placebo in patients completing five years of hormonal therapy consisting of an aromatase inhibitor (AI) or tamoxifen followed by an AI in prolonging disease-free survival in postmenopausal women with hormone receptor-positive breast cancer. *Clin Breast Cancer.* 2006;7:416–421.

43. ABCSG. Annual meeting of the Austrian Breast and Colorectal Study Group (ABCSG). *Breast Care.* 2007;2:47–49.

44. NCT00295620. Secondary adjuvant long term study with Arimidex (SALSA). Available at www.clinical trials.gov.

45. Letrozole Adjuvant Therapy Duration (LEAD) study: standard versus long treatment. A phase III trial in post-menopausal women with early breast cancer. Available at www.oncotech.org/albero/progetti_gim4.asp.

46. NCT00301457. Different durations of adjuvant anastrozole therapy after 2 to 3 years tamoxifen therapy in breast cancer (DATA). Available at www.clinicaltrials.gov.

47. Goldhirsch A, Wood W, Gelber R, et al. Progress and promise: highlights of the international expert consensus on the primary therapy of early breast cancer 2007. *Ann Oncol.* 2007;18:1133–1144.

48. Winer EP, Hudis C, Burstein HJ, et al. American Society of Clinical Oncology technology assessment on the use of aromatase inhibitors as adjuvant therapy for postmenopausal women with hormone receptor-positive breast cancer: status report 2004. *J Clin Oncol* 2005;23:619–629.

49. Hortobagyi GN, Kau S-W, Buzdar AU, et al. What is the prognosis of patients with operable breast cancer (BC) five years after diagnosis? *J Clin Oncol.* 2004;22(14 suppl) (Abstract 585).

Gene Expression Profiling: Personalized Treatment

LEIF W. ELLISEN

DENNIS SGROI

Tumor heterogeneity is a well-recognized, clinically relevant, but poorly understood property of human cancers, including breast cancer. Detailed molecular analysis of tumors provides a window on this heterogeneity while holding the promise of yielding new diagnostic, prognostic, and predictive information to guide clinical decision making. The list of approaches to "tumor molecular profiling" is rapidly expanding as new technologies become both available and adapted for analysis of small quantities of biological specimens. These approaches include RNA analysis (gene expression), DNA-based analyses (copy number assessment and mutational analysis), epigenetic analyses (e.g., DNA methylation patterns), micro-RNA analysis, and various proteomic approaches. Among the most advanced in terms of clinical application are RNA expression profiling approaches, and this chapter therefore will focus on this work. A brief discussion of some of the other techniques and their future promise is included at the end of the chapter.

■ TECHNICAL ASPECTS OF EXPRESSION PROFILING

Each cell contains approximately 30,000 protein-coding genes that are transcribed to produce mRNA transcripts. Current approaches to comprehensive expression profiling rely on hybridization of labeled tumor RNA to gene chips, which contain either oligonucleotide or cDNA probes that are complementary to the sequence of each gene (1). Hybridization of the RNA to the probe on the chip is then detected by optical scanning, with the hybridization signal being proportional to the level of a given transcript in the sample. Depending on the specific microarray platform, the signal generated for each gene is then either normalized to all other genes on the microarray to generate an absolute value or compared to the signal from a reference sample hybridized on the same microarray (1). Of note is the fact that such genome-wide methods of expression profiling rely on the use of frozen (not fixed) tissue as the source of RNA, although newer approaches aim to circumvent this limitation in order to allow the potential for broader diagnostic applications.

■ UNSUPERVISED PROFILING FOR BREAST CANCER CLASSIFICATION

One method for analysis of breast cancer expression profiling is so-called unsupervised clustering, in which tumors are profiled and patterns of gene expression in different tumors are grouped without any specific underlying hypothesis. When applied to a large group of breast cancers, this approach led Perou and colleagues to uncover the "intrinsic gene signatures" that divided breast cancers into groups that correlated remarkably well with clinically recognized breast cancer subtypes (2). These subtypes include luminal A–signature tumors, which express luminal cytokeratins and are most often estrogen receptor–positive (ER+) low-grade tumors. Luminal B–signature tumors express ER but also genes associated with proliferation and are clinically usually high grade. HER2+ tumors also express proliferation genes, as well as HER2 and other genes linked to this genomic locus. Finally, basal-like tumors express cytokeratins and some other factors associated with myoepithelial cells; clinically, these tumors are most commonly ER/progesterone receptor (PR)/HER2–negative (triple negative) (2). These microarray-based intrinsic subtype classifications were shown in multiple retrospective studies to have significant prognostic and predictive power (3–6).

What is the utility of such signatures if they correspond closely to previously clinically recognized breast cancer subtypes? First, these signatures provide a comprehensive analysis of a tumor's biological state that may be a more accurate reflection than single-gene or single-protein markers. Second, these signatures provide an objective assessment of factors that correlate with tumor grade, which is a subjective measure. As discussed below, genes associated with proliferation and with histological grade drive many of the currently useful prognostic signatures, suggesting that molecular determination of tumor grade is an important clinical advance (7). Finally, intrinsic gene signatures can be used to identify new and relevant subcategories of clinically recognized breast cancer subtypes. For example, triple-negative tumors are a heterogeneous group consisting of basal-like and non-basal-like tumors. These two signature-defined subcategories of triple-negative tumors appear to have significantly different clinical behavior (8) and may require the development of different clinical approaches.

■ PROGNOSTICATION THROUGH TOP-DOWN PROFILING

A second approach to generating useful profiles of breast tumors is to compare profiles of tumors from otherwise matched patients who experienced different clinical outcomes. This is a type of supervised approach; however, it does not involve specific hypotheses about the genes to be identified and has been referred to as a "top-down" strategy (9). The Netherlands Cancer Institute Group used this approach to develop a 70-gene signature (now known as MammaPrint) from node-negative patients who did not receive adjuvant systemic treatment and either did or did not suffer a recurrence within 5 years of diagnosis (10). This signature then was validated in an independent cohort of similarly untreated patients (11). In this validation set, the signature had a sensitivity of 84% and a specificity of 42% in predicting relapse. By comparison, standard clinical criteria for prognostication using the Adjuvant!Online algorithm yielded 82% sensitivity and 29% specificity. In this analysis, the signature and Adjuvant!Online criteria were discordant 29% of the time. In these cases, the signature appeared to perform better than the clinical criteria because patients who were rated as high risk by the signature but low risk by Adjuvant!Online had a significantly worse overall survival than patients rated as low

risk by the signature but high risk by Adjuvant!Online criteria (11). These and other data recently led to this signature being cleared by the Food and Drug Administration (FDA) for clinical use. Several caveats remain with this approach, however. Most notably, the utility of this signature in patients who have received adjuvant therapy is not clear. In addition, MammaPrint requires fresh or frozen tissue, which is not routinely collected in many institutions, particularly in the United States. Furthermore, the signature has not been tested in a prospective fashion. As discussed below, the clinical utility of the MammaPrint assay as well as a second signature (Onco*type* DX) is now being tested in independent prospective clinical trials (Table 16.3).

A different top-down comparison was performed by our group in collaboration with bioTheranostics. The goal was to generate a signature that predicted outcome following hormonal therapy by comparing a uniform cohort of node-negative patients treated with adjuvant tamoxifen who either did or did not experience distant tumor recurrence within 10 years. Ultimately, a two-gene ratio, *HOXB13* and *IL17RB* (H/I ratio), was found to be prognostic in this cohort (12). The initial patient cohort matched tumors for grade, and therefore, not surprisingly, the resulting signature was found to be independent of grade. Subsequent studies have demonstrated that the signature has both prognostic and predictive value in the setting of tamoxifen treatment (13,14). In addition, the signature performance was found to be improved by the addition of a five-gene molecular grade index (MGI) (15). Although *HOXB13* and *IL17RB* had not been previously linked to human cancer, emerging data suggest

---

■ Table 16.3 Commercially available multigene prognostic signatures

Signature	MammaPrint	Onco*type* DX	Theros	MapQuant DX
Vendor	Agendia	Genomic Health	Biotheranostics	Ipsogen
Parameter tested	70-gene signature	21-gene recurrence score	Expression ratio of HOXB13 to IL17BR plus 5-gene grade index (MGI)	97-gene grade index (GGI)
Tissue required	Fresh or frozen	FFPE	FFPE	Fresh or frozen
Assay platform	DNA microarray	QRT-PCR	QRT-PCR	DNA microarray
Current indication	To predict high risk/low risk of recurrence for stage 1 and 2, node-negative tumors	To predict recurrence rates and chemotherapy benefit following tamoxifen therapy for ER+, node-negative tumors	To predict high risk/low risk of recurrence following endocrine therapy for ER+, node– tumors	To stratify grade 2, ER+ tumors into high risk and low risk of recurrence
Availability	Europe and United States	Europe and United States	United States	Europe

Abbreviations: ER+, estrogen receptor–positive; FFPE, formalin-fixed, paraffin-embedded; GGI, gene expression grade index; MGI, molecular grade index; QRT-PCR, quantitative real-time polymerase chain reaction.

that they may play a relatively direct role in estrogen signaling (16).

BOTTOM-UP PROGNOSTIC SIGNATURES BASED ON PREDETERMINED BIOLOGICAL PROPERTIES

A third approach to profiling involves the generation of a signature focused on a predefined biological property of the tumor cell. This approach, termed "bottom-up" profiling, therefore rests on a specific hypothesis regarding the association of the biological property with prognosis. This strategy was used to generate the gene expression/genomic grade index (GGI), comprising 97 genes found to be differentially expressed between low-grade (grade 1) and high-grade (grade 3) tumors (17). Consistent with the view that this molecular grade is superior to subjective tumor grading, this signature was able successfully to classify intermediate (grade 2) tumors into two groups with differences in clinical outcomes similar to grade 1 and 3 tumors. Conceptually similar bottom-up approaches have been used to derive hormone-related signatures. In one case an endocrine sensitivity index (SET index) signature was derived on the basis of genes that correlated with ER-alpha expression in primary breast cancer. This signature was found to be predictive in tamoxifen-treated patients but did not provide prognostic information in patients who received no adjuvant therapy (18). In another study a signature was first generated on the basis of exposure of MCF7 cells, an ER+ tumor-derived line, to estrogen. This gene set was then used to derive a prognostic signature for ER/PR+ tumors (19).

A variation on the bottom-up strategy is the 21-gene recurrence score (Onco*type* DX), a multigene assay developed as a continuous variable to predict recurrence in tamoxifen-treated, node-negative patients enrolled in the National Surgical Adjuvant Breast Project (NSABP) B-14 trial (20). Unlike with the other signatures, the development of this signature involved direct selection of genes thought to be of prognostic value, which include *ER, PR, HER2,* and *Ki67*. In addition, this is a reverse-transcription/polymerase chain reaction (RT-PCR)–based rather than a microarray-based assay, and therefore, it can be performed on formalin-fixed, paraffin-embedded tissue, eliminating the need for fresh-frozen tissue. Subsequently, the signature was validated in a second cohort, the NSABP B-20 trial, which included women treated with tamoxifen with or without cytoxan, methotrexate, and 5-fluorouracil (CMF) chemotherapy (21). In this setting, the recurrence score predicted not only prognosis but also a benefit from chemotherapy in patients with a high recurrence score, whereas patients with a low recurrence score derived essentially no benefit from the addition of chemotherapy. Additional data suggest that the recurrence score is also prognostic in certain ER+, node-positive patients (22). Prospective validation of this signature awaits the results of the TAILORx trial (Trial Assigning Individualized Options for Treatment), discussed below.

COMPARISONS AMONG DIFFERENT PROGNOSTIC SIGNATURES

The gene expression signatures described above consist of fairly unique gene sets with very little overlap, yet they all share an ability to predict breast cancer outcome. For example, an independent Dutch group developed a 76-gene prognostic signature from a population similar to that used for the 70-gene signature (node-negative patients who did not receive adjuvant therapy) (23). These two signatures have similar predictive power, even though only three genes are shared between the two signatures. An important issue therefore is whether combining several of these signatures would provide more accurate risk assessment. In one comparative study by Fan and colleagues, four signatures (the intrinsic subtypes, the 70-gene signature, the 21-gene signature, and a "wound response" signature) were found to be highly concordant in classifying patients into low- and high-risk groups (7). Combining these four signatures did not yield significant improvement in predictive accuracy, suggesting that the prognostic information provided by these signatures is largely overlapping and likely reflects a common biological principle. Notably, all four signatures were significantly correlated with tumor grade, and this observation, together with other comparative analyses, suggests that this common principle involves molecular pathways centered on cell proliferation and cell cycle regulation. In support of this view, Sotiriou and colleagues recently performed an unbiased comparison of the 70-gene and 76-gene expression signatures with the GGI in the TRANS-BIG (Translating Molecular Knowledge into Early Breast Cancer Management—Breast International Group) clinical trial series. This analysis demonstrated that GGI, a pure tumor grade–based gene expression biomarker, possessed prognostic performance highly similar to both the 70-gene and the 76-gene expression signatures (24). An additional study by Sotiriou's group demonstrated that GGI and the 21-gene signature had similar prognostic performance (25), whereas our group recently demonstrated that the simple 5-gene MGI biomarker possesses prognostic equivalence to the more complex 97-gene GGI assay (15). Two conclusions can be drawn from these analyses. First, these studies reinforce the utility of an objective measurement of tumor grade or proliferation. Second, they suggest that new approaches may identify complementary, functionally independent signatures (e.g.,

H/I ratio) that could provide additional, independent prognostic information.

■ SIGNATURES PREDICTING CHEMOTHERAPY RESPONSE

In the practical management of breast cancer, much of the usefulness of the signatures described above is the identification of patients who may benefit from the addition of adjuvant chemotherapy to standard hormonal therapy. Depending on how these signatures were derived, however, these signatures do not address the issue of which chemotherapy agents might be most effective for an individual patient. In order to identify such predictors, several groups have utilized patient cohorts treated with neoadjuvant chemotherapy, which provides a rapid readout of clinical response. The group from the MD Anderson Cancer Center derived predictive signatures associated with pathological complete response (pCR) to neoadjuvant paclitaxel and fluorouracil, doxorubicin, and cyclophosphamide (T/FAC) chemotherapy (26). A 30-gene predictor yielded higher sensitivity (92%) than clinical parameters (age, grade, ER status), with high negative predictive value (96%). In another approach, investigators used expression profiles of cancer-derived cell lines (the National Cancer Institute NCI-60 panel) to derive a signature of chemotherapy response that had statistically significant predictive power in small cohorts of patients treated with docetaxel or doxorubicin (27). Other groups have used similar approaches based on in vitro chemosensitivity; however, these findings have not been validated in large trials (28,29).

Even though they may predict chemoresponsiveness, it remains plausible that such signatures in fact predict responsiveness to chemotherapy in general rather than to specific agents. This feature relates in part to the fact that they were derived on the basis of response to a polychemotherapy regimen (e.g., T/FAC) rather than from a comparison of regimens or specific agents. Similarly, the in vitro–derived chemotherapy response signatures were for the most part designed on the basis of response profiles to multiple chemotherapy agents, so it is not surprising that they reflect general chemotherapy responsiveness. Ongoing investigation into DNA damage response pathways that mediate the response to specific agents in different breast cancer subtypes may provide new predictive markers for specific chemotherapy agents. As one example, work in our group and others has identified a pathway for response to cisplatin chemotherapy, but not other chemotherapy agents, in triple-negative tumors (30). This response is mediated by the p53-related proteins p63 and p73, which have been proposed as clinical markers specifically of platinum sensitivity in breast cancer (30,31). Ongoing clinical trials are currently testing this hypothesis.

An effective analysis of any drug response must consider patient-specific genetic factors as well as tumor-specific factors. An emerging example of this principle is the assessment of polymorphisms in the cytochrome P450 subunit 2D6 (CYP2D6), which is involved in the rate-limiting step converting tamoxifen to its active metabolite. Approximately 10% of the population is homozygous for a CYP2D6 variant with severely decreased ability to metabolize tamoxifen, and retrospective data suggest that these patients may experience an inferior outcome when treated with tamoxifen (32). While the adoption of this test as a part of routine clinical practice awaits further validation (33), it is clear that improving the ability to predict clinical response to specific agents will require assessment of both host-specific and tumor-specific factors.

■ CLINICAL APPLICATION OF EXPRESSION SIGNATURES

There are many unanswered questions regarding the optimal use of expression profiles to guide breast cancer treatment decisions. One major issue concerns the applicability of the signatures across breast cancer subtypes. For example, the majority of HER2+ and triple-negative tumors are classified histologically as high grade. Since many of the expression signatures discussed above measure largely proliferation genes that correlate with grade, it is perhaps not surprising that these signatures perform well as prognostics only in the ER+/HER2– breast cancer subset. Indeed, a recent report suggests that functionally distinct (non-proliferation-associated) gene sets related to immune response and invasion are associated with prognosis in HER2+ and triple-negative subsets (34). These findings suggest that new signatures may need to be developed to improve prognostication and prediction in these subsets.

Another major issue is how these signatures should be integrated with clinicopathological parameters. Since these signatures were derived in specific patient populations (for the most part node-negative, T1 or T2 tumors), it is logical that tumor size and nodal status should be taken into consideration to produce optimal prediction (35). In addition, it is critical to assess whether in fact the signatures provide information that improves upon optimal clinicopathological determinations. While a body of retrospective data supports the independent value of signatures, including the 70-gene signature and the recurrence score, other analyses have failed to show an improvement in predictive accuracy (36). Two large, independent randomized trials are now under way that use distinctly different designs to test two of the most prominent signatures, the 70-gene signature (MammaPrint, Agendia) and the 21-gene recurrence score signature (Oncotype DX, Genomic Health).

The 70-gene signature will be assessed in the MINDACT (microarray in node-negative and 1 to 3 positive lymph node disease may avoid chemotherapy) trial, which was organized by the European Organisation for Research and Treatment of Cancer (EORTC) and will enroll 6,000 women with node-negative or node-positive disease (37). All patients will be evaluated by prescribed clinical criteria (Adjuvant!Online) and by the 70-gene signature. All ER+ patients will receive hormonal therapy, and those for whom the evaluations are discordant (high risk by clinical criteria and low risk by gene signature or vice versa) will then receive chemotherapy or not on the basis of their randomization to either clinical or gene signature assessment. While the primary endpoint is metastasis-free survival, the randomized groups will not be compared with each other. Instead, the signature will be considered successful if acceptable metastasis-free survival (92%) is observed for the patients judged to be low risk by signature and high risk by clinical criteria who are not treated with chemotherapy. The trial will therefore address whether chemotherapy might be safely avoided in a subset of patients who might have received chemotherapy on the basis of clinical prognostication alone. The design of the trial was challenging, and the conclusions may therefore be limited (38). Nevertheless, this trial is likely to provide important information regarding both logistic and clinical issues surrounding the application of this signature.

The trial incorporating the 21-gene recurrence score (TAILORx) aims to study a more restricted patient population: ER+, node-negative, HER2– patients (22). In this Eastern Cooperative Oncology Group (ECOG)–sponsored trial, patient assignment will be based not on discordance between clinical and signature assessment but on recurrence score alone. Thus patients with a low score (below 11) will receive hormonal therapy alone, those with a high score (above 25) will receive hormonal therapy plus chemotherapy, and those with intermediate recurrence scores of 11 to 25 will be randomized to receive chemotherapy or not. The objective is to demonstrate noninferiority for the primary endpoint, disease-free survival, between hormonal therapy and hormonal therapy plus chemotherapy treatment for patients with intermediate recurrence scores. Projected enrollment for this trial is 10,500 patients, with approximately 4,000 expected to be randomized. Results from either of these trials may not be available for several years, at which time new and potentially improved diagnostics may be available.

■ INTEGRATION OF MOLECULAR PROFILING TECHNIQUES WITH TARGETED THERAPY

While predicting chemotherapy response will be a clinically important goal for years to come, the emergence of new, targeted therapeutics will ultimately change the nature of breast cancer prognostication and therapeutic response prediction. Specifically, it is likely that as therapies become more pathway-specific, the ability to predict therapeutic response will become more robust. It also appears likely that much of this analysis may involve genome (DNA)–based rather than gene expression–based tests. The most prominent example of this principle is, of course, the use of genomic HER2 amplification as a single marker to predict the clinical response to trastuzumab therapy. Other examples of tumor-specific genomic (DNA) abnormalities linked to clinical response are now emerging. For example, mutations within the EGFR gene predict response to gefitinib therapy in lung cancer, with mutation-negative patients deriving little, if any, benefit (39). In addition, KRAS mutations in colon cancer predict a lack of response to cetuximab and panitumumab, a finding that led to a provisional clinical opinion by the American Society of Clinical Oncology (ASCO) stating that tumors of all patients eligible for such therapy should undergo such testing (40). In breast cancer, mutation of the phosphatidyl inositol-3 kinase (PI3K) subunit gene PIK3CA, which occurs in approximately 30% of cases, has been linked both to poor prognosis and to resistance to trastuzumab and lapatinib in preclinical studies (41,42). Given these findings and the number of clinical inhibitors of the PI3K pathway under development, it is highly likely that mutational analysis of this gene will be integrated into clinical practice for breast and other cancers.

In the same way that single gene expression–based assays have given way to multigene expression profiles, clinical testing for tumor genomic abnormalities may ultimately involve broad profiles of DNA copy number changes and mutations. The technology currently exists for copy number profiling using microarrays that are conceptually similar to those used for gene expression analysis. Extensive mutational analysis using advanced next generation sequencing platforms is still prohibitively expensive for routine clinical application. However, intermediate-scale tumor mutational profiling approaches, which can assess dozens to hundreds of mutations, are being developed and carried out at multiple major centers. Given increasing evidence supporting the use of DNA-based predictors of response to targeted therapeutics, near-term efforts are focused on developing genomic testing platforms that can be integrated into clinical practice.

In addition to helping guide clinical decision making for use of FDA-approved agents, the application of molecular profiling technologies promises to improve the efficiency of clinical testing of new agents. Thus it has been proposed that *prescreening* of patients for specific pathway abnormalities (e.g., HER2 amplification or PIK3CA mutation) as an entry criterion for clinical trial enrollment is the most effective way to conduct trials with specific inhibitors (e.g., lapatinib or new PI3K inhibitors, respectively) (43). Fewer patients would therefore need to be treated in order to demonstrate a treatment effect, and patients who are unlikely to respond can proceed directly to alternative options. While not all agree with the value of tumor profiling as prescreening for clinical trial enrollment, several trials with such design are currently being conducted, and their number is likely to increase in the future.

■ SUMMARY

- Gene expression profiling of primary breast cancers provides multiple insights into this disease. Expression profiles are capable of classifying breast cancers into biological subtypes, as well as providing prognostic and predictive information that complements standard clinical parameters.

- Although many different signatures have been developed, several have similar predictive power, which is associated with measurement of a common biological property of cellular proliferation.

- While the precise clinical utility of these signatures has not been tested in prospective clinical trials, such trials are under way and will help guide future application of these signatures.

- Challenges for the future include developing signatures that are predictive for specific therapies, particularly in *HER2+* and triple-negative subsets, and integrating DNA-based genomic and other molecular approaches to improve prognostication and therapeutic decision making.

■ REFERENCES

1. Gershon D. DNA microarrays: more than gene expression. *Nature.* 2005;437(7062):1195–1198.
2. Perou CM, Sorlie T, Eisen MB, et al. Molecular portraits of human breast tumours. *Nature.* 2000;406(6797):747–752.
3. Hu Z, Fan C, Oh DS, et al. The molecular portraits of breast tumors are conserved across microarray platforms. *BMC Genomics.* 2006; 7:96.
4. Sorlie T, Perou CM, Tibshirani R, et al. Gene expression patterns of breast carcinomas distinguish tumor subclasses with clinical implications. *Proc Natl Acad Sci USA.* 2001;98(19):10869–10874.
5. Sorlie T, Tibshirani R, Parker J, et al. Repeated observation of breast tumor subtypes in independent gene expression data sets. *Proc Natl Acad Sci USA.* 2003;100(14):8418–8423.
6. Sotiriou C, Neo SY, McShane LM, et al. Breast cancer classification and prognosis based on gene expression profiles from a population-based study. *Proc Natl Acad Sci USA.* 2003;100(18):10393–10398.
7. Fan C, Oh DS, Wessels L, et al. Concordance among gene-expression-based predictors for breast cancer. *New Engl J Med.* 2006;355(6):560–569.
8. Rakha EA, Elsheikh SE, Aleskandarany MA, et al. Triple-negative breast cancer: distinguishing between basal and nonbasal subtypes. *Clin Cancer Res.* 2009;15(7):2302–2310.

9. Desmedt C, Ruiz-Garcia E, Andre F. Gene expression predictors in breast cancer: current status, limitations and perspectives. *Eur J Cancer.* 2008;44(18):2714–2720.
10. van't Veer LJ, Dai H, van de Vijver MJ, et al. Gene expression profiling predicts clinical outcome of breast cancer. *Nature.* 2002; 415(6871):530–536.
11. Buyse M, Loi S, van't Veer L, et al. Validation and clinical utility of a 70-gene prognostic signature for women with node-negative breast cancer. *J Natl Cancer Inst.* 2006;98(17):1183–1192.
12. Ma XJ, Wang Z, Ryan PD, et al. A two-gene expression ratio predicts clinical outcome in breast cancer patients treated with tamoxifen. *Cancer Cell.* 2004;5(6):607–616.
13. Goetz MP, Suman VJ, Ingle JN, et al. A two-gene expression ratio of homeobox 13 and interleukin-17B receptor for prediction of recurrence and survival in women receiving adjuvant tamoxifen. *Clin Cancer Res.* 2006;12(7 Pt 1):2080–2087.
14. Ma XJ, Hilsenbeck SG, Wang W, et al. The HOXB13:IL17BR expression index is a prognostic factor in early-stage breast cancer. *J Clin Oncol.* 2006;24(28):4611–4619.
15. Ma XJ, Salunga R, Dahiya S, et al. A five-gene molecular grade index and HOXB13:IL17BR are complementary prognostic factors in early stage breast cancer. *Clin Cancer Res.* 2008;14(9):2601–2608.
16. Wang Z, Dahiya S, Provencher H, et al. The prognostic biomarkers HOXB13, IL17BR, and CHDH are regulated by estrogen in breast cancer. *Clin Cancer Res.* 2007;13(21):6327–6334.
17. Sotiriou C, Wirapati P, Loi S, et al. Gene expression profiling in breast cancer: understanding the molecular basis of histologic grade to improve prognosis. *J Natl Cancer Inst.* 2006;98(4):262–272.
18. Tordai A, Wang J, Andre F, et al. Evaluation of biological pathways involved in chemotherapy response in breast cancer. *Breast Cancer Res.* 2008;10(2):R37.
19. Oh DS, Troester MA, Usary J, et al. Estrogen-regulated genes predict survival in hormone receptor-positive breast cancers. *J Clin Oncol.* 2006;24(11):1656–1664.
20. Paik S, Shak S, Tang G, et al. A multigene assay to predict recurrence of tamoxifen-treated, node-negative breast cancer. *New Engl J Med.* 2004;351(27):2817–2826.
21. Paik S, Tang G, Shak S, et al. Gene expression and benefit of chemotherapy in women with node-negative, estrogen receptor-positive breast cancer. *J Clin Oncol.* 2006;24(23):3726–3734.
22. Sparano JA, Paik S. Development of the 21-gene assay and its application in clinical practice and clinical trials. *J Clin Oncol.* 2008;26(5):721–728.
23. Wang Y, Klijn JG, Zhang Y, et al. Gene-expression profiles to predict distant metastasis of lymph-node-negative primary breast cancer. *Lancet.* 2005;365(9460):671–679.
24. Haibe-Kains B, Desmedt C, Piette F, et al. Comparison of prognostic gene expression signatures for breast cancer. *BMC Genomics.* 2008;9:394.
25. Loi S, Haibe-Kains B, Desmedt C, et al. Definition of clinically distinct molecular subtypes in estrogen receptor-positive breast carcinomas through genomic grade. *J Clin Oncol.* 2007;25(10):1239–1246.
26. Hess KR, Anderson K, Symmans WF, et al. Pharmacogenomic predictor of sensitivity to preoperative chemotherapy with paclitaxel and fluorouracil, doxorubicin, and cyclophosphamide in breast cancer. *J Clin Oncol.* 2006;24(26):4236–4244.
27. Bonnefoi H, Potti A, Delorenzi M, et al. Validation of gene signatures that predict the response of breast cancer to neoadjuvant chemotherapy: a substudy of the EORTC 10994/BIG 00–01 clinical trial. *Lancet Oncol.* 2007;8(12):1071–1078.
28. Lee JK, Havaleshko DM, Cho H, et al. A strategy for predicting the chemosensitivity of human cancers and its application to drug discovery. *Proc Natl Acad Sci USA.* 2007;104(32):13086–13091.
29. Staunton JE, Slonim DK, Coller HA, et al. Chemosensitivity prediction by transcriptional profiling. *Proc Natl Acad Sci USA.* 2001;98(19):10787–10792.

30. Leong CO, Vidnovic N, DeYoung MP, Sgroi D, Ellisen LW. The p63/p73 network mediates chemosensitivity to cisplatin in a biologically defined subset of primary breast cancers. *J Clin Invest.* 2007;117(5):1370–1380.

31. Rocca A, Viale G, Gelber RD, et al. Pathologic complete remission rate after cisplatin-based primary chemotherapy in breast cancer: correlation with p63 expression. *Cancer Chemother Pharmacol.* 2008;61(6):965–971.

32. Schroth W, Antoniadou L, Fritz P, et al. Breast cancer treatment outcome with adjuvant tamoxifen relative to patient CYP2D6 and CYP2C19 genotypes. *J Clin Oncol.* 2007;25(33):5187–5193.

33. Higgins MJ, Rae JM, Flockhart DA, Hayes DF, Stearns V. Pharmacogenetics of tamoxifen: who should undergo CYP2D6 genetic testing? *J Natl Compr Canc Netw.* 2009;7(2):203–213.

34. Desmedt C, Haibe-Kains B, Wirapati P, et al. Biological processes associated with breast cancer clinical outcome depend on the molecular subtypes. *Clin Cancer Res.* 2008;14(16):5158–5165.

35. Wirapati P, Sotiriou C, Kunkel S, et al. Meta-analysis of gene expression profiles in breast cancer: toward a unified understanding of breast cancer subtyping and prognosis signatures. *Breast Cancer Res.* 2008;10(4):R65.

36. Dunkler D, Michiels S, Schemper M. Gene expression profiling: does it add predictive accuracy to clinical characteristics in cancer prognosis? *Eur J Cancer.* 2007;43(4):745–751.

37. Cardoso F, Van't Veer L, Rutgers E, Loi S, Mook S, Piccart-Gebhart MJ. Clinical application of the 70-gene profile: the MINDACT trial. *J Clin Oncol.* 2008;26(5):729–735.

38. Koscielny S. Critical review of microarray-based prognostic tests and trials in breast cancer. *Curr Opin Obstet Gynecol.* 2008; 20(1):47–50.

39. Hida T, Ogawa S, Park JC, et al. Gefitinib for the treatment of non-small-cell lung cancer. *Expert Rev Anticancer Ther.* 2009; 9(1):17–35.

40. McNeil C. K-Ras mutations are changing practice in advanced colorectal cancer. *J Natl Cancer Inst.* 2008;100(23):1667–1669.

41. Eichhorn PJ, Gili M, Scaltriti M, et al. Phosphatidylinositol 3-kinase hyperactivation results in lapatinib resistance that is reversed by the mTOR/phosphatidylinositol 3-kinase inhibitor NVP-BEZ235. *Cancer Res.* 2008;68(22):9221–9230.

42. Lai YL, Mau BL, Cheng WH, Chen HM, Chiu HH, Tzen CY. PIK3CA exon 20 mutation is independently associated with a poor prognosis in breast cancer patients. *Ann Surg Oncol.* 2008; 15(4):1064–1069.

43. Garber K. Trial offers early test case for personalized medicine. *J Natl Cancer Inst.* 2009;101(3):136–138.

Future Directions in Breast Cancer Clinical Trials

RACHEL A. FREEDMAN

ERIC P. WINER

Investigators launched the first modern clinical trials for patients with breast cancer more than five decades ago. Since that time, the nature and design of breast cancer research have evolved considerably. Many of the first studies focused on local therapy—surgery and radiation—and found that the use of less extensive surgery was feasible and as effective as more debilitating procedures. Importantly, these randomized trials altered the treatment approach that had been developed outside of controlled trials over the course of a half-century. Studies of systemic therapy also began almost 50 years ago, and these trials have evolved over time as our knowledge of breast cancer biology has advanced. Increasingly, trials in the twenty-first century are testing the use of targeted agents in highly selected patient populations. Indeed, one of the challenges we currently face is how to harmonize these new approaches with standards of treatment that have evolved from older studies.

As we consider the development of future trials, multidisciplinary management and correlative science will become progressively more important. Our goal should be to maximize what we can learn from each and every trial. Over the next decade, clinical trials should be based on biological principles and translational science, with the hope of enhancing treatment benefit and minimizing toxicity for selected patient populations. Through a combination of improved patient selection (based on both tumor and patient heterogeneity), the development of more effective targeted therapy, and more thoughtful trial design, we have the ability to transform breast cancer treatment in the next 10 to 20 years.

In this chapter, we will provide a brief historical overview of clinical trials in breast cancer as a basis for addressing the future directions of multidisciplinary and translational breast cancer research.

■ EVOLUTION OF CLINICAL TRIALS IN BREAST CANCER

A series of US Cooperative Group trials performed during the 1970s addressed primary local therapy. These trials examined the feasibility of performing less morbid surgery in women with early stage breast cancer. The National Surgical Adjuvant Breast and Bowel Project (NSABP) B-04 protocol demonstrated the equivalence of total mastectomy with radiation to radical mastectomy (1,2), and NSABP B-06 subsequently showed that breast-conserving surgery with radiation was equivalent to total mastectomy (3,4). The historical and practical significance of these trials cannot be overstated. Prior to these trials, the prevailing view of breast cancer was that dissemination occurred through regional lymphatics and that higher cure rates would be obtained by performing more radical surgery. Within a matter of years, these initial NSABP studies and others led to changes in surgical practice that resulted in far less morbidity for women with breast cancer. The studies suggested an alternative view of breast cancer dissemination and demonstrated the power of randomized trials and the effectiveness of multidisciplinary management.

The earliest systemic therapy trials evaluated the use of empirical single-agent chemotherapy. At that time, little was known about breast cancer biology, although it was well appreciated that women with operable breast cancer were at substantial risk of disease recurrence. The initial pioneering trialists used the best available tools in attempting to break new ground in breast cancer treatment. In the late 1950s, the first multicenter randomized breast cancer clinical trial was initiated by the NSABP and assessed the benefit of adding adjuvant triethylenethiophosphoramide (thiotepa) to radical mastectomy in 826 women (5). This trial demonstrated a progression-free survival (PFS) and overall survival (OS) benefit with postoperative thiotepa and set the stage for subsequent adjuvant therapy trials (5–7). Although anatomical extent of disease was appreciated as a risk factor for recurrence in these early studies, other prognostic factors were not fully appreciated. In particular, the role of estrogen and progesterone receptors in the treatment of breast cancer was not understood.

The next generation of adjuvant cytotoxic therapy trials included combination regimens that were limited to patients who were considered at high risk of disease recurrence on the basis of lymph node involvement. These initial landmark trials with postoperative oral cyclophosphamide in combination with intravenous methotrexate and 5-fluorouracil (CMF) demonstrated a significant disease-free survival (DFS) and OS advantage compared with observation and changed standard clinical practice (8). A second generation of clinical trials using the CMF backbone studied the optimal duration of therapy and also further confirmed the efficacy of this regimen in node-positive patients (9,10). The benefit of adjuvant systemic chemotherapy in node-negative women was eventually confirmed in the late 1980s and early 1990s (11–14).

The results of these node-negative trials led to recommendations for consideration of adjuvant chemotherapy in women with tumors larger than 1 cm regardless of nodal or receptor status (15).

Over the past 15 to 20 years, newer combination chemotherapy regimens have entered clinical practice, most notably anthracycline and anthracycline-taxane regimens. In these regimens, the anthracyclines and taxanes are given either concurrently or sequentially (16). Despite literally dozens of trials evaluating these agents, there are many unresolved questions about their optimal use. Perhaps the most important question is to elucidate which women derive relatively little benefit from these moderately toxic therapies and could be spared some or part of the treatment program. For example, recent data suggest that some women may be treated with non-anthracycline-containing regimens without sacrificing efficacy (17), but additional research is needed. It is sobering that there are, indeed, so many unanswered questions. This knowledge gap is partially a result of our expanding understanding of breast cancer biology and the growing recognition that clinical trials need to be limited to distinct biology subsets of the disease. However, the knowledge gap is also a direct consequence of some poorly designed trials and the failure, at times, to coordinate the questions that are being addressed in different trials.

■ UNDERSTANDING THE BENEFITS OF TREATMENT

As noted above, there are many questions about the relative and absolute benefits from chemotherapy in selected patient populations. Prognostic factors remain important, but there is even greater interest in predictive tests that can help determine whether a particular treatment is going to be effective in specific subgroups of patients. The recognition that breast cancer is a heterogeneous disease has been accompanied by a realization that the benefits of chemotherapy vary greatly across different subgroups of women.

Individual trials, particularly those conducted in the 1970s and 1980s, were often small and had insufficient power to answer conclusively the primary treatment question, let alone the impact of treatment on defined subsets of patients. Meta-analyses involving studies with many thousands of subjects have helped to extract important results from individual trials that were inadequately powered. The Early Breast Cancer Trialists' Collaborative Group (EBCTCG) was established in 1984–1985 (18). The EBCTCG's initial mission was to conduct international meta-analyses of centrally collected data from all randomized trials with at least five-year follow-up. The first publication was in 1988 (19), and updates have been published approximately every 5 years since the EBCTCG's inception. These analyses have served as powerful tools to assess the benefits of systemic therapy in defined subsets of women with breast cancer. The EBCTCG meta-analyses have examined data from dozens of trials and thousands of women and have provided critical insights into breast cancer treatment. Initially, the EBCTCG analyses were partially limited by the absence of consistent testing for estrogen receptor (ER) and human epidermal growth factor receptor 2 (HER2) in older studies. More recent efforts on the part of the EBCTCG have rectified these deficiencies. The collaboration has now focused a great deal of attention on the differential benefits of systemic treatments in women with ER-positive and ER-negative disease.

■ INCORPORATION OF TUMOR BIOLOGY AND TARGETED AGENTS

Although the initial characterization and isolation of the estrogen receptor occurred in the 1960s, its prognostic and therapeutic significance was not appreciated until much later (20). In fact, the presence of ER expression was not required for eligibility in the initial adjuvant and metastatic disease trials with tamoxifen and other endocrine therapies (21–23). It was not until the mid-1990s that endocrine therapy was unequivocally demonstrated to be ineffective in patients with hormone receptor–negative disease (24–26). Over time, endocrine therapy has become the cornerstone of treatment for essentially all hormone receptor–positive cancers, with broadened indications for premenopausal and postmenopausal patients as well as early stage disease. ER-directed therapy serves as the fundamental and first example of successful targeted therapy with limited toxicity. Although some investigators in the 1970s thought that ER-positive and ER-negative disease represented highly distinct entities (27–29), this view has become widely accepted only over the past several years.

More recently, our approach to adjuvant therapy in patients with ER-positive and ER-negative disease has diverged as we have come to understand that the benefits of adjuvant chemotherapy vary considerably across these two patient populations. Our latest challenge has focused on identifying the subgroup of patients with ER-positive disease who derive a considerable benefit from adjuvant chemotherapy, while sparing the remaining patients from the toxicity of treatment.

Our appreciation of breast cancer heterogeneity has now moved beyond a simple categorization of breast cancer subtype based on ER status. We now view breast cancer as a family of diseases, although it remains unclear how many distinct family members will be identified. Gene array analyses have revealed at least four or five intrinsic breast cancer subtypes, likely arising from at least two distinct cells of origin (30,31). Since clinicians do not perform gene array analysis to characterize breast cancers in routine practice, we commonly use a combination of hormone receptors (estrogen and progesterone) as well as HER2 status to divide tumors into distinct categories. Increasingly, a new generation of clinical trials is focused on these distinct subtypes. In some cases, additional biological classifiers, such as the 21-gene recurrence score (Oncotype DX) (32), the 70-gene prognosis signature (MammaPrint) (33), or predictors based on gene expression profiles, are incorporated into clinical trials. Finally, despite the emphasis on the biological features, tumor stage remains important from a prognostic standpoint and is critical both from the clinical perspective and in clinical decision making. Recent data suggest that both genomic profiles and clinical staging independently inform the assessment of risk of recurrence following primary surgical management.

Although we know that hormonal therapy significantly reduces the risk of recurrence for women with endocrine-sensitive disease, we have begun to understand that a spectrum of endocrine sensitivity exists. In recent years, previous characterizations of ER-positive tumors have been challenged by the observation that at least two subgroups, termed luminal A and B, exist, each with a distinct gene expression profile (31). Although the two subgroups likely differ in terms of response to both chemotherapy and endocrine therapy, our current endocrine therapy guidelines do not take into account these differences, nor is it fully clear how they should be incorporated into treatment recommendations. There is also growing evidence that a woman's ability to metabolize and respond to tamoxifen may depend on the presence of specific genetic polymorphisms of the CYP2D6 enzyme pathway (34–37).

There are still many questions about the optimal antiestrogen therapy and the duration of administration for both premenopausal and postmenopausal women. For premenopausal women, these questions have led to large international randomized trials to examine the worth of ovarian suppression and aromatase inhibitor therapy above that of tamoxifen (i.e., the Suppression of Ovarian Function Trial and the Tamoxifen and Exemestane Trial). The optimal duration and sequence of hormonal therapy in postmenopausal women is also under study, with examination of both duration and sequencing questions and strategies. One of the challenges in addressing these questions is that many women included in endocrine therapy trials are, fortunately, going to do extremely well as a result of early diagnosis and favorable tumor biology. As a result, thousands of women must be observed over an extended period of time before progression and survival questions can be adequately answered.

The ability of novel therapies to alter biological targets with less toxicity to normal tissues than traditional anticancer therapy is best represented by the identification of the HER2-positive breast cancer subtype. The treatment of HER2-positive disease represents a model that we hope to replicate many times over. The HER2/neu gene was discovered in 1983 (38), and its importance in breast cancer was elucidated by Slamon and colleagues in 1987 (39). The ability to identify HER2-positive breast cancers and, more important, to use targeted therapies directed against the HER2 protein has changed the natural history of this breast cancer subtype. Initial trials in the metastatic setting demonstrated the activity of trastuzumab in the treatment of HER2-positive disease (40,41). Multiple adjuvant trials have since confirmed the substantial efficacy in regards to recurrence and survival (42,43), and trastuzumab has now been incorporated into standard neoadjuvant, adjuvant, and metastatic treatment regimens. A new generation of HER2-directed therapies has since been under intense investigation, and this remains one of the most active areas of breast cancer research today. Lapatinib, the first of these agents to be commercially approved for patients with metastatic breast cancer, has already been incorporated into large adjuvant trials.

Unfortunately, a substantial minority of patients have a subtype of breast cancer referred to as triple-negative, because they neither express estrogen or progesterone receptors nor overexpress HER2. There is substantial but incomplete overlap between these triple-negative tumors and the basal-like cancers that have been identified on gene array analyses (30,31). Triple-negative tumors of the basal subtype tend to be aggressive and are typically of high histological grade. They are more common in younger women, and recent studies suggest that they are more common in the African American population, particularly among younger women (44). While these cancers can be highly sensitive to chemotherapy, they are associated with a higher risk of recurrence and a relatively short survival in the metastatic setting (45,46). The recognition of this subset of breast cancers and the appreciation of the poor overall outcome compared with other subgroups have stimulated ongoing interest in improving outcomes, especially given the lack of identifiable targeted therapies. Recent observations of the sensitivity of triple-negative tumors to platinum-based therapy (47) have led to multiple trials investigating these agents. There is also a great deal of interest in inhibitors of angiogenesis and, more recently, the potential role of poly (ADP-ribose) polymerase (PARP) inhibitors for this group of patients.

Inhibitors of vascular endothelial growth factor (VEGF) such as bevacizumab have shown activity in breast cancer and recently obtained Food and Drug Administration approval in metastatic breast cancer when administered with chemotherapy. The exact role of these targeted agents will be determined by future study. To examine the additional benefit these agents provide to standard chemotherapy and endocrine regimens, various VEGF inhibitors are now being incorporated into adjuvant and neoadjuvant trials for all breast cancer subtypes. Although these agents are promising additions to our systemic therapy armamentarium, elucidating which patient populations and breast cancer subtypes will benefit from novel therapies is critical, especially given their expense and potential toxicity.

■ CURRENT MODELS FOR MULTIDISCIPLINARY TRIALS

As our understanding of tumor biology has continued to evolve, current breast cancer clinical trial design has transitioned to incorporate more focused biological questions in women with specific subtypes of disease. In addition to clinical endpoints, current trials typically include correlative science endpoints. There is also an increased emphasis on quality of life, survivorship issues, adherence, and patterns of care. While complex trials can be challenging for both the study team and the participant, the goal is to maximize what can be achieved with each and every trial.

Many multidisciplinary programs are investing a great deal of effort implementing novel clinical trials that take advantage of treatment in the preoperative setting. In clinical practice, the use of preoperative therapy for women with operable breast cancer has become quite common, offering the opportunity to perform a variety of correlative scientific studies. Randomization between preoperative and postoperative chemotherapy has demonstrated equivalent DFS and OS in one major US trial (48). Outside of a clinical trial, however, the primary advantage of preoperative therapy is that it can increase the proportion of women who can undergo conservative surgery. Within the context of clinical trials, preoperative therapy offers a number of clear advantages, including (a) the ability to assess in vivo response, (b) the possibility to obtain serial tissue samples, and (c) the potential to answer therapeutic questions with a smaller number of study participants. Preoperative research can advance our understanding of resistance mechanisms, pharmacogenomics, and a range of correlative questions, all of which have the potential to accelerate our progress in breast cancer research. By definition, preoperative clinical trials require multidisciplinary involvement and a high level of communication between the multiple specialists in many disciplines who care for women with breast cancer.

Cancer and Leukemia Group B (CALGB) protocol 40601 illustrates many of the principles described above. This trial involves the use of preoperative therapy with paclitaxel in conjunction with either (a) trastuzumab, (b) trastuzumab with lapatinib, or (c) lapatinib, followed by surgery and adjuvant chemotherapy. This study will not only test practical applications of *HER2*-directed therapy but also contains multiple, correlative studies of biological and predictive markers as well as surgical practice pattern analysis. A similar design is also planned with the upcoming CALGB 40603 protocol in triple-negative patients, which utilizes a 2 × 2 factorial trial examining the addition of carboplatin or bevacizumab, or both, to neoadjuvant paclitaxel followed by surgery and adjuvant chemotherapy. In both cases, the trials are focused on a defined subset of patients with incorporation of biologically driven targeted therapies. Multiple correlative questions are also embedded in each trial. These analyses have the potential to characterize the biological diversity that exists within breast cancer subtypes, which will have to be considered as we move forward with the next generation of targeted therapy trials. Within the CALGB and other cooperative groups, the opportunity to study surgical patterns of care in the setting of preoperative treatment now presents itself as well.

■ FUTURE DIRECTIONS

There is great excitement about our expanding understanding of breast cancer biology and the range of biological therapies that will be available in the years ahead. On the one hand, we need to ensure that future trials are designed with both thought and precision, taking advantage of all opportunities and disciplines to answer relevant questions. To accomplish this goal, studies must be designed with broad input from a multidisciplinary group of physicians, scientists, statisticians, and advocates. On the other hand, we need to move the process forward with appropriate haste, since unnecessary delays slow progress and may ultimately cost lives. These concerns are of even greater relevance given the challenges in research funding over the past several years. As National Institutes of Health funding has become more competitive, industry-sponsored trials have grown in number and breadth. As a result, partnerships that involve academia, federal agencies, and pharmaceutical researchers are more important than ever before in order to ensure that proper priority is assigned to the most crucial and pressing questions.

Over the past decades, significant advances have been made in the treatment of breast cancer. Clinical trials have brought us to where we are today, and they will continue to move the field forward. As we transition into the next generation of clinical trials, we must build on this knowledge base. Importantly, we must work to avoid both overtreatment and undertreatment. There are clearly patients who need more effective therapy, and there are others who would do well with less treatment (and fewer side effects) than they presently endure. Trials that involve minimizing treatment are often complex to design but in many ways are as important as trials that seek to include additional therapies. Ultimately, the goal is to personalize breast cancer treatment such that each patient receives the necessary treatment without having to undergo more than is necessary. We must also be cognizant that while clinical trials provide invaluable data to inform treatment decisions, careful poststudy observation in clinical practice and review of long-term toxicities and outcomes will continue to be critical in guiding treatment decisions.

As we attempt to design trials to minimize toxicity and increase efficacy, several additional concerns must be addressed. First, trials must enroll a diverse group of patients who represent the broad spectrum of patients with breast cancer. Too often, clinical trials of the past have inadvertently excluded patients who were of advanced age or were members of racial and ethnic minorities, leaving unanswered questions in these populations. In addition, clinical investigators need to consider how the results of treatment studies will be disseminated and implemented outside of trials. With the growing cost of medical care and the extraordinary costs of the new generation of targeted therapy, economic considerations cannot be ignored. Our society as well as others around the world does not have unending resources, and thus cost-effectiveness is now crucially important to consider. It is inevitable that government and insurance providers will need to implement restrictions on the use of expensive therapies. Expensive treatments that provide minimal benefit will ultimately be replaced by more cost-effective approaches.

The future is bright. There is, however, much work to be done. Breast cancer clinicians, investigators, and advocates need to work closely together to develop treatment approaches that will result in improved disease outcomes and less toxicity. Progress will require insight, hard work, collaboration, commitment, and a willingness to take bold steps. Finally, we must all be advocates for research funding, since without the necessary financial resources, progress, or at least rapid progress, cannot occur.

■ SUMMARY

- Over the past decades, significant advances have been made in the treatment of breast cancer.
- Current breast cancer clinical trial design has transitioned to incorporate more focused biological questions in women with specific subtypes of disease.
- As we consider the development of future trials, multidisciplinary management and correlative science will become progressively more important.
- Through a combination of improved patient selection (based on both tumor and patient heterogeneity), the development of more effective targeted therapy, and more thoughtful trial design, we have the ability to transform breast cancer treatment in the next 10 to 20 years.

■ REFERENCES

1. Fisher B, Montague E, Redmond C, et al. Comparison of radical mastectomy with alternative treatments for primary breast cancer. A first report of results from a prospective randomized clinical trial. *Cancer.* 1977;39(6 Suppl):2827–2839.
2. Fisher B, Redmond C, Fisher ER, et al. Ten-year results of a randomized clinical trial comparing radical mastectomy and total mastectomy with or without radiation. *New Engl J Med.* 1985; 312(11):674–681.
3. Fisher B, Anderson S, Bryant J, et al. Twenty-year follow-up of a randomized trial comparing total mastectomy, lumpectomy, and lumpectomy plus irradiation for the treatment of invasive breast cancer. *New Engl J Med.* 2002;347(16):1233–1241.
4. Fisher B, Bauer M, Margolese R, et al. Five-year results of a randomized clinical trial comparing total mastectomy and segmental mastectomy with or without radiation in the treatment of breast cancer. *New Engl J Med.* 1985;312(11):665–673.
5. Fisher B, Slack N, Katrych D, Wolmark N. Ten year follow-up results of patients with carcinoma of the breast in a co-operative clinical trial evaluating surgical adjuvant chemotherapy. *Surg Gynecol Obstet.* 1975;140(4):528–534.
6. Fisher B, Ravdin RG, Ausman RK, Slack NH, Moore GE, Noer RJ. Surgical adjuvant chemotherapy in cancer of the breast: results of a decade of cooperative investigation. *Ann Surg.* 1968; 168(3):337–356.
7. Fisher B, Redmond C, Fisher ER, Wolmark N. Systemic adjuvant therapy in treatment of primary operable breast cancer: National Surgical Adjuvant Breast and Bowel Project experience. *NCI Monogr.* 1986(1):35–43.
8. Bonadonna G, Brusamolino E, Valagussa P, et al. Combination chemotherapy as an adjuvant treatment in operable breast cancer. *New Engl J Med.* 1976;294(8):405–410.
9. Bonadonna G, Moliterni A, Zambetti M, et al. 30 years' follow up of randomised studies of adjuvant CMF in operable breast cancer: cohort study. *Br Med J.* 2005;330(7485):217.
10. Tancini G, Bonadonna G, Valagussa P, Marchini S, Veronesi U. Adjuvant CMF in breast cancer: comparative 5-year results of 12 versus 6 cycles. *J Clin Oncol.* 1983;1(1):2–10.
11. Fisher B, Dignam J, Mamounas EP, et al. Sequential methotrexate and fluorouracil for the treatment of node-negative breast cancer patients with estrogen receptor-negative tumors: eight-year results from National Surgical Adjuvant Breast and Bowel Project (NSABP) B-13 and first report of findings from NSABP B-19 comparing methotrexate and fluorouracil with conventional cyclophosphamide, methotrexate, and fluorouracil. *J Clin Oncol.* 1996;14(7):1982–1992.
12. Fisher B, Dignam J, Wolmark N, et al. Tamoxifen and chemotherapy for lymph node-negative, estrogen receptor-positive breast cancer. *J Natl Cancer Inst.* 1997;89(22):1673–1682.
13. Fisher B, Jeong JH, Dignam J, et al. Findings from recent National Surgical Adjuvant Breast and Bowel Project adjuvant studies in stage I breast cancer. *J Natl Cancer Inst Monogr.* 2001(30): 62–66.
14. Mansour EG, Gray R, Shatila AH, et al. Survival advantage of adjuvant chemotherapy in high-risk node-negative breast cancer: ten-year analysis—an intergroup study. *J Clin Oncol.* 1998; 16(11):3486–3492.
15. Eifel P, Axelson JA, Costa J, et al. National Institutes of Health Consensus Development Conference Statement: adjuvant therapy for breast cancer, November 1–3, 2000. *J Natl Cancer Inst.* 2001;93(13):979–989.
16. Citron ML, Berry DA, Cirrincione C, et al. Randomized trial of dose-dense versus conventionally scheduled and sequential versus concurrent combination chemotherapy as postoperative adjuvant treatment of node-positive primary breast cancer: first report of Intergroup Trial C9741/Cancer and Leukemia Group B Trial 9741. *J Clin Oncol.* 2003;21(8):1431–1439.

17. Slamon DJ, Mackey J, Robert N, et al. Cancer International Research Group (CIRG), Emonton, AB, Canada. Role of anthracycline-based therapy in the adjuvant treatment of breast cancer: efficacy analyses determined by molecular subtypes of the disease. Presented at the 30th Annual San Antonio Breast Cancer Symposium, San Antonio, Texas, December 13–16, 2007 (Abstract 13).

18. Review of mortality results in randomised trials in early breast cancer. *Lancet.* 1984;2(8413):1205.

19. Early Breast Cancer Trialists' Collaborative Group. Effects of adjuvant tamoxifen and of cytotoxic therapy on mortality in early breast cancer. An overview of 61 randomized trials among 28,896 women. Early Breast Cancer Trialists' Collaborative Group. *New Engl J Med.* 1988;319(26):1681–1692.

20. DeSombre ER. Estrogens, receptors and cancer: the scientific contributions of Elwood Jensen. *Prog Clin Biol Res.* 1990;322:17–29.

21. Cole MP, Jones CT, Todd ID. A new anti-oestrogenic agent in late breast cancer. An early clinical appraisal of ICI46474. *Br J Cancer.* 1971;25(2):270–275.

22. Lerner HJ, Band PR, Israel L, Leung BS. Phase II study of tamoxifen: report of 74 patients with stage IV breast cancer. *Cancer Treat Rep.* 1976;60(10):1431–1435.

23. Ward HW. Anti-oestrogen therapy for breast cancer: a trial of tamoxifen at two dose levels. *Br Med J.* 1973;1(5844):13–14.

24. Fisher B, Anderson S, Tan-Chiu E, et al. Tamoxifen and chemotherapy for axillary node-negative, estrogen receptor-negative breast cancer: findings from National Surgical Adjuvant Breast and Bowel Project B-23. *J Clin Oncol.* 2001;19(4):931–942.

25. Hutchins LF, Green SJ, Ravdin PM, et al. Randomized, controlled trial of cyclophosphamide, methotrexate, and fluorouracil versus cyclophosphamide, doxorubicin, and fluorouracil with and without tamoxifen for high-risk, node-negative breast cancer: treatment results of Intergroup Protocol INT-0102. *J Clin Oncol.* 2005;23(33):8313–8321.

26. Early Breast Cancer Trialists' Collaborative Group. Tamoxifen for early breast cancer: an overview of the randomised trials. *Lancet.* 1998;351(9114):1451–1467.

27. Lippman M, Bolan G, Huff K. The effects of estrogens and antiestrogens on hormone-responsive human breast cancer in long-term tissue culture. *Cancer Res.* 1976;36(12):4595–4601.

28. Lippman ME, Allegra JC, Thompson EB, et al. The relation between estrogen receptors and response rate to cytotoxic chemotherapy in metastatic breast cancer. *New Engl J Med.* 1978;298(22):1223–1228.

29. Lippman ME, Allegra JC. Quantitative estrogen receptor analyses: the response to endocrine and cytotoxic chemotherapy in human breast cancer and the disease-free interval. *Cancer.* 1980;46(12 Suppl):2829–2834.

30. Perou CM, Sorlie T, Eisen MB, et al. Molecular portraits of human breast tumours. *Nature.* 2000;406(6797):747–752.

31. Sorlie T, Perou CM, Tibshirani R, et al. Gene expression patterns of breast carcinomas distinguish tumor subclasses with clinical implications. *Proc Natl Acad Sci USA.* 2001;98(19):10869–10874.

32. Paik S, Shak S, Tang G, et al. A multigene assay to predict recurrence of tamoxifen-treated, node-negative breast cancer. *New Engl J Med.* 2004;351(27):2817–2826.

33. van 't Veer L, Dai H, van de Vijver M, et al. Gene expression profiling predicts clinical outcome of breast cancer. *Nature.* 2002;415(6871):530–536.

34. Borges S, Desta Z, Li L, et al. Quantitative effect of CYP2D6 genotype and inhibitors on tamoxifen metabolism: implication for optimization of breast cancer treatment. *Clin Pharmacol Ther.* 2006;80(1):61–74.

35. Lim HS, Ju Lee H, Seok Lee K, Sook Lee E, Jang IJ, Ro J. Clinical implications of CYP2D6 genotypes predictive of tamoxifen pharmacokinetics in metastatic breast cancer. *J Clin Oncol.* 2007;25(25):3837–3845.

36. Sachse C, Brockmoller J, Hildebrand M, Muller K, Roots I. Correctness of prediction of the CYP2D6 phenotype confirmed by genotyping 47 intermediate and poor metabolizers of debrisoquine. *Pharmacogenetics.* 1998;8(2):181–185.

37. Stearns V, Johnson MD, Rae JM, et al. Active tamoxifen metabolite plasma concentrations after coadministration of tamoxifen and the selective serotonin reuptake inhibitor paroxetine. *J Natl Cancer Inst.* 2003;95(23):1758–1764.

38. Schechter AL, Stern DF, Vaidyanathan L, et al. The neu oncogene: an erb-B-related gene encoding a 185,000-Mr tumour antigen. *Nature.* 1984;312(5994):513–516.

39. Slamon DJ, Clark GM, Wong SG, Levin WJ, Ullrich A, McGuire WL. Human breast cancer: correlation of relapse and survival with amplification of the HER-2/neu oncogene. *Science.* 1987;235(4785):177–182.

40. Slamon DJ, Leyland-Jones B, Shak S, et al. Use of chemotherapy plus a monoclonal antibody against HER2 for metastatic breast cancer that overexpresses HER2. *New Engl J Med.* 2001;344(11):783–792.

41. Vogel C, Cobleigh MA, Tripathy D, et al. First-line, single-agent Herceptin (trastuzumab) in metastatic breast cancer: a preliminary report. *Eur J Cancer.* 2001;37(Suppl 1):S25–S29.

42. Piccart-Gebhart MJ, Procter M, Leyland-Jones B, et al. Trastuzumab after adjuvant chemotherapy in HER2-positive breast cancer. *New Engl J Med.* 2005;353(16):1659–1672.

43. Romond EH, Perez EA, Bryant J, et al. Trastuzumab plus adjuvant chemotherapy for operable HER2-positive breast cancer. *New Engl J Med.* 2005;353(16):1673–1684.

44. Carey LA, Perou CM, Livasy CA, et al. Race, breast cancer subtypes, and survival in the Carolina Breast Cancer Study. *JAMA.* 2006;295(21):2492–2502.

45. Early Breast Cancer Trialists' Collaborative Group. Effects of chemotherapy and hormonal therapy for early breast cancer on recurrence and 15-year survival: an overview of the randomised trials. *Lancet.* 2005;365(9472):1687–1717.

46. Haffty BG, Yang Q, Reiss M, et al. Locoregional relapse and distant metastasis in conservatively managed triple negative early-stage breast cancer. *J Clin Oncol.* 2006;24(36):5652–5657.

47. Tassone P, Tagliaferri P, Perricelli A, et al. BRCA1 expression modulates chemosensitivity of BRCA1-defective HCC1937 human breast cancer cells. *Br J Cancer.* 2003;88(8):1285–1291.

48. Fisher B, Bryant J, Wolmark N, et al. Effect of preoperative chemotherapy on the outcome of women with operable breast cancer. *J Clin Oncol.* 1998;16(8):2672–2685.

Index

Abdominal tissue-based breast
    reconstruction, 180–182
Accelerated partial breast irradiation
    (APBI), 105, 303–304
Access, in multidisciplinary program, 40
Access nurse, 38
Acellular dermal sheet, 179
ACRIN 6666 trial, 33
Adjuvant chemotherapy
    anthracycline-based therapy, 136
    benefit, 136
    dose density, 138
    patient selection, 138–139
    taxane-containing regimens, 136–138
Adjuvant endocrine therapy
    clinical investigations of, 135
    postmenopausal women, 133–135
    premenopausal women, 132–133
Adjuvant!Online, 139
Adjuvant therapy
    extended using tamoxifen, 308
    locally advanced breast cancer
        (LABC), 170
    NCIC MA.17 trial, 308–312
    ongoing trials, 312
    recurrence risk and need for
        extended, 308
Adjuvant Zoledronic Acid to Reduce
    Recurrence (AZURE) trial, 141
Adriamycin, 243
Alprazolam, 274
American College of Radiology
    (ACR), 18
American College of Radiology Imaging
    Network (ACRIN), 24
Anastrozole, 89, 114
Anastrozole (Arimidex), 209
Ancillary tests, 50
Antidepressants, 271–273
Anxiety disorders, in breast cancer
    patients. See Psychiatric issues,
    in breast cancer
ARCOSEIN trial, 126
Aromatase inhibitors, 89
Aromatase inhibitors (AIs), 133
Atypical ductal hyperplasia (ADH),
    33, 57
    in biopsy specimens, 88–89
    incidence, 83

laterality of subsequent breast cancer,
    85–86
    risk of breast cancer, 83–84
    risk parameters, 84–85
    surgical management, 86
    time course, 85
Atypical lobular hyperplasia (ALH), 33
    in biopsy specimens, 88–89
    incidence, 83
    laterality of subsequent breast
        cancer, 85–86
    risk of breast cancer, 83–84
    risk parameters, 84–85
    surgical management, 86
    time course, 85
Austrian Breast & Colorectal Cancer
    Study Group (ABCSG)–12
    trials, 135
Axilla, surgical management of
    axillary dissection, 122
    in elderly, 122
    sentinel node biopsy, 121–122
        eligibility, 122
    surgical staging of the axilla, 117
Axillary lymph nodes, pathological
    assessment of, 58
Axillary tail, 52

Benign breast lesions, 60
Benzodiazepines, 273–274
Bevacizumab, 141
Biases, in mammography sampling
    lead-time, 25
    length, 25
    overdiagnosis and
        "pseudodisease," 25
    selection, 25–26
Biopsy technique
    cysts, 44
    and failure to identify, 42
    multidisciplinary considerations, 47
    percutaneous
        advantages, 41
        fine-needle aspiration, 41
        management considerations, 45–47
        MRI-guided core needle, 45
        of palpable breast lesions, 41

preprocedural evaluation, 41
    stereotactic core needle, 42–44
    ultrasound-guided core needle, 44
specimen orientation, 47
specimen radiography, 43, 47
surgical
    considerations, 47
    indications, 47
    needle localization and
        surgical excision, 47
Bisphosphonates, 141
Bone metastases, 202–203
Brain metastases, 204–205
BRCA1 and BRCA2 gene mutation, 32
BRCA1 and BRCA2 mutations, 3–4
    male BRCA mutation carriers, 11
    NCCN guidelines, 11
    probability of detecting, 4
    techniques, 8
    timing of testing, 8–9
BRCA2-associated breast cancers, 9–10
BRCA2 999del5 mutation,
    in Iceland, 10
BRCA2 6174delT mutation, 10
BRCAPRO model, of identifying
    BRCA mutation, 4
BRCA1-related breast cancers, 9–10
Breast cancer-specific mortality, 1
Breast cancer treatment, evolution, 1
Breast conservation, eligibility for
    margins, 118
    nodal status, 118
    patient preference issues, 119
    preoperative imaging, 118–119
    risk factors, 118
    tumor size, 117–118
Breast-conserving surgery (BCS),
    100–101
    oncoplastic approaches, 293–294
Breast-conserving therapy (BCT),
    100–101
Breast density, 23
Breast Imaging Reporting and Data
    System (BIRADS), 20–23
Breast oncology, 1
Breast reconstruction
    abdominal tissue-based
        reconstruction, 180–182
    adjuvant radiation therapy, 184–185

[Breast reconstruction]
 autologous flap reconstructive
  techniques, 191–192
 chemotherapy, 184
 disadvantages of the two-stage
  implant reconstruction, 179
 effect of reconstruction on radiation
  technique, 193
 free-flap, 182–183
 general considerations
  aspects of the mastectomy
   operation, 178
  autologous flap complications, 178
  frequency of operations, 178
  patient factors and risk profiles, 177
  patient's BMI, 177–178
  tobacco use, 177
 latissimus dorsi musculocutaneous
  flap, 183
 minimizing deleterious interactions
  between radiotherapy and
  reconstructive surgery, 193
 mixed prosthesis/flap reconstructive
  techniques, 192
 multidisciplinary considerations, 185
 nipple reconstruction, 185
 preferred patient for a single-stage
  implant reconstruction, 179–180
 prosthesis-based methods,
  178–180, 191
 risk of complications after
  reconstruction, 192–193
 symmetry procedures, 185
 timing, 183–184
Breast self-examination (BSE), 31
Breast-specific gamma imaging, 292
Breast tomosynthesis, 291
Bupropion, 71

CALGB 9741, 136–138
CALGB 9344 (anthracycline), 138
Cancer and Leukemia Group B
 (CALGB) 9344 trial, 167
Cancer and Leukemia Study Group B
 (CALGB) study, 236
Cancer genetics professional, 5
Cardiomyopathy, 2
CA-125 technique, 11
CDH1 mutation, 4
Chemotherapy-related amenorrhea
 (CRA), 77
Claus model of risk prediction, 3–4
Clinical Laboratory Improvement
 Amendments (CLIA), 7
Clinical testing laboratories, in
 United States, 7
Clinical trials, for breast cancer
 benefits, 323
 evolution, 322–323
 future directions, 325–326

incorporation of tumor biology and
 targeted agents, 323–325
 models, 325
Cognitive behavioral
 therapy (CBT), 271
Colloid carcinoma, 55
Community-based care, of breast cancer
 patients
 axillary lymph node dissection
  (ALND), 283
 economics, 287
 growth of partial breast
  irradiation, 284
 mortality rate, 283
 radiation oncology, 284
 role of multidisciplinary clinics
  ASCO guidelines, 284–285
  breast navigator, 285
  in coordinating care, 284–285
  National Cancer Center Network
   (NCCN) guidelines, 285
  in promoting quality, 285–287
  referral to, 285
  St. Gallen guidelines, 285
  use of breast navigator, 285
  vs in academic settings, 284
Community Clinical Oncology Program
 (CCOP), 287
Contralateral breast cancer, risk of
 a, 10
Core biopsies, of breast, 51
Cowden's syndrome (CS), 12–13, 32
 trichilemmomas with, 6
Cryoablation, 291
Cyclophosphamide, 73, 77, 156
Cyclophosphamide (AC), 136
Cyclophosphamide (TC), 136
Cytochrome 3A inducers, 275
Cytotoxic chemotherapy, 135
Cytoxan (AC), 243
Cytoxan (TAC), 243

Danish Breast Cancer Cooperative
 Group trial, 156
Deep inferior epigastric perforator
 (DIEP) flap, 192
Depression, in breast cancer patients.
 See Psychiatric issues, in breast
 cancer
Digital breast tomosynthesis (DBT), 34
Digital Mammographic Imaging
 Screening Trial (DMIST), 24
Digital mammography, 23–24
Diphenhydramine, 71
Directional vacuum-assisted biopsy
 (DVAB) device, 43–44
Disease-free survival (DFS), 132
Distant metastases, detection of, 55–56
Docetaxel, 136
Doxorubicin, 73, 136

Ductal carcinoma in situ
 adjuvant medical treatment for, 112
 detection, 111
 diagnosis, 93
 histological study of, 56
 incidence and natural history, 93
 lumpectomy vs mastectomy, 94
  margins on lumpectomy, 94–95
  nipple-sparing mastectomy, 96
  skin-sparing mastectomy, 95–96
  total mastectomy, 95
 multidisciplinary considerations, 96
 multidisciplinary treatment of, 114
 natural history of, 111
 pathological classification of, 99
 radiation treatments
  accelerated partial breast
   irradiation (APBI), 105
  clinical presentation, 99–100
  dose and fractionation, 104–105
  epidemiology and risk factors, 99
  hormonal therapy, 105–107
  importance of surgical
   margins, 103
  management, 100–103
  multidisciplinary approach, 107
  pathology factors, 99
  screening mammography, 99–100
  side effects, 105
  for whole breast radiation
   therapy, 104
 risk factors, 111
 risk of recurrence, 111
 sentinel lymph node biopsy for, 96
 surgical treatment options, 93
 Surveillance, Epidemiology and End
  Results (SEER) database
  reviews, 93
Duloxetine, 274

Early breast cancer, treatment of
 eligibility for breast conservation,
  117–119
 lumpectomy treatment
  considerations, 120
  incision placement, 119
  oncoplastic approaches, 120
  specimen orientation, 119–120
 lumpectomy vs mastectomy, 117
 mastectomy treatment of
  efficacy of skin-sparing
   mastectomy, 121
  electron intraoperative therapy
   (ELIOT), 121
  extent of breast tissue removed, 120
  and immediate reconstruction, 120
  with immediate reconstruction,
   120–121
  nipple-sparing mastectomy, 121
  technical considerations, 120

[Early breast cancer, treatment of]
    multidisciplinary considerations,
        122–123
    perioperative considerations, 122
    surgical management of the axilla,
        121–122
Early Breast Cancer Trialists'
    Collaborative Group (EBCTCG)
    meta-analysis, 126, 153
Early Breast Cancer Trialists'
    Collaborative Group (EBCTCG)
    meta-analysis, 132
Eastern Cooperative Oncology Group
    trial (ECOG 5194), 103, 201
E-cadherin, by
    immunohistochemistry, 57
E-cadherin gene (CDH1), 13
ECOG 5103 trial, 141
Education and information resources, in
    multidisciplinary program, 40
Endocrine therapy, 132
Estrogen receptor-positive
    breast cancer, 2
European Organisation for Research
    and Treatment of Cancer
    (EORTC) 10853 trial, 101
Everolimus (Certican), 216
Excisional biopsy, 52
Exemestane (Aromasin), 209

Family history, as screening modality, 6
Fanconi's anemia, 11
Fibroadenomas, pathological assessment
    of, 57–58
Fine-needle aspiration techniques,
    41, 72–73
Fluorodeoxyglucose-positron emission
    tomography staging, of
    the axilla, 293
Fluoroquinolones, 274
5-fluorouracil, 77
Fluorouracil (CMF) plus
    irradiation, 156
Fluoxetine, 71
Follow-up care, longitudinal, 2
Formalin fixation, 52
Fulvestrant, 209

Gadolinium-enhanced breast
    MRIs, 31
Gail model of risk prediction, 3–4, 89
Gene profiling
    "bottom-up" profiling, 317
    comparison of prognostic signatures,
        317–318
        clinical applications, 318–319
        in predicting adjuvant
            chemotherapy, 318

integration of molecular profiling
    techniques with targeted therapy,
    319–320
technical aspects, 315
"top-down" strategy, 316–317
unsupervised clustering for
    classification, 315–316
Genetic counseling and risk
    assessment, 5–6
    criteria for referral to a genetics
        professional, 5
Genetic testing process, 6–8
    American Society of Clinical
        Oncology (ASCO)
        recommendations, 6
    for APC mutations, 5
    clinical testing laboratories, 7
    importance of maintaining
        communication between the
        health care provider and the
        patient, 8
    magnetic resonance imaging (MRI)
        screening, 11
    timing, 8–9
    turnaround time for, 7–8
Genomic profiling of tumors, 1–2
German Breast Cancer Study
    Group-Gynecological Adjuvant
    Study Group Germany
    (GBSG-GABGG) trial, 244
GnRH-a, 79

HER2+ breast cancer treatment,
    139–141
Hereditary breast and ovarian cancer
    syndrome (HBOCS), 9–11
Hereditary breast cancer syndromes
    Cowden's syndrome (CS), 12–13
    hereditary breast and ovarian cancer
        syndrome (HBOCS), 9–11
    hereditary diffuse gastric carcinoma
        syndrome (HDGCS), 13–14
    Li-Fraumeni syndrome (LFS), 11–12
Hereditary diffuse gastric carcinoma
    syndrome (HDGCS), 13–14
HER2/neu amplification, 1
HER2-positive breast cancer, treatment,
    169
HER-2 profiles, of breast cancers,
    58–59
High-risk patients, identification
    breast cancer of 2.0, 10
    empirical models of prediction, 3–4
    genetic counseling and risk
        assessment, 5–6
    genetic testing process, 6–8
    timing, 8–9
    hereditary breast cancer syndromes
        Cowden's syndrome (CS), 12–13
[High-risk patients, identification]

hereditary breast and ovarian
    cancer syndrome (HBOCS), 9–11
hereditary diffuse gastric carcinoma
    syndrome (HDGCS), 13–14
Li-Fraumeni syndrome (LFS), 11–12
of individuals, 5
informed consent, 8
in Jewish women, 10–11
lifetime risk, 10
likelihood of risk, 3
moderate-risk alleles, 10
setting up of risk assessment
    criteria, 5
Hodgkin's disease, 2
Hodgkin's lymphoma, 32
HOPES program, 65
Hormonal therapy. See Adjuvant
    therapy
Hormone receptor studies, of breast
    cancers, 58–59
Hypnotic drugs, 274
Hypofractionation, 104–105
    use in whole breast radiation,
        302–303

Integrated breast cancer care program,
    development of an, 65
Intensity-modulated proton therapy
    (IMPT), 300
International Breast Cancer Intervention
    Study (IBIS)-II trial, 89
International Breast Cancer
    Study Group (IBCSG)
    trials V and VI, 77
Intracystic papillary carcinomas, 55
Invasive breast carcinoma, histological
    tumor grade for, 53–54
Invasive lobular carcinoma,
    histological differentiation
    of, 55
I-SPY trial, 175

Lagios criteria, for tumors, 111
Laser ablation technique, 291
Leptomeningeal metastases, 205
Lesions, warranting special
    consideration
    atypical ductal hyperplasia
        (ADH), 46
    chemoprevention, 89
    lobular neoplasia, 46
    papillary lesions, 46
    radial scars, 46–47
Letrozole, 209, 311
Letrozole (Femara), 209
Letrozole 024 study, 175
Li-Fraumeni-like syndrome (LFLS), 11
Li-Fraumeni syndrome (LFS), 11–12, 32

Lobular carcinoma in situ (LCIS), 33
  in biopsy specimens, 88–89
  incidence, 86
  laterality of developing breast
      cancer, 87
  risk of breast cancer, 87
  surgical management, 87–88
  time course, 87
Lobular carcinomas, histological
      differentiation of, 55
Lobular neoplasia, 46, 57
Locally advanced breast cancer (LABC)
  adjuvant therapy, 170
  chemotherapy
      endocrine receptor-positive/HER2-
          negative breast cancer, 168–169
      HER2-positive breast cancer, 169
      triple-negative breast cancer, 169
  diagnosis and staging evaluation, 165
  endocrine-responsive tumors, therapy
      for, 170–171
  follow-up and recurrent disease, 171
  inflammatory breast cancer,
      treatment of, 169–170
  neoadjuvant chemotherapy, 166–167
  polychemotherapy, 167
  translational studies in, 174–176
  treatment overview, 165–166
Locally recurrent disease,
      management of
  axillary recurrence, 233
  in the BRCA1 and BRCA2 gene
      mutation carriers, 236
  breast-conserving therapy (BCT), 229
  chest wall recurrence, 233
  considerations for medical
      oncologist, 241
  of DCIS, 235
  in the elderly, 235–236
  heterogeneity of prognosis of
      patients, 242
  importance of distinguishing a true
      recurrence from a second primary
      cancer, 243–244
  ipsilateral breast tumor recurrences
      (IBTRs), 229–233, 240
  multidisciplinary approach, 236–237
  NCCN recommendations, 229
  in the previously irradiated
      breast, 230–233
  in the previously nonirradiated
      breast, 230
  prognostic significance of, 240
  role of systemic therapy, 240–241
      clinical trials and future prospects,
          244–245
      in individual patient, 242–243
      suggested guidelines, 244
  sentinel node biopsy for, 233–235
Low grade precursor lesions, 57
Lumpectomy treatment, 52
  of early breast cancer

  considerations, 120
  incision placement, 119
  oncoplastic approaches, 120
  specimen orientation, 119–120
Lymphedema, evaluation and treatment
  Avon Foundation Comprehensive
      Breast Evaluation Center
      information sheet, 262
  definition and measurement, 258–259
  management
      complex decongestive therapy
          (CDT) approach, 263
      compression strategies, 264–265
      manual lymphatic drainage, 265
      role of exercise, 264
      skin care, 263–264
  monitoring of, 261
  multidisciplinary approach, 260
      implementation, 265–266
  risk factors and incidence, 259–260
  and sentinel lymph node biopsy
      (SLNB), 260
Lymphotrophic nanoparticle-enhanced
      MRI (LN-MRI), 300
Lymph vessel invasion, diagnosis of, 54

MA17 clinical trial, 279
MA27 clinical trial, 279
Magnetic resonance imagining (MRI),
      18, 31–33, 72, 292
  ACS recommendations, 33
  of axilla, 293
  DCIS, 93
  recommendations for supplemental
      MRI screening and high-risk
      women, 31–32
  scientific data supporting, 33
Mammalian target of rapamycin
      (mTOR), 316
Mammographic Quality Standards
      Act (MQSA), 20–21
Mammography screening, 291–292
  age at screening, arguments for and
      against, 29–31
  batch reading, 19
  best age for, 20
  BIRADS certification, 20–23
  breast density, 23
  controversies, 28–29
  DCIS, 99–100
  digital mammography, 23–24
      benefit of, 24
  efficacy of cancer screening test
      biases, 24–26
      randomized, controlled trials, 26
  efficient method, 18–19
  evidences supporting, 26–28
  of fibroglandular breast tissues, 23
  and general population, 28–29
  MQSA certification, 20–21

  radiation risks, 29
  randomized controlled trials of, 27
  recommendations, 18–20
  risk factors, 29
  screening standardization and
      reporting, 20–23
  in United States, 18
  use of computer-aided detection
      (CAD) software, 24
MammoPrint, 304
Margin evaluation, in pathological
      study, 53
Massachusetts General Hospital
      Breast Cancer Multidisciplinary
      Program, 64–65
Mastectomy, of DCIS, 101
Mastectomy specimens, 52–53
Mastectomy treatment, of early breast
      cancer
  efficacy of skin-sparing
      mastectomy, 121
  electron intraoperative therapy
      (ELIOT), 121
  extent of breast tissue removed, 120
  and immediate reconstruction, 120
  with immediate reconstruction,
      120–121
  nipple-sparing mastectomy, 121
  technical considerations, 120
Mediolateral oblique (MLO) view only
      modality, 18
Medulloblastoma, 11
Members, of the multidisciplinary
      team, 37–38
Menopause Specific Quality of Life
      Questionnaire (MENQOL),
      310–311
Metaplastic carcinomas, 55
Metastatic breast cancer
  biological therapy
      antiangiogeneic agents, 214
      lapatinib, 213–214
      polyADP-ribose polymerase 1
          (PARP-1) inhibitors, 214
      traztuzumab, 212–213
  bone metastases, 202–203
  and brain metastases, 204–205
  chemotherapy
      anthracycline-based and
          taxane-based therapy,
          combined, 210–212
      capecitabine, 212
      epothilones, 212
      nab-paclitaxel (Abraxane), 212
      triple-negative disease, 209–210
  goal of treatment, 202
  and leptomeningeal
      metastases, 205
  life expectancy, 225
  novel therapeutic
      strategies, 216
  and ocular metastases, 205–206

[Metastatic breast cancer]
palliative care
advance care planning, 224
communication with patients and
families, 224
disease trajectory in advanced
breast cancer, 221
family meetings, 224–225
historical perspective, 221
and hospice care, 222
interdisciplinary care, 222–223
last weeks of life, 227
psychosocial and spiritual needs,
223–224
SPIKES protocol for delivering
bad news, 225
symptom management, 225–227
principles of, 202
radiation therapy (RT), 202–205
selected metastatic sites and
associated symptoms, 226
and spinal cord compression,
203–204
supportive interventions
brain metastases, 215
radiofrequency ablation, 215–216
surgical management of
studies of primary tumor resection
in patients, 198
surgical resection of the primary
breast cancer, 198–201
survival in patients, 197
surgical ovarian ablation therapy, 208
treatment for estrogen-responsive
breast cancer
aromatase inhibitors (AIs), 208–209
selective estrogen response modulator
(SERM) tamoxifen, 208
Methotrexate, 77, 154
Michigan Breast Reconstruction
Outcome study, 193
Micropapillary carcinomas, 55
Mirtazapine, 271
MRI-guided core needle biopsy, 45
Multidisciplinary administrative
coordinator, 37–38
Multidisciplinary breast cancer
evaluations, 1
Multidisciplinary breast cancer
programs, 1
clinical information needed prior to
initial appointment, 38
core members of the multidisciplinary
team, 37–38
role of surgeon, 294–295
and decision making, 2
diagnosis, 68
imperatives of specialists, 2
initial appointment guidelines for, 38
initial evaluation following diagnosis
assessment of modifiable lifestyle
factors, 71

clinical trials, 74
cryopreservation of ovarian
tissue, 74
dietary intervention, 71
fertility preservation, 73–74
further evaluation for risks of
treatment, 73–74
gene expression profiling, 71–72
history, physical exam, and
laboratory studies, 68–72
imaging to evaluate for
metastatic disease, 73
initial imaging studies, 72–73
laboratory studies, 71
multiple-gated acquisition (MUGA)
scans, 73
neurological examination, 71
physical activity, 71
positron-emission tomography
(PET) scans, 73
radionucleotide bone scan, 73
vitamin D levels, 71
integration of new services, 67
limitations to, 2
longitudinal follow-up care, 2
Massachusetts General Hospital
Breast Cancer Multidisciplinary
Program, 64–65
medical education perspective, 66
multidisciplinary visit, 38–40
origin, 2
patient satisfaction/program
evaluation, 40
patients' perspective, 65–66
physicians' perspective, 66
research perspective, 66–67
staging, 68–70
vs standard approach, 37
Myoepithelial cells, 56
Myriad Genetics labs, 8

National Comprehensive Cancer
Network (NCCN), 5
National Surgical Adjuvant Breast and
Bowel Project (NSABP P-1), 89
National Surgical Adjuvant Breast and
Bowel Project (NSABP)/RTOG
trial, 303
National Surgical Adjuvant Breast
and Bowel Project (NSABP)
trials, 156
NSABP B-39/RTOG 0413 phase III
randomized trial, 304
NSABP B-17 study, 101
NSABP B-22 study, 138
NSABP B-24 study, 106–107,
112–113
NSABP B-25 study, 138
NSABP B-35 study, 107, 114
NSABP B-06 trial, 125, 127

NSABP B-14 trial, 132, 279
NSABP B-27 trial, 168
NSABP B-37 trial, 244
NSABP B-39 trial, 232
NSABP B-42 trial, 312
NCI-sponsored Clinical Trials Support
Unit (CTSU), 287
Neoadjuvant chemotherapy, 55
Nipple-sparing mastectomy, 294
DCIS, 96
Nipple-sparing mastectomy specimen,
52–53
Norton–Simon hypothesis, 138
NSABP follow-up prevention trial Study
of Tamoxifen and Raloxifene
(STAR), 280

Ocular metastases, 205–206
Oncotype DX testing, 139, 304
Oophorectomy, 1
Ovarian tumors, borderline, 10

Paclitaxel, 138
Papillary lesions, 46
Paroxetine, 71
PARP1 protein inhibitors, 10
Patient experience and satisfaction, with
multidisciplinary progarm, 40
Patients' perspective, on
multidisciplinary breast cancer
programs, 65–66
Phlebotomy, in multidisciplinary
program, 40
Phyllodes tumors, 57–58
Platinum salts, 136
P53 mutation, 4
genetic testing for, 9
P53 mutations, 12
Postmastectomy radiotherapy (PMRT),
191–193
Postmastectomy radiotherapy (PMRT),
of locally advanced
breast cancer
benefit of, 155
clinical targets, 156
four or more positive axillary nodes,
153–154
indications, 153–155
for large breast tumors, 155–156
for one to three positive node breast
cancer patients, 155
side effects, 156
Pregnancy, after breast cancer
algorithm for considering fertility
issues in women, 76
impact of treatment on fertility and,
77–78
methods of fertility preservation, 79

[Pregnancy, after breast cancer]
oocyte cryopreservation and ovarian tissue cryopreservation, 79
predicting future fertility, 78
risk of chemotherapy-related amenorrhea with common treatment regimens, 77–78
safety, 76–77
Preoperative chemotherapy, 55
Prophylactic mastectomy specimen, 52
Prosthesis-based methods, breast reconstruction, 178–180
Psychiatric issues, in breast cancer diagnosis of, 269–270
somatic etiologies, 270–271
suicidal thoughts, 271
treatment, 271–275
Psychosocial issues, in multidisciplinary program, 40
PTEN mutation, 4, 12

Quality of life and multidisciplinary approach
addressing the needs of young women with breast cancer, 249–250
body image and sexuality, 250–251
considerations for geriatric patients, 254
coping behavior with genetic risk, 253–254
definitions and measurement, 247–248
and living with cancer, 254–255
longitudinal care, 255
morbidity secondary to physical and cognitive symptoms, 252–253
parenting concerns, 251–252
from research to practice, 249
screening for distress, 248–249

Racial disparity, in breast cancer survival
in clinical trial participation, 280
in medical oncology chemotherapy, 278–279
endocrine therapy, 279
in radiation therapy, 278
in surgery
breast-conserving surgery (BCS), 277–278
mastectomy, 277–278
option of breast reconstruction, 278
use of sentinel lymph node biopsy, 277
Radial scars, 46–47
Radiation boost, 105
Radiation techniques, 2
advances in diagnostic radiology

accelerated partial breast irradiation (APBI), 303–304
cardiac sparing techniques, 302
intensity-modulated radiation therapy, 300
target definition, 298–300
use of hypofractionation in whole breast radiation, 302–303
use of molecular profiles and tumor receptors, 304
use of protons beams, 301–302
value of multidisciplinary approach, 304
of early-stage breast cancer
age factor, 125
contraindications to breast-conserving surgery, 126
hypofractionated accelerated courses, 128
lumpectomy-site boost, 128–129
and mortality, 126–127
multidisciplinary approach, 129
omission of, 127–128
prognostic factors, 125–126
risk of local recurrence, 126
sequencing of radiation and systemic therapy, 126
surgical margin, 125
of locally advanced breast cancer
impact of systemic therapy on locoregional control, 153
inflammatory breast cancer (IBC), 158–159
inoperable, 157–158
multidisciplinary approach, 159
operable, 152–153
postmastectomy radiotherapy (PMRT), 153–156
risk factors for locoregional recurrence, 152–153
Radiation Therapy Oncology Group and Cancer and Leukemia Group (RTOG 9804/CALGB 49801), 103
Raloxifene, 3, 89
RF ablation, of breast masses, 290–291
RING finger motif, 10
Risk, of developing cancer, models, 3–4
Risk-reducing bilateral salpingo-oophorectomy (RRBSO), 11

Saline implants, 178–179
Screening modalities, 1
alternative and supplementary methods
breast self-examination (BSE), 31
digital breast tomosynthesis (DBT), 34
MRI, 31–33
ultrasound, 33–34
use of radioactive tracers, 34

empirical models, 3–4
family history questionnaire, 6
preoperative breast imaging modalities, limitations, 94
rudimentary screening program, 5–6
Selective estrogen receptor modulators (SERMs), 89
Sentinel lymph node biopsy (SLNB), 101
Sentinel lymph nodes, mapping and excision of, 58
S428F mutant, 10
Silicone implants, 178–179
Skin-sparing mastectomy, 52
DCIS, 95–96
Southwest Oncology Group (SWOG) trial, 139
Specimen radiography, 43, 47, 52, 95
Spinal cord compression and breast cancer, 203–204
Stereotactic breast biopsy
clinical considerations, 43–44
directional vacuum-assisted biopsy sampling, 43
fine-needle, 42–43
large-core automated sampling, 43
technical considerations, 42
Supportive psychotherapy, 271
Suppression of Ovarian Function Trial (SOFT), 133
Surgical biopsy, 47
Surgical pathological findings, for breast specimens
core biopsies, 51
excisions, 52
histological examples
benign findings, 57–58
ductal carcinoma in situ, 56
invasive carcinoma, 53–56
low grade precursor lesions, 57
immunohistochemistry
hormone receptor and HER-2 profiles, 58–59
intraoperative consultations and frozen sections, 59
margin evaluation, 53
mastectomy specimens, 52–53
multidisciplinary considerations, 60
pathological tumor characteristics, 50–51
quality assurance and control, 59–60
Swiss Group for Clinical Cancer Research SAKK trial, 241–242

Tamoxifen, 3, 73, 77, 89, 105, 112–114, 132–135, 209
Taxanes, 167–168
Taxotere, 243
Telephone, in multidisciplinary program, 40

Three-dimensional treatment planning (3D-CRT), 299
Transvaginal ultrasound, 11
Transverse rectus abdominis myocutaneous (TRAM) flap, 180–182
Trastuzumab, 73, 112, 139–141
Treatment
  of early breast cancer
    eligibility for breast conservation, 117–119
    lumpectomy considerations, 119–120
    lumpectomy vs mastectomy, 117
    mastectomy considerations, 120–121
    multidisciplinary considerations, 122–123
    perioperative considerations, 122
    surgical management of the axilla, 121–122
  future directions
    impact of advanced imaging approaches in guiding surgery, 291–292
    improved margin assessment, 289
    improving axillary staging, 292–293
    improving cosmetic outcome, 293–294

intraoperative assessment of lumpectomy margins, 289–290
    nonsurgical ablation techniques, 290–291
  of locally advanced breast cancer
    assessment of tumor response after preoperative therapy, 146
    axillary dissection, 148
    breast conservation after neoadjuvant therapy, 146–147
    breast reconstruction, 149–150
    initial evaluation, 145
    inoperable tumors, 145–146
    internal mammary node issues, 148–149
    mastectomy techniques, 149
    multidisciplinary considerations, 150
    operable tumors, 146
    selection of initial therapy in operable patients, 146
    sentinel lymph node biopsy (SLNB) in, 147–148
Triple-negative breast cancer, treatment, 169
Triptorelin with either Exemestane or Tamoxifen (TEXT), 133
Tubular carcinomas, 55

UK Standardisation of Breast Radiotherapy (START) trials, 128
Ultrasound-guided core needle biopsy, 44
Ultrasound screening modalities, 33–34, 291–292
  of axilla, 292–293
United Kingdom, Australia, and New Zealand (UK/ANZ) trial, 113–114
United Kingdom Coordinating Committee on Cancer Research (UKCCCR) trial, 102, 106

Van Nuys classification, for tumors, 111
Van Nuys Prognostic Index (VPNI), 102

Waits and delays, in multidisciplinary program, 40
Wilms' tumors, 11

Zolpidem, 274